Dissemination and Implementation Research in Health

Translating Science to Practice

EDITED BY

Ross C. Brownson
Graham A. Colditz
Enola K. Proctor

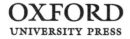

OXFORD
UNIVERSITY PRESS

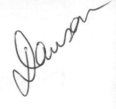

OXFORD
UNIVERSITY PRESS

Oxford University Press, Inc., publishes works that further
Oxford University's objective of excellence
in research, scholarship, and education.

Oxford New York
Auckland   Cape Town   Dares Salaam   Hong Kong   Karachi
Kuala   Lumpur   Madrid   Melbourne   Mexico City   Nairobi
New Delhi   Shanghai   Taipei   Toronto

With offices in
Argentina   Austria   Brazil   Chile   Czech Republic   France   Greece
Guatemala   Hungary   Italy   Japan   Poland   Portugal   Singapore
South Korea   Switzerland   Thailand   Turkey   Ukraine Vietnam

Library of Congress Cataloguing-in-Publication Data
Dissemination and implementation research in health: translating science
to practice / edited by Ross C. Brownson, Graham A. Colditz, Enola K. Proctor.
p. ; cm
Includes bibliographical references and index.
ISBN 978-0-19-975187-7 (hardcover: alk. paper)
I. Brownson, Ross C.   II. Colditz, Graham A.   III. Proctor, Enola K.
[DNLM: 1. Translational Research—methods.   2. Clinical Trials as Topic.
3. Information Dissemination. W 20.55.T7]
610.72'4—dc23
2011037127

1 3 5 7 9 8 6 4 2
Printed in the United States of America
on acid-free paper

Dissemination and Implementation Research in Health

We dedicate this book to our spouses: Carol Brownson, Pat Cox, and Frank Proctor. We are grateful for their loving support and good humor

■ FOREWORD

I write this having just marked my tenth year at the National Institute of Mental Health, the balance of that time spent on efforts to grow the field of dissemination and implementation research. With great enthusiasm, I consider this comprehensive volume that reflects that progress the field has made and the significant challenges that lie ahead. It has been a privilege to see the development of the theories, frameworks, and empirical data captured by the authors. We can see a dramatic shift from an era in which dissemination and implementation processes were considered to be beyond science to the current state, in which diverse scientists, practitioners, and policymakers are actively pursuing knowledge on how to accrue the most public health benefit from our scientific discoveries.

From my perspective, the origins of dissemination and implementation research lie in a number of key developments in the last century: Archibald Cochrane's efforts, highlighted by his landmark monograph *Effectiveness and Efficiency*,[1] to derive empirical support for health care treatments and the subsequent development of the Cochrane Collaboration, which systematized the process for considering evidence sufficient enough to warrant widespread use of health interventions; Andrew Oxman and colleagues' 1995 paper, "No Magic Bullets to Change,"[2] which systematically assessed a large number of studies targeting clinical behavior change, finding better results with active (not passive) strategies, and discussing the necessity of a comprehensive approach to maximize the likelihood of change; David Sackett's 1996 paper heralding the arrival of modern "Evidence-Based Medicine," where clinical practice could be optimized by the "judicious use of evidence" in concert with medical acumen.[3] Around the same time, public health and other related disciplines were formalizing tenets of evidence-based practice and policy.[4] The popularization of Everett Rogers's Diffusion of Innovations theory,[5] which originated from his own experience as a farmer and then as an investigator of the spread of agricultural innovations, was another important development and one from which health researchers learned a great deal about spread of evidence-based interventions.

Each was an important stepping-stone toward the significant advancement of the field. Quite relevant to me in drafting the first NIMH program announcement on Dissemination and Implementation Research (2002)[6] was the work of Jonathan Lomas, whose 1993 paper sought to clarify concepts of Diffusion, Dissemination, and Implementation as related to transferring knowledge into health care practice.[7] This framework described the different levels of intensity through which the goals could be achieved, and continues to be the source for NIH's working definitions for the field.

In contemplating the growth of dissemination and implementation research, I find myself returning to a basic theory of behavior change quite present in D&I discussions—the Transtheoretical Model of Change.[8] Prochaska and DiClemente's model provides a helpful heuristic for me to frame the dramatic shifts in thinking. Certainly not everyone has traversed the stages from precontemplation to maintenance (perhaps to termination), but I find that an increasing contingent of health researchers have not only progressed but also become agents of change themselves.

Precontemplation (pre-1990s):

For many years, there was no field of dissemination and implementation research. The linear model from research to practice of most treatment or preventive interventions proceeded from intervention development to efficacy studies (less frequently to effectiveness studies) and then to the literature, destined to be a paperweight or reliant on a microfilm projector to be further disseminated. The biomedical research community seemed to assume that the journals that they published in were fully digested by clinicians, and thus the work to get science to the masses was accomplished. Few considered that publication was not the golden path to full integration of interventions within health systems.

Contemplation (1990s–2000):

The 1990s saw a significant rise in a discussion of dissemination and implementation as conferences, commentaries, special issues, and federal and independent reports underscored the ineffectiveness of the publication as a tool to change clinical practice. The rise of evidence-based medicine and evidence-based public health, first in the UK and then elsewhere, popularized the notion that scientific findings should be more comprehensively implemented within typical practice, filling the gulf (or "Quality Chasm" as the IOM depicted).[9] The Agency for Health Care Policy Research (later AHRQ) began to fund a series of evidence-based practice centers around the country to improve the "translation of research to practice," and articles appeared by the truckload, identifying many facilitators and barriers to the diffusion of innovations. There was recognition that the path from research to practice was a messy and frequently futile one, but little organized inquiry into the "how" and "why" existed. In short, the field was heavy on contemplation and light on action. For many of us, the culmination of this period was the Balas and Boren (2000) article in the *Yearbook of Medical Informatics,* which quantified this path from research to practice at 17 years after which some 14% of findings filtered into clinical use.[10]

Preparation (2000–2003)

By the end of the last century, we had reached the dawn of a new stage in our field. Well recognized were the diverse and multiple barriers and facilitators to disseminate research findings and implement effective interventions. The next step was figuring out what to do about it. These next few years saw more organized calls for research, from federal agencies, foundations, and states. Many researchers still remained hesitant to jump fully into the fray, but an increasing number of study ideas began to emerge. We saw an influx of reports, chronicling multiple demonstration projects targeting the uptake of effective interventions, but frequently focusing more on "what happened" and less on "how do get something good to happen." The dissemination and implementation strategies were crafted with experience and expertise behind them but rarely tested in a way to bring knowledge about how to do better.

Action (2003–Present)

Recently, we have seen a true explosion in the quantity and quality of dissemination and implementation research in health. Attendance at the annual NIH conferences has quadrupled, and the rigor and ambitiousness of ongoing studies has significantly advanced. Many conceptual frameworks have been developed and are being tested, measures of key constructs (e.g., organizational readiness, fidelity, reach, culture and climate, clinician acceptability of innovations) have been validated, and we are seeing more comparative effectiveness studies of active strategies to disseminate health information and implement evidence-based interventions. We are in a golden age for dissemination and implementation research, helped through capacity building of multiple research centers and networks, and with comprehensive texts that summarize much of the learning of the last generation. Action is upon us.

Maintenance (The Future):

So with this book as a tool, and perhaps a divining rod, we look ahead to a bright future. The capacity of the field has grown, but while progress has been made, we have not yet reached a status in which perceived value of this science is ubiquitous and unchallenged. Scientifically, we have yet to progress to a long-term view of dissemination and implementation. The next generation of studies to get us there will address the sustainable integration of interventions within dynamic health care delivery systems and the implementation of evidence-based systems of care rather than the individual intervention. We will rely on improved quality and specificity of methods and measures, and more available data to look at the ultimate impact of dissemination and implementation efforts on population health. Our science will embrace the increased globalization of health care research and encompass the application of dissemination and implementation across the world.

Reflecting this exciting journey, this book brings together much of what is currently known about dissemination and implementation, priming readers with all levels of familiarity and expertise. Within our field, necessary expertise typically transcends the bounds of any individual; this book orients us to what we know, and what we don't. With this volume as a marker of progress to this point, it is even more exciting to gaze ahead and see what the next decade will bring.

— David Chambers, D.Phil.
Associate Director, Dissemination and Implementation Research
National Institute of Mental Health
National Institutes of Health

REFERENCES

1. Cochrane AL. *Effectiveness and efficiency. Random reflections of health services* (new edition). London: RSM Publishing, 1999.
2. Oxman AD, Thomson MA, Davis DA, Haynes RB. No magic bullets: a systematic review of 102 trials of interventions to improve professional practice. *CMAJ*. Nov 15 1995;153(10):1423–1431.
3. Sackett DL, Rosenberg WM, Gray JA, Haynes RB, Richardson WS. Evidence based medicine: what it is and what it isn't. *BMJ*. January 13 1996;312(7023):71–2. PMID 8555924.
4. Satterfield JM, Spring B, Brownson RC, et al. Toward a transdisciplinary model of evidence-based practice. *Milbank Q.* Jun 2009;87(2):368–390.
5. Rogers, Everett M. *Diffusion of innovations.* 5th edition. New York: Free Press, 2003.
6. NIMH. PA-02-131: Dissemination and Implementation Research in Mental Health. Accessed at http://grants.nih.gov/grants/guide/pa-files/PA-02-131.html on July 30, 2011.
7. Lomas, J. Diffusion, dissemination, and implementation: who should do what? *Ann N Y Acad Sci.* 1993;703: 226–237.
8. Prochaska, JO, DiClemente, CC. *The transtheoretical approach: crossing traditional boundaries of therapy.* Homewood, IL: Dow Jones-Irwin; 1984. ISBN 087094438X.
9. Institute of Medicine. *Crossing the quality chasm: a new health system for the 21st century.* Washington, DC: National Academy Press, 2001.
10. Balas EA, Boren SA. Managing clinical knowledge for health care improvement. In: Bemmel J, McCray AT, eds. *Yearbook of medical informatics.* Stuttgart: Schattauer; 2000:65–70.

■ PREFACE

Decades of support by governmental and private sources has produced a remarkable foundation of knowledge in all disciplines related to public health, mental health, and health care. The discovery of new knowledge should not occur in large measure to satisfy the curiosity of scientists; rather, the goal must be to improve the human condition (lower morbidity and mortality, enhance quality of life). Yet the gap between care that *could be*, were health care informed by scientific knowledge, and the care *that is* in routine practice has been characterized as a "chasm" by the Institute of Medicine. The lack of ability to apply research findings has sometimes been equated to a leaky or broken pipeline between discovery and application.

To understand and begin to fill these leaks, an exciting new science is emerging. It goes by numerous titles, including: translational research, knowledge translation, knowledge exchange, technology transfer, and dissemination and implementation (D&I) research. Although the terminology can be cumbersome and changing existing practices complex, the underlying rationale is simple: too often, discovery of new knowledge begets more discovery (the next study) with little attention on how to apply research advances in real-world public health, social service, and health care settings. The early efforts in D&I research focused on ways to increase the use of evidence-based guidelines among practitioners. The subsequent research has shown that in efforts to disseminate practice guidelines using passive methods (e.g., publication of consensus statements, mass mailings), adoption has been relatively low, resulting in only small changes in the uptake of a new evidence-based practice.

A return on investment of the billions spent on basic and clinical research requires a marked increase in translational research, including the development of its tools, and analytic approaches. These efforts have been receiving much greater attention in mainline medical and public health journals. There also is a small set of journals dedicated to D&I research, notably *Implementation Science* (begun in 2006) and *Translational Behavioral Medicine* (begun in 2011). Similarly, federal agencies and foundations are beginning to support D&I research more fully. For example, recent funding announcements from the National Institutes of Health (NIH) show the higher priority being placed on translational research. While NIH is placing renewed emphasis on T1 research from bench to bedside (first in human studies as defined by Collins in July 2011), we place emphasis on methods and research opportunities for moving from scientific discovery of efficacy to population-wide benefits.

There are tangible examples where the D&I gap has been shortened. This may be best illustrated over the 20th century in the United States where life expectancy rose from 49 years in 1900 to 77 years in 2000. In large part, this increasing longevity was due to the application of discoveries on a population level (e.g., vaccinations, cleaner air and water). Yet for every victory, there is a parallel example of progress yet to be realized. For example, effective treatment for tuberculosis has been available since the 1950s, yet globally, tuberculosis still accounts for 2 million annual deaths with 2 billion people infected. In many ways, the chapters in this book draw on successes (e.g., what works in tobacco control) and remaining challenges (e.g., how to address translational research challenges in populations with health disparities).

What needs to happen to shorten the translational research gap?

• First, priorities need to shift. Of the U.S. annual health expenditures, only about 0.1% is spent on health services research (where D&I research is nested). This shift in priorities requires political will and a need for social change.
• Second, capacity for finding and implementing evidence-based practice needs to improve among numerous practitioner audiences. For example, most individuals working in public health practice have no formal training in a public health discipline—which suggests the need for more and better on-the-job training.
• Third, the science of D&I research needs further development. The range of research needs is vast and covered extensively in this volume.
• Fourth, capacity for conducting D&I research needs to be advanced through training. This training can occur in government agencies, academic institutions, and nongovernmental organizations (such as the World Health Organization).
• And finally, to build this science and capacity, institutional support and incentives are needed. For example, academic institutions need to shift priorities for faculty to reward time spent in conducting D&I research.

We have organized the book in a format that covers the major concepts for D&I researchers and practitioners. It draws on the talents of some of the top D&I scholars in the world—crossing many disciplines, health topics, and intervention settings. Our book has four sections. The first section provides a rationale for the book, highlights core issues needing attention, and begins to develop the terminology for D&I research. In the second section, we highlight the historical development of D&I research and describe several key analytic tools and approaches. Some of the tools are well developed with a rich literature (e.g., economic evaluation, participatory approaches) and others are relatively new, developing fields (e.g., comparative effectiveness, systems thinking). This section also emphasizes the need to better plan interventions for dissemination and think creatively about how lessons from business and marketing can be applied to health. The third section is devoted to design and analysis of D&I studies. It covers core principles of study design, measurement and outcomes, and evaluation. In addition, this section highlights the concepts of fidelity and external validity, which are fundamental to D&I science. The final section of the book focuses on settings and populations. Since D&I research occurs in places where people live their lives (communities, schools) or receive care (health care, social service agencies), we devote chapters to specific settings. This section also recognizes the importance of policy influences on health, the need for cultural adaptation, and the science of addressing health disparities. Our book concludes with a short chapter on emerging issues and future research directions.

The target audience for this text is broad and includes researchers and practitioners across many different disciplines, including epidemiology, biostatistics, behavioral science, medicine, social work, psychology, and anthropology. It seeks to inform practitioners in health promotion, public health, health services, and health systems. We anticipate this book will be useful in academic institutions, state and local health agencies, federal agencies, and health care organizations. Although the book is intended primarily for a North American audience, there are authors and examples drawn from various parts of the world, and we believe that much of the information covered will be applicable in both developed and developing countries. The challenges of moving research to practice and policy appear to be universal, so future progress calls for collaborative partnership and cross-country research.

Our book documents that in a time of increasing pressure on scientific and public resources, researchers must continue to meet the implied obligation to the public that the billions of dollars invested in basic science will yield specific and tangible benefits to their health. Taxpayers have paid for many new discoveries, yet these are not being translated into better patient care, public policy, and public health programs. We believe that applying the principles in this volume will begin to bridge the chasm between discovery and practice.

R. C. B.
G. A. C.
E. K. P.

■ ACKNOWLEDGMENTS

We are grateful to numerous individuals who contributed to the development of this book.

We particularly wish to thank the outstanding team of authors who contributed chapters. Their exceptional knowledge and dedication is reflected in the chapters, providing an up-to-date snapshot of dissemination and implementation science. Four reviewers provided valuable comments that allowed us to revise and improve the manuscript. We also appreciate the assistance from Lauren Carothers, Linda Dix, Katie Duggan, Nora Geary, Wes Gibbert, and Nosa Osazuwa-Peters.

Development of this book was supported by the following awards: (1) UL1 RR024992, Clinical and Translational Science Award (CTSA) program of the National Center for Research Resources; (2) Cooperative Agreement Number U48/DP001903 from the Centers for Disease Control and Prevention, Prevention Research Centers Program; (3) Grant Number 1R01CA124404–01 from the National Cancer Institute at the National Institutes of Health, (4) P30 MH 068579, Advanced Centers for Interventions and Services Research; (5) R25 MH080916, National Institute of Mental Health; (6) a grant to Graham Colditz to Build Prevention and Control Research at Siteman Cancer Center from Barnes-Jewish Hospital Foundation, St Louis; and (7) the American Cancer Society Clinical Research Professorship CRP-03–194-07 CCE.

We acknowledge the leadership of Washington University's George Warren Brown School of Social Work, Institute for Public Health, Alvin J. Siteman Cancer Center, Institute for Clinical and Translational Science, and Department of Surgery (Division of Public Health Sciences) for fostering an environment in which transdisciplinary and translational science are valued and encouraged. Finally, we are indebted to Maura Roessner and Nicholas Liu, Oxford University Press, who provided valuable advice throughout the production of this edition.

■ CONTENTS

SECTION THREE ■ Design and Analysis

SECTION FOUR ■ Setting- and Population-Specific
Dissemination and Implementation

CONTRIBUTORS

Gregory A. Aarons, PhD
Department of Psychiatry
University of California, San Diego
Child and Adolescent Services
Research Center
Rady Children's Hospital San Diego
San Diego, California

Jennifer D. Allen, ScD, MPH
Center for Community-Based
Research and
Phyllis F. Cantor Center for
Research in Nursing & Patient
Care Services
Dana-Farber Cancer Institute
Boston, Massachusetts
Harvard Medical School
Boston, Massachusetts

LaShawnta Bell-Lewis, DrPH
UCLA Kaiser Permanente Center for
Health Equity
Department of Health Services
School of Public Health
University of California,
Los Angeles
Division of Cancer Prevention and
Control Research
Jonsson Comprehensive
Cancer Center
University of California, Los Angeles
Los Angeles, California

Jennifer L. Bellamy, PhD
School of Social Service
Administration
University of Chicago
Chicago, Illinois

Jay M. Bernhardt, PhD, MPH
Department of Health Education
and Behavior
College of Health and Human
Performance
University of Florida
Gainesville, Florida

Allan Best, PhD
InSource Research Group
West Vancouver, British Columbia,
Canada

C. Hendricks Brown, PhD
Department of Epidemiology
and Public Health
School of Medicine
University of Miami
Miami, Florida

Ross C. Brownson, PhD
Prevention Research Center in
St. Louis
George Warren Brown School
of Social Work
Washington University
in St. Louis
St. Louis, Missouri

Division of Public Health
Sciences, Department of
Surgery and
Alvin J. Siteman Cancer Center
Washington University School of
Medicine
Washington University
in St. Louis
St. Louis, Missouri

Christopher M. Casey, MPH
Health Communication Research
Laboratory
George Warren Brown School
of Social Work
Washington University in St. Louis
St. Louis, Missouri

Patricia Chamberlain, PhD
Oregon Social Learning Center
Eugene, Oregon

Graham A. Colditz, MD, DrPH
Division of Public Health Sciences,
Department of Surgery
Washington University School of
Medicine
St. Louis, Missouri

Sara Czaja, PhD
Departments of Psychiatry &
Behavioral Sciences and Industrial
Engineering
University of Miami
Miami, Florida

James W. Dearing, PhD
Kaiser Permanente Colorado
Denver, Colorado

Lauren R. Dlugosz, BA
Department of Psychiatry
University of California, San Diego
Child and Adolescent Services
Research Center
Rady Children's Hospital San Diego
San Diego, California

Elizabeth A. Dodson, PhD, MPH
Prevention Research Center in St.
Louis
George Warren Brown School of Social
Work
Washington University in St. Louis
St. Louis, Missouri

Mariah Dreisinger, MPH
School of Medicine
University of Missouri
Columbia, Missouri

Elizabeth Eakin, PhD
Baker IDI Heart and Diabetes
Institute
Melbourne, Victoria, Australia

Mark G. Ehrhart, PhD
Department of Psychology
San Diego State University
San Diego, California

Karen M. Emmons, PhD
Center for Community-Based
Research
Dana-Farber Cancer Institute
Boston, Massachusetts

Department of Society, Human
Development, and Health
Harvard School of Public Health
Boston, Massachusetts

Diane T. Finegood, PhD
Department of Biomedical Physiology
and Kinesiology
Simon Fraser University
Burnaby, British Columbia, Canada

Brianna Fjeldsoe, PhD
Cancer Prevention
Research Centre
School of Population Health
University of Queensland
Brisbane, Queensland, Australia

Chandra L. Ford, PhD
Department of Community Health
Sciences
School of Public Health
University of California, Los Angeles
Los Angeles, California

Bridget Gaglio, PhD, MPH
Mid-Atlantic Permanente Research
Institute
Mid-Atlantic Permanente Medical
Group
Rockville, Maryland

Russell E. Glasgow, PhD
Institute for Health Research
Kaiser Permanente Colorado
Denver, Colorado

Division of Cancer Control and
Population Sciences
National Cancer Institute
National Institutes of Health
Rockville, Maryland

Beth A. Glenn, PhD
UCLA Kaiser Permanente Center for
Health Equity
Department of Health Services
School of Public Health
University of California, Los Angeles

Division of Cancer Prevention and
Control Research
Jonsson Comprehensive Cancer Center
University of California, Los Angeles
Los Angeles, California

Jeremy D. Goldhaber-Fiebert, PhD
Department of Medicine and the
Centers for Health Policy
and Primary Care and Outcomes
Research
Stanford University
Stanford, California

Ana Goode, MPH
Cancer Prevention
Research Centre
School of Population Health
University of Queensland
Brisbane, Queensland, Australia

Steven Gortmaker, PhD
Department of Society, Human
Development, and Health
Harvard School of Public Health
Boston, Massachusetts

Lawrence W. Green, DrPH
Department of Epidemiology and
Biostatistics
School of Medicine
University of California at San
Francisco
San Francisco, California

Bev J. Holmes, PhD
Michael Smith Foundation for Health
Research
Vancouver, British Columbia, Canada

Jonathan D. Horowitz, PhD
Department of Psychiatry
University of California, San Diego

Child and Adolescent Services
Research Center
Rady Children's Hospital San Diego
San Diego, California

Sarah McCue Horwitz, PhD
Department of Pediatrics and
Centers for Health Policy and Primary
Care and Outcomes Research
Stanford University
Stanford, California

Kerk F. Kee, PhD
Chapman University
Orange, California

Jon F. Kerner, PhD
Canadian Partnership
Against Cancer
Toronto, Ontario, Canada

Matthew W. Kreuter, PhD, MPH
Health Communication Research
Laboratory
George Warren Brown School of
Social Work
Washington University in St. Louis
St. Louis, Missouri

John Landsverk, PhD
Child and Adolescent Services
Research Center
Rady Children's Hospital San Diego
San Diego, California

Rebekka Lee, ScM
Department of Society, Human
Development, and Health
Harvard School of Public Health
Boston, Massachusetts

Laura A. Linnan, ScD
Department of Health Behavior
and Health Education
Gillings School of Global
Public Health
University of North Carolina
Chapel Hill, North Carolina

Lineberger Comprehensive Cancer
Center
Chapel Hill, North Carolina

Douglas A. Luke, PhD
Center for Tobacco Policy Research
George Warren Brown School
of Social Work
Washington University
St. Louis, Missouri

Curtis McMillen, PhD
School of Social Service
Administration
University of Chicago
Chicago, Illinois

Meredith Minkler, DrPH, MPH
School of Public Health
University of California, Berkeley
Berkeley, California

Brian S. Mittman, PhD
VA Center for Implementation Practice
and Research Support
U.S. Department of Veterans
Affairs
Los Angeles, California

Mona Nasser, DDS
Peninsula Dental School
University of Plymouth
Plymouth, England,
United Kingdom

Mitsunori Ogihara, PhD
Department of Computer Science
University of Miami
Miami, Florida

Neville Owen, PhD
Baker IDI Heart and
Diabetes Institute
Melbourne, Victoria, Australia

Lawrence Palinkas, PhD
School of Social Work
University of Southern
California
Los Angeles, California

Child and Adolescent Services
Research Center
Rady Children's Hospital San Diego
San Diego, California

Enola K. Proctor, PhD
George Warren Brown School
of Social Work
Washington University in St. Louis
St. Louis, Missouri

Borsika A. Rabin, PhD, MPH
Cancer Research Network Cancer
Communication Research Center
Institute for Health Research
Kaiser Permanente Colorado
Denver, Colorado

Ramesh Raghavan, MD, PhD
George Warren Brown School of Social
Work and
Department of Psychiatry, School of
Medicine
Washington University in St. Louis
St. Louis, Missouri

Barbara L. Riley, PhD
Propel Centre for Population Health
Impact
University of Waterloo
Waterloo, Ontario, Canada

Jennifer A. Rolls Reutz, MPH
Child and Adolescent Services
Research Center
Rady Children's Hospital San Diego
San Diego, California

Alicia L. Salvatore, DrPH, MPH
Stanford Prevention
Research Center
Stanford University School of Medicine
Stanford, California

Katherine A. Stamatakis, PhD, MPH
Division of Public Health Sciences,
Department of Surgery and
Alvin J. Siteman Cancer Center
Washington University School of
Medicine
Washington University in St. Louis
St. Louis, Missouri

John F. Steiner, MD, MPH
Institute for Health Research
Kaiser Permanente Colorado
Denver, Colorado

Takemi Sugiyama, PhD
Baker IDI Heart and Diabetes Institute
Melbourne, Victoria, Australia

Cynthia A. Vinson, MPA
Division of Cancer Control and
Population Sciences
National Cancer Institute
Bethesda, Maryland

Stephen M. Weiss, PhD, MPH
Department of Psychiatry and
Behavioral Sciences
Miller School of Medicine
University of Miami
Miami, Florida

Antronette (Toni) Yancey, MD, MPH
UCLA Kaiser Permanente Center for
Health Equity
Department of Health Services
School of Public Health
University of California, Los Angeles

Division of Cancer Prevention and
Control Research
Jonsson Comprehensive
Cancer Center
University of California, Los Angeles
Los Angeles, California

Luis H. Zayas, PhD
George Warren Brown School of Social
Work and
School of Medicine
Washington University in St. Louis
St. Louis, Missouri

■ SECTION ONE
Background

1

The Promise and Challenges of Dissemination and Implementation Research

■ GRAHAM A. COLDITZ

To him who devotes his life to science, nothing can give more
happiness than increasing the number of discoveries, but his cup of
joy is full when the results of his studies immediately find practical
applications.   LOUIS PASTEUR

The ability of science to deliver on its promise of practical and timely
solutions to the world's problems does not depend solely on research
accomplishments but also on the receptivity of society to the
implications of scientific discoveries.   AGRE AND LESHNER[1]

■ INTRODUCTION

Dissemination and implementation of research findings into practice are necessary
to achieve a return on investment in our research enterprise and to apply research
findings to improve outcomes in the broader community. At the level of molecular
biology and pathogenesis of disease, parallel issues arise with the call from the NIH
Director, Francis Collins, seeking more rapid translation from discovery of recep-
tors or pathways to first in patient studies.[2] Whether we are focusing on genomic
discovery or evidence that treatment of a condition improves outcomes, moving
from scientific discovery to broader application brings society the full return on
our collective investment in research. In 2008, it is estimated that the biomedical
research expenditures in the United States exceeded $100 billion on health-related
research.[3,4] Within this commitment, spending on health services research, models
of care, and service innovations, represented only approximately 1.5% of biomedical
research funding.[5] Perhaps reflecting the low priority of research on implementation
of scientifically proven approaches to care, in 2001, the Institute of Medicine noted
a substantial gap between care that could be delivered if health care was informed
by scientific knowledge and the care that is delivered in practice—defining this gap
as a chasm.[6] What then is dissemination and implementation research (D&I)?

To paraphrase Rubenstein and Pugh, implementation research is active and supports movement of evidence-based effective health care and prevention strategies
or programs from the clinical or public health knowledge base into routine use.[7]
The Canadian Institutes of Health Research (http://www.cihr-irsc.gc.ca/e/27904.
html) use the following definition for knowledge translation: "the exchange,

synthesis, and ethically-sound application of knowledge—within a complex set of interactions among researchers and users—to accelerate the capture of the benefits of research for Canadians through improved health, more effective services and products, and a strengthened health care system." Along these lines, the CDC has defined implementation research as "the systematic study of how a specific set of activities and designated strategies are used to successfully integrate an evidence-based public health intervention within specific settings" (RFA-CD-07-005).[8] The National Cancer Institute (NCI) in a "Request For Applications" (RFA) has defined implementation research as "the use of strategies to adopt and integrate evidence based health interventions and change practice patterns within specific settings." Despite these definitions, a recent survey of readers in *Nature Medicine* showed little agreement and understanding of translational research.[9] In Chapter 2 we outline terminology to help move to common understanding of disciplines in D&I.

While the translation of evidence-based interventions into practice to improve population health outcomes is a common theme of government agencies, the *process* for distribution of scientific findings, materials, and associated resources to support interventions is less developed. Dissemination is defined in NIH program announce-ments as "the targeted distribution of information and intervention materials to a specific public health or clinical practice audience." Rabin et al. are more specific calling for an active approach of spreading evidence-based interventions to the tar-get audience via determined channels using planned strategies.[10] These definitions are similar to that of Lomas[11,12] but contrast some with the approach of Curry,[13] who defines dissemination as a push-pull process. Those who adopt innovations must want them or be receptive (pull) while there is systematic effort to help adopters imple-ment innovations (push). The intent of *dissemination research* is to spread knowledge and the associated interventions, building understanding of approaches to increased effectiveness of dissemination efforts. In understanding these approaches, numer-ous studies have shown that dissemination of evidence-based interventions using passive methods (e.g., publication of consensus statements in professional journals, mass mailings) has been ineffective, resulting in only small changes in the uptake of a new practice.[14] Therefore, more targeted, active approaches to D&I are needed that take into account many factors including the characteristics and needs of users, types of evidence needed, and organizational climate and culture. These definitions and other terms used in the field are described in more detail in Chapter 2.

One useful model of translation of discovery to applications that will gener-ate population health benefits comes from a thoughtful review by Bowen and colleagues. Reviewing the application of discovery to prevention of cancer, Bowen and colleagues note, "Our previous 30 years have taught us that dissemination does not just happen if we wait for it. New information is often needed to make it happen. Let's consider this a call to action to gather the new information in support of making it happen."[15(p.483)] The challenges in D&I are broad and apply far beyond health and health care systems. In fact, early examples, as we will see, come from other fields of learning. For example, much research in education has addressed the application of new knowledge to improve outcomes in children's learning.[16–18] The rapidly expanding field of D&I research has some common themes and lessons that this book will help bring together so that a more uniform understanding of the principles of D&I research methods and applications may help speed us to achieve the potential to improve population health. First, some key questions arise from the review that Bowen and colleagues conducted that are applicable to the broader field of D&I research, across health, education, and technology.

- How will we gather this information on effective interventions to form the evidence base?
- Will interventions be applicable to our setting?
- What methods should we use to decide what to disseminate or implement?
- Which strategies will give us the greatest impact on population health?
- What outcomes should be tracked to know if we are making progress?
- How long will it take to show progress, or when will it be observed?

These are but a few of the questions raised by the call to action from Bowen and colleagues.[15] Other authors address specific questions in translation from clinical trials to policy and practice.[19,20] Through this book, we aim to lay out many options to help guide the field as it matures, thus speeding our progress toward improved health for all. This introductory chapter seeks to place D&I research in context, and to identify the challenges in moving forward, and the pressure to increase the emphasis on this aspect of knowledge translation and research utilization.

■ THE CHALLENGE IN TRANSLATING RESEARCH TO PRACTICE

Moving from discovery to application brings society the full return on our collective investment in research. It is estimated that between 9 and 25% of the 30 billion NIH component was expended on prevention research[21,22]—that is, the direct and immediate application of effective intervention strategies to benefit the public's health (p.93).[23] Despite this low priority, the NIH maintains an active program in "dissemination" research, though the level of funding is extremely low. Farquhar has estimated that 10% or less of prevention research is focused on dissemination.[21] Across all funding sources through 2008—federal and foundations—spending on health services research, models of care, and service innovations represented only approximately 1.5% of biomedical research funding.[5] While Moses and colleagues use broad classification categories to assess trends in funding of pharmaceutical research over time (pre-human and preclinical, Phases 1–3, Phase 4, approval and regulatory, other and unclassified), D&I does not fall into any clear category for this or other analyses.[24] Rather, D&I research spans all areas from translating discoveries to bedside and broader clinical applications, to health services interventions to implement effective approaches to care. In global health it also spans from innovation in technology for extremely low-cost delivery systems to implementation in field settings.

Another way to gauge the volume of D&I research is to examine the types of articles appearing in the peer-reviewed literature. To illustrate this, three reviews showed the extent of dissemination and institutionalization of effective interventions. In a content analysis of 1,210 articles from twelve prominent public health journals, 89% of published studies were classified as basic research and development.[25] The authors classified another 5% of studies as innovation development, less than 1% as diffusion, and 5% as institutionalization. Similarly, Sallis and colleagues conducted a content analysis of four journals and found 2 to 20%

of articles fell in a phase defined as "Translate research to practice."[26] In another review of three health promotion journals, dissemination research was poorly represented despite editorials calling for more D&I research.[27] This publication record follows funding priorities.

What are the outcomes for progress in dissemination and implementation of discoveries? These can be counted as more effective health services, better prevention, reduction in health disparities, or in nonhealth settings impact on the underlying root causes of population health—such as social services, better schooling for our children, or employment opportunities. The methods and issues may appear to differ across fields of study. Like statistics, which has a long history of development in agriculture (the leading industry of the time—Cochran wrote on meta-analysis of results from agriculture trial plots in 1937 and helped define modern approaches[28]), D&I research also grew from agriculture to guide thinking in this field.[29] The history of dissemination and implementation science is presented in more detail in Chapter 3. With health care expenditures consuming an ever-increasing portion of national and state budgets in the developed world, methods to maximize our societal benefit must be refined and accessible to end users—and will likely be developed and refined most quickly in the context of health and wellness. In fact, data from the Organization for Economic Co-operation and Development (OECD) indicate that the average ratio of health expenditure to GDP has risen from 7.8% in 2000 to 9.0% in 2008 and is at 16.0% for the United States and 10.4% for Canada.[30] There is no shortage of academic research, but how do we sift through studies and draw inference to disseminate and implement effective programs and policies more broadly? A recurring question as we approach D&I research is "Will the evidence and intervention be applicable to the new setting?"

Delay in adoption of scientific discoveries is not a new phenomenon. We can look at Bayesian methods used in statistics in the 1960s to evaluate the authorship of the Federalist papers.[31] In the process, described in detail by Fred Mosteller in his autobiography, an empirical test of the Bayesian approach gave new insight to manuscript classification.[32] Mosteller also presented on using Bayesian approaches to combine means (Lake Junaluska, North Carolina, 1946—see pp. 186–187; also see "On pooling data"—JASA 1948).[33] These statistical methods have only much more recently been adapted to widespread use with modern computer technology supporting this application. So advances in statistical methods development did not achieve widespread application for decades perhaps, in part, due to technical difficulty of implementing these approaches (lack of technology), but also reluctance on the part of investigators (intrapersonal factors). Both individual and structural barriers impeded implementation, reflecting a complex interplay of barriers to implementation of innovations.

How can the principles and methods we see presented in this book help us move more quickly to build on research findings and apply them to improve health? Do we need new ways of thinking, conducting, and reporting research, or can we take our existing approaches and through consensus apply what is known more rapidly? The challenge of implementation extends along the continuum from discovery of biologic phenomena to clinical application in research settings and the broader application in the population at large. While a range of approaches to describing this continuum has been developed, perhaps more pertinent from the D&I perspective is the perspective summarized by Green and colleagues as a leaky pipeline from research to practice.[34] Across these approaches to defining stages of translation and application, some common themes emerge: discovery on its own does not lead to use of knowledge; evidence of impact does not lead to uptake of new strategies; organizations often do not support the culture of evidence-based practice; and maintenance of change is often overlooked, leading to regression of system-level changes back to a prior state. The focus of an intervention for implementation, whether at the individual level or up through to system-level changes or policies, determines in part the breadth of change toward improved population outcomes. The lag from discovery to application (implementation of effective programs and practices) may vary across disciplines. Examples from public health include the gap from perfecting the Papanicolaou test in 1943 to the establishment of screening programs in all U.S. states in 1995, and the delay from the 1964 Surgeon General's report on smoking to effective statewide tobacco control programs.[35] Of course, early applications will be in place to varying degrees before full widespread programs are implemented and sustained. As Collins notes, many false starts or failures may be needed before successful translation of discoveries to human applications.[2]

A frequently quoted statement about the total attrition in the funnel and the lapse between research and medical practice indicates that it takes 17 years to turn 14% of original research to the benefit of patient care, and is attributed to Balas and Boren.[36] The leakage or loss of medical-clinical research from the pipeline at each stage from completed research through submission, publication, indexing, and systematic reviews that produce guidelines and textbook recommendations for best practices, to the ultimate implementation of those practices in health care settings, all contribute to these estimates. Changing technologies and priorities of publishing, bibliographic data management, and systematic reviews and disseminating evidence-based guidelines will lead to different estimates over time and in different fields. Green and colleagues depict this flow of information as a leaky funnel. In it they identify many leakage points in the scientific process (see Figure 1–1).[34]

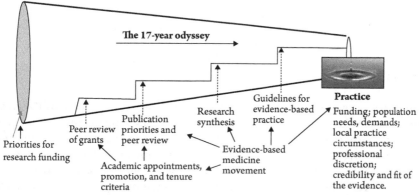

Figure 1–1. The funnel depicts loss in the pipeline from research to practice. From Green et al.[34]

Looked at from the other end of the funnel, identifying major advances in engineering that have improved quality of life in the 20th century, the National Academy of Engineering included electricity, electric motors, and imaging—each with a long line of scientific discovery and application before broader social impact was achieved.[37] The path from scientific discovery to social benefit from broad implementation has common challenges across many scientific disciplines.

■ CASE STUDIES: FROM BENCH TO BEDSIDE TO POPULATIONS

Several case studies can help in illustrating the real-world challenges and successes in moving from research to practice. Of course, we learn from both successful translation of research to practice and also from failures.

Penicillin

Fleming discovered penicillin in 1928 (though others are attributed with noticing the effect of mold on bacteria in research laboratories). Use of penicillin was not implemented for more than 15 years, when an Australian Rhodes Scholar, Howard Florey, then in the Pathology Department at Oxford, evaluated penicillin in humans and with a team of scientists developed methods for mass production, leading to widespread military use for infected soldiers.[38] Clearly the burden of infection reduced the military capability of the United Kingdom and allied forces in WWII, and increased the priority for effective antibiotics to be available. Only after the War did civilian use become available, first in Australia and then more broadly. The time delay from discovery to clinical application is typical of the lag we still see today. Of course, war has a long history for development of new methods in trauma surgery and other areas of clinical medicine, but our focus in this book is broader application of scientific advances. This example includes several steps from discovery to clinical application during WWII and then broader community-level application for effective health care, but it exemplifies how delays happen and how innovation is motivated by exceptional circumstances (unfortunately all too often war leads to major innovations in technology for destruction and for sustaining lives). Systems for large-scale production were not available, and the market forces did not support commercialization, until after WWII.

Insulin

Insulin offers another extreme example we do not see replicated today. Pancreas extract was evaluated in dogs in physiology laboratories in numerous medical centers in the early 1900s. After only 6 or so months of experimentation, Banting and Best moved from their physiology laboratory and animal studies in the Medical Building at the University of Toronto to the delivery to humans at Toronto General Hospital.[39] The clinical condition favored rapid translation to practice since patients routinely had a steady decline after onset of Type 1 or insulin-dependent diabetes, following standard therapies such as starvation and ultimately dying from metabolic imbalances.[40] Rapid physiologic evidence of response to pancreatic extract in terms of blood sugar and urinary ketones led to demand for pancreas extract outstripping supply. Few medical discoveries have had such a huge effect that they move so quickly from bench to bedside and broader application in clinics across North America. In fact, the will of the patients and their providers outpaced the slower development of approaches to large-scale production. Eli Lilly had a major interest from even before the discovery of the extraction methods in Toronto[41] reinforcing the influence of market forces on implementation. More recent experience with HIV and the social forces brought to bear by AIDS activists, along with speeding of the drug approval process, and marketing show faster developments from identification of a new disease condition to effective treatment. This time line spans from detection of AIDS cases in California and New York in 1981, to the viral cause identified in 1984, AZT as first drug for treating AIDS in 1987, a U.S. national education campaign in 1988, and combination antiretroviral therapy that is highly effective against HIV in 1996. Like diabetes the political will generated by a patient population garnered support for scientific advances at exceptional speed with clear success, making efforts in cancer and other chronic disease management pale in comparison.

Smallpox

Smallpox epidemics raged in Boston in 1690 and 1702; inoculation was a folk remedy that was shown to be effective, but political leaders forbade the use of inoculation as it was deemed to spread the disease rather than prevent it. The 1721 epidemic had a major controversy as Reverend Cotton Mather and the Boston physician William Douglass disagreed as to the utility of inoculation. Reverend Mather had inoculated his son and was an advocate while the Boston physicians argued that inoculation spread the disease. Furthermore, church leaders also debated the value of this medical intervention—Mather arguing that inoculation was a gift from God, while those opposed to inoculation claimed the epidemic afflicted people for divine reasons, and so did not want to interfere with the will of God.[42] Thus, political will alone was not sufficient to implement a potentially major preventive strategy. In 1966, the World Health Organization established a goal to interrupt smallpox transmission throughout the world by the end of 1976.[43] Because of the development of the Jenner vaccine (in 1796) and a worldwide campaign to eradicate smallpox, the last known smallpox cases were observed near the 1976 goal—a case in Somalia in October 1977 and two laboratory infections in England in 1978.[44] The WHO certified that smallpox was eradicated from the world in December 1979. The enormous global public health commitment to achieve this goal of eradication was achieved after more than 150 years of less cohesive public health activity.

These examples of translating discovery to widespread application in varying time frames demonstrate the enormous variation in implementation and some of the social and political factors that may facilitate implementing effective programs and practices. We must balance timely implementation with the caution that pervades the scientific process; too rapid implementation of ineffective or even harmful technologies will have deleterious consequences for population health. Tempering such caution is evidence from public health, where use of lead in petroleum (gasoline) was opposed by Alice Hamilton as early as 1925 because of the expected adverse health effects. Tobacco smoking continues to show just how slow we can be to implement effective prevention strategies when commercial interests oppose development of cohesive political will to advance population health. We contend, and the chapters in this book illustrate, that stronger methods for D&I research can help reduce this gap and bring us population benefits.

■ WHAT IS DISSEMINATION AND IMPLEMENTATION RESEARCH, AND WHY DOES IT MATTER?

Given these historical examples, how do we conceptualize D&I research and classify it in relation to other systems or types of research? Growing emphasis on the pace of advances in medical systems leads to a number of approaches to classifying the continuum from discovery to delivery and the improvement of the health of the population. Classification of the research continuum from bench to bedside and use of population health metrics are now post hoc and continue to evolve. Briefly, the language to describe these steps and procedures has evolved over the past decade (see Chapter 2). Furthermore, the methods research to understand the limitations of research synthesis to gather information on effective interventions and inform next steps continues to provide caution in planning and evaluation of programs.[19,20] The Institute of Medicine has defined implementation research as an important component of the framework for clinical research, and Zerhouni called for reengineering the clinical research enterprise, but we are more broadly focused, including clinical research, health systems, and prevention.[45] The roadmap[46] defines T1 as moving from basic science to clinical applications (translation to humans); T2 as clinical research (up to Phase 3 trials) moving to broader clinical practice (translation to patients); and T3 as D&I research following development of guidelines for practice, moving research into health practice through diffusion, dissemination, and delivery research (translation to practice) (see Figure 1–2). T4 research has now been added to evaluate real-world outcomes from applying discoveries and bringing them to practice (translation to population). No doubt further subdivisions will be proposed in coming years. Public health approaches may broadly be defined as practice based (though health departments and social marketing strategies for health promotion may be beyond most people's vision for practice-based research).[47] Accordingly, our methods must be robust and adaptive to the situation that they are applied in.

A number of proposed models for D&I research are discussed in multiple chapters in this book. Some are "source based" (i.e., they view D&I from the lens of researchers pushing out science) (also see Chapter 11). Others are community centered, focusing on bringing research into practice settings. Systems approaches are also proposed to conceptualize the overall framework for D&I.[48] Underlying these approaches the body of scientific evidence must be sufficient to justify moving from individual studies to broader practice (i.e., an evidence-based practice). How this is determined, through systematic synthesis, subgroup analysis, or other approaches, continues to be debated. However, to move forward with an intervention one needs a strong scientific evidence base, political will to allocate resources to achieve the

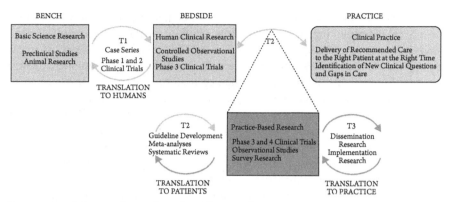

Figure 1–2. "Blue Highways" on the NIH Roadmap.

goal of implementation, and a social strategy that defines a plan of action to achieve the health goals.[49,50] We noted in our examples earlier in the chapter that lack of political will may hinder the uptake of effective public health interventions such as smallpox vaccination.

Scientific Evidence Base

In moving forward with dissemination and implementation research, we can start with the first of these three dimensions: the scientific evidence base. Here we see confusion in the field over when we have a sufficient scientific evidence base to be more broadly implemented.[51] In Chapter 15, Green and Nasser highlight how the emphasis on internal validity in our research enterprise drives us to restricted populations and narrowly defined interventions. Do these interventions work? Will they work in a different setting? Will results from trials hold up with further evaluation?[20] The tension of priority on internal validity against external validity and the associated evidence to support broader applications of scientific findings continue within the scientific process.[52] Much of the evidence synthesis "industry" focuses on narrowing evidence to specific finite questions. In medicine and public health, this began by meta-analysis even excluding nonrandomized trials from study.[53] In an early application of research synthesis and meta-analysis to observational public health data, Berlin and Colditz evaluated quality of exposure measure and used regression methods to predict future health benefits from increases in physical activity.[54] Can stronger use of existing approaches to prediction (e.g., meta-regression) help us understand when interventions will work and how large a benefit we might ultimately see? What range of benefits will fit within the distribution of findings to date?

The scope of synthesis has broadened over time—from consensus and review articles[55] to rigorous panel (systematic review) methods such as those used by the U.S. and Canadian Preventive Services[56] and the CDC community guide. The GRADE system has been developed to more explicitly guide panel decision making.[57–59]

While reporting standards have focused on the internal validity of clinical trials and observational studies,[60] new approaches to make features of study design most relevant to effectiveness have been proposed (PRECIS).[61] By making explicit a number of dimensions such as flexibility of the comparison condition and experimental intervention, practitioner expertise, eligibility criteria participant compliance, and so forth, approaches such a meta-regression[62] may be implemented to draw on these contextual factors to better understand if results can be applied in different settings. Furthermore, regression can then be used to predict what level of benefit may be seen in future applications (as has been done in the meta-analysis of BCG vaccine for prevention of tuberculosis).[63,64] While one often thinks of meta-analysis as driving for a common single answer to a clinical or public health problem, regression approaches and using meta-analysis to understand sources of heterogeneity highlight the many potentially untapped ways in which data can be synthesized to better inform policy and clinical decision making.[65]

Bero has studied the delay in implementation of clinical practices—guidelines are typically published and sit on a bookshelf.[14] Practice does not change. She reviews a range of effectiveness for approaches that are commonly used. Importantly, while the field of health care has moved substantially to accepting a role for research synthesis over the past quarter century, the study of how to implement the effective approaches to health and public health practice has been far less rigorous. Approaches to synthesis of strategies that work[66] could strengthen the field. In addition, Anderson and colleagues adapted some of the Bero factors as they apply to public health settings (Table 1–1).[67]

As in any field, a thorough review of evidence may provide a summary of where the field is or identify gaps that require further research.[68] Reviewing evidence in service organizations, Greenhalgh and colleagues[69] provide a model for diffusion of innovations in health service organizations, summarize methodology for review

TABLE 1-1. *Factors Influencing Dissemination among Health Administrators, Policy Makers, and the General Public*

Category	Influential Factor
Information	• Sound scientific basis, including knowledge of causality
	• Source (e.g., professional organization, government, mass media, friends)
Clarity of contents	• Formatting and framing
	• Perceived validity
	• Perceived relevance
	• Cost of intervention
	• Strength of the message (i.e., vividness)
Perceived values, preferences, beliefs	• Role of the decision maker
	• Economic background
	• Previous education
	• Personal experience or involvement
	• Political affiliation
	• Willingness to adopt innovations
	• Willingness to accept uncertainty
	• Willingness to accept risk
	• Ethical aspect of the decision
Context	• Culture
	• Politics
	• Timing
	• Media attention
	• Financial, or political constraints

Sources: adapted from Bero et al.[14] and Anderson et al.[67]

of evidence in this setting, and identify gaps to focus research on. They argue that research on diffusion of innovations should be theory driven, process rather than package oriented, ecological, collaborative, multidisciplinary, detailed, and participatory. They distinguish between "letting it happen," "helping it happen," and "making it happen" as related to diffusion and dissemination. "Letting or helping it happen" relies on the providers or consumers to work out how to use the science, in contrast with "making it happen," which places accountability for implementation on teams of individuals who may coach, support, or guide the implementation. Minkler and Salvatore describe the value of participatory research in speeding implementation of research findings (see Chapter 10).

Policy and Politics (Political Will)

The framework of Kingdon[70] is useful in illustrating the policy-making process and its impact on D&I research. Kingdon argues that policies move forward when elements of three "streams" come together. The first of these is the definition of the problem (e.g., a high cancer rate, or synthesis of the scientific knowledge base). The second is the development of potential policies to solve that problem (e.g., identification of policy measures to achieve an effective cancer control strategy). Finally, there is the role of politics, political will, and public opinion (e.g., interest groups supporting or opposing the policy). Policy change occurs when a "window of opportunity" opens and the three streams push policy change through.

But how do we summarize the stream of evidence to improve support to get resources allocated for implementation research or knowledge translation? Does the form of the evidence summary interact with the rate of uptake by end users, including policy makers? Lack of consistent approaches may again hinder the allocation of resources to these activities. Academic debate about the appropriateness of data, study populations, and the like distracts from cohesion and a decision to move forward. The U.S. Preventive Services Task Force separates the level of evidence from the magnitude of expected benefit when synthesizing data. They use a hierarchy of study designs to classify the source of evidence. This approach was expanded by the Institute of Medicine in their reports on vaccines[71] and health effects of Agent Orange[72] (see Mosteller and Colditz for descriptions).[68] It was adapted to a range of epidemiologic evidence on causes of cancer to guide risk assessment and prevention strategies.[73] Brownson and colleagues add to these design-level considerations of the research base contextual variables that inform implementation and adoption: individual, interpersonal, organizational, sociocultural, and political and economic.[74] Further research is needed to better understand the interplay of methods for research synthesis, presentation of summary data, and subsequent translation of research findings to policy and practice.

Prevention is lower on the priority list for public health funding at the NIH and CDC than the discovery of new therapies with emphasis on the research priority end of the Green funnel and limited attention to practitioner needs and applications.[75] In contrast with best communication practices that include promotion with repeat messages, the CDC rewards new approaches to prevention rather than sustain effective programs as exemplified by the contrast between the Australian Sun Smart program running for decades[76] and the CDC continuing to fund "novel" approaches to prevention of excess sun exposure. Quantifying improvements in population health contrasts with disease-focused treatment programs where individuals can self-identify demanding services and measurable outcomes. This identifiable bene-factor (patient) contrasts with the beneficiaries of public health, who are largely unknown.[75] Systems innovations to improve delivery-of-care equity and access to state-of-the-art therapies all receive less support or are valued less by the population than services that are regarded as personal. The time frame for benefits of knowl-edge translation—D&I research—is in the future and runs counter to public policy and planning, conflicting with pressure to deliver services today.[75] In contrast with disease (e.g., breast cancer) and exposure advocacy groups (e.g., those focusing on environmental contaminants; or unions and related occupational exposures), pre-vention does not have a voice from those who benefit. Despite the apparent priority of tobacco control efforts since the 1964 Surgeon General's report, we have only halved the rate of smoking in the United States. While this reduction in smoking may have prevented more cancer deaths than all adult cancer therapy advances over the same time frame, it leaves us with an enormous lack of accomplishment when the full burden of smoking is summed up. Where are all those who quit smoking or never started and are not suffering or dying prematurely from lung cancer and many other chronic diseases? A lack of voice leads to limited political will and lack of resource allocation to achieve the benefits of translating research to practice.

Social Strategy

Richmond defined social strategy in the context of health—guiding Healthy People 1980, and nutrition guidelines for a nation.[49] He proposed changes to promote health through health care providers, through regulations, and through community (individual and organizational changes).

Now we may expand this concept to incorporate the D&I elements—the inno-vation, the communication channel, the time, and the social system.[15] Proctor[77] proposes a model of implementation research that defines the intervention (from the evidence base) and the implementation strategy (systems environment, organizational, group/learning, supervision, and individual providers/consumers); see Figure 1–3.

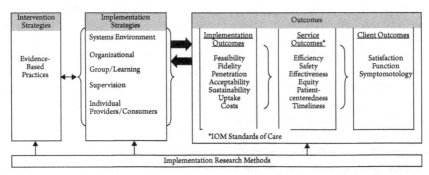

Figure 1–3. Proctor conceptual model of implementation research.

Here Proctor specifically defines the levels of change that an intervention is addressing: the larger system or environment, the organization, a group or team, or the individual. This is not unlike Richmond, who focused on policy-level changes, provider-level changes, and individual- and community-level changes to promote health.[49] One can ask, "Is there a parallel model for dissemination research addressing all these levels"?

■ WHAT IS MISSING — OUR SOCIAL CONTEXT FOR TRANSLATING RESEARCH INTO PRACTICE

Funding—NIH, CDC, AHRQ, and Canadian Priorities

Growing emphasis through funding adds credibility to the area of research implementation and evaluation. RFAs from the NIH, CDC, and the Agency for Health Care Research and Quality (AHRQ) attest to the growing commitment of resources in the United States. The Canadian Institutes of Health Research have also increased emphasis on funding of D&I, or knowledge translation. Priority for methods development and application is included in these funding opportunities, and for many institutions provides the building block on which junior faculty members are themselves promoted (holding grants in addition to scientific productivity are often key components of promotion criteria).

Academic Rewards

Priority has historically been placed on novel contributions to science—in other words, discovery. Even at the Nobel Prize level of recognition, debate was substantial regarding the role of Florey in moving from discovery of penicillin to the refinement of methods for mass production. From the point of view of impact, it was clearly the application of methods leading to broad use that saved lives during WWII, not the discovery years earlier that lay dormant in a journal article. So how do we change our academic reward system to acknowledge that application of knowledge or translation to practice is an essential component of effective and affordable health and welfare services? Accountability given the high levels of government funding for research in the United States and many other countries does not on its own shift the reward system. In fact, Moses and Martin call for sweeping changes in the way we conduct research in academic medical centers and reward scientists to more efficiently translate research to practice.[78] We need models that are implemented and evaluated within our major academic centers to show that the translation of science to practice is an academic discipline with its methods and outcomes that can be evaluated like any other discipline. However, if junior investigators do not have options for a career path in these disciplines, then again the growth of this area will be retarded. The Roadmap changes from the NIH altering the structure of support for research through the Clinical Translational Science Awards is one such endeavor to transform the research and training environment.[45,79] As another example, academic primary care has supported leading researchers at Dartmouth and Case Western to develop strategies for increased use of evidence-based preventive services, testing subsequent widespread implementation[80–83] and recognition at the level of membership in the Institute of Medicine in the National Academy. Broader recognition across health sciences disciplines will support methods development and applications to improve population health.

Innovation versus Replication (Delivery of Effective Programs)

Again the criteria for funding of grants and the promotion of faculty often hinge on innovation and discovery. Moving a discovery from bench to clinical application or from one health department to a statewide intervention may not appear to be as innovative as a more focused basic science contribution. We might argue it is, however, far more complex and less likely to succeed! Can we refine metrics that will help us estimate lives saved or improvement in quality-adjusted life years to summarize the public health impact of D&I research? How should we quantify the contextual factors that moderate the effectiveness of implementation? As Titler asks,[84] can we become consistent in approaches to circumstances and setting in which implementation or translation to practice is effective, and define mechanisms for effective interventions?

Systems to Quantify Benefits of Effective Programs (Outcomes)

How do we sum up the benefits of implementation and effective programs being delivered to broad sectors of the population? Ginexi and Hilton propose that focusing on evidence-based best practices may help bridge the gap from research to practice.[85] They argue that best and worst practice can inform practice improvement. How we quantify program fidelity and implementation remains at the core of the challenge. Proctor and colleagues[77] now propose a taxonomy of eight conceptually distinct implementation outcomes—acceptability, adoption, appropriateness, feasibility, fidelity, implementation cost, penetration, and sustainability—along with their nominal definitions. Further, they propose using a two-pronged agenda for research on implementation outcomes. Conceptualizing and measuring implementation outcomes (or process evaluation measures in the European framework) will advance understanding of implementation processes, enhance efficiency in implementation research, and pave the way for studies of the comparative effectiveness of implementation strategies. As we note in this book, several novel approaches are proposed, but coming to agreement on when these measures are most helpful will require further study.

New methods are needed, and consistency across programs will add to the overall advance of the field. The magnitude of benefit, the proportion of the population reached, and the degree to which a program is sustained all impact the long-term population benefit. Proctor defines steps in the model of implementation, noting that conceptualizing and measuring implementation outcomes will advance understanding of implementation processes, enhance efficiency in implementation research, and pave the way for studies of the comparative effectiveness of implementation strategies.[77] The RE-AIM (reach, effectiveness, adoption, implementation, and maintenance) approach to evaluation is also summarized in Chapter 16. Other approaches that apply across settings will make for a more robust area of inquiry.

SUMMARY

Given the growing emphasis on D&I as a means to increase the efficiency of the research enterprise, public policy, and the services with which we work, refining methods that will facilitate translation and implementation are imperative. Cultural changes within the academy and in linking researchers and practitioners will be necessary adjuncts to effective progress. Bringing the D&I research community to a common understanding of answers to our overarching questions will be a necessary step. Then we can more consistently answer the questions: How will we gather this information on effective interventions to form the evidence base? Will interventions be applicable to our setting? What methods should we use to decide what to disseminate or implement? Which strategies will give us the greatest impact on population health? What outcomes should be tracked to know if we are making progress? How long will it take to show progress, or when will it be observed? The methods outlined in this book will help us in answering these and other important questions.

SUGGESTED READINGS

Glasziou P, Chalmers I, Altman DG, et al. Taking healthcare interventions from trial to practice. *BMJ.* 2010;341:c3852.

Improved reporting of details of trials will enable use of results in practice. An example of this is illustrated, and a call for increased reporting of intervention details to improve replication and use in practice.

Green LW, Ottoson JM, Garcia C, Hiatt RA. Diffusion theory and knowledge dissemination, utilization, and integration in public health. *Annu Rev Public Health.* Apr 29 2009;30:151–174.

Rigorous review of public health implications of diffusion, dissemination, and implementation to improve public health practice and guide design of future research.

Ioannidis JP, Karassa FB. The need to consider the wider agenda in systematic reviews and meta-analyses: breadth, timing, and depth of the evidence. *BMJ.* 2010;341:c4875.

Thoughtful critique of limitations of meta-analysis of clinical interventions, the narrow scope of practice they cover, and the potential to draw misleading conclusions from systematic reviews and meta-analysis.

Proctor E, Silmere H, Raghavan R, et al. Outcomes for implementation research: Conceptual distinctions, measurement challenges, and research agenda. *Adm Policy Ment Health.* Oct 19 2010;38(2):65–76.

Ground-breaking summary of issues in design and evaluation of implementation research, setting out a model that defines steps in the process an discusses a model for quantifying benefits of program implementation.

Woolf SH. The meaning of translational research and why it matters. *JAMA.* Jan 9 2008;299(2):211–213.

An important contribution defining stages of research and the importance of translation from bench to bedside and from reseach clinic to population-wide applications. Also calls for research funding to be directed to improving population health outcomes.

SELECTED WEBSITES AND TOOLS

Cancer Control P.L.A.N.E.T. http://cancercontrolplanet.cancer.gov/index.html. Cancer Control P.L.A.N.E.T. acts as a portal to provide access to data and resources for designing, implementing, and evaluating evidence-based cancer control programs. The site provides five steps (with links) for developing a comprehensive cancer control plan or program.

Dissemination and Implementation Research Core at Washington University in St. Louis, Enola Proctor, Director. http://cmhsr.wustl.edu/PractitionersResearchers/ DIRC/Pages/DIRC.aspx. The Dissemination and Implementation Research Core (DIRC) provides methodological expertise to advance translational research that moves efficacious health practices from clinical knowledge into routine, real-world use—a process called Dissemination and Implementation research (DIR). The DIRC focuses on the second of two areas of translational research, as defined by the NIH: research to inform the adoption of best practices in the community.

Task Force on Community Preventive Services. http://www.thecommunityguide.org. The Community Guide provides a repository of the 200+ systematic reviews conducted by the Task Force, an independent, interdisciplinary group with staff support by the Centers for Disease Control and Prevention. Each review gives attention to the "applicability" of the conclusions beyond the study populations and settings in which the original studies were conducted.

Cochrane Collaboration. http://www.cochrane.org/. The Cochrane Collaboration prepares Cochrane Reviews and aims to update them regularly with the latest scientific evidence. Members of the organization (mostly volunteers) work together to assess evidence to help people make decisions about health care practices and policies. Some people read the health care literature to find reports of randomized controlled trials; others find such reports by searching electronic databases; others prepare and update Cochrane Reviews based on the evidence found in these trials; others work to improve the methods used in Cochrane Reviews; others provide a vitally important consumer perspective.

RE-AIM. http://www.RE-AIM.org. The acronym refers to Reach, Effectiveness, Adoption, Implementation, and Maintenance, all important dimensions in the consideration of D&I research and in the external validity or applicability of research results in original studies for the alternative settings and circumstances in which they might be applied. These were applied in the development of a set of guidelines for assessing and reporting external validity in reference 29 below.

D-cubed. http://www.tedi.uq.edu.au/dissemination/. A review of dissemination strategies used by projects funded by the Australian Learning and Teaching Council promotes dissemination strategies that have facilitated effective dissemination. A useful framework for dissemination and guide to use is provided.

■ REFERENCES

1. Agre P, Leshner AI. Bridging science and society. *Science.* Feb 19 2010; 327(5968):921.
2. Collins FS. Reengineering translational science: the time is right. *Sci Transl Med.* Jul 6 2011;3(90):90cm17.
3. Dorsey ER, de Roulet J, Thompson JP, et al. Funding of US biomedical research, 2003–2008. *JAMA.* Jan 13 2010;303(2):137–143.

4. Office of Management and Budget. *Budget: Department of Health and Human Services.* Washington, DC: The Executive Office of the President; 2010.
5. Woolf SH. The meaning of translational research and why it matters. *JAMA.* Jan 9 2008;299(2):211–213.
6. Institute of Medicine. *Crossing the quality chasm: a new health system for the 21st century.* Washington, DC: National Academy Press; 2001.
7. Rubenstein LV, Pugh J. Strategies for promoting organizational and practice change by advancing implementation research. *J Gen Intern Med.* Feb 2006;21(Suppl 2): S58–64.
8. United States Department of Health and Human Services. Improving Public Health Practice through Translational Research. 2007; http://grants.nih.gov/grants/guide/ rfa-files/rfa-cd-07–005.html. Accessed November 14, 2011.
9. Anonymous. Lost in clinical translation. *Nat Med.* Sep 2004;10(9):879.
10. Rabin BA, Brownson RC, Haire-Joshu D, Kreuter MW, Weaver NL. A glossary for dissemination and implementation research in health. *J Public Health Manag Pract.* Mar–Apr 2008;14(2):117–123.
11. Lomas J, Sisk JE, Stocking B. From evidence to practice in the United States, the United Kingdom, and Canada. *Milbank Q.* 1993;71(3):405–410.
12. Lomas J. Diffusion, dissemination, and implementation: who should do what? *Ann N Y Acad Sci.* Dec 31 1993;703:226–235; discussion 235–227.
13. Curry SJ. Organizational interventions to encourage guideline implementation. *Chest.* Aug 2000;118(2 Suppl):40–46S.
14. Bero L, Grillr R, Grimshaw J, Harvey E, Oxman AD, Thompson M. Closing the gap between research and practice: an overview of systematic reviews of interventions to promote the implementation of research findings. *BMJ.* 1998;317:465–468.
15. Bowen DJ, Sorensen G, Weiner BJ, Campbell M, Emmons K, Melvin C. Dissemination research in cancer control: where are we and where should we go? *Cancer Causes Control.* May 2009;20(4):473–485.
16. Crandall D. Implementation aspects of dissemination. *Science Communication.* 1989;11(1):79–106.
17. Huberman M. Research utilization: the state of the art. *Knowledge, Technology & Policy.* 1991;7(4):13–33.
18. Huberman AM, Levinson NS, Havelock RG, Cox PL. Interorganizational arrangements. An approach to education practice improvement. *Knowledge: Creation, Diffusion, Utilization.* 1981;3(1):5–22.
19. Glasziou P, Chalmers I, Altman DG, et al. Taking healthcare interventions from trial to practice. *BMJ.* 2010;341:c3852.
20. Ioannidis JP, Karassa FB. The need to consider the wider agenda in systematic reviews and meta-analyses: breadth, timing, and depth of the evidence. *BMJ.* 2010;341:c4875.
21. Farquhar JW. The case for dissemination research in health promotion and disease prevention. *Can J Public Health.* Nov–Dec 1996;87(Suppl 2):S44–49.
22. Harlan WR. Prevention research at the National Institutes of Health. *Am J Prev Med.* May 1998;14(4):302–307.
23. Institute of Medicine. *Linking research to public health practice. A review of the CDC's program of Centers for Research and Demonstration of Health Promotion and Disease Prevention.* Washington, DC: National Academy Press; 1997.
24. Moses H, 3rd, Dorsey ER, Matheson DH, Thier SO. Financial anatomy of biomedical research. *JAMA: the journal of the American Medical Association.* Sep 21 2005;294(11):1333–1342.

25. Oldenburg BF, Sallis JF, Ffrench ML, Owen N. Health promotion research and the diffusion and institutionalization of interventions. *Health Educ Res.* Feb 1999;14(1): 121–130.

26. Sallis JF, Owen N, Fotheringham MJ. Behavioral epidemiology: a systematic framework to classify phases of research on health promotion and disease prevention. *Ann Behav Med.* Fall 2000;22(4):294–298.

27. Rychetnik L, Nutbeam D, Hawe P. Lessons from a review of publications in three health promotion journals from 1989 to 1994. *Health Educ Res.* Dec 1997;12(4): 491–504.

28. Cochran W. Problems arising in the analysis of a series of similar experiments. *J R Stat Soc Suppl.* 1937;4:102–118.

29. Rogers E. *Diffusion of innovations.* 3rd ed. London: The Free Press; 1993.

30. OECD. *OECD Health Data 2010: Statistics and Indicators.* Paris: Organisation for Economic Co-operation and Development (OECD); 2010.

31. Mosteller F, Wallace D. *Inference and disputed authorship: The Federalist.* Reading, MA: Addison-Wesley Publishing Company; 1964.

32. Mosteller F. *The pleasures of statistics. The autobiography of Frederick Mosteller.* New York: Springer; 2010.

33. Mosteller F. On pooling data. *J Am Stat Assoc.* 1948;43:231–242.

34. Green LW, Ottoson JM, Garcia C, Hiatt RA. Diffusion theory and knowledge dissemination, utilization, and integration in public health. *Annu Rev Public Health.* Apr 29 2009;30:151–174.

35. Brownson RC, Bright FS. Chronic disease control in public health practice: looking back and moving forward. *Public Health Rep.* May–Jun 2004;119(3):230–238.

36. Balas EA, Boren SA. Managing clinical knowledge for health care improvement. In: Bemmel J, McCray A, editors. *Yearbook of medical informatics 2000: patient-centered systems.* Stuttgart, Germany: Schattauer; 2000;65–70

37. Goodwin I. Engineers proclaim top achievements of 20th century, but neglect attributing feats to roots in physics. *Physics Today.* 2000;53:48–49.

38. Bickell L. *Howard Florey: the man who made penicillin (Australian Lives series).* Melbourne: Melbourne University Press; 1996.

39. Banting FG, Best CH. The internal secretion of the pancreas. 1922. *Indian J Med Res.* Mar 2007;125(3):251–266.

40. Banting FG, Best CH, Collip JB, Campbell WR, Fletcher AA. Pancreatic extracts in the treatment of diabetes mellitus. *Can Med Assoc J.* Mar 1922;12(3):141–146.

41. Bliss M. *The discovery of insulin.* 25th anniversary edition ed. Chicago: University of Chicago Press; 2007.

42. Anonymous. The Boston Smallpox Epidemic, 1721. 2010; http://ocp.hul.harvard.edu/contagion/smallpox.html. Accessed December 5, 2010.

43. World Health Organization. *Handbook of Resolutions and Decisions of the World Health Assembly and the Executive Board.* Geneva: WHO; 1971.

44. Breslow L. The future of public health: prospects in the United States for the 1990s. *Annu Rev Public Health.* 1990;11:1–28.

45. Zerhouni E. Medicine. The NIH Roadmap. *Science.* Oct 3 2003;302(5642):63–72.

46. Westfall JM, Mold J, Fagnan L. Practice-based research—"Blue Highways" on the NIH roadmap. *JAMA.* Jan 24 2007;297(4):403–406.

47. Frieden TR. A framework for public health action: the health impact pyramid. *Am J Public Health.* Apr 2010;100(4):590–595.

48. Wandersman A, Duffy J, Flaspohler P, et al. Bridging the gap between prevention research and practice: the interactive systems framework for dissemination and implementation. *Am J Community Psychol.* Jun 2008;41(3–4):171–181.

49. Richmond J, Kotelchuck M. Coordination and development of strategies and policy for public health promotion in the United States. In: Holland W, Detel R, Know G, eds. *Oxford textbook of public health.* Vol 1. Oxford: Oxford University Press; 1991.

50. Atwood K, Colditz GA, Kawachi I. From public health science to prevention policy: placing science in its social and political contexts. *Am J Public Health.* Oct 1997;87(10):1603–1606.

51. Petticrew M, Tugwell P, Welch V, et al. Better evidence about wicked issues in tackling health inequities. *J Public Health.* Sep 2009;31(3):453–456.

52. Lavis J, Davies H, Oxman A, Denis JL, Golden-Biddle K, Ferlie E. Towards systematic reviews that inform health care management and policy-making. *J Health Serv Res Policy.* Jul 2005;10(Suppl 1):35–48.

53. Sacks H, Berrier J, Reitman D, Ancona-Berk V, Chalmers T. Meta-analysis of randomized controlled studies. *N Engl J Med.* 1987;316:450–455.

54. Berlin J, Colditz G. A meta-analysis of physical activity in the prevention of coronary heart disease. *Am J Epidemiol.* 1990;132:612–628.

55. Bastian H, Glasziou P, Chalmers I. Seventy-five trials and eleven systematic reviews a day: how will we ever keep up? *PLoS Med.* 2010;7(9):e1000326.

56. Preventive Services Task Force. *Guide to clinical preventive services.* 2nd ed. Baltimore: Williams and Wilkins; 1996.

57. Schunemann HJ, Oxman AD, Brozek J, et al. GRADE: assessing the quality of evidence for diagnostic recommendations. *Evid Based Med.* Dec 2008;13(6): 162–163.

58. Jaeschke R, Guyatt GH, Dellinger P, et al. Use of GRADE grid to reach decisions on clinical practice guidelines when consensus is elusive. *BMJ.* 2008;337:a744.

59. Guyatt GH, Oxman AD, Vist GE, et al. GRADE: an emerging consensus on rating quality of evidence and strength of recommendations. *BMJ.* Apr 26 2008; 336(7650):924–926.

60. Moher D, Schulz KF, Altman DG. The CONSORT statement: revised recommendations for improving the quality of reports of parallel-group randomized trials. *Ann Intern Med.* Apr 17 2001;134(8):657–662.

61. Thorpe KE, Zwarenstein M, Oxman AD, et al. A pragmatic-explanatory continuum indicator summary (PRECIS): a tool to help trial designers. *CMAJ.* May 12 2009;180(10):E47–57.

62. Berkey CS, Hoaglin D, Mosteller F, Colditz GA. A random-effects regression model for meta-analysis. *Stat Med.* 1995;14:395–411.

63. Colditz GA, Brewer TF, Berkey CS, et al. Efficacy of BCG vaccine in the prevention of tuberculosis. Meta-analysis of the published literature. *JAMA.* Mar 2 1994;271(9):698–702.

64. Colditz GA, Berkey CS, Mosteller F, et al. The efficacy of bacillus Calmette-Guerin vaccination of newborns and infants in the prevention of tuberculosis: meta-analyses of the published literature. *Pediatrics.* Jul 1995;96(1 Pt 1):29–35.

65. Colditz G, Burdick E, Mosteller F. Heterogeneity in meta-analysis of data from epidemiologic studies: a commentary. *Am J Epidemiol.* 1995;142:371–382.

66. Proctor EK, Landsverk J, Aarons G, Chambers D, Glisson C, Mittman B. Implementation research in mental health services: an emerging science with

conceptual, methodological, and training challenges. *Adm Policy Ment Health.* Jan 2009;36(1):24–34.

67. Anderson LM, Brownson RC, Fullilove MT, et al. Evidence-based public health policy and practice: promises and limits. *Am J Prev Med.* Jun 2005;28(5 Suppl):226–230.

68. Mosteller F, Colditz G. Understanding research synthesis (meta-analysis). *Ann Rev Public Health.* 1996;17:1–32.

69. Greenhalgh T, Robert G, Macfarlane F, Bate P, Kyriakidou O. Diffusion of innovations in service organizations: systematic review and recommendations. *Milbank Q.* 2004;82(4):581–629.

70. Kingdon JW. *Agendas, alternatives, and public policies.* New York: Addison-Wesley Educational Publishers, Inc; 2003.

71. Institute of Medicine. *Adverse effects of pertussis and rubella vaccines.* Washington, DC: National Academy Press; 1991.

72. Institute of Medicine. *Veterans and Agent Orange. Health effects of herbicides used in Vietnam.* Washington, DC: National Academy Press; 1994.

73. Colditz G, Atwood K, Emmons K, et al. Harvard Cancer Risk Index. *Cancer Causes Control.* 2000;11:477–488.

74. Brownson RC, Fielding JE, Maylahn CM. Evidence-based public health: a fundamental concept for public health practice. *Annu Rev Public Health.* Apr 21 2009; 30:175–201.

75. Hemenway D. Why we don't spend enough on public health. *N Engl J Med.* May 6 2010;362(18):1657–1658.

76. Dobbinson SJ, Wakefield MA, Jamsen KM, et al. Weekend sun protection and sunburn in Australia trends (1987–2002) and association with SunSmart television advertising. *Am J Prev Med.* Feb 2008;34(2):94–101.

77. Proctor E, Silmere H, Raghavan R, et al. Outcomes for implementation research: conceptual distinctions, measurement challenges, and research agenda. *Adm Policy Ment Health.* Oct 19 2010;38(2):65–76.

78. Moses H, 3rd, Martin JB. Biomedical research and health advances. *N Engl J Med.* Feb 10 2011;364(6):567–571.

79. Zerhouni EA. Clinical research at a crossroads: the NIH roadmap. *J Investig Med.* May 2006;54(4):171–173.

80. Dietrich A, Carney P, Winchell C, et al. An office systems approach to cancer prevention in primary care. *Cancer Practice.* 1997;5:375–381.

81. Dietrich AJ, Tobin JN, Cassells A, et al. Telephone care management to improve cancer screening among low-income women: a randomized, controlled trial. *Ann Intern Med.* Apr 18 2006;144(8):563–571.

82. Dietrich AJ, Tobin JN, Cassells A, et al. Translation of an efficacious cancer-screening intervention to women enrolled in a Medicaid managed care organization. *Ann Fam Med.* Jul–Aug 2007;5(4):320–327.

83. Stewart EE, Nutting PA, Crabtree BF, Stange KC, Miller WL, Jaen CR. Implementing the patient-centered medical home: observation and description of the national demonstration project. *Ann Fam Med.* 2010;8(Suppl 1):S21–32; S92.

84. Titler MG. Translation science and context. *Res Theory Nurs Pract.* 2010; 24(1):35–55.

85. Ginexi EM, Hilton TF. What's next for translation research? *Eval Health Prof.* Sep 2006;29(3):334–347.

2 Developing the Terminology for Dissemination and Implementation Research

■ BORSIKA A. RABIN AND
ROSS C. BROWNSON

■ BACKGROUND

Dissemination and implementation (D&I) research is increasingly recognized as an important function of academia and is a growing priority for major health-related funding agencies (e.g., the National Institute of Health [NIH], the Centers for Disease Control and Prevention [CDC]), the National Institute on Disability and Rehabilitation Research (NIDRR), the Canadian Institutes of Health Research (CIHR), and the World Health Organization (WHO).[1-7] One challenging aspect of D&I research is the lack of standardized terminology.[8-12] As noted by Ciliska and colleagues: "closing the gap from knowledge generation to use in decision-making for practice and policy is conceptually and theoretically hampered by diverse terms and inconsistent definitions of terms."[13] A survey conducted by *Nature Medicine* on how their readers define the term "translational research" found substantial variation in interpretation by respondents. Some definitions were consistent with the NIH definition ("the process of applying ideas, insights and discoveries generated through basic scientific inquiry to the treatment or prevention of human disease"), others believed that only research that leads to direct clinical application should be defined as translational research, and only a small group emphasized the bidirectional nature of the process (i.e., bench to bedside and back).[14] This phenomenon can be partly explained by the relatively new appearance of D&I research on the health research agenda and by the great diversity of disciplines that made noteworthy contributions to the understanding of D&I research.[15-17] Some of the most important contributions originate from the nonhealth fields of agriculture, education, marketing, communication, and management.[18] The primary health-related areas presently contributing to D&I research include health services research, HIV prevention, school health, mental health, nursing, cancer control, violence prevention, and disability and rehabilitation.[15,19-23] Further complexity is injected by the variation in terminology and classification of terms across countries. This book uses the term "dissemination and implementation research" to denote the newly emerging field in the United States; however, other countries and international organizations (e.g., the United Kingdom, Canada, the WHO) commonly use the terms "knowledge translation and integration," "population health intervention research," or "scaling up" to define this area of research.[7,24-26] Furthermore, Graham and colleagues identified 29 distinct terms referring to the some aspect of the D&I (or knowledge translation) process when they looked at the terminology used by 33 applied research funding agencies in nine countries.[26]

Definitions presented in this chapter reflect the terminology used in the most frequently cited manuscripts and reports on D&I research in health and in funding announcements of major federal funding agencies (e.g., NIH, CDC, NIDRR, CIHR). To identify terms and definitions, an initial search of the English language literature was conducted to identify peer-reviewed manuscripts and documents from governmental agencies (i.e., gray literature). Further papers and documents were identified from reference lists and expert recommendations using snowball sampling.[27] This chapter builds on a previously published article that used an expert discussion to select definitions to be included from a list of 106 definitions. Additional terms and their definitions were included based on recommendations from the authors and review of each chapter of this book. For each definition, the most relevant publications and chapters from this book were included so that readers may consult the literature for a more in-depth discussion of the term and its application.

To facilitate the thinking and discussion on D&I research, terms were organized under five major sections. The first section ("Foundation Concepts") provides definition for the most commonly used terms in D&I research. The second section ("Types of Research") identifies stages of the research process continuum and their relationship to D&I-related activities and defines varieties of Type 1 and 2 research. In the third section ("Models, Theories, and Frameworks"), the most commonly used models and frameworks that can inform planning and evaluation activities in D&I research are discussed. The fourth section ("Factors Influencing Dissemination and Implementation Processes") defines key factors that are related to the success, speed, and extent of D&I. Finally, the fifth section ("Evaluation of the D&I Process") summarizes important concepts of study design and measurement that should be considered when evaluating D&I research.

■ FOUNDATION CONCEPTS

Evidence-Based Intervention

The objects of D&I activities are interventions with proven efficacy and effectiveness (i.e., evidence-based). Interventions within D&I research should be defined broadly and may include programs, practices, processes, policies, and guidelines.[28] More comprehensive definitions of evidence-based interventions are available elsewhere.[29-33] In D&I research, we often encounter complex interventions (e.g., interventions using community-wide education) where the description of core intervention components and their relationships involve multiple settings, audiences, and approaches.[19,34] For a more detailed discussion of complex interventions, refer to Hawe et al.[34]

Additional terms denoting the objects of D&I activities include best practices or evidence-based practices (EBPs), evidence-based processes, and empirically supported treatments (ESTs).[35,36]

Innovation

The term *innovation* can refer to "an idea, practice, or object that is perceived as new by an individual or other unit of adoption."[18(p.12)] Some authors use this term interchangeably with the term *evidence-based intervention*.

Types of Evidence

The types of evidence available for decision making in health can be classified as Type 1, Type 2, and Type 3 evidence.[37] These evidence types differ in their characteristics, scope, and quality.

Type 1 evidence

Type 1 evidence defines the cause of a particular outcome (e.g., health condition). This type of evidence includes factors such as magnitude and severity of the outcome (i.e., number, incidence, prevalence) and the actionability of the cause (i.e., preventability or changeability) and often leads to the conclusion that *"something should be done."*[31,37]

Type 2 evidence

Type 2 evidence focuses on the relative impact of a specific intervention to address a particular outcome (e.g., heath condition). This type of evidence includes information on the effectiveness or cost effectiveness of a strategy compared with others and points to the conclusion that *"specifically, this should be done."*[31] Type 2 evidence (interventions) can be classified based on the source of the evidence (i.e., study design) as evidence based, efficacious, promising, and emerging interventions.[37]

Type 3 evidence

Type 3 evidence is concerned with the type of information that is needed for the adaptation and implementation of an evidence-based intervention.[29] This type of evidence includes information on how and under which contextual conditions interventions were implemented and how they were received, and addresses the issue of *"how* something should be done." Type 3 is the type of evidence we have the least of and derives from the context of an intervention.[37]

Diffusion

Diffusion is the passive, untargeted, unplanned, and uncontrolled spread of new interventions. Diffusion is part of the diffusion–dissemination–implementation continuum, and it is the least focused and intense approach.[38,39]

Dissemination

Dissemination is an active approach of spreading evidence-based interventions to the target audience via determined channels using planned strategies.[38,39]

Dissemination Strategy

Dissemination strategies describe mechanisms and approaches that are used to communicate and spread information about interventions to targeted users (see also Chapter 13).[40] Dissemination strategies are concerned with the packaging of the information about the intervention and the communication channels that are used to reach potential adopters and the target audience. Passive dissemination strategies include mass mailings, publication of information including practice guidelines, and untargeted presentations to heterogeneous groups.[28] Active dissemination strategies include hands-on technical assistance, replication guides, point-of-decision prompts for use, and mass media campaigns.[28] It is consistently stated in the literature that dissemination strategies are necessary but not sufficient to ensure widespread use of an intervention.[41,42]

Implementation

Implementation is the process of putting to use or integrating evidence-based interventions within a setting.[40]

Implementation Strategy

Implementation strategies refer to the systematic processes, activities, and resources that are used to integrate interventions into usual settings (see also Chapter 13).[43] Some authors refer to implementation strategies as core implementation components or implementation drivers and list staff selection, preservice and in-service training, ongoing consultation and coaching, staff and program evaluation, facilitative administrative support, and systems interventions as components.[9,42]

Adoption

Adoption is the decision of an organization or community to commit to and initiate an evidence-based intervention.[18,44,45]

Sustainability

Sustainability describes the extent to which an evidence-based intervention can deliver its intended benefits over an extended period of time after external support from the donor agency is terminated.[46] Most often sustainability is measured through the continued use of intervention components; however, Scheirer and Dearing suggest that measures for sustainability should also include considerations of maintained community- or organizational-level partnerships, maintenance of organizational or community practices, procedures, and policies that were initiated during the implementation of the intervention, sustained organizational or community attention to the issue that the intervention is designed to address, and efforts for program diffusion and replication in other sites.[47] As discussed below, three operational indicators of sustainability are: (1) *maintenance* of a program's initial health benefits, (2) *institutionalization* of the program in a setting or community, and (3) *capacity building* in the recipient setting or community.[46]

Maintenance

Maintenance refers to the ability of the recipient setting or community to continuously deliver the health benefits achieved when the intervention was first implemented.[46]

Institutionalization

Institutionalization assesses the extent to which the evidence-based intervention is integrated within the culture of the recipient setting or community through policies and practice.[45,46,48] Three stages that determine the extent of institutionalization are: (1) *passage* (i.e., a single event that involves a significant change in the organization's structure or procedures such as transition from temporary to permanent funding), (2) *cycle or routine* (i.e., repetitive reinforcement of the importance of the evidence-based intervention through including it into organizational or community procedures and behaviors, such as the annual budget and evaluation criteria), and (3) *niche saturation* (the extent to which an evidence-based intervention is integrated into all subsystems of an organization).[46,49,50] Niche saturation is also referred to as **penetration** in the literature as described by Proctor and colleagues in Chapter 13 of this book.[51]

Capacity Building

Any activity (e.g., training, identification of alternative resources, building internal assets) that builds durable resources and enables the recipient setting or community to continue the delivery of an evidence-based intervention after the external support from the donor agency is terminated.[46,49,52]

Other terms that are commonly used in the literature to refer to program continuation include incorporation, integration, local or community ownership, confirmation, durability, stabilization, and sustained use.[50]

Knowledge-for-Action Terms

The terms **knowledge translation, knowledge transfer, knowledge exchange, and knowledge integration** are commonly used, especially outside of the United States, to refer to the entire or some aspects of the D&I process. This chapter uses definitions coined by the CIHR, Graham and colleagues, and Best and colleagues to define these terms.[5,26,53] As Best and colleagues suggested, these terms can be classified as linear (knowledge translation and transfer), relationship (knowledge exchange), or systems (knowledge integration) models of D&I.[53]

Knowledge translation

Knowledge translation is the term used by the CIHR to denote "a dynamic and iterative process that includes synthesis, dissemination, exchange and ethically sound application of knowledge."[5] Knowledge translation occurs within a complex social system of interactions between researchers and knowledge users and with the purpose of improving population health, providing more effective health services and products, and strengthening the health care system.[5,26]

Knowledge transfer

Knowledge transfer is a commonly used term both within and outside of the health care sector and is defined as the process of getting (research) knowledge from producers to potential users (i.e., stakeholders).[26,53] This term is often criticized for its linear (unidirectional) notion and its lack of concern with the implementation of transferred knowledge.[26]

Technology transfer

Technology transfer is closely related to (some suggest that it is a subset of) knowledge transfer, and it refers to the process of sharing technological developments with potential users.[54,55] While knowledge transfer often refers to individuals as the recipients of the knowledge, technology transfer more often focuses on transfer to larger entities such as organizations, countries, or the public at large.[55] The object of technology transfer is often defined broadly as a process, product, know-how, or resource, but its focus is still narrower than the focus of the more encompassing knowledge transfer.[55]

Knowledge exchange

Knowledge exchange is the term used by the Canadian Health Services Research Foundation and describes the interactive and iterative process of imparting meaningful knowledge between knowledge users (i.e., stakeholders) and producers, such that knowledge users (i.e., stakeholders) receive relevant and easily usable information and producers receive information about users' research needs.[26,53] This term was introduced to, in contrast to the terms *knowledge translation* and *knowledge transfer*, highlight the bi- or multidirectional nature of the knowledge transmission process (relationship model).[26,53,56]

Knowledge integration

The term was introduced by Best and colleagues as the systems model for the knowledge transmission process and is defined as "the effective incorporation of knowledge into the decisions, practices and policies of organizations and systems."[53] The key assumptions around the knowledge integration process are that (1) it is tightly woven within priorities, culture, and context; (2) it is mediated by complex relationships; (3) it needs to be understood from a systems perspective (i.e., in the context of organizational context and strategic processes); (4) it requires the integration with the organization(s) and its systems.[53]

Knowledge utilization

Knowledge utilization refers to the use of broadly defined knowledge including not only research evidence but also scholarly practice and programmatic interventions. It can be regarded as an overarching term that encompasses both research utilization and evidence-based practice.[57,58]

Research utilization

Research utilization is a form of knowledge utilization, and it has long traditions in the nursing literature and refers to "the process by which specific research-based knowledge (science) is implemented in practice."[58,59] Research utilization, similarly to knowledge translation and knowledge transfer, follows a linear model and is primarily concerned with moving research knowledge into action.[26]

Knowledge brokering

Knowledge brokering has emerged from the understanding that there is a belief, value, and practice gap between producers (i.e., researchers) and users (i.e., practitioners, policymakers) of knowledge, and it involves the organization of the interactive process between these two groups to facilitate and drive the transfer and implementation of research evidence.[60-63] Specific tasks include synthesis and interpretation of relevant knowledge, facilitation of interaction and setting of shared agendas, building of new networks, and capacity building for knowledge use.[60,61] Knowledge brokering is described as a two-way process that not only aims at facilitating the uptake and use of evidence by practitioners and policymakers but also focuses on prompting researchers to produce more practice-based evidence.[61]

Knowledge broker

A knowledge broker is an intermediary (individual or organization) who facilitates and fosters the interactive process between producers (i.e., researchers) and users (i.e., practitioners, policymakers) of knowledge through a broad range of activities (see "Knowledge Brokering").[60,64] More broadly, knowledge brokers assist in the organizational problem-solving process through drawing analogic links between solutions learned from resolving past problems, often in diverse domains, and demands of the current project. Knowledge brokers also help "make the right knowledge available to the right people at the right time."[64(p.67)]

A more detailed discussion of knowledge brokering and knowledge brokers is provided by Hargadon.[64]

Scale-up and Scaling up

The term is commonly used in the international health and development literature and refers to "deliberate efforts to increase the impact of health service innovations successfully tested in pilot or experimental projects so as to benefit more people and to foster policy and programme development on a lasting basis."[6,65,66] Scaling up most commonly refers to expanding the coverage of successful interventions; however, it can also be concerned with the financial, human, and capital resources necessary for the expansion.[6,67] It is suggested that sustainable scale-up requires a combination of horizontal (e.g., replication and expansion) and vertical (institutional, policy, political, legal) scaling up efforts that benefit from different D&I strategies (i.e., training, technical assistance hands-on support versus networking, policy dialogue, advocacy).[7] Furthermore, some researchers suggest that scale-up has a broader reach and scope than D&I and expands to national and international levels.[68] The National Implementation Research Network uses the term *going to scale* when an evidence-based intervention reaches 60% of the target population that could benefit from it.[42]

Additional terms used to describe some aspect of the D&I process include *knowledge cycle, knowledge management, knowledge mobilization, research transfer, research translation, expansion, linkage,* and *exchange.*[5,7]

■ TYPES OF RESEARCH

Fundamental (or Basic) Research

Fundamental or basic research develops laboratory-based, etiologic models to provide theoretical explanation for generic or more specific phenomena of interest.[44]

Translational research

T1 research

T1 translational research uses discoveries generated through laboratory and/or preclinical research to develop and test treatment and prevention approaches. In other words, T1 clinical research moves science from "the bench" (fundamental research, methods development) to the patient's "bedside" (efficacy research).[44,69]

Efficacy research

Efficacy research evaluates the initial impact of an intervention (whether it does more good than harm among the individuals in the target population) when it is delivered under optimal or laboratory conditions (or in an ideal setting). Efficacy trials typically use random allocation of participants and/or units and ensure highly controlled conditions for implementation. This type of study focuses on internal validity or on establishing a causal relationship between exposure to an intervention and an outcome.[44,70]

T2 research

T2 translational research focuses on the enhancement of widespread use of efficacious interventions by the target audience. This type of research includes effectiveness research, diffusion research, dissemination research, and implementation research[44] and is also referred to as "bedside to (clinical) practice (or trench)" translation.[69,71]

Effectiveness research • Effectiveness research determines the impact of an intervention with demonstrated efficacy when it is delivered under "real-world" conditions. As a result, effectiveness trials often must use methodological designs that are better suited for large and/or less controlled research environments with a major purpose to obtain more externally valid (generalizable) results.[44,70]

Dissemination research • Dissemination research is the systematic study of processes and factors that lead to widespread use of an evidence-based intervention by the target population. Its focus is to identify the best methods that enhance the uptake and utilization of the intervention.[44,72]

Implementation research • Implementation research seeks to understand the processes and factors that are associated with successful integration of evidence-based interventions within a particular setting (e.g., a worksite or school).[73] Implementation research assesses whether the core components of the original intervention were faithfully transported to the real-world setting (i.e., the degree of fidelity of the disseminated and implemented intervention with the original study) and is also concerned with the adaptation of the implemented intervention to local context.[73] Another often overlooked but essential component of implementation research involves the enhancement of readiness through the creation of effective climate and culture in an organization or community.[19,74]

   More recently it was suggested that rather than two types (T1 and T2), four phases of translational research should be distinguished (T1 through T4).[69,75] According to this new classification, (1) T1 translational research is defined as translation of basic research into potential clinical application, which leads to theoretical knowledge about a possible intervention; (2) T2 translational research involves efficacy studies and results in efficacy knowledge about interventions that work under optimal conditions; (3) T3 translational research involves effectiveness, dissemination, and implementation research and leads to applied knowledge about interventions that work in real-world settings; and (4) T4 translational research involves outcomes assessment at the population level and results in public health knowledge at the population level.[75,76]

Mode I and II Science

A similar model for the classification of research (knowledge production) established by Gibbons and colleagues was considered by the National Cancer Institute of Canada Working Group on Translational Research and Knowledge Transfer.[53,77] This model suggests the distinction of **Mode I** and **Mode II science**. **Mode I science** refers to traditional investigator-initiated scientific methods designed to produce discipline-based generalizable knowledge and is characterized by a clear hypothesis, transparent methods, and replicability. **Mode II science** is defined as *"science in the context of its application"* and is described as context-driven, problem-focused research with the production of interdisciplinary knowledge.[53] Mode II science is concerned with contextual factors such as organizational structure, geography, attitudes, economics, and ethics.[53] Graham Harris introduces the concept of **Mode III science** that is not only done "in the context of its application but which also influences the context and application through engagement in a contextual and recursive debate." He further suggests that "to achieve this aspirational goal requires the establishment of a collaborative 'magic circle', a creative collaboration linking the worlds of science, governance, industry, the media and the community."[78]

Science-to-service gap

Science-to-service gap refers to the phenomenon when the interventions that are adopted by individuals and organizations are not the ones that are known to be effective and hence most likely to benefit the target population.[42,79]

Implementation gap

Implementation gap refers to the phenomenon when the interventions that are adopted by individuals and organization are not implemented with sufficient fidelity and consistency to produce optimal benefits.[42,79]

Assimilation gap

Assimilation gap refers to the population-level (or public health) impact of interventions and describes the phenomenon when interventions that are adopted by individuals or organizations are not deployed widely (e.g., population level) and/or not sustained sufficiently at the individual or organizational level.[79–81]

Population Health Intervention Research

Population health intervention research (PHIR) emerged from the work of Hawe and colleagues and is supported by the CIHR through their Population Health Intervention Research Initiative for Canada (PHIRIC).[82] PHIR uses scientific methods to produce knowledge on interventions operating either within or outside the health sector with potential to impact health at the population level.[24] Population health interventions include programs, policies, and resource distribution processes and are often aimed at multiple systems, use multiple strategies, and are implemented both within and outside of the health sector into dynamic and complex systems.[82] PHIR integrates the components of evaluation research and community-based intervention research into traditional intervention research and is concerned with multiple aspects of an intervention, including efficacy and effectiveness, processes by which change is brought about, contextual factors that favor desirable outcomes, reach, differential uptake, dissemination, and sustainability.[83] PHIR considers both controlled and uncontrolled intervention designs and produces practice-relevant knowledge for real-world decision making.[83]

Comparative Effectiveness Research to Accelerate Translation (CER-T)

Comparative effectiveness research (CER) is defined as "the conduct and synthesis of research comparing the benefits and harms of different interventions and strategies to prevent, diagnose, treat and monitor health conditions in 'real-world' settings. The purpose of this research is to improve health outcomes by developing and disseminating evidence-based information to patients, clinicians, and other decision-makers, responding to their expressed needs, about which interventions are most effective for which patients under specific circumstances."[84] As defined by Glasgow and Steiner in Chapter 4, **CER-T** refers to CER that is concerned with producing results that will disseminate and translate into population-level change. The linkages between CER and D&I research are discussed in more detail in Chapter 4.

■ MODELS, THEORIES, AND FRAMEWORKS

Stage Models

Stage models propose that D&I of interventions occurs as a series of successive phases rather than as one event.[16,18,85,86] Although different stage models vary in the number and name of the identified stages,[16] all models suggest that D&I does not stop at the level of initial uptake; further steps are necessary to ensure the long-term utilization of an intervention.[87] This chapter identifies the stages as dissemination, adoption, implementation, and sustainability. Other commonly used models are the innovation decision process (knowledge, persuasion, decision, implementation, and confirmation)[18] and the stages of the RE-AIM framework (reach, adoption, implementation, maintenance).[88] The different stages of the D&I process can be thought of as process variables or mediating factors (i.e., factors that lie in the causal pathway between an independent variable [e.g., the exposure to the intervention] and dependent variable [e.g., an outcome such as organizational change]) and require different strategies and are influenced by different moderating variables.[89]

Theories and Frameworks

There are a number of theories, theoretical frameworks, and models that shape the way that we think about D&I research and guide our planning and evaluation activities.[12,72] The most commonly used theories and frameworks include the Diffusion of Innovations theory,[18,87] theories of organizational change,[90] Social Marketing theory,[91] theories of communication,[92] individual and organizational decision making,[93] community organizing models,[94] the RE-AIM framework,[81] the Precede–Proceed model,[95] the Interactive Systems Framework for D&I,[96] and the Practical, Robust Implementation and Sustainability Model (PRISM),[97] the Knowledge-to-Action (KTA) model,[26] and the Promoting Action on Research Implementation in Health Services (PARiHS) framework.[98,99]

In this chapter we discuss one theory (Diffusion of Innovations) and one framework (RE-AIM) that are commonly applied in D&I research in the field of health. More comprehensive discussion of diffusion and D&I theories is available in Chapter 3 by Dearing and Kee.

Diffusion of Innovations

The Diffusion of Innovations theory was proposed by Rogers to explain the processes and factors influencing the spread and adoption of new innovations through certain channels over time.[18] Key components of the diffusion theory are: (1) perceived attributes of the innovation, (2) innovativeness of the adopter, (3) the social system, (4) individual adoption process, and (5) the diffusion system.[43] Some of these key components are discussed later in this chapter.

RE-AIM Framework

The RE-AIM framework developed by Glasgow and colleagues[70,81,100] provides a conceptual model to guide researchers and practitioners in the development of adequate multistage (reach, adoption, implementation, maintenance) and multilevel (individual, setting) indicators when evaluating D&I efforts.[88] A more comprehensive description of the RE-AIM framework and related tools can be found at: http://www.re-aim.org/.

■ FACTORS INFLUENCING THE D&I PROCESS

Designing for Dissemination and Implementation (D4D&I)

Designing for Dissemination and Implementation refers to a set of processes that are considered and activities that are undertaken throughout the planning, development, and evaluation of an intervention to increase its dissemination and implementation potential. Some authors refer to the understanding and consideration of the user context (receiver "pull").[41] D4D&I builds on the premises that (1) effective dissemination of interventions requires an active, systematic, planned, and controlled approach;[28] (2) planning for D&I in the early stage of conceptualization and development of the intervention can increase the success of later D&I efforts;[101] (3) early involvement of and partnership with target users in the conceptualization and development process can increase the likelihood of success for later dissemination and implementation efforts;[41] (4) close understanding of and building on the characteristics, beliefs, norms, and wants of target adopters can positively influence their perception of a new intervention and consequently will increase the likelihood of adoption, implementation, and sustained use of the intervention;[41] (5) study designs and measures that generate practice-relevant evidence facilitate and inform later-stage D&I efforts.[102]

Audience Segmentation

Audience segmentation is the process of distinguishing between different subgroups of users and creating targeted marketing and distribution strategies for each subgroup. Dearing and Kreuter suggest that "segmentation of intended audience members on the basis of demographic, psychographic, situational, and behavioral commonalities" allows for the design of products and messages that are perceived to be more relevant by the intended target audience.[41] A more detailed discussion about marketing approaches for D&I is described in Chapter 11.

Fidelity

Fidelity measures the degree to which an intervention is implemented as it is prescribed in the original protocol.[16,44] Fidelity is commonly measured by comparing the original evidence-based intervention and the disseminated and implemented intervention in terms of: (1) adherence to the program protocol, (2) dose or amount of program delivered, (3) quality of program delivery, and (4) participant reaction and acceptance.[103]

In the case of complex interventions, the measurement of fidelity focuses more on the function and process of the intervention than on the individual components.[34] A more comprehensive discussion of fidelity measurement of complex interventions is found in Hawe et al.[34]

Reinvention/Adaptation

For the success of D&I, interventions often need to be reinvented or adapted to fit the local context (i.e., needs and realities).[7] Reinvention or adaptation is defined as the degree to which an evidence-based intervention is changed or modified by a user during adoption and implementation to suit the needs of the setting or to improve the fit to local conditions.[18] The need for adaptation and understanding of context has been called Type 3 evidence (i.e., the information needed to adapt and implement an evidence-based intervention in a particular setting or population) (see more on this under "Types of Evidence" earlier in this chapter).[29,37] Ideally, adaptation will lead to at least equal intervention effects as is shown in the original efficacy or effectiveness trial. To reconcile the tension between fidelity and adaptation, the **core components** (or essential features) of an intervention (i.e., those responsible for its efficacy/effectiveness) must be identified and preserved during the adaptation process.[104] For a more comprehensive discussion of fidelity and adaptation, see Dearing.[105]

Although in this chapter it is defined differently, *translation* is another term commonly used in the literature to denote the adaptation of relevant research findings to make them useful for a variety of audiences.[106]

Core Elements (or Components)

The term *core elements* or *components* can refer to the intervention (core intervention elements or components) and is defined as the active ingredients of the intervention that are essential to achieving the desired outcomes of the intervention.[9] Some authors differentiate between core intervention elements or components and customizable components; the latter can be modified to local context without harming the effectiveness of the intervention.[47] While understanding of the core elements or components of an intervention or the implementation process can facilitate the adaptation and sustainability of the intervention in a new context (i.e., setting, audience),[47] the identification of these core elements is not always straightforward.[9] Identification can be facilitated by detailed description of the elements or components, but as Fixsen and colleagues noted, "the eventual specification of the core intervention components for any evidence-based program or practice may depend upon careful research and well-evaluated experiential learning from a number of attempted replications."[9(p.26)]

Core elements or components can also refer to the implementation process (Core implementation elements or components) and indicate the drivers of the implementation process that are indispensable for the successful implementation of an intervention.[9]

An extensive discussion of core intervention and implementation components that can be used to successfully implement evidence-based interventions is provided in the report of Fixsen and colleagues.[9]

Factors Associated with the Speed and Extent of D&I

Several factors (i.e., moderators) influence the extent to which D&I of evidence-based interventions occur in various settings.[18] Moderators are factors that alter the causal effect of an independent variable on a dependent variable.[89] In this case, organizational capacity can moderate the effect of an intervention on a desired outcome. These factors can be classified as the characteristics of the intervention, characteristics of the adopter (organizational and individual), and contextual factors. Adoption rate will be influenced by the interaction among the attributes of the innovation, characteristics of the intended adopters, and the given context.[19]

Characteristics of the Intervention

Rogers identifies five perceived attributes of an innovation that are likely to influence the speed and extent of its adoption: (1) relative advantage (effectiveness and cost efficiency relative to alternatives), (2) compatibility (the fit of the innovation to the established ways of accomplishing the same goal), (3) observability (the extent to which the outcomes can be seen); (4) trialability (the extent to which the adopter must commit to full adoption), and (5) complexity (how simple the innovation is to understand).[18,105] Relative advantage and compatibility are particularly important in influencing adoption rates.[18]

Acceptability

Acceptability is related to the ideas of complexity and relative advantage; it refers to a specific intervention and describes whether the potential implementers, based on their knowledge of or direct experience with the intervention, perceive it as agreeable, palatable, or satisfactory.[51]

Appropriateness

Appropriateness is related to the idea of compatibility and is defined as the perceived fit and relevance of the intervention for a given context (i.e., setting, user group) and/or its perceived relevance and ability to address a particular issue. Organizational culture and organizational climate might explain whether an intervention is perceived as appropriate by a potential group of implementers.[51]

The concepts of acceptability and appropriateness are related terms but not identical. While an intervention might be perceived as a good fit to address an issue in question (i.e., appropriate), it might not be perceived as acceptable due to its characteristics and vice versa.

Feasibility

Feasibility is closely related to the concepts of compatibility and trialability and refers to the actual fit, suitability, or practicability of an intervention in a specific setting. Perceived feasibility plays key role in the early adoption process.[51] A more detailed discussion of this concept is provided in Chapter 13.

Implementation cost

Implementation cost (or incremental cost) is defined as the cost impact of an implementation effort and depends on the costs of the particular intervention, the implementation strategy used, and the characteristics of the setting(s) where the intervention is being implemented. Understanding implementation cost can be especially important for comparative effectiveness research.[51]

A more detailed discussion of the concepts of acceptability, appropriateness, feasibility, and implementation cost is provided in Chapter 13.

Characteristics of the Adopters

Characteristics of the adopters can be discussed at the individual and organizational/community level. Attributes of the organization/community include its size, formalization, perceived complexity, and readiness for the implementation of the innovation. The characteristics, attitudes, and behaviors of individuals within an adopting organization (e.g., position in the organization, education, individual concerns and motivations) may also determine the uptake and use of an innovation.[107] Rogers classifies the individual adopters according to their degree of innovativeness into five categories: (1) innovators, (2) early adopters, (3–4) early and late majority, and (5) laggards.[18,105]

Opinion Leader

Opinion leaders are members of a community or organization who have the ability to influence attitudes and behaviors of other members of the organization or community. Opinion leadership is based on perceived competence, accessibility, and conformity to system norms and is not a function of formal position. Opinion leaders serve as models for other members of the organization or community for innovation decisions, and hence they can facilitate or impede the dissemination and adoption process.[18]

Change Agent

Change agents are representatives of change agencies that are external to an organization or community, and their goal is to influence the innovation decisions of members of the organization or community. Change agents often use opinion leaders from an organization or community to facilitate the dissemination and adoption process.[18]

Contextual Factors

Contextual factors may include the political, social, and organizational setting for the implementation of the intervention and include social support, legislations and regulations, social networks, and norms and culture.[28,108] Understanding the delivery context for the intervention is essential for the success of the D&I and closely linked to the concepts of fidelity and adaptation.[109] Recent efforts in the organizational change literature discussed context in terms of the inner (organizational) context, including structural and cultural features, and system readiness and the outer (interorganizational) context, including interorganizational networks and collaborations.[19] They also identified several core aspects of context, including leadership, infrastructure, and unit variability.[110]

Organizational culture

Organizational culture is defined as the organizational norms and expectations regarding how people behave and how things are done in an organization.[111,112] This includes implicit norms, values, shared behavioral expectations, and assumptions that guide the behaviors of members of a work unit.[113] Organizational culture refers to the core values of an organization, its services, or products as well as how individuals and groups within the organization treat and interact with each other. Schein defined it as "the pattern of shared basic assumptions that was learned by a group as it solved its problems of external adaptation and internal integration, and that has worked well enough to be considered valid and, therefore, to be taught to new members as the correct way to perceive, think, and feel in relation to those problems."[114(p. 17)]

Organizational climate

Organizational climate refers to the employees' perceptions of and reaction to the characteristics of the work environment.[115–121]

Organizational readiness for change

Organizational readiness for change is defined as the extent to which organizational members are psychologically and behaviorally prepared to implement a new

intervention. Organizational readiness is widely regarded as an essential antecedent to successful implementation of change in healthcare and social service
organizations.[122–124]

Factors that are associated with organizational readiness for change include
(1) change valence (i.e., the employees' perception of the personal benefit of implemented change), (2) change efficacy (i.e., the perception of their capability of implementing the change), (3) discrepancy (i.e., the employees' belief in the necessity of
change to bridge the gap between the organization's current and desired state), and
(4) principal support (i.e., the employees' perception of the commitment of the formal organizational leaders and opinion leaders to support successful implementation
of change) and are discussed in more detail in Chapter 7.

Chapter 7 provides a detailed discussion of organizational characteristics that
influence D&I efforts.

■ EVALUATION OF THE D&I PROCESS

Traditional randomized controlled trials (RCTs) are not always desirable or feasible for the evaluation of dissemination and implementation programs. To achieve
a greater understanding of external validity, a variety of study designs that take
into count contextual factors should be considered for the evaluation of dissemination and implementation efforts, including quasi-experimental designs, interrupted times series design, and before–after designs, adequacy and plausibility
designs, cluster (or group) randomized designs, participatory research methods,
and pragmatic clinical trials.[125,126] In this chapter we define mixed-methods designs,
pragmatic clinical trials, natural experiments, and plausibility designs. A more
detailed discussion of design-related issues is provided in "Models, Theories, and
Frameworks".

Study Designs

Mixed-methods designs

Mixed-methods designs involve the collection and analysis of multiple, both quantitative and qualitative data in a single study to answer research questions using
a parallel (quantitative and qualitative data collected and analyzed concurrently),
sequential (one type of data informs the collection of the other type), or converted
(data is converted—qualitized or quantitized—and reanalyzed) approach. The
mixed-methods research design can generate rich data from multiple levels and
a number of stakeholders and hence is appropriate to answer complex research
questions (also see "Systems thinking").[127,128]

Pragmatic (or practical) clinical trial (PCT)

PCTs are clinical trials that are concerned with producing answers to questions faced
by decision makers.[129] Tunis and colleagues define PCTs as studies that "(1) select
clinically relevant alternative interventions to compare, (2) include a diverse population of study participants, (3) recruit participants from heterogeneous practice

settings, and (4) collect data on a broad range of health outcomes."[129] PCTs that take into rather than "take out of" (i.e., control for) consideration the large number of mediators and moderators that influence the D&I process are more likely to produce practice-based evidence than their highly controlled counterparts.[125]

Natural experiment

Natural experiment is a form of observational study design and is defined as "naturally occurring circumstances in which subsets of the population have different levels of exposure to a supposed causal factor, in a situation resembling an actual experiment where human subjects would be randomly allocated to groups."[89(p.25)]

Plausibility design

Plausibility design is used to document impact and rule out alternative explanations when RCT approach is not feasible or acceptable (i.e., complexity of intervention, known efficacy or effectiveness in small-scale, ethical concerns). Plausibility studies include comparison groups and also address potential confounders.[126]

Measurement considerations

In the context of measures of the D&I process, three main components should be considered: moderators (i.e., factors associated with the speed and extent of dissemination and implementation), mediators (i.e., process variables), and outcomes. Moderators and mediators are defined in a previous section of this paper. The measurement of moderators and mediators can help to identify the factors and processes that lead to the success or failure of an evidence-based intervention to achieve certain outcomes. To reflect the complexity of interventions and diversity in the interest of potential stakeholders (i.e., policymakers, practitioners, clinicians), in D&I research we commonly measure multiple moderators, mediators, and outcomes and assess their relationship.[130]

Systems thinking

Systems thinking is the process of understanding how things influence one another other within a whole and is based on the premise that societal problems are complex and that the response to these complex problems is only possible by intervening at multiple levels and with the engagement of stakeholders and settings across the different levels including the home, school, workplace, community, region, and country.[131,132] Systems thinking is not only concerned with applying multiple strategies at multiple levels but also focuses on the interrelationships within and across levels and how interventions need to take these relationships into account in their design and implementation.[131,132] Chapter 9 provides a detailed discussion on the concept of systems thinking for D&I.

Outcome variables

Outcome variables, the end results of evidence-based interventions, in D&I research are often different from those in traditional health research and have to be defined broadly, including short- and long-term outcomes, individual and organizational- or population-level outcomes, impacts on quality of life, adverse consequences, and economic evaluation.[28] Although individual-level variables can also be important (e.g., behavior change variables such as smoking or physical activity), outcome measures in D&I research are typically measured at organizational, community, or policy level (e.g., organizational change, community readiness for change).

Implementation outcomes • Implementation outcomes are distinct from system outcomes (e.g., organizational-level measures) and individual-level behavior and health outcomes and are defined as "the effects of deliberate and purposive actions to implement new treatments, practices, and services."[51(p.65)] Implementation outcomes are measures of implementation success, proximal indicators of implementation processes, and key intermediate outcomes of effectiveness and quality of care. The main value of implementation outcomes is to distinguish intervention failure (i.e., when an intervention is ineffective in a new context) from implementation failure (i.e., when the incorrect deployment of a good intervention causes lack of previously documented desirable outcomes).[51]

External validity

External validity is concerned with the generalizability or real-world applicability of findings from a study and determines whether the results and inferences from the study can be applied to the target population and settings.[133,134] Standardized and detailed reporting on factors that influence external validity (such as the ones recommended in the RE-AIM framework) can contribute to more successful D&I efforts.[81,102,133] The concept of external validity is discussed in detail in Chapter 15.

■ CONCLUSION

In order for a field to prosper and thrive, a common language is essential. As is often the case when many disciplines and numerous organizations converge in the development of a field, D&I research is characterized by inconsistent terminology.

When compiling this chapter, we encountered a number of challenges. Our research was limited to English-language documents, so we may have missed important information from non-English-speaking countries. Another challenge was the lack of consensus on the overall classification of terms in the literature that may lead to apparent contradictions. For example, this chapter defines the different stages (dissemination, adoption, implementation, and sustainability) of the process under the umbrella term "D&I research." Other stage models may discuss adoption and sustainability as a distinct stage.[103] Finally, it is important to note that the five-section classification introduced in this chapter was not developed to impose a rigid structure; rather, it is used as an organizing framework that allows us to discuss terms in the domain where they are most commonly applied. At the end of this book, we also include an alphabetized list of terms with respective page numbers to facilitate the search of definitions.

The lack of agreed-upon language for D&I research impedes the systematic analysis and summary of existing evidence in the field and the communication across different stakeholders (i.e., researchers, practitioners, policymakers).[11,135] The purpose of this chapter is not to advocate or argue the superiority of one term or classification scheme over another, but to facilitate communication by beginning to define commonly used terms in D&I research for researchers, practitioners, policymakers, and funding agencies. A common language should help accelerate the scientific progress in D&I research by facilitating comparison of methods and findings, as well as identifying gaps in dissemination knowledge.

We believe that the "state of the art" is not advanced enough to resolve all of the existing inconsistencies, and this chapter represents a starting point rather than the definitive language for D&I research. Given the increased interest and financial support from the NIH, the CDC, CIHR, and the WHO, we anticipate that the terminology and frameworks for D&I research will be refined and expanded to reflect this evolving field. Finally, it is our hope that our definitions, as a first step, will lead to agreed-upon terminology by initiating further dialogue among stakeholders and will ultimately contribute to higher quality D&I research and more effective public health and clinical practice.

SUGGESTED READINGS

Fixsen DL, Naoom SF, Blase KA, Friedman RM, Wallace F. *Implementation research: A synthesis of the literature.* Tampa, FL: National Implementation Research Network, University of South Florida; 2005.

> *A monograph that summarizes findings from the review of the research literature on implementation, including findings from the domains of agriculture, business, child welfare, engineering, health, juvenile justice, manufacturing, medicine, mental health, nursing, and social services. The authors organize and synthesize critical lessons regarding implementation from these domains and provide definitions for constructs and processes.*

Khoury MJ, Gwinn M, Yoon PW, Dowling N, Moore C, Bradley C. The continuum of translation research in genomic medicine: how can we accelerate the appropriate integration of human genome discoveries into health care and disease prevention? *Genetics in Medicine.* 2007;9(10):665–674.

> *This article introduces concepts of T3 and T4 research in this key emerging area of public health genomics. It emphasizes the need to focus on the need to conduct research and programs that will lead to better care and will have public health impact.*

Ottoson JM, Hawe P, eds. *Knowledge utilization, diffusion, implementation, transfer, and translation: Implications for evaluation.* Vol. 124. San Francisco: Jossey-Bass and the American Evaluation Association; 2009.

> *A monograph on issues and terminology for knowledge utilization, diffusion, implementation, transfer, and translation. The authors recommend more consideration of background, contextual factors that may influence a policy or program, and how this impacts evaluation efforts.*

World Health Organization. *Practical guidance for scaling up health service innovations.* Geneva, Switzerland: WHO Press; 2009.

> *A practical guide on how to perform the scale up of effective health services innovations in an international context. The document identifies general principles and provides concrete suggestions and is organized around an action oriented framework and is illustrated by case studies.*

Glasgow RE, Vogt TM, Boles SM. Evaluating the public health impact of health promotion interventions: the RE-AIM framework. *Am J Public Health.* Sep 1999; 89(9):1322–1327.

In this seminal article, Glasgow et al. evaluate public health interventions using the RE-AIM framework. The model's five dimensions (reach, efficacy, adoption, implementation, and maintenance) act together to determine a particular program's public health impact. The article also summarizes the model's strengths and limitations, and suggests that failure to evaluate on all five dimensions can result in wasted resources.

Feldstein AC, Glasgow RE. A practical, robust implementation and sustainability model (PRISM) for integrating research findings into practice. *Jt Comm J Qual Patient Saf.* 2008;34(4):228–243.

This article describes the Practical, Robust Implementation and Sustainability Model (PRISM), a comprehensive approach to implementation science. The model emphasizes the importance of considering worker perspectives, building partnerships, and providing for program sustainability.

Wandersman A, Duffy J, Flaspohler P, et al. Bridging the gap between prevention research and practice: the interactive systems framework for dissemination and implementation. *Am J Community Psychol.* Jun 2008;41(3–4):171–181.

Wandersman et al. describe the gap between research and practice and the need for new approaches to close this gap. Their design, the Interactive Systems Framework for Dissemination and Implementation (ISF), can be used by a wide variety of stakeholders to recognize the various needs and resources of different systems.

Graham ID, Logan J, Harrsion MB, et al. Lost in knowledge translation: time for a map? *J Contin Educ Health.* 2006;26:13–24.

Graham et al. review the terms used to describe the knowledge-to-action (KTA) process, and describe a framework for conceiving of this process. They stress the importance of relationships to facilitate the knowledge-to-action process, as well as a common definition of how KTA works.

Kitson A, Harvey G, McCormack B. Enabling the implementation of evidence based practice: a conceptual framework. *Qual Health Care.* Sep 1998;7(3):149–158.

This article proposes three elements that influence the translation of research into practice: the level of the evidence, the context of the research, and how the research is conducted. These are considered to be of equal importance in the implementation process.

Rycroft-Malone J, Kitson A, Harvey G, et al. Ingredients for change: revisiting a conceptual framework. *Qual Saf Health Care.* Jun 2002;11(2):174–180.

Rycroft-Malone et al. refine an existing framework to improve the translation of research to practice. A better understanding of the relationships between elements of the framework will contribute to more effective implementation methods.

■ ACKNOWLEDGMENTS

The authors are thankful to Ms. Shannon Keating for her assistance with the preparation of this chapter.

An earlier version of this chapter was published in the *Journal of Public Health Management and Practice* in 2008 and was coauthored by Drs. Debra Haire-Joshu, Matthew Kreuter, and Nancy Weaver. We appreciate the contribution from these coauthors.

Partial support for the preparation of this chapter was provided through the National Cancer Institute CRN Cancer Communication Research Center (1P20 CA137219)

■ REFERENCES

1. National Cancer Institute. *The National Cancer Institue Strategic Plan for Leading the Nation.* Bethesda, MD: National Institutes of Health; 2006.
2. National Cancer Institute. *Designing for dissemination.* http://cancercontrol.cancer.gov/d4d/. Accessed on August 9, 2010.
3. National Institute for Occupational Safety and Health. *Communication and information dissemination.* http://www.cdc.gov/niosh/programs/cid/. Accessed on August 9, 2010.
4. National Institute on Disability and Rehabilitation Research. *NIDRR's core areas of research.* http://www2.ed.gov/rschstat/research/pubs/core-area.html#kdu. Accessed on August 9, 2010.
5. Canadian Institutes of Health Research. *Knowledge translation at CIHR.* http://www.cihr-irsc.gc.ca/e/33747.html. Accessed on November 9, 2011.
6. Mangham LJ, Hanson K. Scaling up in international health: what are the key issues? *Health Policy Plan.* 2010;25:85–96.
7. World Health Organization. *Practical guidance for scaling up health service innovations.* Geneva, Switzerland: World Health Organization Press; 2009.
8. National Center for the Dissemination of Disability Research. *A review of the literature on dissemination and knowledge utilization.* Austin, TX: Author; 1996.
9. Fixsen DL, Naoom SF, Blase KA, Friedman RM, Wallace F. *Implementation research: a synthesis of the literature.* Tampa, FL: National Implementation Research Network, University of South Florida; 2005.
10. Kerner J, Rimer B, Emmons K. Introduction to the special section on dissemination: dissemination research and research dissemination: how can we close the gap? *Health Psychol.* Sep 2005;24(5):443–446.
11. Glasgow RE, Marcus AC, Bull SS, Wilson KM. Disseminating effective cancer screening interventions. *Cancer.* Sep 1 2004;101(5 Suppl):1239–1250.
12. Crosswaite C, Curtice L. Disseminating research results—the challenge of bridging the gap between health research and health action. *Health Promot Int.* 1994;9(4): 289–296.
13. Ciliska D, Robinson P, Armour T, et al. Diffusion and dissemination of evidence-based dietary strategies for the prevention of cancer. *Nutr J.* Apr 8 2005;4(1):13.
14. Anonymous. Lost in clinical translation. *Nat Med.* Sep 2004;10(9):879.
15. Dobbins M. *Is scientific research evidence being translated into new public health practice?* Toronto, ON: Central East Health Information Partnership; 1999.
16. Mayer JP, Davidson WS. Dissemination of innovations. In: Rappaport J, Seidman E, eds. *Handbook of community psychology.* New York: Plenum Publishers; 2000: 421–438.
17. Green LW, Johnson JL. Dissemination and utilization of health promotion and disease prevention knowledge: theory, research and experience. *Can J Public Health.* Nov–Dec 1996;87(Suppl 2):S11–S17.
18. Rogers EM. *Diffusion of innovations.* Fifth edition. New York: Free Press; 2003.

19. Greenhalgh T, Robert G, Macfarlane F, Bate P, Kyriakidou O. Diffusion of innovations in service organizations: systematic review and recommendations. *Milbank Q.* 2004;82(4):581–629.

20. Solomon J, Card JJ, Malow RM. Adapting efficacious interventions: advancing translational research in HIV prevention. *Eval Health Prof.* Jun 2006;29(2): 162–194.

21. Proctor EK, Landsverk J, Aarons G, Chambers D, Glisson C, Mittman B. Implementation research in mental health services: an emerging science with conceptual, methodological, and training challenges. *Adm Policy Ment Health.* 2009;36(1): 24–34.

22. Saul J, Duffy J, Noonan R, et al. Bridging science and practice in violence prevention: addressing ten key challenges. *Am J Community Psychol.* 2008;41(3–4):197–205.

23. Bowen DJ, Sorensen G, Weiner BJ, Campbell M, Emmons K, Melvin C. Dissemination research in cancer control: where are we and where should we go? *Cancer Causes Control.* May 2009;20(4):473–485.

24. Hawe P, Potvin L. What is population health intervention research? *Can J Public Health.* 2009;100(1 Suppl): I8–I14.

25. Tetroe J. *Knowledge Translation at the Canadian Institutes of Health Research: A Primer.* Austin, TX: National Center for the Dissemination of Disability Research; 2007.

26. Graham ID, Logan J, Harrison MB, et al. Lost in knowledge translation: time for a map? *J Cont Educ Health Prof.* 2006;26:13–24.

27. Balbach ED. *Using case studies to do program evaluation.* Sacramento, CA: California Department of Health Services; 1999.

28. Rabin BA, Brownson RC, Kerner JF, Glasgow RE. Methodologic challenges in disseminating evidence-based interventions to promote physical activity. *Am J Prev Med.* Oct 2006;31(4 Suppl):S24–S34.

29. Rychetnik L, Hawe P, Waters E, Barratt A, Frommer M. A glossary for evidence based public health. *J Epidemiol Community Health.* Jul 2004;58(7):538–545.

30. Sackett DL, Rosenberg WM, Gray JA, Haynes RB, Richardson WS. Evidence based medicine: what it is and what it isn't. *BMJ.* Jan 13 1996;312(7023):71–72.

31. Brownson RC, Baker EA, Leet TL, Gillespie KN. *Evidence-based public health.* New York: Oxford University Press; 2003.

32. Guyatt G, Rennie D, eds. *Users' guides to the medical literature. A manual for evidence-based clinical practice.* Chicago, IL: American Medical Association Press; 2002.

33. Jenicek M. Epidemiology, evidenced-based medicine, and evidence-based public health. *J Epidemiol.* Dec 1997;7(4):187–197.

34. Hawe P, Shiell A, Riley T. Complex interventions: how "out of control" can a randomised controlled trial be? *BMJ.* Jun 26 2004;328(7455):1561–1563.

35. Borkovec TD, Castonguay LG. What is the scientific meaning of empirically supported therapy? *J Consult Clin Psychol.* 1998;66(1):136–142.

36. Gambrill E. Evidence-based practice: Implications for knowledge development and use in social work. In: Rosen A, Proctor E, eds. *Developing practice guidelines for social work intervention.* New York: Columbia University Press; 2003:37–58.

37. Brownson RC, Fielding JE, Maylahn CM. Evidence-based public health: a fundamental concept for public health practice. *Ann Rev Public Health.* 2009;30: 175–201.

38. Lomas J. Diffusion, dissemination, and implementation: who should do what? *Ann N Y Acad Sci.* 1993;703:226–235.

39. MacLean DR. Positioning dissemination in public health policy. *Can J Public Health*. Nov–Dec 1996;87(Suppl 2):S40–S43.
40. National Institutes of Health. *PA-10–038: Dissemination and implementation research in health (R01)*. http://grants.nih.gov/grants/guide/pa-files/PAR-10–038.html. Accessed on November 10, 2011.
41. Dearing JW, Kreuter MW. Designing for diffusion: how can we increase uptake of cancer communication innovations? *Patient Educ Couns*. Dec 2010;81(Suppl):S100–S110.
42. Blase KA, Fixsen DL, Duda MA, Metz AJ, Naoom SF, Van Dyke AK. Implementing and sustaining evidence-based programs: Have we got a sporting chance? PowerPoint presentation presented at Blueprints Conference, University of North Carolina, Chapel Hill. April 8, 2010.
43. National Institutes of Health. *PA-08–166: Dissemination, implementation, and operational research for HIV prevention interventions (R01)*.http://grants.nih.gov/grants/guide/pa-files/PA-08–166.html. Accessed November 10, 2011.
44. Sussman S, Valente TW, Rohrbach LA, Skara S, Pentz MA. Translation in the health professions: converting science into action. *Eval Health Prof*. Mar 2006;29(1):7–32.
45. Hoelscher DM, Kelder SH, Murray N, Cribb PW, Conroy J, Parcel GS. Dissemination and adoption of the Child and Adolescent Trial for Cardiovascular Health (CATCH): a case study in Texas. *J Public Health Manag Pract*. Mar 2001;7(2):90–100.
46. Shediac-Rizkallah MC, Bone LR. Planning for the sustainability of community-based health programs: conceptual frameworks and future directions for research, practice and policy. *Health Educ Res*. Mar 1998;13(1):87–108.
47. Scheirer MA, Dearing JW. Agenda for research on sustainability of public health programs. *Am J Public Health*. Nov 2011;101(11):2059–67.
48. Goodman RM, Steckler A. A model for the institutionalization of health promotion programs. *Fam Community Health*. 1989;11(4):63–78.
49. Pluye P, Potvin L, Denis J. Making public health programs last: conceptualizing sustainability. *Eval Program Plan*. 2004;27:121–133.
50. Johnson K, Hays C, Center H, Daley C. Building capacity and sustainable prevention innovations: a sustainability planning model. *Eval Program Plann*. 2004;27:135–149.
51. Proctor E, Silmere H, Raghavan R, et al. Outcomes for implementation research: conceptual distinctions, measurement challenges, and research agenda. *Adm Policy Ment Health*. 2011;38:65–76.
52. Community Partnership for Healthy Children. Spotlight: funding alternatives. A Sierra Health Foundation initiative. Sacramento, CA: Author; 2002;4(3):1–4.
53. Best A, Hiatt RA, Norman CD. Knowledge integration: conceptualizing communications in cancer control systems. *Patient Educ Couns*. 2008;71(3):319–327.
54. National Science Board. *Science and engineering indicators 2006*. Arlington, VA: Author; 2006.
55. Oliver ML. The transfer process: Implications for evaluation. In: Ottoson SM, Hawe P, eds. *Knowledge utilization, diffusion, implementation, transfer, and translation: Implications for evaluation*. Vol 124. San Francisco: Jossey-Bass and the American Evaluation Association; 2009:61–73.
56. Mitton C, Adair CE, McKenzie E, Patten SB, Perry BW. Knowledge transfer and exchange: review and synthesis of the literature. *Milbank Q*. 2007;85(4):729–768.
57. Loomis ME. Knowledge utilization and research utilization in nursing. *Image J Nurs Sch*. Spring 1985;17(2):35–39.

58. Estabrooks CA. The conceptual structure of research utilization. *Res Nurs Health.* Jun 1999;22(3):203–216.
59. Estabrooks CA, Wallin L, Milner M. Measuring knowledge utilization in healthcare. *International Journal of Policy Evaluation & Management.* 2003;1:3–36.
60. Ward VL, House AO, Hamer S. Knowledge brokering: exploring the process of transferring knowledge into action. *BMC Health Serv Res.* 2009;9:12.
61. van Kammen J, de Savigny D, Sewankambo N. Using knowledge brokering to promote evidence-based policy-making: the need for support structures. *Bull World Health Organ.* Aug 2006;84(8):608–612.
62. Lomas J. Using 'linkage and exchange' to move research into policy at a Canadian foundation. *Health Aff (Millwood).* May–Jun 2000;19(3):236–240.
63. Caplan N. The two-communities theory and knowledge utilization. *Am Behav Sci.* 1979;22(3):459–470.
64. Hargadon AB. Brokering knowledge: linking learning and innovation. *Res Organ Behav.* 2002;24:41–85.
65. Simmons R, Fajans P, Ghiron L. Introduction. In: Simmons R, Fajans P, Ghiron L, eds. *Scaling up health service delivery: from pilot innovations to policies and programmes.* Geneva: World Health Organization; 2007:vii–xvii.
66. Johns B, Torres TT. Costs of scaling up health interventions: a systematic review. *Health Policy Plan.* 2005;20(1):1–13.
67. Hanson K, Cleary S, Schneider H, Tantivess S, Gilson L. Scaling up health policies and services in low- and middle-income settings. *BMC Health Serv Res.* 2010; 10(Suppl 1):I1.
68. Norton WE, Mittman B. *Scaling-up health promotion/disease prevention programs in community settings: barriers, facilitators, and initial recommendations.* Report submitted to Patrick and Catherine Weldon Donaghue Medical Research Foundation Hartford, CT; 2010.
69. Woolf SH. The meaning of translational research and why it matters. *JAMA.* 2008;299:211–213.
70. Glasgow RE, Lichtenstein E, Marcus AC. Why don't we see more translation of health promotion research to practice? Rethinking the efficacy-to-effectiveness transition. *Am J Public Health.* Aug 2003;93(8):1261–1267.
71. National Institute of Health. *Roadmap for medical research.* Bethesda, MD: Author; 2002.
72. Johnson JL, Green LW, Frankish CJ, MacLean DR, Stachenko S. A dissemination research agenda to strengthen health promotion and disease prevention. *Can J Public Health.* Nov–Dec 1996;87(Suppl 2):S5–S10.
73. National Institutes of Health. *PA-10–040: Dissemination and implementation research in health (R21).* http://grants.nih.gov/grants/guide/pa-files/PAR-10–040.html. Accessed on November 10, 2011.
74. Center for Mental Health in Schools at UCLA. *Systemic change and empirically-supported practices: The implementation problem.* Los Angeles, CA: School Mental Health Project, Department of Psychology, UCLA; 2006.
75. Szilagyi PG. Translational research in pediatrics. *Acad Pediatr.* 2009;9(2):71–80.
76. Khoury MJ, Gwinn M, Yoon PW, Dowling N, Moore C, Bradley C. The continuum of translation research in genomic medicine: how can we accelerate the appropriate integration of human genome discoveries into health care and disease prevention? *Genet Med.* 2007;9(10):665–674.

77. Gibbons M, Limoges C, Nowotny H, Schwartzman S, Scott P. *The new production of knowledge: the dynamics of science and research in contemporary societies.* London: Sage; 1994.
78. Harris G. Wicked meso-scale problems and a new kind of science. *Seeking sustainability in an age of complexity.* First edition: Cambridge, Cambridge University Press. 2007:162–174.
79. Panzano P. *Images of Implementation.* http://www.screencast.com/users/MGrossman/folders/VCBH/media/073c8f7b-4176–447f-a442-a4c677d1dd30. Accessed on November 10, 2011.
80. Fichman RG, Kemerer CF. The illusory diffusion of innovation: an examination of assimilation gaps. *Inform Syst Res.* 1999;10(3):255–275.
81. Glasgow RE, Vogt TM, Boles SM. Evaluating the public health impact of health promotion interventions: the RE-AIM framework. *Am J Public Health.* Sep 1999;89(9): 1322–1327.
82. Canadian Institutes of Health Research. *Population health intervention research.* http://www.cihr-irsc.gc.ca/e/33503.html. Accessed on November 9, 2011.
83. Institute of Population and Public Health. *Population health intervention research. Spotlight on research.* Toronto, ON: Author; 2007.
84. Pawson R, Greenhalgh T, Harvey G, Walshe K. Realist review: a new method of systematic review designed for complex policy interventions. *J Health Serv Res Policy.* 2005;10:S21–S39.
85. Goodman RM, Tenney M, Smith DW, Steckler A. The adoption process for health curriculum innovations in schools: a case study. *J Health Educ.* 1992;23: 215–220.
86. Brownson RC, Ballew P, Dieffenderfer B, et al. Evidence-based interventions to promote physical activity: what contributes to dissemination by state health departments. *Am J Prev Med.* 2007;33(1 Suppl):S66–S73; quiz S74–S68.
87. Oldenburg B, Glanz K. Diffusion of innovation. In: Glanz K, Rimer BK, Viswanath K, eds. *Health behavior and health education.* Fourth edition: John Wiley & Sons, Inc.; 2008:313–334.
88. Dzewaltowski DA, Estabrooks PA, Glasgow RE. The future of physical activity behavior change research: what is needed to improve translation of research into health promotion practice? *Exerc Sport Sci Rev.* Apr 2004;32(2):57–63.
89. Last JM. *A dictionary of epidemiology.* Fourth edition. New York: Oxford University Press; 2001.
90. Butterfoss FD, Kegler MC, Francisco VT. Mobilizing organizations for health promotion: theories of organizational change. In: Glanz K, Rimer BK, Viswanath K, eds. *Health behavior and health education.* Fourth edition: John Wiley & Sons, Inc.; 2008:335–362.
91. Storey JD, Saffitz GB, Rimon JG. Social marketing. In: Glanz K, Rimer BK, Viswanath K, eds. *Health behavior and health education.* Fourth edition: John Wiley & Sons, Inc.; 2008:435–464.
92. Finnegan JRJ, Viswanath K. Communication theory and health behavior change: the media studies framework. In: Glanz K, Rimer BK, Viswanath K, eds. *Health behavior and health education.* Fourth edition: John Wiley & Sons, Inc.; 2008:363–388.
93. Kegler MC, Glanz K. Perspectives on group, organization, and community interventions. In: Glanz K, Rimer BK, Lewis FM, eds. *Health behavior and health education.* Fourth edition: John Wiley & Sons, Inc.; 2008:389–404.

94. Bracht NK, Rissel C. A five stage community organization model for health promotion: empowerment and partnership strategies. In: Bracht N, ed. *Health promotion at the community level: new advances.* Thousand Oaks, CA: Sage Publications; 1999:83–116.

95. Green LW, Kreuter M. *Health program planning: an educational and ecological approach.* Fourth edition. New York, NY: McGraw-Hill; 2005.

96. Wandersman A, Duffy J, Flaspohler P, et al. Bridging the gap between prevention research and practice: the interactive systems framework for dissemination and implementation. *Am J Community Psychol.* Jun 2008;41(3–4):171–181.

97. Feldstein AC, Glasgow RE. A practical, robust implementation and sustainability model (PRISM) for integrating research findings into practice. *Jt Comm J Qual Patient Saf.* 2008;34(4):228–243.

98. Kitson A, Harvey G, McCormack B. Enabling the implementation of evidence based practice: a conceptual framework. *Qual Health Care.* Sep 1998;7(3):149–158.

99. Rycroft-Malone J, Kitson A, Harvey G, et al. Ingredients for change: revisiting a conceptual framework. *Qual Saf Health Care.* Jun 2002;11(2):174–180.

100. Glasgow RE, Klesges LM, Dzewaltowski DA, Bull SS, Estabrooks P. The future of health behavior change research: what is needed to improve translation of research into health promotion practice? *Ann Behav Med.* Feb 2004;27(1):3–12.

101. Kerner JF, Guirguis-Blake J, Hennessy KD, et al. Translating research into improved outcomes in comprehensive cancer control. *Cancer Causes Control.* Oct 2005;16(Suppl 1):27–40.

102. Green LW, Glasgow RE. Evaluating the relevance, generalization, and applicability of research: issues in translation methodology. *Eval Health Prof.* 2006;29(1): 126–153.

103. Rohrbach LA, Grana R, Sussman S, Valente TW. Type II translation: transporting prevention interventions from research to real-world settings. *Eval Health Prof.* Sep 2006;29(3):302–333.

104. Castro FG, Barrera M, Jr., Martinez CR, Jr. The cultural adaptation of prevention interventions: resolving tensions between fidelity and fit. *Prev Sci.* Mar 2004;5(1): 41–45.

105. Dearing JW. Evolution of diffusion and dissemination theory. *J Public Health Manag Pract.* Mar–Apr 2008;14(2):99–108.

106. Brownson RC, Kreuter MW, Arrington BA, True WR. Translating scientific discoveries into public health action: how can schools of public health move us forward? *Public Health Rep.* 2006;121:97–103.

107. Elliott JS, O'Loughlin J, Robinson K, et al. Conceptualizing dissemination research and activity: the case of the Canadian Heart Health Initiative. *Health Educ Behav.* 2003;30(3):267–282.

108. Waters E, Doyle J, Jackson N, Howes F, Brunton G, Oakley A. Evaluating the effectiveness of public health interventions: the role and activities of the Cochrane Collaboration. *J Epidemiol Community Health.* Apr 2006;60(4):285–289.

109. Bauman LJ, Stein RE, Ireys HT. Reinventing fidelity: the transfer of social technology among settings. *Am J Community Psychol.* Aug 1991;19(4):619–639.

110. Stetler CB, Ritchie J, Rycroft-Malone J, Schultz A, Charns M. Improving quality of care through routine, successful implementation of evidence-based practice at the bedside: an organizational case study protocol using the Pettigrew and Whipp model of strategic change. *Implement Sci.* 2007;2:3.

111. Gilson L, Schneider H. Managing scaling up: what are the key issues? *Health Policy Plan.* 2010;25:97–98.
112. Verbeke W, Volgering M, Hessels M. Exploring the conceptual expansion within the field of organizational behaviour: organizational climate and organizational culture. *J Manage Stud.* 1998;35:303–330.
113. Cooke RA, Rousseau DM. Behavioral norms and expectations: a quantitative approach to the assessment of organizational culture. *Group Organ Stud.* 1988;13: 245–273.
114. Schein E. *Organizational culture and leadership.* Third edition. San Francisco: Jossey-Bass; 2004.
115. Glisson C, James LR. The cross-level effects of culture and climate in human service teams. *J Organ Behav.* 2002;23:767–794.
116. James LR, Hater JJ, Gent MJ, Bruni JR. Psychological climate: implications from cognitive social learning theory and interactional psychology. *Pers Psychol.* 1978;31:783–813.
117. James LR, Sells SB. Psychological climate: theoretical perspectives and empirical research. In: Magnusson D, ed. *Toward a psychology of situations: an international perspective.* Hillsdale, NJ: Erlbaum; 1981:275–295.
118. Litwin G, Stringer R. *Motivation and organizational climate.* Cambridge, MA: Harvard University Press; 1968.
119. Hellriegel D, Slocum JWJ. Organizational climate: measures, research and contingencies. *Acad Manage J.* 1974;17:255–280.
120. Reichers A, Schneider B. Climate and culture: an evolution of constructs. In: Schneider B, ed. *Organizational climate and culture.* San Francisco: Jossey-Bass; 1990.
121. Schneider B. Organizational climate: an essay. *Pers Psychol.* 1975;28(4):447–479.
122. Lehman WE, Greener JM, Simpson DD. Assessing organizational readiness for change. *J Subst Abuse Treat.* Jun 2002;22(4):197–209.
123. Weiner BJ. A theory of organizational readiness for change. *Implement Sci.* 2009;4:67.
124. Weiner BJ, Amick H, Lee SY. Conceptualization and measurement of organizational readiness for change: a review of the literature in health services research and other fields. *Med Care Res Rev.* Aug 2008;65(4):379–436.
125. Rabin BA, Glasgow RE, Kerner FJ, Klump MP, Brownson RC. Dissemination and implementation research on community-based cancer prevention: a systematic review. *Am J Prev Med.* 2010;38(4):443–456.
126. Victora C, Habicht J, Bryce J. Evidence-based public health: moving beyond randomized trials. *Am J Public Health.* 2004;94(3):400–406.
127. Tashakkori A, Teddlie C. *Handbook of mixed methods in the social and behavioral research.* Second edition. Thousand Oaks, CA: Sage Publications; 2010.
128. Johnson RB, Onwuegbuzie AJ. Mixed methods research: a research paradigm whose time has come. *Educational Researcher.* 2004;33(7):14–26.
129. Tunis SR, Stryer DB, Clancy CM. Practical clinical trials: increasing the value of clinical research for decision making in clinical and health policy. *JAMA.* Sep 24 2003;290(12):1624–1632.
130. Glasgow RE. What outcomes are the most important in translational research? PowerPoint presentation at the From clinical science to community: The science of translating diabetes and obesity research Conference,Bethesda, MD. January 12–13, 2004.

131. Leischow SJ, Best A, Trochim WM, et al. Systems thinking to improve the public's health. *Am J Prev Med.* Aug 2008;35(2 Suppl):S196–S203.
132. Trochim WM, Cabrera DA, Milstein B, Gallagher RS, Leischow SJ. Practical challenges of systems thinking and modeling in public health. *Am J Public Health.* Mar 2006;96(3):538–546.
133. Rothwell PM. External validity of randomised controlled trials: "to whom do the results of this trial apply?" *Lancet.* Jan 1–7 2005;365(9453):82–93.
134. Rothman KJ, Greenland S. Precision and validity of studies. In: Rothman KJ, Greenland S, eds. *Modern epidemiology.* Second edition: Lippincott Williams and Wilkins; 1998:115–135.
135. Cunningham-Sabo L, Carpenter WR, Peterson JC, Anderson LA, Helfrich CD, Davis SM. Utilization of prevention research: searching for evidence. *Am J Prev Med.* Jul 2007;33(1 Suppl):S9–S20.

Section TWO

Theory and Approaches

3 Historical Roots of Dissemination and Implementation Science

JAMES W. DEARING AND KERK F. KEE

▪ INTRODUCTION

A worldwide science of dissemination and implementation is emerging, driven by new media, the interests of philanthropies and the needs of government agencies, and the persistent and growing applied problems that have been addressed but not solved by the dominant research paradigms in disciplines such as psychology, sociology, and political science. Dissemination science is being shaped by researchers in the professional and applied fields of study, including public health, health services, communication, marketing, resource development, forestry and fisheries, education, criminal justice, and social work. The U.S. Centers for Disease Control and Prevention has formed an implementation science working group tying together program officers and staff across disparate centers and divisions. The Bill & Melinda Gates Foundation has founded a cross-cutting diffusion and dissemination work group in its global health program and hosted, in 2011, a convening about diffusion of innovations and developing countries.[1] At least 10 peer-reviewed journals[2-11] have since 2004 devoted special issues/sections to the topic of dissemination or implementation of evidence-based practices.

Research about dissemination and implementation (D&I) is a response to a general acknowledgment that successful, effective practices, programs, and policies resulting from clinical and community trials, demonstration projects, and community-based research as conducted by academicians very often do not affect the services that clinical staff, community service providers, and other practitioners fashion and provide to residents, clients, patients, and populations at risk. In any one societal sector (populated, for example, by planners for health care delivery, or city-level transportation and parkway planners), the state of the science (what researchers collectively know) and the state of the art (what practitioners collectively do) co-exist more or less autonomously, each realm of activity having little effect on the other. In the United States, this situation has been referred to as a "quality chasm" by the U.S. Institute of Medicine.[12]

Dissemination science is the study of how evidence-based practices, programs, and policies can best be communicated to an interorganizational societal sector of potential adopters and implementers to produce uptake and effective use. For example, public middle school nurses in U.S. southern states can comprise a societal sector. This definition means that dissemination embeds the objectives of both *external validity*, the replication of positive effects across dissimilar settings and conditions, and *scale-up*, the replication of positive effects across similar settings and conditions.[13] A *potential adopter* is someone who is targeted by a change agency to make a decision about whether to try an *innovation*, an idea, practice, program, policy, or technology that is perceived to be new. In public health or health care delivery, the innovation may be an evidence-based intervention that shows the potential to improve the well-being of a population.

Whereas dissemination concerns what the sources or sponsors of innovations do to reach and affect the decisions of potential adopters, implementation concerns the response of those targeted. *Implementation science* is the study of what happens after adoption occurs, especially in organizational settings. Implementation is one stage (after awareness and adoption, and before sustained use) in the over-time process of diffusion. An *implementer* is someone who will actually change his or her behavior to use an innovation in practice. In organizations, the people who make the decision to adopt an innovation are often not the users of innovations. The extent and quality of implementation and client or constituent responses to it have become dependent variables of study just as important, and sometimes more important, than initial adoption. Implementation researchers have not studied sustainability much, which may be even more important than implementation, though this is beginning to change.[13] So dissemination science and implementation science merge the study and objectives of marketing and diffusion with those of organizational change. For example, public health researchers or practitioners can conduct combined D&I studies that target many county departments of public health with a new disease prevention program (a dissemination study objective) and then focus on understanding what is done with the program in a purposively derived sample of all adopting departments (an implementation study objective). The questions by public health researchers and practitioners about dissemination and implementation can lead to rather different but perhaps equally fascinating projects, including questions such as:

- For a given public health program, does the change agency target types of organizations that are the most logical adopters serving the most needy clients or populations, or does the change agency simply target convenient or familiar organizations that they can easily contact because of a preexisting database or established relationships?
- Does the change agency develop messages about the new program based on systematic formative evaluation?
- To what extent does the change agency strategically consider *when* to introduce the new program, or do they just disseminate information as it becomes available?
- What is the competition for attention from the proponents of other similar programs and how does this change over time?
- What proportion of organizations targeted with dissemination messages respond by contacting the change agency for more information?
- How many try the new program (which might qualify them as adopters) of all those targeted (a measure of *reach*)?
- Was the program truly new conceptually to decision makers in the adopting organizations, or were they already experimenting with similar programs?
- Do some organizations invest resources in adoption (taking the time to learn about the program, pay licensing fees, attend trainings, order booklets and

train-the-trainer materials, become certified as coaches, etc.) but then never implement the program?

- What proportion of adopting organizations actually offers the program but then discontinues it?
- How many organizations stay in a holding pattern of adopting/not implementing/not discontinuing?
- What proportion of implementers offer the program as its designers intended with the same content, same number of modules, same behavior stimuli, same support and checks on enrollee or client performance?
- What types of adaptations to the program are made by implementers? Do they offer all the program's core components? Are they true to the program's theory of behavior change? Do they drop some components, customize others, and/or create their own to better suit their organization and their clients?
- Does the implementing organization change in ways unanticipated by the program designers? Does learning the one program serve as a trigger or precipitating event for organizational decision makers to adopt other, consonant or complementary public health programs?
- Do implementers think they are offering the program as the designers intended but, in practice, do something quite different?
- What is the client or enrollee yield? How many individuals sign up? How many complete all modules or classes? How many people actually do the variety of behavior changes—wearing pedometers, meeting in groups, writing in diaries, coming to class, completing their workbook, monitoring their progress—as suggested (and tested in efficacy trials) by the program designers?
- Is the public health program sustained by the organization? Do clients or enrollees continue their participation, too? Is fidelity or adaptation a better predictor of sustainability?
- What are the individual outcomes (weight loss, muscle tone, etc.) and public health impacts (for example, proportion of obese people in intervention communities)?

Given this range of dissemination science and implementation science questions that can be studied, it can be argued that these foci represent a most important type of diffusion of innovations study. The key, we suggest, is the stimulation of or tapping into intrinsic motivation of the staff in public health organizations and among their clients and program enrollees in communities. Certain innovations are met with enthusiasm, open arms, and eager learners who go on to champion new programs and advocate them to others. Innovations spread rapidly when people want them and can access them.

Where does the current emphasis on dissemination and implementation science come from? How are new media altering the diffusion of new practices, programs, and beliefs? We turn to the diffusion of innovations paradigm to address these questions.

■ THE CLASSICAL DIFFUSION PARADIGM

Diffusion is the process through which an innovation is communicated through certain channels over time among the members of a social system.[14] For example,

Barker[15] reports on three international development efforts in relation to diffusion concepts. In Haiti, a United States Agency for International Development (USAID) effort to conduct HIV prevention education in rural villages identified and recruited village voodoo practitioners, who are almost always considered credible and trusted sources of advice by Haiti villagers, to encourage villagers to participate in village meetings with USAID change agents. Meeting attendance exceeded campaign objectives by 124%. In Nepal, where vitamin A deficiency contributes to very high rates of infant and maternal mortality, the innovation of kitchen gardens was diffused among households through neighbor social modeling, resulting in heightened knowledge, positive attitudes, increased vegetable and fruit growing and consumption, and improvements in vitamin A nutrition. In Mali in 1999, a study of 500 Malian youth evaluated their information-seeking behavior and perceptions of source credibility concerning reproductive health. A lack of accurate knowledge among youth was attributed to their most trusted sources of information being friends and siblings; youth did not consider information sources such as health agents and teachers to be accessible enough or trustworthy. In all three cases, the innovations of HIV prevention education, kitchen gardens, and reproductive health information are unlikely to impact Haitian villagers, Nepali infants and mothers, and Malian youths if the diffusion process is not stimulated by accessing trusted, informal opinion leaders.

Diffusion studies have demonstrated a mathematically consistent sigmoid pattern (the S-shaped curve) of over time adoption for innovations that are perceived to be consequential by potential adopters, when the decisions to adopt are voluntary as opposed to them being compulsory, and with attendant logically related propositions, qualifying this literature as a theory of social change.[17] Many studies have shown a predictable over-time pattern when an innovation spreads, the now familiar S-shaped cumulative adoption curve. The "S" shape is due to the engagement of informal opinion leaders (as in Barker's study reported above) in talking about and modeling the innovation for others to hear about and see in action (Figure 3–1). For any given consequential innovation, the rate of adoption tends to begin slow, accelerate because of

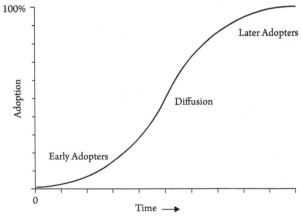

Figure 3–1. The generalized cumulative curve that describes the curvilinear process of the diffusion of innovations.

the activation of positive word-of-mouth communication and social modeling by the 5–8% of social system members who are sources of advice (i.e., opinion leaders) for subsequent other adopters, and then slow as system potential is approached.

Key components of diffusion theory are:

1. The *innovation*, and especially potential adopter perceptions of its *attributes* of cost, effectiveness, compatibility, simplicity, observability, and trialability (see Table 3–1);
2. The *adopter*, especially each adopter's degree of *innovativeness* (earliness relative to others in adopting the innovation);
3. The *social system*, such as a geographic community, a distributed network of collaborators, a professional association, or a province or state, especially in terms of the *structure* of the system, its informal *opinion leaders*, and potential adopter perception of *social pressure* to adopt;
4. The *individual adoption process*, a stage-ordered model of awareness, persuasion, decision, implementation, and continuation;[18]
5. The *diffusion system*, especially an external *change agency* and its paid *change agents* who, if well trained, correctly seek out and intervene with the client system's opinion leaders and paraprofessional aides, and support the enthusiasm of unpaid emergent innovation champions.

Diffusion occurs through a combination of (1) the need for individuals to reduce personal uncertainty when presented with information about an innovation, (2)

TABLE 3-1. *Classic Innovation Attributes, Their Definitions, and Application to the Context of Public Health and Health Care Delivery*

Innovation Attributes	Definitions	Application to Public Health and Health Care Delivery
Cost	Perceived cost of adopting and implementing an innovation	How much time and effort are required to learn to use the innovation and routinize its use? How long does recouping of costs take?
Effectiveness	The extent to which the innovation works better than that which it will displace	Does a gain in performance outweigh the downsides of cost? Do different stakeholders agree on the superiority of the innovation? What is the scientific evidence of effect?
Simplicity	How simple the innovation is to understand	How easy is an evidence-based program for adopters/implementers to understand? How easy is it to use?
Compatibility	The fit of the innovation to established ways of accomplishing the same goal	How much/little would an evidence-based program disrupt the existing routine and/or workflow of the adopting/implementing organization? To what extent is the innovation and the context adaptable to achieve a best fit?
Observability	The extent to which outcomes can be seen	How much and/or how quickly will the results of an evidence-based program become visible to an implementing organization, its clients, funders, and peer organizations?
Trialability	The extent to which the adopter must commit to full adoption	Can the innovation be implemented first at small scale? Is investment necessarily sunk and thus lost if the implementer decides to discontinue use?

the need for individuals to respond to their perceptions of what specific credible others are thinking and doing, and (3) to general, felt social pressure to do as others have done. Uncertainty in response to an innovation typically leads to a search for information and, if the potential adopter believes the innovation to be interesting and with the potential for benefits, a search for evaluative judgments of trusted and respected others (informal opinion leaders). This advice-seeking behavior is a heuristic that allows the decision maker to avoid comprehensive information seeking, reflecting Herbert Simon's seminal insight about the importance of everyday constraints in "bounding" the rationality of our decision making.[19]

Needs or motivations differ among people according to their degree of innovativeness (earliness in adoption relative to others): The first 2.5% to adopt (*innovators*) tend to do so because of novelty and having little to lose; the next 13.5% to adopt (*early adopters*, including the subset of about 5–7% informal opinion leaders) do so because of an appraisal of the innovation's attributes; the subsequent 34% of early majority adopters and 34% of late majority adopters do so because others have done so. They come to believe that adoption is the right thing to do (an imitative effect rather than a carefully reasoned rational judgment). The last 16% to adopt do so grudgingly with reservations. Their recalcitrance is sometimes later proven to be well justified since new programs can have undesirable consequences.

One's orientation to an innovation and time of adoption are related to and can be predicted by each adopter's structural position in the network of relations that tie a social system such as a school, community, or even a far-flung professional network together. When viewed sociometrically (especially who-seeks-advice-from-whom within a social network) in two-dimensional space as in Figure 3–2, the pattern of diffusion begins on the periphery of a network as the first to try the innovation experiment with it; central members of the network—informal opinion leaders who are a special subset of early adopters—then adopt if they judge the innovation to have important advantages over current practices; the many others then follow, who pay attention to what these sociometrically central and highly connected network members do and advise.[20]

This outside-inside-outward progression of adoption, when graphed as the cumulative number of adoptions over time, can reflect an S-shaped diffusion curve (as seen previously in Figure 3–1).

Forefathers of the Diffusion Model

The French judge cum sociologist Gabriel Tarde explained diffusion as a societal-level phenomenon of social change in his 1902 book, *The Laws of Imitation*, including the identification of an S-shaped curve in cumulative adoptions over time, the role of conversation in producing mimicry, and the importance of informal opinion leaders in jump-starting the S-shaped curve. As a judge, Tarde had taken note of the way people coming before the bench used new slang and wore new clothing fashions as if on cue. In Germany at the same time, Georg Simmel, a political philosopher, was writing about how individual thought and action was structured by the set of interpersonal relations to which a person was subject. Tarde's perspective was the forerunner for the macro, social system perspective on diffusion as the means

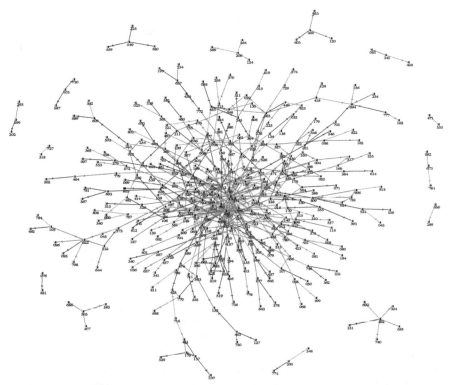

Figure 3-2. A sociogram of reported advice-seeking by judges and probation officers in Pennsylvania in 2006 in response to the question: "Whom do you look to for new ideas in juvenile justice?"

by which cultures and societies changed and progressed. Simmel's contribution, explicated in his book, *Conflict: The Web of Group Affiliations,* was the forerunner for understanding how social network position affects what individuals do in reaction to innovations, and when. Together, these perspectives provided an explanation for how system-level effects pressured the individual to adopt new things, and how individuals can affect change through their relationships in social networks.

Following Tarde and Simmel, European anthropologists seized on diffusion as a means to explain the continental drift of people, ideas, means of social organization, and primitive technologies. American anthropologists such as Alfred Kroeber in the 1920s also conducted historical studies, but they confined their analyses—for the first time called *diffusion* study—to more discrete innovations in smaller social systems such as a community or a region of the country. Anthropologists studying diffusion focused not only on spread of innovations but also on how cultures in turn shaped those innovations[21] by giving them new purposes and by adapting them to suit local needs—the beginnings of what we now call implementation science. The studies of these early diffusion researchers encouraged sociologists to take up diffusion work in contemporary 1920s and 1930s society, focusing on informal communication in friendship or social support networks as an explanation for the city-to-rural spread of innovations, the importance of jurisdictions as barriers to diffusion, and the importance of proximity to the spread of ideas.[22] And diffusion was not only understood as a one-way process: The American sociologist Pitirim Sorokin saw diffusion as inherently recursive. More developed countries extract raw materials from developing countries and sent back finished goods; classical music composers, for example, absorb ideas from folk tunes into the creation of symphonies.[20] Public health and health care can be interpreted recursively, too: Epidemiologic data about communities and practice-based research results are "diffused" to researchers who develop new public health and health care interventions and seek to disseminate them back to those same practitioner systems and communities.[23]

A landmark event for diffusion science occurred in 1943 with a report on the diffusion of hybrid seed corn in two Iowa communities.[24] This seminal article set the paradigm for many hundreds of future diffusion studies by emphasizing individuals as the locus of decision, adoption as the key dependent variable, a centralized innovation change agency that employed change agents, and the importance of different communication channels for different purposes at different times in the individual innovation-decision process. The Ryan and Gross article propelled diffusion study to center stage among rural sociologists. It also made the application of diffusion concepts a key set of tools in the work of agricultural extension agents. Rural sociologists were closely wedded to the extension services for funding and for providing the distribution system by which diffusion study ideas could be tested. The academics were practice oriented. From 1954 to 1969, key faculty in the Iowa State University Department of Sociology gave an estimated 600 presentations about the diffusion process, many to extension service groups. In 1958 alone, there were 35 publications reporting diffusion data collected in the United States by rural sociologists. Six years later, rural sociology publications about diffusion in less developed countries reached a peak of 20.[25] Diffusion studies by rural sociologists began to wane in 1969, but by that time scholars in sociology, medical sociology, education, communication, and public health had begun diffusion research, such as Coleman, Katz, and Menzel's classic study of physician's drug-prescribing behavior as a result of social network ties.[26]

Synthesizing the Diffusion Paradigm

The diffusion of innovations paradigm began to synthesize its approaches, central challenges, and lessons learned beginning in the 1960s. Internationally, an "invisible college" of rural sociologists had formed based in the American Midwest, drawn together both by intellectual questions and funding opportunities for research into a coauthorship, collaborative, and competitive network.[27] As these questions were answered by rural sociologists, diffusion research became fashionable to scholars in other disciplines and fields who conceptualized somewhat different problems, especially concerning policymakers as adopters and the conditions of innovation and spread in complex organizations. Yet diversification did not limit the centrality of diffusion scholarship as it importantly related to the growing paradigms of knowledge utilization and technology transfer studies and then to the evidence-based medicine movement.[28]

Everett M. Rogers, trained as a rural sociologist at Iowa State University, defended his dissertation in 1957 after growing up poor on an Iowa farm.[29,30] While the dissertation was ostensibly about the diffusion of 2-4-D weed spray among farmers, Rogers's real interest was in drawing generalizations that he believed were warranted on the basis of commonalities he had discovered by reading diffusion studies being published in different fields. The authors of the studies were not aware that other researchers were studying diffusion in fields different from theirs. Rogers expanded his Chapter 2 literature review into the 1962 seminal book, *Diffusion of Innovations*, which synthesized what was known about diffusion in general terms. His modeling of diffusion as an over-time social process and, at the individual level, as a series of stages that a person passes through in relation to an innovation would soon come to be recognized across fields of study as the diffusion-of-innovations paradigm. Though Rogers[31] would remain for decades the single most recognizable name associated with the diffusion of innovations, many other scholars were studying diffusion. And many diffusion scholars took a slightly different approach than Rogers. Many of these scholars were former students and colleagues of his; their contributions continue to push the paradigm forward and outward. In particular, some working in the paradigm took a macrostructural perspective on diffusion, especially those in population planning, demography, economics, and international relations. Anthropologists studying the spread of culture and linguists studying the spread of language also preferred a structural perspective on diffusion, which conceptualized waves of innovations washing over societies. To these structuralists, the study of diffusion was the study of social change writ large. For them, units of adoption are countries or cultures.

This macroorientation to diffusion was highly enticing to scholars because of its deductive and parsimonious potential based in a simple mathematical law of nature that describes a logistic (S-shaped or exponential) growth curve. Marketing scientists, epidemiologists, demographers, and political scientists instantly appreciated the predictive potential and eloquence of the population perspective on diffusion. Mathematical modeling formed the basis of this work, most of which continues today in fields such as family planning apart from more qualitatively informed microlevel studies of diffusion.[32]

So a major part of Rogers's contribution was in persuasively showing how macrolevel processes of system change could be linked to microlevel behavior. These ideas harkened back to Simmel and Tarde that individuals were influenced by system norms, and system structure and rules were the cumulative results of individual actions. Diffusion was one of the very few social theories that persuasively linked macro- with microlevel phenomena.

■ KNOWLEDGE UTILIZATION AND TECHNOLOGY TRANSFER

The agricultural extension model, with its basis in the training of social change concepts to full-time staff who were experts in areas such as cherry blight, zebra mussel eradication, and pine beetle control, was critical to the popularity of the diffusion-of-innovations paradigm. It was also important in the genesis of two closely related bodies of research. *Knowledge utilization* has been a robust paradigm for 40 years; its central problem was not how a new practice came to be voluntarily adopted by many people, but rather how knowledge in the form of prior results of a social program (the effectiveness of school busing, or of curbside recycling, or of business enterprise zones in cities) affected the subsequent decisions of elected representatives and policy staff in government. This is another route to social change, one that relies more on policy action by formal authorities followed by the compulsory adoptions of others than the traditional diffusion attention to informal influence. Were ineffective programs phased out by policymakers while effective programs were replicated and expanded? Did the social and education programs that managed to spread across the American states deserve to spread? The key intellectual contributor to this paradigm was the education scholar, Carol H. Weiss.[33] Weiss's studies of policy decision making showed that rational expectations between evidence and program continuation/expansion were not supported by social science study. And beyond the expectation of a rational outcomes-to-funding relationship, Weiss and other knowledge utilization researchers of the policy-making process showed that any direct program evaluation-to-policy decision link was rare; rather, policy making was inherently political.[34] Many more factors besides evidence of program effectiveness factored into decision making.[35] When program evidence did affect subsequent decisions by policymakers, it did so through circuitous cumulative learning by policymakers and staff as they became "enlightened" over time in terms of general programming lessons. In a gradual, accretionary way, indirect and partial knowledge diffusion did occur.

From the perspective of knowledge utilization, Blake and Ottoson[36] maintain that dissemination is the process of moving information from one source to another (as from program evaluators to policymakers), and the ultimate purpose of dissemination should be utilization by users. When utilization by users is achieved, information/knowledge has impact. This perspective has evolved with the field of knowledge utilization studies, through "waves" of research from the empirical studies in the 1940s by rural sociologists to studies of international development and family planning in the 1970s, to research in the 1990s about how research could improve human services in health and education.[37,38]

Researchers studying *technology transfer* identified a different problem. Beginning with Mansfield in the 1960s, scholars such as Leonard-Barton and von Hippel focused on the firm, especially complex organizations such as multinational corporations that partly by virtue of their size exhibited problems of coordination, knowledge sharing, and even knowing what was going on across its many divisions let alone having a managerial system for knowing which practices were more effective than others.[39] Whereas diffusion was about innovations that usually began with a single source and then spread broadly, technology transfer was one-to-one or "point-to-point." How can an innovative workflow redesign or unit-based team approach to scheduling that produces huge productivity gains in Argentina be applied to improve the same company's productivity in Canada? What sorts of adaptation might be necessary?[40]

Contrary to the technology transfer label, Dunn, Holzener, and Zaltman[41(p.120)] argued that "Knowledge use is transactive. Although one may use the analogy of 'transfer,' knowledge is never truly marketed, transferred or exchanged. Knowledge is really negotiated between the parties involved." Similarly, Estabrooks and colleagues[42(p.28)] clarify that the Canadian Institutes of Health Research defines knowledge translation as the "exchange, synthesis and ethically sound application of knowledge—within a complex system of interactions among researchers and users." In other words, the notions of transaction, negotiation, interactions, and synthesis are key to the conceptualization of transfer (and dissemination/diffusion) of information/knowledge from producers to users. In health research and organizational technology transfer, one needs to understand what is being transferred, by whom, to which targets, through what process, and with what outcomes.[43] So effective transfer has knowledge utilization at its core.[35]

■ EVIDENCE-BASED MEDICINE AND EVIDENCE-BASED PUBLIC HEALTH

Literatures about diffusion of innovations, knowledge utilization, and technology transfer have found new application and expansion in the fields of medicine and public health. *Evidence-based medicine* is the conscientious, explicit, and judicious use of current best evidence in making decisions about the care of individual patients. The practice of evidence-based medicine means integrating individual clinical expertise with the best available external clinical evidence from systematic research.[44]

Evidence-based medicine is an approach to medical practice that emphasizes the role of research literature (new information, latest knowledge) usually in the form of clinical practice or medical guidelines (increasingly based on comparative effectiveness research) over prior training and clinical experiences such that each becomes an input in decision making about each particular patient's health. Although evidence-based medicine has been controversial among some medical professionals[45] and somewhat misunderstood as a movement to displace traditional practices in medicine, advocates[46] argue for augmentation rather than displacement. Clinical epidemiology, for example, has become infused with evidence-based knowledge generation, rapid critical appraisal of evidence, efficient storage and retrieval, and evidence synthesis.[47] When all four components are effectively practiced, the quality of patient care increases.

The desire for valid and generalizable evidence to inform decisions also has been applied to the domain of public health. Brownson and colleagues[48] proposed the following attributes as key to defining evidence-based public health: (1) Decisions are guided by best available peer-reviewed evidence and literature from a range of methodologies, (2) evidence-based public health approaches systematically make use of data and information systems, (3) its practice frameworks for program planning come from theories rooted in behavioral science, (4) the community of users are involved in processes of decision making and assessment, (5) evidence-based public health approaches carry out sound evaluation of programs, and (6) lessons learned are shared with stakeholder groups and decision makers. Glasgow and Emmons[49] additionally emphasize contextual factors as key in matching practice refinements to local conditions.

During the dissemination of evidence-based practices, we believe that it is useful to consider the interplay between the technical rationalities of knowledge producers or change agencies, and users' narrative rationalities, whether those users are patients and community members or health care providers and public health professionals. Technical rationalities are based on logics that are predictive, instructive, and technocratic while narrative rationalities are stories of experiences that are interpretive, contextual, and dynamic.[50] Narratives can be illuminating to program planners as well as inform ongoing attempts to improve care and public health practice.[51,52] New media and emerging technologies can facilitate the access to and use of both technical rationalities (guideline content) and narrative rationalities (for example, clinical practitioners' perspectives about how they have implemented such guidance given the realities of their practices).

■ NEW (AND NEWER) MEDIA

What are the effects of new information and communication technologies on dissemination activities by change agencies, the social diffusion processes that may result as potential adopters consider an innovation, and how implementation in organizations unfolds?

Collective knowledge of the diffusion-of-innovations paradigm has given way to a focus on those paradigmatic concepts that can be operationalized in purposive tests of how to best disseminate and implement evidence-based health practices, programs, and policies.[53] This has long been an objective in trying to spread effective innovations for improved global health as well as for domestic health care and public health.[54,55] New media, in the ways in which they affect the dissemination of information by change agencies, the subsequent diffusion process among targeted adopters, and the resultant critical stage of implementation of evidence-based practices in organizations, are iteratively changing how we work and how targeted adopters respond to change initiatives. D&I researchers and practitioners are well advised to be agile.

The traditional notion of an innovation as predesigned by centralized change agents is increasingly inaccurate. Increasingly, innovations are malleable and coproduced by researchers, practitioners, and those persons who adopt them, whether the researchers in question have this intention or not. Such a perspective on change has the advantage of enabling learning from those persons who are best positioned to make insightful and applicable real-time improvements to an innovation: users themselves.[56] This shift in emphasis to utilization by users would wed source perspectives on change with those of innovation users-as-creators. Utilization properly involves both the logics of innovation producers and the experiential expertise of users who are sensitized to issues of context and compatibility.

Technologies can facilitate information access and knowledge creation in the context of dissemination. In terms of information access, it is clear that information technologies and certain new media accelerate our ability to disseminate information worldwide.[57] Do they also accelerate diffusion (that is, resultant decision making) among those health care and public health practitioners whom we sometimes try to reach and affect?[58] Technologies increase the dissemination of knowledge about innovations and expand reach in terms of health promotion,[59] disease prevention,[60] health compliance, telehealth,[61,62] and cybermedicine.[63] Technologies allow easy access to new information and latest knowledge via specialized knowledge management systems (such as medical literature databases) that health care providers can use to inform their medical practice, and general knowledge management systems (such as public Web-based search engines) to help patients make better health-related choices in life.[64]

Furthermore, technologies may intensify the diffusion process among connected adopters whom change agents may target for change.[65] Traditionally and still today, diffusion is facilitated by mass media and interpersonal networks among people. In today's wired societies and more specifically in our networked market segments that are organized by common interests and professions, new media create new online social communities that are critical to the facilitation of information knowledge dissemination beyond geographically/temporally bound communities of the past. Technologies intensify the dissemination process by elevating social media platforms and their amateur broadcasters as well as new networks among people who do not know each other except through online communities[66] to an emerging position of intermediary, thus giving information/knowledge another push for dissemination throughout social systems.[67]

In terms of knowledge creation, technologies are enabling new and expanded professional networks among health care providers and public health professionals, leading to interorganizational sharing and cross-fertilization of information and knowledge about common challenges.[68] New media make coproduction of knowledge between producers and users easier to achieve because of the low cost and high speed for feedback and ongoing communication.[69] Technologies support automatic and cumulative data acquisition (including electronic medical records in health care organizations and online data mining) for computations and analyses that, in turn, can produce more knowledge. In this way, the use of technologies demonstrates Sorokin's view that diffusion is inherently recursive. We surmise that if potential adopters of innovations feel that they have been involved in the creation of or refinement of an innovation, their adoption and implementation is more likely. If new media lead to the experience of broader participation in knowledge creation, then those media will stimulate not only dissemination but diffusion, too.

We have tried to show the evolution of the diffusion-of-innovations theory, and how concepts from that paradigm as well as knowledge utilization and technology transfer research have contributed to the evidence-based medicine and evidence-based public health emphases in dissemination and implementation. We suggest that D&I researchers and practitioners will continue to find relevance and applicability in these former research traditions as they seek ways to study and apply new information and communication technologies to the challenges of dissemination activity by innovation proponents, diffusion responses by adopters, and then subsequent implementation and sustained use.

SUGGESTED READINGS

Dearing JW. Evolution of diffusion and dissemination theory. *J Public Health Manag Pract.* 2008;14(2):99–108.

Dearing describes changes in diffusion of innovations research and suggests applying what is known about diffusion to design more effective dissemination interventions. He also discusses the need to consider the impact of contextual factors on implementation efforts.

Estabrooks C, Derksen L, Winther C, et al. The intellectual structure and substance of the knowledge utilization field: A longitudinal author co-citation analysis, 1945 to 2004. *Implement Sci.* 2008;3(1):49.

This article is a bibliographic analysis of the knowledge utilization field between World War II and the present and how it has evolved in that time. The authors cite the emergence of evidence-based medicine during this time period, a major advance with significant influences on models of evidence-based practice in other fields, including public health.

Green LW, Ottoson JM, Garcia C, Hiatt RA. Diffusion theory and knowledge dissemination, utilization, and integration in public health. *Annu Rev Public Health.* 2009;30:151–174.

Green et al. provide a rigorous review of the public health implications of diffusion, dissemination, and implementation to improve public health practice and guide the design of future research. The article suggests a decentralized approach to dissemination and implementation, as well as ways diffusion may be combined with other theories.

Rogers EM. *Diffusion of innovations.* 5th ed. New York: Free Press; 2003.

Rogers's classic text on how new ideas, beliefs, practices and technologies diffuse over time through various communication channels and networks. Because many new ideas involve taking a risk, people seek out others whom they know and trust for advice. Propositions about a generalized process of diffusion are included.

SELECTED WEBSITES

www.research-practice.org. This site lists hundreds of recent publications in dissemination and implementation, and catalogues a variety of tools that can help practitioners and researchers with the challenges of dissemination in order to elicit diffusion.

■ REFERENCES

1. Achieving Lasting Impact at Scale: Behavior Change and the Spread of Family Health Innovations in Low-Income Countries. Seattle, WA: Bill & Melinda Gates Foundation; November 1–2, 2011.
2. *Health Psychol* 24;5: 2005.
3. *Acad of Manage Exec* 19;2:2005.
4. *J Health Commun* 9;Suppl 1:2004.
5. *Metropolitan Universities* 17;4:2006.
6. *Am J Public Health* 96;2:2006.
7. *Am J Prev Med* 31;4S:2006.
8. *AIDS Educ Prev* 18;Suppl A:2006.
9. *J Public Health Manag Pract* 2008;14(2):2008.
10. *Res Soc Work Pract* 19;5:2009.
11. *New Dir Eval* 124;Winter:2009.
12. Institute of Medicine. *Crossing the Quality Chasm: A New Health System for the 21st Century.* Washington, DC: Author; 2001.
13. Moffitt RA. Forecasting the effects of scaling up social programs: An economics perspective. In: Schneider B, McDonald S, editors. *Scale-up Education.* Volume 1 ed. Lanham, MD: Rowman & Littlefield; 2007. 173–186.
14. Scheirer MA, Dearing JW. An agenda for research on the sustainability of public health programs. *Am J Public Health.* 2011;101:2059–2067. .
15. Rogers EM. *Diffusion of Innovations.* 5th ed. New York: The Free Press; 2003.

16. Barker K. Diffusion of innovations: A world tour. *J Health Commun* 2004;9:131–137.
17. Green LW, Gottlieb NH, Parcel GS. Diffusion theory extended and applied. *Advances in Health Education and Promotion* 1991;3:91–117.
18. Brownson RC, Ballew P, Brown KL et al. The effect of disseminating evidence-based interventions that promote physical activity to health departments. *Am J Public Health* 2007;97(10):1900–1907.
19. Gigerenzer G, Reinhard S. *Bounded Rationality: The Adaptive Toolbox*. Cambridge, MA: The MIT Press; 2001.
20. Kerckhoff AC, Back KW, Miller N. Sociometric patterns in hysterical contagion. *Sociometry* 1965;28(1):2–15.
21. Katz E. Theorizing diffusion: Tarde and Sorokin revisited. *Ann Am Acad Pol Soc Sci* 1999;566:144–155.
221. Katz E, Levin ML, Hamilton H. Traditions of research on the diffusion of innovation. *Am Sociol Rev* 1963;28(2):237–252.
23. Orleans CT. Increasing the demand for and use of effective smoking-cessation treatments reaping the full health benefits of tobacco-control science and policy gains—in our lifetime. *Am J Prev Med* 2007;33(6 Suppl):S340–S348.
24. Ryan B, Gross NC. The diffusion of hybrid seed corn in two Iowa communities. *Rural Sociol* 1943;8(1):15–24.
25. Valente TW, Rogers EM. The origins and development of the diffusion of innovations paradigm as an example of scientific growth. *Sci Commun* 1995;16(3):242–273.
26. Coleman JS, Katz E, Menzel H. The diffusion of an innovation among physicians. *Sociometry* 1957;20:253–270.
27. Crane D. *Invisible Colleges: Diffusion of Knowledge in Scientific Communities*. Chicago: University of Chicago Press; 1972.
28. Estabrooks CA, Derksen L, Winther C et al. The intellectual structure and substance of the knowledge utilization field: A longitudinal author co-citation analysis, 1945 to 2004. *Implement Sci* 2008;3:49.
29. Rogers EM. A conceptual variable analysis of technological change. *PhD Dissertation* 1957; Ames, IA (Iowa State University).
30. Rogers EM. *The Fourteenth Paw: Growing Up on an Iowa Farm in the 1930s*. Singapore: Asian Media Information and Communication Centre; 2008.
31. Singhal A, Dearing JW. *Communication of Innovations: A Journey with Ev Rogers*. New Delhi, India: Sage Publications, Inc.; 2006.
32. Montgomery MR, Casterline JB. The diffusion of fertility control in Taiwan: Evidence from pooled cross-section time-series models. *Popul Stud (NY)* 1993;47(3): 457–479.
33. Weiss CH, Bucuvalas MJ. *Social Science Research and Decision-Making*. New York: Columbia University Press; 1980.
34. Kingdon JW. *Agendas, Alternatives, and Public Policies*. New York: Longman; 2003.
35. Anderson LM, Brownson RC, Fullilove MT et al. Evidence-based public health policy and practice: Promises and limits. *Am J Prev Med* 2005;28(5 Suppl):226–230.
36. Blake SC, Ottoson JM. Knowledge utilization: Implications of evaluation. *New Dir Eval* 2009;124:21–34.
37. Backer TE. Knowledge utilization: The third wave. *Knowledge: Creation, Diffusion, Utilization* 1991;12(3):225–240.
38. Green LW, Ottoson JM, Garcia C, Hiatt RA. Diffusion theory and knowledge dissemination, utilization, and integration in public health. *Annu Rev Public Health* 2009;30:151–174.

39. O'Dell C, Grayson CJ. If Only We Knew What We Know: Identification and transfer of internal best practices. *Calif Manage Rev* 1998;40(3):154–174.
40. Leonard-Barton D. Implementation as mutual adaptation of technology and organization. *Res Policy* 1988;17(5):251–267.
41. Dunn WN, Holzener B. Knowledge in society: anatomy of an emergent field. *Knowledge in Society: The International Journal of Knowledge Transfer* 1988;1:3–26.
42. Estabrooks CA, Thompson DS, Lovely JJE, Hofmeyer A. A guide to knowledge translation theory. *J Contin Educ Health Prof* 2006;26(1):25–36.
43. Lavis JN, Robertson D, Woodside J, McLeod CB, Abelson J. How can research organizations more effectively transfer research knowledge to decision makers? *The Milbank Q* 2003;81(2):221–248.
44. Sackett DL, Rosenberg WMC, Gray JAM, Haynes RB, Richardson WS. Evidence based medicine: What it is and what it isn't. *Br Med J* 1996;312:71–72.
45. Mykhalovskiy E, Weir L. The problem of evidence-based medicine: Directions for social science. *Soc Sci Med* 2004;59(5):1059–1069.
46. Haynes RB. What kind of evidence is it that Evidence-Based Medicine advocates want health care providers and consumers to pay attention to? *BMC Health Serv Res* 2002;2(1):3.
47. Sackett DL. Clinical epidemiology. What, who, and whither. *J Clin Epidemiol* 2002;55(12):1161–1166.
48. Brownson RC, Fielding JE, Maylahn CM. Evidence-based public health: A fundamental concept for public health practice. *Annu Rev Public Health* 2009;30:175–201.
49. Glasgow RE, Emmons KM. How can we increase translation of research into practice? Types of evidence needed. *Annu Rev Public Health* 2007;28:413–433.
50. Browning LD. Lists and stories as organizational communication. *Commun Theory* 1992;2:281–302.
51. Greene JD. Communication of results and utlization in participatory program evaluation. *Eval Program Plann* 1988;11(4):341–351.
52. Doolin B. Narratives of change: Discourse, technology and organization. *Organization* 2003;10(4):751–770.
53. Dearing JW. Evolution of diffusion and dissemination theory. *J Public Health Manag* 2008;14(2):99–108.
54. Rogers EM. *Communication Strategies for Family Planning.* New York: Free Press; 1973.
55. Office of Behavioral and Social Sciences Research. *Putting Evidence into Practice: The OBSSR Report of the Working Group on the Integration of Effective Behavioral Treatments into Clinical Care.* Washington, DC: Author; 1997.
56. von Hippel E. *Democratizing Innovation.* Cambridge, MA: The MIT Press; 2005.
57. Edejer TT. Disseminating health information in developing countries: The role of the internet. *BMJ* 2000;321(7264):797–800.
58. Dearing JW, Maibach E, Buller DB. A convergent diffusion and social marketing approach for disseminating proven approaches to physical activity promotion. *Am J Prev Med* 2006;1–13.
59. Korp P. Health on the Internet: Implications for health promotion. *Health Educ Res* 2006;21(1):78–86.
60. Atherton H, Huckvale C, Car J. Communicating health promotion and disease prevention information to patients via email: A review. *J Telemed Telecare* 2010;16(4):172–175.

61. Tuerk PW, Fortney J, Bosworth HB et al. Toward the development of national telehealth services: The role of Veterans Health Administration and future directions for research. *Telemed J E Health* 2010;16(1):115–117.

62. Dellifraine JL, Dansky KH. Home-based telehealth: A review and meta-analysis. *J Telemed Telecare* 2008;14(2):62–66.

63. Eysenbach G, Sa ER, Diepgen TL. Shopping around the Internet today and tomorrow: Towards the millenium of cybermedicine. *Br Med J* 1999;319(7220):1294.

64. Jadad AR, Haynes RB, Hunt D, Browman GP. The Internet and evidence-based decision-making: A needed synergy for efficient knowledge management in health care. *CMAJ* 2000;162(3):362–365.

65. Dearing JW, Kreuter MW. Designing for diffusion: How can we increase uptake of cancer communication innovations? *Patient Educ Couns* 2010; 81S:100–110.

66. Hawn C. Take two aspirin and tweet me in the morning: How Twitter, Facebook, and other social media are reshaping health care. *Health Aff (Millwood)* 2009;28(2): 361–368.

67. Shirky C. *Here Comes Everybody: The Power of Organizing without Organizations.* New York: Penguin Press; 2009.

68. Eysenbach G. Medicine 2.0: Social networking, collaboration, participation, apomediation, and openness. *J Med Internet Res* 2008;10(3):e22.

69. Griffiths F, Lindenmeyer A, Powell J, Lowe P, Thorogood M. Why are health care interventions delivered over the internet? A systematic review of the published literature. *J Med Internet Res* 2006;8(2):e10.

4 Comparative Effectiveness Research to Accelerate Translation: Recommendations for an Emerging Field of Science

■ RUSSELL E. GLASGOW AND
JOHN F. STEINER

■ INTRODUCTION

The term "comparative effectiveness research (CER)" is a new way of describing a research field with a long intellectual tradition. The U.S. Federal Coordinating Council for CER defines it as "the conduct and synthesis of research comparing the benefits and harms of different interventions and strategies to prevent, diagnose, treat and monitor health conditions in 'real-world' settings. The purpose of this research is to improve health outcomes by developing and disseminating evidence-based information to patients, clinicians, and other decision makers, responding to their expressed needs, about which interventions are most effective for which patients under specific circumstances."[1,2] While other organizations such as the Institute of Medicine and the Agency for Healthcare Research and Quality have proposed slightly different definitions, there are clear points of congruence among them. These funding agencies and researchers in the field are approaching consensus on what is and is not included in CER.

Among the many areas of agreement are: (1) CER involves the comparison of strategies for prevention, diagnosis, treatment, or delivery system designs that are feasible in the day to day practice of clinical medicine or public health. (2) A wide array of research designs may be used, including conventional or novel randomized trials, quasi-experimental evaluations, observational studies using existing databases, and modeling or simulation studies. (3) Because the outcomes are varied, multiple data sources may be required to conduct these studies. Primary data collected for a CER study can be augmented by data from electronic medical records, administrative claims, patient reports, and other sources. (4) The outcomes assessed in CER should be those that patients and practitioners value and can readily use to assess the effectiveness of the strategy. As a result, a wide array of outcomes generally must be measured.

Conventional biomedical research has long been dominated by the paradigm of the "Phase III" randomized clinical trial, in which two therapeutic options—usually medications—are compared in highly selected patients and a carefully controlled research environment.[3,4] All definitions of CER dramatically expand the range of research possibilities. Although it is likely that, in practice, the bulk of CER research will focus on pharmacological therapies, medical devices, or clinical procedures, all definitions emphasize that CER includes behavioral interventions, evaluation of alternative systems of care for delivery of public health services, clinical preventive services, or treatments, and new strategies for early diagnosis or individualization of treatment, such as genomic testing. Though rarely stated, these definitions also imply that CER can expand to examine and compare the effectiveness of environmental and policy interventions. Some observers feel that all CER research will be focused at relatively narrow levels comparing one drug or device to another. We do not share this view, and think that, especially with opportunities soon to become announced through the Patient Reported Outcomes Research Institute (http://www.pcori.org/), there is an important opportunity for implementation science and population-based research with public health implications to be included.

Despite this expansive mandate, CER is vulnerable to the same problem that has beset prior health research—the long delay between demonstration that a strategy is effective and its widespread dissemination and implementation (D&I) in practice.[5] Our purpose in this chapter is to review developments in this rapidly evolving area, and to discuss the opportunities and issues relevant to the D&I of CER.

Without a strong commitment to D&I and to rapid learning paradigms,[6] the field of CER will not achieve its lofty goal of contributing to comprehensive reform of personal and public health care delivery systems. Meaningful change on this scale will likely require simultaneous intervention at multiple levels—the organ system, the person, the social network, the care delivery organization, and the broader policy and community environment. This emphasis on the critical importance of context is central to D&I research.[7-9] In addition, CER is explicitly intended to help policymakers, clinicians, patients, and community members to make shared decisions. Since these different decision makers are likely to see a problem from different perspectives, different outcomes and strategies for D&I are likely to be necessary to engage them all.

The overall goal of this chapter is to summarize D&I issues involved in CER. In this introductory section, core elements that all major stakeholders agree are included in CER are discussed. In subsequent sections, evolving content and scope issues are covered in more detail, such as research design, comparison conditions, and rapid learning paradigms from networks of settings. Finally, we discuss some of the controversies within this young field, such as the role and types of economic analyses[10] and recommendations for future research needed to enhance D&I and produce CER results that will disseminate and translate into population-based change.

■ TYPES OF CER AND CORRESPONDING ROLES FOR D&I

Many implications flow from the four essential attributes of CER (feasible implementation, flexible research designs, rich data sources, and relevant outcomes) defined in the previous section. The first consequence is that CER studies directly compare two or more real-world alternatives, rather than contrast a preferred intervention to no treatment or placebo controls—comparisons that are not relevant for practice.[3] Second, CER includes a wide range of efforts to redesign care delivery systems, such as different approaches to operationalize elements of the Chronic Care Model,[11,12] and systems approaches to multilevel community interventions.[13] Third, CER includes evaluation of alternative strategies for D&I itself. In other words, D&I can be the subject of CER, not just an approach to publicize the findings of CER. For example, one could compare different methods to promote adoption of the results of research, such as online training in guidelines implementation versus academic detailing. Currently, this effort to disseminate CER is limited in scope, although entities such as the AHRQ-funded Eisenberg Center for promoting the uptake of evidence-based guidelines are conducting work in this area.

The spectrum of interventions amenable to CER is summarized in Table 4–1. In the eyes of many proponents, the intent of CER is primarily to evaluate devices, procedures, and alternative medication treatment strategies. "Big ticket" CER studies of devices (such as implantable cardiac defibrillators for individuals with heart failure) or procedures (such as robotic versus traditional surgery for individuals with prostate cancer) primarily involve individuals with established and advanced diseases, specialist clinicians, and substantial technological complexity that make intensive demands on delivery and payment systems. As a result, the outcomes of these studies are of substantial interest to large payers and delivery systems, which may be required to make large investments to support the more effective treatment alternative.[14] In this situation, D&I research must define the essential infrastructure, the appropriate training of the practitioner(s) (e.g., how many procedures are necessary to achieve competence and safety),[15] and related issues such as whether these services should be regionalized or can be safely distributed to small communities.

Although studies of one-time high-tech interventions are conceptually the simplest type of CER, the most common use of CER to date has been to evaluate alternative medication treatments (or treatment strategies) for chronic health conditions. As Table 4–1 indicates, the role of the practitioner and the patient/citizen changes dramatically in these situations. The role of the practitioner is to recommend a course of treatment, while the patient recipient retains "veto power" over that recommendation through his or her decision whether or not to adhere to treatment. Indeed, strategies to improve adherence with effective medications in individuals at high risk of adverse outcomes may have a greater public health impact than providing treatment to a large population of individuals at lower risk.[16]

In the decision whether to have a surgical procedure, the recipient requires information and one-time consent; in the decision whether to accept a long-term medication, the recipient also must initiate long-term behavior change. Often (and most obviously in the elderly), such behavior change may require the support of individuals in the recipient's social environment. CER-T (comparative effectiveness research that is likely to translate) studies of medications should at the very least describe the evaluation settings and the strategies that are used to promote adherence. Further, CER-T studies of strategies to enhance adherence in routine practice with complex patients are sorely needed.[17] D&I efforts for medications found to be effective should articulate the social context, the attributes of the practitioner or team, and the system prerequisites (such as providing larger supplies of long-term medications, limiting copayments, or providing uncapped drug benefits) for supporting adherence.[18,19]

As shown in the third intervention type in Table 4–1, CER to assess behavioral interventions to prevent or treat psychosocial concerns makes even greater demands on recipients, practitioners, and delivery systems. The demands on D&I research in this area are correspondingly greater. Interventions to address problems such as depression, posttraumatic stress disorder, or domestic violence require a mix of strategies that include collaborative goal setting, behavior change, and social supports, and in some cases medications. The success of such efforts is impossible to assess without ongoing measurement of the behavior itself or of the distress caused by that behavior. While brief, useful tools for assessment of problems such as depression and distress are readily available,[20,21] they are rarely used systematically to assess the response to treatment, and even more rarely included in the large datasets often used in CER. Thus, D&I for mental health and related disorders must also address issues of measurement and capture of relevant information to assess treatment outcomes.

Recent definitions of CER have recognized the critical role of system-level interventions to improve care outcomes. In so doing, they build on over a decade of research using the Chronic Care Model, which has emphasized the many system prerequisites for successful care of individuals with chronic health conditions.[11,12,22] Measuring the attributes of care delivery systems that promote or impede successful interventions is difficult, and rigorous evaluation of strategies for changing organizational structure or behavior are relatively uncommon within the public health or health services research literature.[23–25] To support D&I of successful interventions, the research community needs to import measures from fields other than health care, such as business or organizational psychology, and engage complex issues in the financing of care. CER that assesses different approaches to facilitate policy interventions, such as getting legislatures or worksites to adopt clean indoor air (nonsmoking) polices would fall in between such system change strategies and the community intervention at the bottom of Table 4–1.

Finally, CER-T can and should address community-level health concerns among individuals who may have limited interaction with the health care system. An example of current concern is prevention and treatment of obesity. Medical interventions such as gastric bypass surgery, or medications to encourage weight loss, address only the "tip of the iceberg" of this public health problem, although they are likely to be the most commonly studied interventions in CER. CER-T will require strategies for the promotion of healthy eating and active living, "counterdetailing" to the pervasive effects of advertising for high-calorie foods, and recruitment of mutually reinforcing social networks to support appropriate behaviors.[26] Public health practitioners should lead in this effort, while the role of clinical practitioners may be relatively small and supportive (Table 4–1). CER-T for obesity prevention will also require careful assessment of the environmental and social factors, as well as personal determinants of successful behavior change.

TABLE 4–1. *Types of Interventions Studied in CER*

Type of Intervention	Role of Care Recipient	Role of Practitioner (Clinician or Public Health)	Role of System	Implications for D and I
Device, procedure	Informed consent; often a one-time decision	Carry-out procedure	Create physical and staffing environment to support effective and safe installation of device or conduct of procedure	Needs to assess required organizational infrastructure, technical skills, and training requirements for practitioners
Medication treatment	Informed decision, ongoing adherence	Recommend intervention, provide ongoing support for adherence	Supplement "front-line" practitioner in ongoing monitoring and follow-up support for maintenance of behavior change	Identify contextual factors that promote adherence
Behavior change (e.g. mental health; health behaviors)	Informed decision, ongoing adherence	May recommend intervention, provide ongoing support for adherence, assess patient-centered outcomes	Supplement "front-line" practitioner in ongoing monitoring and follow-up support for maintenance of behavior change, develop approaches to measure and report patient-centered outcomes	Identify environmental and other contextual factors that promote adherence and ability to measure relevant patient-level outcomes
System change	May be largely invisible to recipients	Align individual efforts with larger teams and organizations	Establish infrastructure, support teams and coordinate approaches to achieve outcomes	Detailed assessment of organizational predictors of successful intervention
Community intervention	Person, not patient—lifestyle modification, participate in environmental and policy change actions	Support efforts at more distal levels	Integration across multiple systems and levels	Document environmental, political, and social context of particular importance

Designs for CER-T: Pragmatic Philosophies and Research Strategies

For intervention studies of comparative effectiveness, researchers must make a fundamental decision—whether to design and conduct a "pragmatic" versus an "explanatory" trial.[27-29] Also known as "practical trials," pragmatic research designs are concerned with answering real-world questions of relevance to practitioners, policymakers, administrators, and citizens, in contrast to conventional "explanatory" or "efficacy" trials, whose purpose is to evaluate interventions under optimal conditions that maximize treatment fidelity and adherence, and exclude individuals with complex problems or competing demands.[30,31] The ongoing debate about the relative merits of explanatory versus pragmatic trials[3,32] is beyond the scope of this chapter, but a core issue of contention concerns whether the fundamental purpose of evaluation should be to isolate intervention effects and determine general conclusions about the efficacy of a treatment while controlling for or standardizing conditions of observation (explanatory approach) or to study the impact of interventions under different conditions on different outcomes for different subgroups (pragmatic approach). The later realist[1,33,34] or contextualist[8,35] approach argues that it is generally not possible to identify interventions that are robust or consistently effective across all the dimensions where such an intervention might reasonably be applied in practice. As discussed in detail in Chapter 15, it is misleading to test an intervention under optimal conditions (highly motivated patients, expert clinicians, highly resourced academic settings) and expect these results to generalize to quite different and more complex patients and settings.

At its foundation, this debate reflects fundamental differences in philosophy of science, in particular the extent to which it is possible and desirable to control and hold constant factors that might "confound" interventions. Several of these issues have to do with variations in intervention settings, staff, and delivery conditions. Explanatory trials[36] strive for homogeneity on these factors as well as patient characteristics to eliminate unwanted variance, which is often conceived of as "noise," whereas a pragmatic or realist approach advocates explicitly investigating the impact of variations in these and other dimensions on outcomes.

A recent development that may help to bridge the chasm between pragmatic and explanatory research groups and shed light on this often contentious issue concerns transparent and nonjudgmental reporting of specific conditions under which research is conducted.[36-38] The recent publication of the PRECIS[28,36] framework by the CONSORT group (http://www.consort-statement.org)[28,36] proposes that investigators summarize the extent to which a trial is pragmatic versus explanatory on 10 evaluation dimensions (see Chapter 16). By recognizing that a given trial may have both explanatory and pragmatic design elements, the PRECIS criteria should help improve reporting and increase available information for systematic reviews, most of which find inadequate data on external validity.[3,39] The intent of the PRECIS rating criteria is not to judge or conclude that one approach or the other is superior, but rather to objectively and transparently report the extent to which a study is explanatory (more close to the origination point in Figure 4–1) or pragmatic (further from the center of Figure 4–1) on all 10 dimensions.

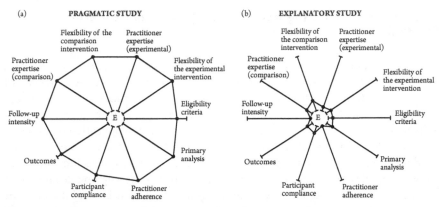

Figure 4–1. Comparison of pragmatic and exploratory studies.

Our thesis is that CER trials and observational studies that are more pragmatic, are more representative, and more transparently report results (see point 7 below) will be more likely to translate more completely and quickly to practice, policy, and public health applications (www.re-aim.org).[37] We term such research "CER-T." Such research is needed to advance application and relevance,[40] and accelerate translation of research to practice and policy.

Key Characteristics of CER-T

Table 4–2 summarizes the key features of CER-T, each of which we discuss in the following section. While many of the characteristics are very similar to those of D&I, or practical trials research,[29] items listed as points B, C, and D most emphatically separate CER-T from other types of translational research and thus can be seen as required elements of CER-T.

Evaluation of representativeness and/or variation across settings, clinicians, delivery conditions, and patient subgroups[41] is one of the cardinal indicators of likelihood of D&I success. Studies that either randomly sample, or use purposeful selection[41] to include diverse settings, clinicians, and patients, and are able to demonstrate robust effects across these strata, are most likely to have large-scale applicability.

Comparison conditions in CER-T, as in practical trials,[29,42] should be real-world alternatives, rather than placebo, attention control, or no-treatment conditions. This is one of the quintessential characteristics of research intended to have practical consequences. We especially recommend that the alternative treatment be the current standard treatment for a given condition or problem. For example, novel treatments for common illnesses such as high blood pressure should be compared with standard, low-cost medications of proven effectiveness rather than with placebos. We further recommend studies to identify "MINC"[43]—the Minimal Intervention Needed for Change (R. Croyle and B. Rimer, personal communication, 2010) for a given problem, given the pressing need to reduce health care delivery costs.

Particularly if novel treatments are compared to effective, standard, and low-cost alternatives, an evaluation of costs seems implicit in the purpose of CER.

TABLE 4-2. *Key Characteristics of CER-T: Research That Will Translate*

Characteristic	Translational Purpose of This Feature
A. Pragmatic[a] or practical	To answer questions from patients, practitioners, and policymakers to inform real-world decision making.
B. Evaluates participation and representativeness[b]	To determine breadth of applicability. Assesses participation rate and representativeness of participants, settings, staff, and subgroups.
C. Comparison condition(s) are real alternatives	To address practical questions in context of currently available (and usually less expensive) alternatives.
D. Collects costs and economic data	To provide information on resources needed to adopt and replicate in different settings.
E. Assesses multiple outcomes using mixed methods	To provide results that recognize the different priorities of multiple audiences—e.g., behavior change, quality of life/functioning, health care use, impact on health disparities, unintended consequences.
F. Uses flexible research design to fit question	To consider and addresses key threats to internal *and* external validity.
G. Transparent reporting[a,b,c]	To include information on implementation and modifications; numerators and denominators of settings, staff, patients invited, participating, and completing treatment.

[a] Thorpe et al.[36]
[b] Glasgow et al.[4,9]
[c] DesJarlais[37]

The inclusion of cost considerations in CER has become extremely politicized, out of concern that if the novel treatment is not cost effective, it might be denied to patient subgroups that could derive benefit. Of course, this concern can be mitigated in part by the prospective definition of such subgroups and their inclusion in the trial design (as discussed in point A above). Described in Chapter 5 on economic evaluation, it is beyond the scope of this chapter to discuss the political issues other than to note the controversies over cost and cost-effectiveness analyses (CEA) in CER.[44] From our perspective, if we wish to truly inform decision makers, it is imperative to assess the costs of delivering an intervention, to estimate the costs due to development, recruitment, training, supervision, staff time, equipment or technology, and other costs, and to conduct sensitivity analyses[45] to evaluate the scalability and the impact of variations in sample size, conditions or administration, and other factors on cost and cost effectiveness.[10]

The problems for which we need CER are complex, and it is overly simplistic to assume that there is only a single important outcome for these important questions. Thus, CER-T studies should generally have multiple outcomes. The relative importance of different outcomes may vary with "the eye of the beholder,"[46] and the perspectives of multiple stakeholders, including policymakers, patients, practitioners, administrative decision makers, and others should be considered. Also which outcomes—and which costs—are important to and borne by respective parties also varies across important CER settings including industry, employers, health plans, CMS, and so on. For CER-T, we recommend consideration of quality-of-life outcomes; behavior change of patients, staff, and organizations; health care risk indicators (e.g., BMI, lipids, blood pressure, etc., and/or utilization) relevant to the condition being studied; as well as relevant economic outcomes. Finally, we also recommend reporting unanticipated consequences—both positive and negative, resulting from interventions or procedures studied. The expectation of multiple outcomes imposes additional concerns in trial design, since the sample size must be sufficient to address multiple outcomes. Further, the outcomes should be measured independently, rather than aggregated into a "composite" outcome (such as death or hospitalization for heart failure) that mixes different outcome domains.[47]

To enable CER to be more relevant for D&I science, researchers will often need to employ qualitative data and mixed-methods designs.[48] Particularly for CER studies that assess behavior change, system change, or community interventions (Table 4–1), the means by which an intervention is implemented and outcomes come about may be based on important contextual factors that are rarely reported in conventional clinical trials. For example, a study that uses laypersons to help disadvantaged individuals with cancer "navigate" the complex process of evaluation and treatment may critically depend on the interpersonal skills and networking ability of the navigator. Unless such potential contextual factors are described, the effect of the intervention may be incorrectly estimated. Similarly, it may be helpful to collect "representative stories" of study participants who experience relevant outcomes, since these narratives are often much more influential than quantitative data when presenting to a wide array of audiences such as patients and families, organizational policymakers, and legislators.[49] The inclusion of stories in CER-T is not a reversion to an earlier time of decision making by anecdote. Rather, it is an attempt to complement the quantitative findings of rigorous research with information that can give decision makers insight into the human consequences of that decision.[50]

More broadly, qualitative methods may have a role in every stage of CER-T. In the formative and design phases of research, insights from qualitative observations of the conduct of an intervention may help "get the intervention right." To facilitate implementation and dissemination, stories can be collected to help illustrate main findings for nontechnical audiences, as noted previously. Finally, if the outcomes of a study are unexpected or contradict extant knowledge, qualitative information can help with the sense making or "postmortem examination" of a research study. For example, an unexpectedly "negative" trial of a reminder recall system for childhood immunizations in a disadvantaged population led to qualitative discussions with the staff of the clinic where the intervention took place, and then in turn to further quantitative analyses that demonstrated several critical components of clinic infrastructure that had prevented the intervention from being successful.[51] The results of a well-designed study should be informative whether "positive" or "negative"—a "postmortem examination" of a negative RCT can identify important barriers to D&I.

Other chapters discuss D&I design issues, and we will not repeat that information here other than to state that, in our view, CER-T does not have to, and in many cases cannot, use a randomized design. Useful designs for CER-T include multiple baseline across settings, patients, or time;[42,52–54] natural experiments; careful observational studies in real-world settings, a series of sequential small RCTs,[55] noninferiority or preference designs,[56] and even "n of 1" studies.[57] The research design should be appropriate and tailored to the question or interest, what is known at the time, and the specific likely threats to internal and external validity. Every design has advantages and disadvantages, and the question should determine the design—not vice versa.[53,54,58] A key point is that in CER-T it is important to maximize both internal and external validity.

Rapid learning health care systems. Etheredge and colleagues[6,59] have argued that the increasing availability of electronic medical records, especially as interoperability increases, adds a new data source for CER data. Such data will provide real-time information on hundreds of thousands (or possibly even millions depending on the question) of patients being treated in real-world settings with interventions implemented under usual care conditions. If health care organizations are appropriately structured and have capacity to carefully analyze and interpret these data, taking into account the impact of potential confounding factors, the opportunities for "rapid learning" are enormous. Such studies, especially when conducted across settings in collaborations such as managed-care networks, the U.S. Veteran's Administration system, or practice-based research networks[60,61] also provide data for investigation of variation in practices and their impact.[62]

■ SUMMARY

The goal of CER-T is to produce evidence that is relevant, practical, and actionable.[63] Possibly most important, CER-T contributes knowledge on contextual factors important for realist systematic reviews, decision making, and understanding of complex health issues.[1,34,63] CER-T demands much more complete and transparent reporting of factors such as setting and patient-level recruitment and participation (Figure 4-2). Two efficient ways to facilitate such transparent reporting are the PRECIS criteria (Figure 4-1),[36,64] and use of an "extended CONSORT Figure" such as that in Figure 4-2 to describe recruitment of settings and staff, and to document sustainability after a research project concludes (www.re-aim.org).[38]

Generalization across several important factors, including robustness of results across the "3 S's" of Settings, Staff, and Subgroups, is especially important in CER-T. For example, a CER-T question might be: "Do incentives and patient navigator programs for increasing medication adherence work equally well when delivered by community health workers compared to nurses, for individuals with low versus high incomes, and for individuals with low vs. high health numeracy?" Such information about the subgroups most likely to benefit from an intervention has direct implications for addressing health disparities [65] and for guiding the most efficient use of limited health care resources. The related and frequently underemphasized issue of replication[4,66] is an important dimension of causality that deserves greater attention in all types of health care research. Replication across settings, staff, and key patient subgroups, and replication by different research groups, adds confidence that CER-T results are worth taking to scale. Ironically, multiple—and at times superfluous—efficacy trials have often been conducted for pharmaceutical treatments, whereas replication of "real-world" effectiveness studies is seldom seen.

As illustrated in Figures 4-1 and 4-2, transparent reporting of implementation—including how programs are adapted over time, in different settings, and by different staff, is critically important. Even in closely monitored multisite efficacy trials, implementation always varies, and we need more transparent

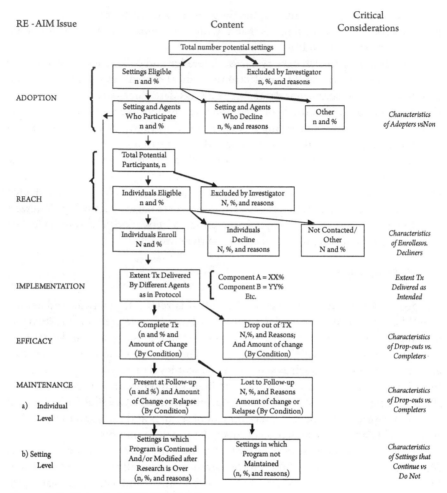

Figure 4–2. Extended CONSORT diagram.

reporting of such variation. The fidelity adaptation issue is discussed in detail in Chapter 14, but our position is that rather than being inherently bad, variation in implementation is inevitable and instructive, especially in real-world settings. Some of this variation undoubtedly has adverse impacts on outcomes, but other adaptations are likely appropriate and may well enhance participation, engagement, or outcomes. Rather than suppress reporting of variation, it needs to be transparently reported so that program developers and evaluators can learn from it using both quantitative and qualitative methods of inquiry.[4,62]

Even more than most health research, CER-T requires true transdisciplinary teams.[67] To thoroughly evaluate and understand the results and implications of CER-T, teams from multiple disciplines are needed, including health services research, behavioral science, health economics, biostatistics and modeling, community-based participatory research, medical anthropology and sociology, psychology, public health, social work, and clinical disciplines (e.g., medicine, pharmacy, nursing), in addition to study and content-specific subject matter experts who can learn from each other. The complex and challenging issues for which CER-T is needed demand that teams of professionals engage in respectful and emergent dialogue with key stakeholders and policymakers using community-based participatory and partnership research principles[68,69] throughout the research process.[68,69]

Limitations. The entire field of CER, and especially CER-T, is new and rapidly evolving. The traditional paradigm of conducting explanatory trials has evolved over the last 60 years—in contrast, CER-T is in its infancy. As a result, many of the suggestions we make in this chapter are based on limited experience in the research community, which will undoubtedly render some of these ideas outdated as more CERT-T studies are designed, implemented, and reported. In particular, we yet know little about whether resolving the current barriers to translation of research will, in fact, motivate stakeholders to incorporate CER-T findings into their decisions more rapidly, or to base decisions on the evidence derived from these studies. In the meantime, we hope that this chapter can be a useful guide to those venturing into this new high-priority area, and that D&I researchers will wrestle with, use, and improve upon the ideas presented.

A few specific limitations deserve mention. First, this discussion applies primarily to intervention studies; the issues we discuss apply less well to observational studies or statistical modeling simulations, both of which will be an important part of CER-T and rapid-learning health care systems.[6,29,59] We hope that some of the points we raise can be generalized or adapted to other areas, such as public health genomics.[70,71] Second, the conduct of CER-T calls for fairly radical departures from business as usual in research.[4] We anticipate the objection that such studies will be too costly because (for example) the sample size for the study is enlarged by the necessity of detecting significant differences in multiple, individual outcome measures. An additional objection is that it is not possible to do some of what we recommend. Investigators are not trained to do research this way; it will take longer to truly involve community members and stakeholders in research, and so on. Our response is that something dramatically different is needed. If CER follows the usual path of traditional drug efficacy studies, the vast number of soon-to-be-funded CER studies will simply not translate into practice or inform policy, and the few that do will take an embarrassingly long time to translate.[4] Congress, the public, and key government, business, and health care decision makers need answers soon to the pressing health and budgetary problems facing us. Business as usual will not get the job done: something fundamentally different is needed.[4]

Finally, CER-T can be characterized as complexity upon complexity. CER-T, by design, is the *study of complex patients with complex problems and complex health care (or public health) teams embedded in complex systems, and the goal is to evaluate complex and multifaceted outcomes (intended and unintended) of complex interventions.*[8,13,72,73] Answers to these issues will not come from research paradigms that are designed to simplify and decontextualize issues.[4] Rather, the goal of CER-T should be "to determine which intervention or policy, administered under what conditions is most effective for which subgroups—on what outcomes, and how does this come about?"[1,63,74]

Even though CER-T research questions are complex and "wicked," as defined by Kreuter—this is not a reason to avoid CER-T.[75] This new field demands new approaches and requires rethinking what many of us were taught about research design. For example, to produce actionable, generalizable results, one would not use run-in periods to exclude less motivated or complex patients; exclude patients with comorbidities; or only study interventions when delivered by world experts in the most advanced and state-of-the-science settings. Indeed, CER-T conducted under typical and generalizable conditions will be likely to reduce effects sizes and result in increased variation, and requires increased sample sizes. But it will also give practitioners, patients, and policymakers a better idea of the effects they can expect from implementation and dissemination of programs in their settings (see Chapter 15).[4,63]

How might these concepts be applied in an actual intervention trial? Assume that a research group decides to design a study to improve adherence among individuals with high cholesterol who are prescribed 3-hydroxy-3methylglutaryl co-enzyme A reductase inhibitors ("statins"). It is clearly an important clinical and public health issue, given the benefit of statins in reducing the risk of cardiovascular events in appropriate populations,[76,77] and the repeated observation that only about 50% of individuals prescribed a statin continue to take it one year later.[78] Further assume that this research group decides to try a novel outreach method—delivering periodic SMS text message reminders to patients after their first statin prescription, with a trained clinical pharmacist available to provide back-up for patients who wish to call or reply by text with questions or concerns. Given this broad framework, the study can be designed and implemented either as an explanatory or efficacy trial, or as a CER-T study. Some (although by no means all) of the contrasts between those designs are summarized in Table 4–3.

Examination of the differences in intervention design between the explanatory/efficacy trial and the pragmatic CER-T study in Table 4–3 illustrates many of the messages in this chapter. To those trained in traditional methods of trial design or used to conducting FDA approval trials, the decisions made in the efficacy trial would appear likely to lead to a "cleaner" design. The message of this chapter, however, is that a clean design in a "dirty, complex, contextual" world (where D&I research occurs) may not give us the information we need to decide whether this treatment strategy is feasible, worthwhile, or generalizable. The efficacy design is likely to be more efficient, use a shorter period of follow-up, and produce a greater intervention effect size. However, almost every design decision for the efficacy trial excludes those clinics, clinicians, and subjects who are less likely to be adherent (and are often most in need or could most benefit). In other words, the efficacy design selects for a study environment that is unrepresentative of the very issue—the likelihood of treatment adherence—that is being studied. Given this, such a study is likely to substantially overestimate the impact of such an intervention in a "real-world" setting, as well as fail to detect unanticipated consequences such as adverse reactions for complex patients, and so on.

Finally, such a study imposed on the busy "microculture" of an office practice can have many effects that cannot be predicted. The need to provide more follow-up care for individuals on statins may take time away from other important clinical issues. Alternatively, initial effectiveness of this program may encourage generalization of

TABLE 4-3. *Efficacy (or Explanatory) Trial versus CER-T Trial for Promoting Adherence with "Statin" Medications*

Design Decision	Efficacy Trial	CER-T Trial
Which clinics to approach?	Highly motivated site(s) within high-performing systems having excellent EMR resources	Randomly selected site(s) from multiple, diverse delivery systems
Which clinicians to approach?	Highly motivated clinicians within those sites	All clinicians within those sites
Which patients to enroll?	Highly motivated patients with minimal comorbidity	All patients newly prescribed a statin, regardless of comorbid physical or psychosocial problems
What level of comfort with cell phones to select for?	Comfortable using wide range of cell phone features	No cell phone (need to provide one and instruct), or wide range of comfort with cell phone features
How frequently to send text messages?	Frequently; isolated from workflow in clinic, close highly individualized intensive monitoring	Less frequently, but consistent with workflow patterns in clinic
What level of training to require from supporting clinical pharmacist?	Single individual, highly experienced, trained in motivational interviewing	Multiple clinical pharmacists with standard training in patient counseling
What kind of advice protocol to provide?	Highly scripted, standardized	Unscripted or general guidelines and suggestions for adapting
How to monitor implementation of advice protocol?	Careful assessment of fidelity to protocol, and intensified intervention if not optimal	Qualitative assessment of advice actually delivered by pharmacists
How to monitor adherence?	Active, continuous assessment with electronic medication monitors	Surveillance by patient self-report and/or prescription refill records
How to monitor impact on cholesterol?	Fasting cholesterol levels drawn at prespecified intervals during additional visits for that purpose	Fasting cholesterol levels drawn in the course of routine practice visits
Which patient subgroups to monitor for differences in effectiveness?	Few subgroups assessed (due to exclusions in recruitment), homogeneous patients not on other medications	Multiple, prespecified subgroups (particularly for subgroups that might be excluded in an efficacy trial, e.g., individuals with multimorbidity or limited cell phone comfort), low–health literacy/numeracy participants
Duration of follow-up?	Short-term (e.g., 3–6 months), allowing identification of individuals who soon stop treatment	Long-term (12–24 months), allowing identification of individuals who later restart treatment
Continuation of intervention?	To end of grant funding	Long-term incorporation into clinic operations
Does this intervention have any effects, positive or negative, on clinic operations?	Not relevant to assess Not assessed	Critical to assess through staff interviews, observations, and qualitative assessments
Cost of intervention		Assessed from perspective of adopting organization and patient, includes cost-effectiveness indices

the adherence strategy to related problems such as adherence with antihypertensive medications. A traditional efficacy trial would generally not assess these contextual effects, whereas CER-T researchers would devote substantial attention to them, particularly expanding the program to other adherence problems, including cost effectiveness.

■ FUTURE DIRECTIONS

These are exciting times for science and for CER; we need to embrace new opportunities to conduct research that will make a difference in the daily lives of patients and populations. However, we also need to keep the purpose of CER-T in mind. Doing so will demand that we learn new and unorthodox approaches—and that we unlearn old habits.[4,79] The need is too great and too urgent not to act. CER-T research that will actually translate, breaking the cycle of studies that lead only to more similar studies, provides many exciting opportunities. Among them are:

1. Investigations of key ways to use electronic medical records and patient portals as intervention vehicles. For example, such research might utilize natural language processing and patient report outcomes to provide clinicians with feedback on patient-centered counseling and health behavior change skills.

2. Rapid learning research networks—such as those created by AHRQ practice-based research networks, the VA QUERI program[25,80,81] (http://www.queri.research.va.gov), the HMO (http://www.hmoresearchnetwork.org) and CRN research networks (http://crn.cancer.gov), HRSA community health centers (http://bphc.hrsa.gov/about), prevention research centers (www.cdc.gov/prc),[60,82] and CTSA collaboratives (http://www.ctsi.mcw.edu/index.php?id=80). Such networks sharing common electronic databases can rapidly study contextual effects on interventions and study the impact of variations in care on health outcomes. KT Canada is a similar collaboration among D&I scientists across Canada. Much can also be learned from networks such NICE in the U.K. (http://www.nice.org.uk) and German CER-related efforts (www.iqwig.de/index.2.en.html)

3. Public health genomics[70,83,84] offers numerous opportunities such as comparative studies of new genomic assessments versus family history approaches to genetic counseling; and the influence of different health communication strategies on genetic testing rates and risk perceptions.

4. Community-based studies of different policy/environmental change programs (such as recent stimulus funding from the U.S. government on CER and practice-based research networks being funded by RWJF [http://www.publichealthsystems.org/pbrn/PBRNCoordinatingCenter]) can help inform these community decisions on resource allocation.

5. The identification of health disparities presents many opportunities and challenges for dissemination and translation of CER-T, such as questions about whether an intervention is culturally appropriate, or likely to be "lost in translation." We need much more research on whether studies proven efficacious with majority populations will work with low-income, minority, and less economically advantaged groups and settings.

6. CER-T studies of interventions for low–health literacy and numeracy populations,[85-87] as well as more commonly studied groups suffering from health inequities, are needed to ensure that CER helps to reduce rather than exacerbate health disparities.

■ CONCLUSIONS

Unlike some of the more developed areas discussed in other chapters, the field of translational CER-T is just beginning. The success of CER-T, whether or not it takes the forms described in this chapter, will be a key to both the long-term success of the overall national investment in CER and, more importantly, whether the national investment in health research will pay dividends in terms of care that reaches more people and is safe, timely, effective, patient centered, efficient, and equitable, as the Institute of Medicine has articulated.[88]

The overall field of CER and its companion field of "precision medicine"[89] (a terminology now preferred by some to patient-centered medicine and genomic medicine) have great potential to either improve care and reduce adverse health outcomes or to vastly increase expenses and health disparities.[70,83] Attention to the above CER-T issues will help keep this train going down the former track.

We are confident that the translational research area of CER-T will continue to evolve. We are particularly encouraged by recent developments such as the CONSORT focus on pragmatic trials[36,64] and the PRECIS criteria,[36] which along with other efforts to enhance transparency of reporting should advance the relevance and usefulness of our science.

CER-T is primed to take on the complex and "wicked problems"[75] facing health care and medicine today. To make progress on such questions, a realist approach capable of addressing complex interventions[1,72,73] in their social cultural-political-historical context[63] is necessary. We provide resources below for investigators interested in this evolving field of CER-T and look forward to being able to review research contributions and the state of the CER-T science in 5–10 years, instead of having to rely upon informed hunches and lessons from what has not worked in the past.[4]

SUGGESTED READINGS

An Engelberg Center for Health Care Reform and Hamilton Project Event, Brookings Institution. Implementing comparative effectiveness research: priorities, methods, and impact. June 9, 2009. http://www.brookings.edu/events/2009/0609_health_care_cer.aspx. Accessed 11–10–11.

Compiled by the Engleberg Center for Healthcare Reform at the Brookings Institution, in partnership with The Hamilton Project, this compendium of thought pieces on comparative effectiveness research (CER) includes discussions of implementation and design issues by leaders in the field.

Glasgow RE, Emmons KM. How can we increase translation of research into practice? Types of evidence needed. *Annu Rev Public Health.* 2007;28:413–433.

Glasgow and Emmons offer a summary and review of what is needed to facilitate more and faster uptake of research. The authors use the RE-AIM model and community partnership perspectives to discuss current status and future needs.

Institute of Medicine. The Learning Healthcare System: Workshop Summary. Washington, DC: The National Academies Press. April 2, 2007.

This is a summary of the work of Lynn Etheredge and other leaders concept of need for rapid-learning health care systems, and types of research this would involve. These data provide real-time information on thousands (or hundreds of thousands depending on condition) of patients in real-world settings and discuss how these data can be used for decision making.

Jha AK, Perlin JB, Kizer KW, Dudley RA. Effect of the transformation of the Veterans Affairs Health Care System on the quality of care. *N Engl J Med.* 2003;348:2218–2227.

This article summarizes primary results of CER applied to the Veterans Affairs system through their QUERI approach. The Veterans Affairs has dramatically improved their quality of care over the past decade using the approaches outlined in this article.

Khoury MJ, Gwinn M, Yoon PW, Dowling N, Moore CA, Bradley L. The continuum of translation research in genomic medicine: how can we accelerate the appropriate integration of human genome discoveries into health care and disease prevention? *Genet Med.* 2007;9:665–674.

This article introduces concepts of T3 and T4 research in this key emerging area of public health genomics. It emphasizes the need to focus on the need to conduct research and programs that will lead to better care and will have public health impact.

Luce BR, Kramer JM, Goodman SN et al. Rethinking randomized clinical trials for comparative effectiveness research: the need for transformational change. *Ann Intern Med.* 2009;151:206–209.

This article discusses the "out-of-the-box" type of thinking necessary to make a difference in comparative effectiveness research (CER), and how research design needs to fit the setting and the question. The authors identify three key issues—operational efficiency, analytical efficiency, and pragmatic approaches to trial design—that have the potential to produce more valid and broadly applicable evidence.

Pawson R, Greenhalgh T, Harvey G, Walshe K. Realist review: a new method of systematic review designed for complex policy interventions. *J Health Serv Res Policy.* 2005;10:S21–S39.

Pawson et al. suggest an alternative approach to systematic reviews and evidence that emphasizes context and external validity. This approach to evidence review seeks to answer questions such as: which intervention, for which problem, for which set of patients is the intervention most effective, and for producing what outcome?

SELECTED WEBSITES AND TOOLS

Cancer Control P.L.A.N.E.T. (http://cancercontrolplanet.cancer.gov/index.html). Cancer Control P.L.A.N.E.T. acts as a portal to provide access to data and resources for designing, implementing, and evaluating evidence-based cancer control programs. The site provides five steps (with links) for developing a comprehensive cancer control plan or program.

RE-AIM online training. (http://www.center-trt.org/index.cfm?fa=webtraining.reaim). RE-AIM Online is a web-based training module available through the Center of Excellence for Training and Research Translation (Center-TRT). The module includes four lessons that provide instruction on the five dimensions of the RE-AIM framework and that use case examples to illustrate the application of RE-AIM to behavior change and policy/environmental change interventions. This training is appropriate for anyone interested in considering the overall public health impact of health promotion interventions including researchers, program planners, evaluators, funders, and policymakers.

Institute of Medicine. The Learning Healthcare System. Washington, D.C.: National Academies Press, 2007. This book summarizes perspectives from leaders in the emerging field of rapid learning healthcare systems and covers issues such as the use of electronic health records, systems design, patient-centeredness, and feedback system.

■ REFERENCES

1. Pawson R, Greenhalgh T, Harvey G, Walshe K. Realist review: A new method of systematic review designed for complex policy interventions. *Journal of Health Services Research and Policy* 2005;10:S21–S39.
2. Institute of Medicine of the National Academies. Initial National Priorities for Comparative Effectiveness Research. *www.iom.edu/Reports/2009/Comparative EffectivenessResearchPriorities.aspx* [serial online] 2009;Accessed 7-26-11.
3. Rothwell PM. Factors that can affect the external validity of randomised controlled trials. *PLoS Clin Trials* 2006;1:e9.
4. Kessler R, Glasgow RE. A proposal to speed translation of healthcare intervention research into practice: Dramatic change is needed. *Am J Prev Med* 2011;40: 637–644.
5. Zerhouni EA. Translational and clinical science—time for a new vision. *N Eng J Med* 2005;353:1621–1623.
6. Etheredge LM. A rapid-learning health system: What would a rapid-learning health system look like, and how might we get there? *Health Affairs* 2007;Web Exclusive Collection:w107–w118.
7. Glass TA, McAtee MJ. Behavioral science at the crossroads in public health: Extending horizons, envisioning the future. *Soc Sci Med* 2006;62:1650–1671.
8. Schensul JJ. Community, culture and sustainability in multilevel dynamic systems intervention science. *Am J Community Psychol* 2009;43:241–256.
9. Glasgow RE, Emmons KM. How can we increase translation of research into practice? Types of evidence needed. *Ann Rev Public Health* 2007;28:413–433.
10. Ritzwoller DP, Sukhanova A, Gaglio B, Glasgow RE. Costing behavioral interventions: A practical guide to enhance translation. *Ann Behav Med* 2009;Apr 37: 218–227.
11. Bodenheimer TS, Wagner EH, Grumbach K. Improving primary care for patients with chronic illness. The Chronic Care Model, Part 2. *JAMA* 2002;288:1909–1914.
12. Wagner EH, Austin BT, Davis C, Hindmarsh M, Schaefer J. Improving chronic illness care: Translating evidence into action. *Health Aff* 2001;20:64–78.
13. Breslau E, Dietrich AJ, Glasgow RE, Stange KC. State-of-the-art and future directions in multilevel interventions across the Cancer Control Continuum. *J Natl Cancer Inst.* In press.
14. Sedrakyan A, Marinac-Dabic D, Normand SL, Mushlin A, Gross T. A framework for evidence evaluation and methodological issues in implantable device studies. *Med Care* 2010;48:S121–S128.
15. Neumayer L, Giobbie-Hurder A, Jonasson O et al. Open mesh versus laparoscopic mesh repair of inguinal hernia. *N Engl J Med* 2004;350:1819–1827.
16. Shroufi A, Powles JW. Adherence and chemoprevention in major cardiovascular disease: A simulation study of the benefits of additional use of statins. *J Epidemiol Community Health* 2010;64:109–113.
17. McDonald HP, Garg AX, Haynes RB. Interventions to enhance patient adherence to medication prescriptions: Scientific review. *JAMA* 2002;288:2868–2879.

18. Batal HA, Krantz MJ, Dale RA, Mehler PS, Steiner JF. Impact of prescription size on statin adherence and cholesterol levels. *BMC Health Serv Res* 2007;7:175.
19. Hsu J, Price M, Huang J et al. Unintended consequences of caps on Medicare drug benefits. *N Engl J Med* 2006;354:2349–2359.
20. Kroenke K, Spitzer RL, Williams JB. The PHQ-9: Validity of a brief depression severity measure. *J Gen Intern Med* 2001;16:606–613.
21. Fisher L, Glasgow RE, Mullan JT, Skaff MM, Polonsky WH. Development of a brief diabetes distress screening instrument. *Ann Fam Med* 2008;6:246–252.
22. Berwick DM. A user's manual for the IOM's "Quality Chasm" report: Patients' experience should be the fundamental source of the definition of "quality." *Health Aff* 2002;21:80–90.
23. Berwick DM. Disseminating innovations in health care. *JAMA* 2003;289: 1969–1975.
24. Berwick DM. The science of improvement. *JAMA* 2008;299:1182–1184.
25. Yano EM. The role of organizational research in implementing evidence-based practice: QUERI Series. *Implement Sci* 2008;3:29.
26. Christakis NA, Fowler JH. *Connected: The surprising power of our social networks and how they shape our lives*. New York: Little, Brown and Company, 2009.
27. Green LW, Glasgow RE. Evaluating the relevance, generalization, and applicability of research: Issues in external validity and translation methodology. *Eval Health Prof* 2006;29:126–153; PMID16510882.
28. Zwarenstein M, Treweek S, Gagnier JJ et al. Improving the reporting of pragmatic trials: An extension of the CONSORT statement. *Br Med J* 2008;11 November; 337:a2390 (doi: 10.1136/bmj).
29. Tunis SR, Stryer DB, Clancey CM. Practical clinical trials: Increasing the value of clinical research for decision making in clinical and health policy. *JAMA* 2003;290: 1624–1632; PMID 14506122.
30. Flay BR. Efficacy and effectiveness trials (and other phases of research) in the development of health promotion programs. *Prev Med* 1986;15:451–474.
31. Greenwald P, Cullen JW. The new emphasis in cancer control. *J Natl Cancer Inst* 1985;74:543–551.
32. Glasgow RE, Lichtenstein E, Marcus AC. Why don't we see more translation of health promotion research to practice? Rethinking the efficacy to effectiveness transition. *Am J Public Health* 2003;93:1261–1267.
33. Pawson R, Tilley N. *Realistic evaluation*. Thousand Oaks, CA: Sage Publications, 1997.
34. Greenhalgh T, Robert G, Macfarlane F, Bate P, Kyriakidou O. Diffusion of innovations in service organizations: Systematic review and recommendations. *Milbank Q* 2004;82:581–629.
35. Biglan A. *Changing cultural practices: A contextualist framework for intervention research*. Reno, NV: Context Press, 1995.
36. Thorpe KE, Zwarenstein M, Oxman AD et al. A pragmatic-explanatory continuum indicator summary (PRECIS): A tool to help trial designers. *CMAJ* 2009;180: E47–E57.
37. Des Jarlais DC, Lyles C, Crepaz N, TREND Group. Improving the reporting quality of nonrandomized evaluations of behavioral and public health interventions: The TREND statement. *Am J Public Health* 2004;94:361–366.
38. Glasgow RE. HMC research translation: Speculations about making it real and going to scale. *Am J Health Behav* 2009;Nov–Dec;34:833–840.

39. Glasgow RE, Klesges LM, Dzewaltowski DA, Bull SS, Estabrooks P. The future of health behavior change research: What is needed to improve translation of research into health promotion practice? *Ann Behav Med* 2004;27:3–12; PMID 14979358.
40. Rothwell PM. External validity of randomised controlled trials: To whom do the results of this trial apply? *Lancet* 2005;365:82–93.
41. Cook TD, Campbell DT. *Quasi-experimentation: Design and analysis issues for field settings.* Chicago: Rand McNally, 1979.
42. Glasgow RE, Magid DJ, Beck A, Ritzwoller D, Estabrooks PA. Practical clinical trials for translating research to practice: Design and measurement recommendations. *Med Care* 2005;43:551–557; PMID 15908849.
43. Brownson RC, Fielding JE, Maylahn CM. Evidence-based public health: A fundamental concept for public health practice. *Annu Rev Public Health* 2009;30: 175–201.
44. Luce BR, Drummond M, Jonsson B et al. EBM, HTA, and CER: Clearing the confusion. *Milbank Q* 2010;88:256–276.
45. Gold MR, Siegel JE, Russell LB, Weinstein MC. *Cost-effectiveness in health and medicine.* New York: Oxford University Press, 2003.
46. Kerner JF. Integrating research, practice, and policy: What we see depends on where we stand. *J Public Health Manag Pract* 2008;14:193–198.
47. Tomlinson G, Detsky AS. Composite endpoints in randomized trials: There is no free lunch. *JAMA* 2010;303:267–268.
48. Greene J, Benjamin L, Goodyear L. The merits of mixing methods in evaluation. *Evaluation* 2001;7:25–44.
49. Steiner JF. The use of stories in clinical research and health policy. *JAMA* 2005;294: 2901–2904.
50. Steiner JF, Nowels CT, Main DS. Returning to work after cancer: Quantitative studies and prototypical narratives. *Psychooncol* 2010;19:115–124.
51. Kempe A, Lowery NE, Pearson KA et al. Immunization recall: Effectiveness and barriers to success in an urban teaching clinic. *J Pediatr* 2001;139:630–635.
52. Biglan A, Ary D, Wagenaar AC. The value of interrupted time-series experiments for community intervention research. *Prev Sci* 2000;1:31–49.
53. Sanson-Fisher RW, Bonevski B, Green LW. Limitations of the randomized controlled trial in evaluating population-based health interventions. *Am J Prev Med* 2007;33: 162–168.
54. Mercer SM, DeVinney BJ, Fine LJ, Green LW. Study designs for effectiveness and tranlsation research: Identifying trade-offs. *Am J Prev Med* 2007;33:139–154.
55. Daley MF, Steiner JF, Kempe A et al. Quality improvement in immunization delivery following an unsuccessful immunization recall. *Ambul Pediatr* 2004;4:217–223.
56. Glasgow RE, Edwards LL, Whitesides H, Carroll N, Sanders TJ, McCray BL. Reach and effectiveness of DVD and in-person diabetes self-management education. *Chronic Illn* 2009;5:243–249; PMID 19933245.
57. Kravitz RL, Duan N, Niedzinski EJ, Hay MC, Subramanian SK, Weisner TS. What ever happened to N-of-1 trials? Insiders' perspectives and a look to the future. *Milbank Q* 2008;86:533–555.
58. Luce BR, Kramer JM, Goodman SN et al. Rethinking randomized clinical trials for comparative effectiveness research: The need for transformational change. *Ann Intern Med* 2009;151:206–209.

59. Institute of Medicine. A foundation for evidence-driven practice: A rapid learning system for cancer care. Workshop summary, National Cancer Policy Forum, *NAS Press* June 4, 2010.

60. Nutting PA, Beasley JW, Werner JJ. Practice-based research networks answer primary care questions. *JAMA* 1999;281:686–689.

61. Stetler CB, Mittman BS, Francis J. Overview of the VA Quality Enhancement Research Initiative (QUERI) and QUERI theme articles: QUERI Series. *Implement Sci* 2008;3:8.

62. Selby JV, Schmittidiel JA, Lee J et al. Meaningful variation in performance: What does variation in quality tell us about improving quality? *Med Care* 2010;Feb;48: 133–139.

63. Glasgow RE. What types of evidence are most needed to advance behavioral medicine? *Ann Behav Med* 2008;35:19–25.

64. Treeweek S, Zwarenstein M. Making trials matter: Pragmatic and explanatory trials and the problem of applicability. *Trials* 2009;10:37.

65. Woolf SH, Johnson RE, Fryer GE, Jr., Rust G, Satcher D. The health impact of resolving racial disparities: An analysis of US mortality data. *Am J Public Health* 2008;98:S26–S28.

66. Sidman M. *Tactics of scientific research: Evaluating experimental data in psychology.* 5th ed. New York: Basic Books, Inc., 1960.

67. Stokols D, Hall KL, Taylor BK, Moser RP. The science of team science: Overview of the field and introduction to the supplement. *Am J Prev Med* 2008;35:S77–S89.

68. Minkler M, Wallerstein N, Wilson N. Improving health through community organization and community building. In: Glanz K, Rimer BK, Viswanath K, Eds. *Health behavior and health education.* 4th Ed. San Francisco, CA: John Wiley; 2008;287–312.

69. Mercer SL, MacDonald G, Green LW. Participatory research and evaluation: From best practices for all states to achievable practices within each state in the context of the Master Settlement Agreement. *Health Promot Pract* 2004;5:167S–178S.

70. Khoury MJ, Gwinn M, Yoon PW, Dowling N, Moore CA, Bradley L. The continuum of translation research in genomic medicine: How can we accelerate the appropriate integration of human genome discoveries into health care and disease prevention? *Genet Med* 2007;9:665–674.

71. Valdez R, Yoon PW, Qureshi N, Green RF, Khoury MJ. Family history in public health practice: A genomic tool for disease prevention and health promotion. *Annu Rev Public Health* 2010;31:69–87.

72. Anderson R. New MRC guidance on evaluating complex interventions. *Br Med J* 2008;337:a1937.

73. United Kingdom. Medical Research Council. *http://www.mrc.ac. uk/Utilities/ Documentrecord/index htm?d=MRC004871* [serial online] 2010;Accessed 6–23-10.

74. Paul GL. Behavior modification research: Design and tactics. In: Franks CM, ed. *Behavior therapy: Appraisal and status.* New York: McGraw-Hill; 1969;29–62.

75. Kreuter MW, DeRosa C, Howze EH, Baldwin GT. Understanding wicked problems: A key to advancing enviornmental health promotion. *Health Educ Behav* 2004;Aug; 31:441–454.

76. Mills EJ, Rachlis B, Wu P, Devereaux PJ, Arora P, Perri D. Primary prevention of cardiovascular mortality and events with statin treatments: A network meta-analysis involving more than 65,000 patients. *J Am Coll Cardiol* 2008;52:1769–1781.

77. McGinnis B, Olson KL, Magid D et al. Factors related to adherence to statin therapy. *Ann Pharmacother* 2007;41:1805–1811.
78. Benner JS, Glynn RJ, Mogun H, Neumann PJ, Weinstein MC, Avorn J. Long-term persistence in use of statin therapy in elderly patients. *JAMA* 2002;288:455–461.
79. Vogt TM, Aickin M, Ahmed F, Schmidt M. The Prevention Index: Using technology to improve quality assessment. *HSR* 2004;39:511–530.
80. Luck J, Hagigi F, Parker LE, Yano EM, Rubenstein LV, Kirchner JE. A social marketing approach to implementing evidence-based practice in VHA QUERI: The TIDES depression collaborative care model. *Implement Sci* 2009;4:64.
81. Graham ID, Tetroe J. Learning from the U.S. Department of Veterans Affairs Quality Enhancement Research Initiative: QUERI Series. *Implement Sci* 2009;4:13.
82. Chin MH, Drum ML, Guillen M et al. Improving and sustaining diabetes care in community health centers with the health disparities collaboratives. *Med Care* 2007;45:1135–1143.
83. Khoury MJ, Rich EC, Randhawa G, Teutsch SM, Niederhuber J. Comparative effectiveness research and genomic medicine: An evolving partnership for 21st century medicine. *Genet Med* 2009;11:707–711.
84. McBride CM, Bowen D, Brody LC et al. Future health applications of genomics: Priorities for communication, behavioral, and social sciences research. *Am J Prev Med* 2010;38:556–565.
85. Institute of Medicine. *Health Literacy: A prescription to end confusion*. Washington, DC: National Academies Press, 2004.
86. Rothman RL, Montori VM, Cherrington A, Pignone MP. Perspective: The role of numeracy in health care. *J Health Comm* 2008;13:583–595.
87. Schillinger D, Piette JD, Bindman A. Closing the loop: Missed opportunities in communicating with diabetes patients who have health literacy problems. *Arch Intern Med* 2003;163:83–90.
88. Institute of Medicine, Committee on Quality of Health Care in America. *Crossing the quality chasm: A new health system for the 21st Century*. Washington, DC: National Academy Press, 2001.
89. Christiansen CM, Grossman JH, Hwang J. *The innovator's prescription: A disruptive solution for health care*. New York: McGraw-Hill, 2009.

5 The Role of Economic Evaluation in Dissemination and Implementation Research

■ RAMESH RAGHAVAN

■ INTRODUCTION

Over the past several decades, many new and highly efficacious interventions have been developed in health and public health settings thanks to considerable investments in intervention research. Unfortunately, these advances in the development of interventions have not been accompanied by their spread to real-world, community settings. In several health-related disciplines, there is a considerable lag between the ideal, espoused by the science of interventions, and the actual, exemplified by clinical practice in community settings. This lag has led to a state where the Institute of Medicine estimates that only between 10 and 27% of individuals are receiving care consistent with scientific principles,[1] and where it reportedly takes 17 years to incorporate advances in clinical research into everyday practice.[2]

Bridging this gap between science and practice is a principal goal of dissemination and implementation (D&I) research, the former being concerned with increasing the use of evidence-based interventions widely by a target population, and the latter being concerned with the integration of evidence-based interventions within particular service settings such as schools or worksites (please see the Glossary for more formal definitions of these terms). D&I research focuses on processes or strategies by which interventions can be spread to, or adopted by, target audiences. In the field of implementation science, where the study of these processes is more developed, there are several distinct implementation strategies, which are designed to systematize the uptake of an intervention in a provider setting.

The challenge for the target audience of D&I research, whether a population of clinicians or a provider organization, is that many of these processes and strategies are highly complex endeavors and, consequently, are likely to be very expensive to deploy. Most health and public health settings in the community do not have access to research funds, and current reimbursement mechanisms do not cover the costs of disseminating and implementing interventions.

For these reasons, an economic analysis of D&I processes and strategies is required, one that systematically examines what outcomes a strategy—or a set of competing strategies— achieves, and the costs of achieving those outcomes. Once a provider organization knows how much it will cost them to implement an intervention, for example, and what the returns are likely to be of spending those dollars, it can then take an informed decision regarding whether or not to participate in such an implementation. Economic evaluations can also be of use to D&I researchers. A very expensive implementation strategy that produces small improvements in outcomes is likely to be less attractive than another implementation strategy that produces the same improvement but at a fraction of the cost. Conducting economic evaluations of competing implementation strategies is one way in which D&I researchers can justify scaling up the use of their implementation strategy.

This chapter presents an overview of how D&I research can be evaluated from an economic point of view. This chapter does not discuss or evaluate any intervention that may be disseminated and implemented; its efficacy is assumed. Because implementation science has better developed strategies whose costs can be assessed, we accentuate implementation strategies in this chapter and illustrate costing one particular implementation strategy as a case example. This approach, however, can be also extended to quantifying the costs of dissemination processes. D&I researchers are interested in both proximal outcomes—such as fidelity (an implementation outcome), or timeliness of care (a service outcome)—as well as distal outcomes, such as improvements in client health and well-being.[3] Each of these types of outcomes can be subject to an economic evaluation. As a first step, researchers might quantify the relative costs of different implementation strategies and compare changes in an intermediate outcome, such as fidelity, resulting from the use of those strategies. This type of an analysis provides a researcher with the incremental costs of improving the fidelity to an intervention. The next step might be to examine if these improvements in fidelity have resulted in improvements in a distal outcome, such as improved client health. This type of an analysis provides information on whether the costs of implementation are a good value for a provider organization attempting to deploy a given evidence-based intervention.

The chapter begins by providing a brief review of economic concepts and in the next section discusses cost and outcome estimation from a D&I perspective. Using the Breakthrough Series Collaborative as a case study, a suggested approach is outlined to costing this implementation strategy and comparing its costs versus a "usual" implementation. Finally, observations are provided regarding the implications of economic evaluations for the field of D&I research in particular, and for policy in general.

■ BRIEF REVIEW OF ECONOMIC EVALUATIONS

Economic evaluations use a formal methodology to quantify whether or not the money that is spent on the purchase of health care goods and services represents the best use of that money.[4] This kind of information is one among many other factors (such as availability of a good or service, or clinician familiarity with an intervention, for example) that drive decision making. This information is important not only for policymakers but also for administrators, executive directors, and budget managers within hospitals and health care facilities who each day face decisions regarding whether their organizational expenditures are producing the biggest "bang for the buck."

More formally, economic evaluations have been defined as the "...comparative analysis of alternative courses of action in terms of both their costs and

consequences."[4] This definition suggests that economic evaluations are characterized by two features. First, they are *comparative*, requiring a choice between two
proposed alternatives. Second, this comparison between the two proposed alternatives is based on the analysis of the *costs* and *consequences* (or outcomes) of each
alternative. Comparing approach A against approach B is what makes economic
evaluations *incremental*, in that it is the relative difference in costs and consequences
between the two alternatives that is used to drive decision making.

A common type of economic evaluation used in the health care literature is the
cost-effectiveness analysis, which examines the relative costs of different interventions designed to affect a health outcome. A cost-effectiveness analysis expresses its
results in the form of a ratio,

$$\text{Cost-effectiveness ratio} = \frac{\text{Cost}_{\text{Intervention A}} - \text{Cost}_{\text{Intervention B}}}{\text{Outcome}_{\text{Intervention A}} - \text{Outcome}_{\text{Intervention B}}},$$

where the denominator reflects the gain in a health outcome resulting from
Intervention A measured in, say, years of life gained, or reductions in the value of an
abnormally high laboratory test result. The numerator reflects the increased costs
required to procure that gain.[5]

The task for decision makers is easiest if Intervention A is cheaper and produces
better outcomes than Intervention B; in this case Intervention A is the obvious choice
from a cost-effectiveness perspective. If Intervention A is costlier than Intervention
B but produces better outcomes, then administrators have to decide whether those
increased outcomes are worth the added cost. Or, given that Intervention B produces worse outcomes than the more expensive Intervention A, administrators will
have to decide if they and their patients can afford to live with the poorer outcomes
given the lowered costs of Intervention B. It is perhaps obvious that these are not
purely economic decisions, and policymakers have to consider other elements that
go into the making of a decision regarding adopting a given strategy.

A related type of economic evaluation is the *cost–utility analysis*, where the goal
is to measure costs associated with changes in client-level or patient-level health-related quality of life (which incorporates preferences with regard to a health outcome
instead of using the health outcome per se). These preferences are operationalized
and expressed in changes in quality-adjusted life years (QALYs), which forms the
denominator in these types of studies.[6] Another type of economic evaluation,
cost–benefit analysis, examines only those outcomes that can be quantified in dollar
terms. Unlike cost-effectiveness analyses and cost–utility analyses, which allow the
determination of cost-per-unit-outcome, cost–benefit analyses place dollar values
on the outcome and compare whether or not the monetary benefits of an intervention are greater than its costs.[7]

Not all analyses consider costs as well as consequences. Studies frequently deal
with either comparisons or costs or consequences, but not all of these. Studies
may compare alternatives but only consider either cost or consequences. Other
studies examine *cost-offsets*, for example, examining if costs of treating depression
can be partially recouped by reductions in utilization of general medical services

by patients suffering from depression.[8] These types of studies are not considered in this chapter; we confine our discussion to economic evaluations that compare both costs and consequences between two or more competing approaches. Further details on how to perform economic evaluations in health care are available elsewhere.[5, 9–11]

Examples from the Literature

In the field of health care, much of the focus of economic evaluations has been on analyzing *interventions*, a term that we use to encompass activities that are preventative as well as curative in purpose. For example, cost-effectiveness studies have been performed on the use of vaccines to prevent cervical cancer caused by the human papilloma virus (HPV),[12] on screening for maternal depression following childbirth,[13] and on the use of exercise-based treatments in various diseases,[14] among several others. These analyses are designed to provide guidance to health care administrators and payers—to continue the above examples—on whether or not to deploy an immunization program using the HPV vaccine, whether or not to screen for maternal depression following childbirth, or whether or not to add an exercise treatment to extant treatment for individuals suffering from various diseases. In other words, they are all designed to provide an answer to the question, "What intervention makes the most economic sense to deploy?"

■ ECONOMIC EVALUATIONS IN DISSEMINATION AND IMPLEMENTATION RESEARCH

Dissemination and implementation research, however, requires the answer to a slightly different question—"What are the costs of a particular dissemination approach?" or "Does deploying a formal implementation strategy really make the most economic sense?" D&I researchers who develop implementation strategies and organizations considering using an implementation strategy to deploy a desired intervention both want to know whether the money used to deploy that implementation strategy represents the best use of organizational dollars. Is it really necessary to spend the money on a lengthy process to train, evaluate, and supervise clinicians in delivering an intervention? Or will a weekend seminar suffice? Is the added cost of deploying that implementation strategy really that much better than the seminar when it comes to, say, how well clinicians learn to use that intervention (an intermediate outcome), or how well their clients get (the final outcome)?

The answer to this question requires an adaptation to D&I research of the economic evaluation approach described in the previous section. In other words, the purpose of conducting a cost-effectiveness analysis of an implementation strategy, for example, is to quantify the following ratio:

$$\text{Implementation cost-effectiveness ratio} = \frac{\text{Cost}_{\text{Implementation Strategy}} - \text{Cost}_{\text{"Usual" implementation}}}{\text{Outcome}_{\text{Implementation Strategy}} - \text{Outcome}_{\text{"Usual" implementation}}}.$$

Here, "usual" implementation refers to the way an organization routinely supports skill development in its clinicians, whether this involves undergoing a training program, having them read a book and discuss as a group, requiring peer supervision and consultation, or attending the aforementioned weekend seminar. "Implementation Strategy" refers to one of many formal approaches to implement interventions in clinical settings (discussed below). The denominator quantifies the gains in an intermediate or final, clinical outcome; the numerator compares the costs required to achieve those gains; hence, in this equation, a candidate implementation strategy is being compared to usual clinical practice on relative measures of costs and ability to produce outcomes. As in the intervention example in the prior section, the choice for administrators depends on their valuation of the relative costs and outcomes of one implementation strategy over another.

There are several named or "branded" implementation strategies, including leadership facilitation; community development teams[15]; the Breakthrough Series Collaborative[16]; the Translating Initiatives for Depression into Effective Solutions (TIDES) model[17]; the Network for the Improvement of Addiction Treatment model[18]; Cascading Diffusion; Research Practice Partnership; Quality Enhancement Research Initiative (QUERI)[19]; the Availability, Responsiveness, Continuity (or ARC) model[20]; Replicating Effective Programs[21]; the IDEAL model[22]; and several others.[23] The (usually) highly structured nature of these strategies allows them to be subject to an economic evaluation. In contrast, models of diffusion[24] present greater challenges to economic evaluators because each of their elements needs to be operationalized before costs can be attached to them. The overall goal of economic evaluations of D&I approaches is to quantify their incremental costs associated with producing change in intermediate or final outcomes.

Perspective

What costs to capture usually depends on whose perspective is adopted. The cost of a single day of hospital care, for example, is either the amount of money paid to the hospital by the health plan (health plan perspective); the total expenditure undertaken by the hospital on that patient that day, including labor costs, medicines, and overhead (organizational perspective); out-of-pocket payments made to the hospital (patient perspective); or *all* costs associated with the hospital stay, irrespective of who incurs them, including the opportunity costs of all resources donated to the hospital (societal perspective).[10] Economic evaluations of interventions usually take a variety of perspectives, including those of the social planner (societal perspective) as well of the entity making the decision whether or not to adopt the intervention being evaluated (i.e., the payer). The latter perspective is important because the payer is making the decision of whether or not to adopt the intervention; the reason the societal perspective is also important is because the payer may vary by intervention and disease, so results using the societal perspective provide a common metric for comparing all treatments across all disorders across all patient populations.

Implementation studies seem largely to adopt the organizational (or program) perspective, which is likely appropriate given that organizations bear the costs of implementing interventions. Currently, third-party payers do not as yet explicitly resource the costs of implementation in their rate-setting decisions, basing reimbursement either on the intervention or, additionally, on the type of provider delivering the intervention. Given current approaches to the financing of services, such an organizational perspective is probably appropriate for economic evaluations of implementation. Dissemination studies, by corollary, should likely take the perspective of the organization disseminating the information—a not-for-profit entity, a professional society, or some other knowledge purveyor.

Cost Estimations

In this chapter, costs are classified into direct labor, indirect labor, and nonlabor costs.[25] *Direct labor costs* are the costs associated with client contact, for example, the cost of delivering an intervention by a clinician, and are measured by the time cost for the clinician to deliver that intervention. *Indirect labor costs* are also associated with client contact but occur outside of an examination or intervention room, for example, the time cost of scoring a rating instrument. *Nonlabor costs* are overhead and include costs associated with clients (e.g., the actual cost to obtain that rating instrument), as well as costs that cannot be assigned to a particular client (e.g., the cost of utilities, administrative support, and building space that are necessary to deliver interventions). The costs of treatment (i.e., service costs), therefore, are the sum of direct labor costs, indirect labor costs, and nonlabor costs associated with delivering that intervention. The costs of disseminating and implementing that intervention are the sum of indirect labor costs and nonlabor costs associated with all implementation activities. Examples of the indirect labor costs of implementation include the cost of clinician time spent in training and supervision, foregone clinical revenues due to the loss of these clinicians' billable hours, and the time cost of the supervisor assisting the clinicians in delivering the intervention. Examples of nonlabor costs include the costs of tuition and manuals, and the costs of travel, if necessary (please see Table 5–1 for an example of these costs as applied to implementation).

Outcomes

As in economic evaluations of interventions, economic evaluations of D&I are also concerned with the achievement of client-level health outcomes. However, clinical outcomes are but one type of outcome of interest to dissemination and implementation scientists.[26] Proctor and colleagues define implementation outcomes as "...the effects of deliberate and purposive actions to implement new treatments, practices, and services").[3] These outcomes not only encompass distal clinical outcomes, but also more proximal implementation and service outcomes (Figure 5–1). Hence, cost-effectiveness analyses can be conducted on the costs of achieving gains on a measure of clinician fidelity to an intervention (an implementation outcome), or on the costs of achieving gains on a measure of timeliness of care (a service outcome), or both.

Some implementation scientists may want to compare implementation strategies on gains in patient quality-adjusted life years or QALYs (cost–utility analysis). Scientists interested in capturing clinician preferences across competing

TABLE 5-1. *Implementation Costs for the Breakthrough Series Collaborative*

	Time in Hours (a)	Hourly Wage (Inclusive of Fringe Benefits) (b)	Cost (a)*(b) = (c)
Indirect Labor Costs			
Prework			
Clinician			
Online training course			
Familiarization with training methodology			
Readiness assessment			
Initial skills-based training			
Administrator			
Familiarization with training methodology			
Readiness assessment			
Manager/Supervisor			
Familiarization with training methodology			
Readiness assessment			
Learning Session			
Clinician			
Time cost of training			
Administration of instruments			
Scoring of instruments			
Administrator			
Time cost of participation			
Quality assurance			
Manager/Supervisor			
Time cost of participation			
Quality assurance			
Action Period			
Clinician			
Time cost of participation in case conference			
Nonlabor Costs			
Prework			
Tuition costs			
Cost of curriculum (manual and materials)			
Audiotapes, DVDs, and other recording materials			
Travel costs			
Airfare			
Hotel stay			
Meals and other expenses			
Learning Session			
Costs of supervision/case consultation			
Telephone charges			
Travel costs			
Airfare			
Hotel stay			
Meals and other expenses			
Action Period			
Costs of supervision/case consultation			
Telephone charges			
Costs of audiovisual materials (DVDs, etc.)			
Mailing charges			

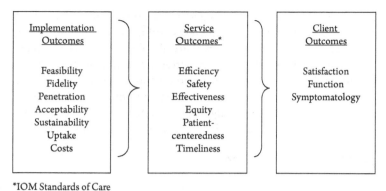

*IOM Standards of Care

Figure 5–1. Implementation outcomes (from Proctor and colleagues[3]).

implementation strategies can use an instrument like the Evidence-Based Practice Attitude Scale.[27] Such studies examining gains in clinician preference across competing implementation strategies may be useful to implementation scholars seeking an alternative way to examine implementation outcomes such as clinician acceptability of an intervention. Clinician-level outcomes can also be measured directly. In mental health, for example, clinician fidelity to an intervention is an important metric. (Fidelity is the extent to which an intervention as implemented resembles the original protocol of the investigators who developed the intervention.[28,29]) Using fidelity as a clinician-level outcome, implementation strategies can be compared with respect to the congruence between the deployed intervention and original protocol, and the costs that are necessary to achieve such congruence.

The field of operationalizing D&I outcomes is relatively new, and more development needs to occur before these can be used in economic evaluations. Conceptually, however, implementation outcomes perhaps are of more relevance to D&I scholars than are clinical outcomes, and future work that conducts economic evaluations using these consequences is necessary.

Time Horizon

A time horizon (or analytic horizon) is a period of time within which all costs and consequences can be expected to occur. Intervention researchers commonly use long time horizons because client outcomes following an intervention may take decades (survival after chemotherapy for a malignancy, for example). If D&I researchers are also examining clinical (patient) outcomes, then the issue of specifying an appropriate time horizon is critical. If, however, D&I researchers are only studying dissemination or implementation or service outcomes, and if these outcomes are coterminous with D&I costs, then the issue of specifying a long time horizon is less critical.

Discounting

Discounting is a way to downwardly adjust future costs and consequences in order to derive their present value. Costs are discounted because the value of receiving $1 today is more than the value of receiving $1 ten years from now. An individual can invest that $1 today, and reinvest any interest earnings and obtain in 10 years a sum of money greater than $1. Health outcomes are also discounted because most people would rather enjoy better health now than better health 10 years from now.[30] If D&I researchers focus on dissemination and implementation costs, and on implementation and service outcomes, all occurring within a short time horizon, then discounting is of lesser relevance. D&I researchers studying client outcomes will need to identify and incorporate appropriate cost and health outcome discounting approaches.

Examples from the Literature

The bulk of the literature on economic analyses of D&I seems to have focused on the implementation of clinical practice guidelines (also known as practice parameters or clinical protocols). Economic evaluations of selected preventive interventions recommended by the Task Force on Community Preventive Services have also been conducted.[31]

A systematic review of guideline implementation studies by Grimshaw and colleagues[32] revealed that 63 of 235 studies (approximately a third) provided information on costs of implementation. Strategies to implement these clinical guidelines varied and included dissemination of educational materials, educational meetings, audit and feedback, and the use of clinical reminders, deployed either singly or in combination. Over half of these 63 studies were cost-outcome studies that did not compare alternative implementation strategies, some were cost descriptions, and 11 were cost-effectiveness studies. Many guideline implementation studies since the date of publication of that review seem to focus on cost analyses,[33,34] although cost-effectiveness and cost–benefit studies offer support for patient-focused educational strategies in the implementation of practice guidelines in diabetic care,[35] and in asthma care.[36]

Researchers publishing in other disciplines have also conducted economic analyses of D&I within their own disciplines. In the field of infectious diseases, for example, researchers have conducted cost descriptions of competing strategies to ensure infection control,[37] have compared competing vaccination strategies with respect to costs and consequences,[38] and have reported cost analyses of alternative strategies to perform screening for a variety of communicable diseases.[39] Researchers have also performed cost descriptions of a Community-Directed Intervention strategy to implement treatments to reduce roundworm infestation,[40] and of a community health worker-based implementation strategy to deploy interventions to reduce malaria.[41] In the field of pharmaceutical services research, scholars have conducted cost analyses of a strategy to optimize use of a certain high-risk class of medications,[42] and a review reported on equivocal results of cost studies designed to implement strategies to reduce prescribing of acid-suppressive medications.[43] Reviews of studies examining implementation of clinical pathways (which are structured intervention protocols also called *care protocols* or *care pathways*) for a variety of illnesses have also reported modest, though highly heterogeneous and variable, reductions in hospital costs.[44]

While few of the above referenced studies are explicitly economic evaluations, several studies currently underway will provide greater information on the economics of implementation. Published protocols on the use of implementation strategies to reduce colorectal cancers among individuals with heightened familial risk of such cancer[45] and cost analysis of an implementation of Dutch national guidelines designed to reduce vaginal breech deliveries[46] are all examples of studies that can provide valuable information once they are completed.

Two principal challenges seem to characterize this burgeoning literature on the economics of implementation. First, there is disagreement in the literature regarding which activities should have costs attached to them when it comes to implementation. In a study of guideline implementation, for example, should the cost of developing the guideline be counted, as some authorities suggest?[47] It is not entirely clear that it should be. In mental health, for example, there is considerable information on the costs of treatment;[48-52] to include all of these costs within the costs of implementation would comingle an economic evaluation of treatment with an economic evaluation of its implementation. One study valued the time spent by teachers, parents, school administrators, and project staff associated with implementing a behavioral intervention for children at risk for conduct problems.[53] While time costs are a critical element of the costs of implementation, equating time costs with the costs of implementation can underestimate the true cost of implementing interventions when there are (expensive) manuals and other nonlabor costs associated with implementing the intervention. Another study of service costs included the costs of quality assurance—a category that included "clinical case review, clinical supervisions, team meetings, and case staffing"[25]—in addition to case management and the costs of treatment, but did not include added costs associated with implementation. Other studies that have examined cognitive behavioral therapy implementation have calculated the time taken to train the clinicians, as well as the costs of ongoing supervision, but not nonlabor costs associated with implementation,[54-56] while other studies have excluded costs of supervision from the costs of implementation.[57] Clearly, some unifying framework for cost estimations is necessary in the field of implementation research. It also seems necessary to distinguish between one-time (fixed) costs, such as the costs of initial training; regularly-scheduled but fixed costs, such as the costs of ongoing supervision; and variable costs that increase incrementally with, say, providing client services, such as the costs of rating instruments and their administration.

Second, many studies examine heterogeneous implementation outcomes. Some focus on clinical (patient) outcomes only,[40] a justifiable outcome given that the ultimate goal of implementation is to improve client or patient well-being. Others examine provider behavior,[43] while others study various other aspects of the implementation enterprise. In order to standardize the economic evaluation of implementation, some agreement on the appropriate outcomes for implementation is necessary.

■ CASE STUDY—COSTING THE BREAKTHROUGH SERIES COLLABORATIVE IMPLEMENTATION STRATEGY

With the above caveats, one suggested approach to assessing the costs of D&I within a short time horizon from an organizational perspective is described below. Table 5–1 displays a worksheet listing the various elements of a typical Breakthrough Series Collaborative (BSC) strategy, which has been primarily used to implement interventions, but which could be adapted to the use of diffusion researchers. Table 5–2 displays elements of a weekend seminar (the "usual" dissemination or implementation approach); costs can be attached to each of the elements listed in the tables. The difference in costs between the BSC and "usual" implementation forms the numerator of a cost-effectiveness analysis for the BSC implementation strategy. Tables 5–1 and 5–2 are largely based on the idea that one way to capture costs associated with D&I is to adapt methods of service costing [9,58] to a D&I approach. This approach assumes that the same intervention can have varying D&I costs depending on whether it is implemented using a weekend seminar or a multimonth implementation strategy. These added costs make one implementation strategy more expensive than another.

Costing a D&I strategy requires a close familiarity with the strategy. A full description of the BSC model is beyond the scope of this chapter, and the reader is referred to overviews of this strategy.[16] *Indirect labor costs* of the BSC model are generated by clinicians, administrators, and supervisors. During the *prework* phase, much of the time of clinicians, administrators, and supervisors is spent in familiarization with the BSC training model (the Institute of Healthcare Improvement requires the formation of three-member teams comprising of clinicians as well as administrative staff). This stage also requires an organizational assessment, which must be completed prior to participation in the model. All of these indirect labor costs can be quantified by using the same approach as used for service costs—they

TABLE 5-2. *Implementation Costs for a Weekend Seminar ("Usual" Implementation)*

	Time in Hours (a)	Hourly Wage (Inclusive of Fringe Benefits) (b)	Cost (a)*(b) = (c)
Indirect Labor Costs			
Prework			
Clinician			
Reading intervention materials			
At the Seminar			
Clinician			
Time cost of training			
Nonlabor Costs			
Prework			
Tuition costs			
Cost of curriculum (manual and materials)			
Audiotapes, DVDs, and other recording materials			
Travel costs			
Airfare			
Hotel stay			
Meals and other expenses			
At the Seminar			
Telephone charges			
Travel costs			
Airfare			
Hotel stay			
Meals and other expenses			

represent time costs of participating in these activities. If the time taken in these tasks by clinicians and other personnel is quantified, this time can be multiplied by wage and fringe information, resulting in the cost of participation.

These three sets of personnel also incur opportunity costs during the *learning session* phase, where teams gather in person to discuss the results of their implementation, establish new goals for treatment, and strategize about ways to overcome observed challenges. These learning sessions lead to *action periods*, where clinicians actually deploy the strategies elicited during the learning session. Implementation costs are incurred by clinicians, supervisors, and administrators during these action periods. The BSC model is cyclical, iterative, and cumulative, with learning sessions leading to action periods, which in turn lead to new learning sessions. Hence, organizations have to be prepared to invest in several iterations of this process in order to successfully achieve implementation.

The BSC model is also associated with *nonlabor costs*. In the *prework* phase, these include the costs of procuring training in the intervention using the BSC model (tuition, and other materials) as well as travel expenses for (minimally) one clinician, an administrator, and a supervisor. Costs of tuition involves two types of costs—the costs of learning about the intervention (which are charged by its developers) and the costs of learning how to implement it using the particular implementation strategy (e.g., the costs of training in the BSC methodology, which are charged by the Institute of Healthcare Improvement). Although organizations bear the costs of learning about the intervention (which is a part of treatment cost), we only suggest counting the costs of implementation here. It may be difficult to disaggregate costs of an implementation strategy from the costs of the treatment that will be deployed using it. In other words, there may be no way to teach the "how" of an intervention without also teaching the "what" of an intervention. (It is, however, possible to do the reverse—teach the "what" of an intervention without teaching the "how" of it.) If researchers find themselves in this quandary, a sensitivity analysis that clearly distinguishes the costs of treatment from the costs of its implementation should be shown.

Implementation costs of the BSC approach during the learning sessions and action periods are largely time costs associated with case consultation, and the material costs associated with developing audiovisual materials of sessions undertaken by trainee psychotherapists (DVDs or videotapes), and then mailing them to trainers. To the extent that some learning sessions occur in person rather than over the telephone, travel costs need to be factored into the indirect nonlabor costs. The estimation of these costs is done in the same manner as for nonlabor costs for the service (treatment). All of these costs unfold over time (since the BSC approach may spill over into a succeeding fiscal year), and with stage of the implementation process (as different elements of the implementation process manifest and recede with implementation). Organizations undertaking their cost estimations will need to be cognizant of these time horizons and use appropriate discounting for complicated, multiyear implementation endeavors.

These cost domains can be easily generalized to other implementation strategies so long as all these strategies require time for learning, ongoing supervision, case consultation, curricula and other materials, and travel. Some types of generic training will require the resourcing of idiosyncratic costs, and provider organizations will need to identify and quantify these idiosyncratic costs in order to accurately capture their overall cost of implementing a treatment.

The denominator of an economic evaluation depends on whether investigators are interested in clinical outcomes, or in a particular intermediate outcome. In the latter instance, to some extent, the denominator also depends on the intervention that is being implemented. Researchers wishing to study client improvement across several mental health interventions can use a generic instrument such as the Child Behavior Check List[59,60] and examine improvements in this measure across the BSC and "usual" implementation conditions. Researchers wishing to study a particular implementation outcome such as fidelity will need to use a fidelity scale developed for a specific intervention—if the intervention is trauma-focused cognitive-behavioral therapy,[61,62] then investigators will need to use the fidelity scale developed for this intervention.[63] The difference in fidelity measures between clinicians participating in the BSC implementation strategy and those participating in the weekend seminar, then, forms the denominator in the cost-effectiveness intervention.

■ IMPROVING THE STATE OF THE ART IN THE ECONOMICS OF DISSEMINATION AND IMPLEMENTATION

The relative paucity of studies reporting on economic evaluations of D&I suggests that researchers are currently focused on developing and refining implementation strategies rather than on evaluating them from an economic perspective. This section outlines some overarching themes emerging from this review.

First, the bearers of the costs of D&I efforts are likely to emerge as its key stakeholders. Provider organizations currently bear much of the costs of implementation, and information purveyors and health communicators bear much of the costs of dissemination. These organizations will need to be cognizant of the added costs imposed as a result of the use of D&I strategies, and clearly distinguish them from intervention costs. As discussed earlier, much of the variations in D&I costs likely result from the complexity of the D&I strategy, and approaches that require a large number of stakeholders and change agents interacting with various individuals within an organization over prolonged periods of time, or approaches that use highly expensive communicative media like television, likely will be very expensive with respect to D&I costs. In contrast, leaner approaches involving fewer personnel who do much of their work using videoconferencing, telephone consultations, and remote viewing of trainee's sessions will incur fewer implementation costs. Provider organizations that do not possess many resources will need to carefully consider their financial ability to implement treatments using expensive D&I approaches, and D&I scholars developing new approaches should provide data on the long-term advantages of their approaches to these various stakeholders.

Second, because D&I approaches have associated costs, this cost information can be used to develop a future research agenda on the comparative cost-effectiveness of D&I strategies. Currently, there seems to be little literature directly comparing one implementation strategy against another on their relative ability to achieve implementation, service, or clinical outcomes. Incorporating costs into the mix will permit researchers to ask not only if a particular implementation strategy works, but also whether its outcomes are worth the money. Those strategies that produce greatest change in outcomes at lowest cost are likely to be the ones that are most practicable in everyday use. Much like for service costs, the costs of D&I are a function of price (the expense of various elements that go into a given approach) and quantity (how long it takes to disseminate or implement a treatment using this strategy, and with what intensity), aggregated over all resources required for the D&I effort. Thus, the most cost-efficient implementation strategies are likely to be the ones that reduce the complexity of the D&I process, the various resources necessary for the strategy, and the total duration of D&I while still producing desirable outcomes.[26]

Third, the rate-limiting step in the economics of D&I research is the nascent operationalization of implementation and service outcomes, and the need for greater development of dissemination processes and outcomes. D&I researchers interested in examining client outcomes can simply adopt the outcomes of cost-effectiveness studies on interventions. Other implementation outcomes such as fidelity, and some service outcomes such as timeliness, can be adequately operationalized given the current state of the science. However, researchers interested in other D&I outcomes will need to wait until many of these are better operationalized and measured.

Delivering a treatment, especially one that comes with expensive D&I costs, is very expensive; high-fidelity implementation requires considerable investment of organizational resources. Because multiprovider organizations are more likely to possess the kinds of resources and the economies of scale required to undertake successful implementation, it is likely that much of the traction in the economics of implementation will occur within large organizations. It also seems apparent that an organization's returns to investment in a treatment are greatest when most of the organization's clients are those who require that particular treatment. To train all clinicians in all treatments is likely to be cost prohibitive. For this reason, the economics of implementation also suggest greater organization and specialization in the health care enterprise.

From a policy perspective, the principal challenge is how to pay for implementation.[64] In health care, there are efforts focused around twin approaches of *value-based purchasing*[65]—assisting health care purchasers to contract with plans that offer greater value rather than merely lower cost—and *pay-for-performance*[66]— which involves tying fiscal and nonfiscal rewards and punishments to a variety of performance outcomes, such as health outcomes, patient satisfaction, scores on quality scorecards, screening rates, prescribing practices, adherence to clinical guidelines, and investments in information strategy, among others. More recently, pay-for-performance approaches have also been proposed for population-level health outcomes such as health inequalities.[67] Scholars have proposed methods for determining the policy cost-effectiveness of implementation, which attempts to provide guidance to policymakers on the relative costs and outcomes of implementation strategies and is expressed as a function of the cost-effectiveness of treatment, and cost-effectiveness of the practice (organization).[68] But in many disciplines, such as in mental health, the data necessary to determine these cost-effectiveness ratios are not extant. Paying for implementation, then, is an alternative to paying for outcomes in such cases where outcomes are very difficult to pay for given problems in assessing risk.[69] If efficacious treatments are identified, then the task for policymakers is to help resource the delivery of these treatments by paying for their implementation.

■ SUMMARY

D&I imposes costs upon knowledge purveyors, provider organizations, public health organizations, and payers. However, whether these added costs will result in improved service delivery and, perhaps more importantly, client outcomes and improvements in population health remains an open question. If emerging studies reveal that defined implementation strategies are more cost effective than "usual" implementation, then policymakers and service providers will need to resource these added costs of implementation in order to assure the success and sustainability of high-quality health services over the long term.

SUGGESTED READINGS

Drummond MF, Sculpher MJ, Torrance GW, O'Brien BJ, Stoddart GL. *Methods for the economic evaluation of health care programmes.* 3rd ed. New York: Oxford University Press; 2005.

This is a standard textbook for economic evaluation in health care. It includes a helpful critical appraisal checklist that can be applied to an intervention study.

Gold MR, Siegel JE, Russell LB, Weinstein MC. *Cost-effectiveness in health and medicine.* New York: Oxford University Press; 1996.

This text is the result of the deliberations of the Panel on Cost-Effectiveness in Health and Medicine. It is a seminal text in providing a clear and consistent set of methods for performing cost-effectiveness analysis.

Kilo CM. A framework for collaborative improvement: lessons from the Institute for Healthcare Improvement's Breakthrough Series. *Quality management in health care.* Sep 1998;6(4):1–13.

This article was used to motivate the Breakthrough Series case. The Breakthrough Series Collaborative is a specific type of implementation strategy, originally developed as a quality improvement tool in manufacturing, that is now widely used in health care settings.

Fixsen DL, Naoom SF, Blase KA, Friedman RM, Wallace F. *Implementation Research: A Synthesis of the Literature.* Tampa, FL: University of South Florida, Louis de la Parte Florida Mental Health Institute, The National Implementation Research Network; 2005.

Proctor EK, Landsverk J, Aarons G, Chambers D, Glisson C, Mittman B. Implementation research in mental health services: an emerging science with conceptual, methodological, and training challenges. *Administration and Policy in Mental Health.* 2009;36(1):24–34.

These are two good overviews of the field of implementation research. The review by Fixsen and colleagues is a comprehensive summary of the literature on implementation science that illustrates several conceptualizations relevant to the field, emphasizes programmatic aspects of the implementation enterprise, and provides recommendations for various stakeholders involved with implementation. The article by Proctor and colleagues conceptualizes implementation from a variety of perspectives and advances the operationalization of implementation outcomes.

Weinstein MC, Siegel JE, Gold MR, Kamlet MS, Russell LB, for the Panel on Cost-Effectiveness in Health and Medicine. Recommendations of the panel on cost-effectiveness in health and medicine. *JAMA*. 1996;276:1253–1258.

A consensus statement that outlines appropriate methodology for the use of cost-effectiveness analyses in health.

SELECTED WEBSITES AND TOOLS

Task Force on Community Preventive Services. Economic Reviews. http://www.the-communityguide.org/about/economics.html#where. The Community Guide provides a repository of the 200+ systematic reviews conducted by the Task Force, an independent, interdisciplinary group with staff support by the Centers for Disease Control and Prevention. This link is for their economic reviews section, which reviews the applications of cost-effectiveness analyses to interventions analyzed by the Community Guide.

■ ACKNOWLEDGMENTS

The assistance of Susan Ettner, PhD, in the conceptualization and writing of this chapter is gratefully acknowledged.

■ REFERENCES

1. Institute of Medicine (U.S.). Committee on Crossing the Quality Chasm: Adaptation to Mental Health and Addictive Disorders. *Improving the quality of health care for mental and substance-use conditions*. Washington, DC: National Academies Press; 2006.
2. Balas EA, Boren SA. Managing clinical knowledge for health care improvement. In: Bemmel J, Cray AT, eds. *Yearbook of medical informatics 2000: Patient-centered systems*. Stuttgart, Germany: Schattauer; 2000:65–70.
3. Proctor E, Silmere H, Raghavan R, et al. Outcomes for implementation research: conceptual distinctions, measurement challenges, and research agenda. *Administration and Policy in Mental Health and Mental Health Services Research*. 2011;38(2):65–76.
4. Drummond MF, Sculpher MJ, Torrance GW, O'Brien BJ, Stoddart GL. *Methods for the economic evaluation of health care programmes*. 3rd ed. Oxford; New York: Oxford University Press; 2005.
5. Gold MR, Siegel JE, Russell LB, Weinstein MC. *Cost-effectiveness in health and medicine*. New York: Oxford University Press; 1996.
6. Dasbach EJ, Teutsch SM. Cost-utility analysis. In: Haddix AC, Teutsch SM, Shaffer PA, Dunet DO, eds. *Prevention effectiveness: A guide to decision analysis and economic evaluation*. New York: Oxford University Press; 1996:130–142.
7. Clemmer B, Haddix AC. Cost-benefit analysis. In: Haddix AC, Teutsch SM, Shaffer PA, Dunet DO, eds. *Prevention effectiveness: A guide to decision analysis and economic evaluation*. New York: Oxford University Press; 1996:85–102.
8. Simon GE, Katzelnick DJ. Depression, use of medical services and cost-offset effects. *Journal of Psychosomatic Research*. 1997;42(4):333–344.
9. Drummond MF, McGuire A. *Economic evaluation in health care: Merging theory with practice*. New York: Oxford University Press; 2001.
10. Petitti DB. *Meta-analysis, decision analysis, and cost-effectiveness analysis: Methods for quantitative synthesis in medicine*. 2nd ed. New York: Oxford University Press; 2000.

11. Warner KE, Luce BR. *Cost-benefit and cost-effectiveness analysis in health care: Principles, practice, and potential.* Ann Arbor, MI: Health Administration Press; 1982.

12. Armstrong EP. Prophylaxis of cervical cancer and related cervical disease: a review of the cost-effectiveness of vaccination against oncogenic HPV types. *Journal of Managed Care Pharmacy.* 2010;16(3):217–230.

13. Paulden M, Palmer S, Hewitt C, Gilbody S. Screening for postnatal depression in primary care: cost effectiveness analysis. *British Medical Journal.* 2009;339:b5203.

14. Roine E, Roine RP, Rasanen P, Vuori I, Sintonen H, Saarto T. Cost-effectiveness of interventions based on physical exercise in the treatment of various diseases: a systematic literature review. *International Journal of Technology Assessment in Health Care.* 2009;25(4):427–454.

15. Evans SW, Green AL, Serpell ZN. Community participation in the treatment development process using community development teams. *Journal of Clinical Child and Adolescent Psychology.* Dec 2005;34(4):765–771.

16. Kilo CM. A framework for collaborative improvement: lessons from the Institute for Healthcare Improvement's Breakthrough Series. *Quality Management in Health Care.* Sep 1998;6(4):1–13.

17. Luck J, Hagigi F, Parker L, Yano E, Rubenstein L, Kirchner J. A social marketing approach to implementing evidence-based practice in VHA QUERI: the TIDES depression collaborative care model. *Implementation Science.* 2009;4(1):64.

18. McCarty D, Gustafson DH, Wisdom JP, et al. The Network for the Improvement of Addiction Treatment (NIATx): enhancing access and retention. *Drug and Alcohol Dependence.* 2007;88(2–3):138–145.

19. Rubenstein LV, Mittman BS, Yano EM, Mulrow CD. From understanding health care provider behavior to improving health care: the QUERI framework for quality improvement. *Medical Care.* Jun 2000;38(6,Suppl1):I129-I141.

20. Glisson C, Schoenwald SK. The ARC organizational and community intervention strategy for implementing evidence-based children's mental health treatments. *Mental Health Services Research.* Dec 2005;7(4):243–259.

21. Kilbourne AM, Neumann MS, Pincus HA, Bauer MS, Stall R. Implementing evidence-based interventions in health care: application of the replicating effective programs framework. *Implementation Science.* 2007;2:42.

22. Solberg LI, Reger LA, Pearson TL, et al. Using continuous quality improvement to improve diabetes care in populations: the IDEAL model. Improving care for Diabetics through Empowerment Active collaboration and Leadership. *The Joint Commission Journal on Quality Improvement.* Nov 1997;23(11):581–592.

23. McLaughlin CP, Kaluzny AD. *Continuous quality improvement in health care: Theory, implementations, and applications.* 3rd ed. Sudbury, MA: Jones and Bartlett; 2006.

24. Lawrence RS. Diffusion of the U.S. Preventive Services Task Force recommendations into practice. *Journal of General Internal Medicine.* 1990;5:S99–103.

25. Zarkin GA, Dunlap LJ, Homsi G. The substance abuse services cost analysis program (SASCAP): a new method for estimating drug treatment services costs. *Evaluation and Program Planning.* 2004;27(1):35–43.

26. Proctor EK, Landsverk J, Aarons G, Chambers D, Glisson C, Mittman B. Implementation research in mental health services: an emerging science with conceptual, methodological, and training challenges. *Administration and Policy in Mental Health.* 2009;36(1):24–34.

27. Aarons GA. Mental health provider attitudes toward adoption of evidence-based practice: The Evidence-Based Practice Attitude Scale (EBPAS). *Mental Health Services Research.* 2004;6(2):61–74.
28. Rabin BA, Brownson RC, Haire-Joshu D, Kreuter MW, Weaver NL. A glossary for dissemination and implementation research in health. *Journal of Public Health Management and Practice.* Mar–Apr 2008;14(2):117–123.
29. Fixsen DL, Naoom SF, Blase KA, Friedman RM, Wallace F. *Implementation Research: A Synthesis of the Literature.* Tampa, FL: University of South Florida, Louis de la Parte Florida Mental Health Institute, The National Implementation Research Network; 2005.
30. Brouwer WB, Niessen LW, Postma MJ, Rutten FF. Need for differential discounting of costs and health effects in cost effectiveness analyses. *British Medical Journal.* 2005;331:446–448.
31. Task Force on Community Preventive Services. Economic Reviews. http://www.thecommunityguide.org/about/economics.html#where. Accessed 1/10/11.
32. Grimshaw JM, Thomas RE, MacLennan G, et al. Effectiveness and efficiency of guideline dissemination and implementation strategies. *Health Technology Assessment.* Feb 2004;8(6):iii–iv, 1–72.
33. Koskinen H, Rautakorpi UM, Sintonen H, et al. Cost-effectiveness of implementing national guidelines in the treatment of acute otitis media in children. *International Journal of Technology Assessment in Health Care.* Fall 2006;22(4):454–459.
34. Hoeijenbos M, Bekkering T, Lamers L, Hendriks E, van Tulder M, Koopmanschap M. Cost-effectiveness of an active implementation strategy for the Dutch physiotherapy guideline for low back pain. *Health Policy.* 2005;75(1):85–98.
35. Dijkstra RF, Niessen LW, Braspenning JCC, Adang E, Grol RTPM. Patient-centred and professional-directed implementation strategies for diabetes guidelines: a cluster-randomized trial-based cost-effectiveness analysis. *Diabetic Medicine.* 2006;23(2):164–170.
36. Tschopp JM, Frey JG, Janssens JP, et al. Asthma outpatient education by multiple implementation strategy. Outcome of a programme using a personal notebook. *Respiratory Medicine.* 2005;99(3):355–362.
37. Mubayi A, Zaleta CK, Martcheva M, Castillo-Chavez C. A cost-based comparison of quarantine strategies for new emerging diseases. *Mathematical Biosciences and Engineering.* Jul 2010;7(3):687–717.
38. Coudeville L, Van Rie A, Getsios D, Caro JJ, Crepey P, Nguyen VH. Adult vaccination strategies for the control of pertussis in the United States: an economic evaluation including the dynamic population effects. *PloS One.* 2009;4(7):e6284.
39. Kania D, Sangare L, Sakande J, et al. A new strategy to improve the cost-effectiveness of human immunodeficiency virus, hepatitis B virus, hepatitis C virus, and syphilis testing of blood donations in sub-Saharan Africa: a pilot study in Burkina Faso. *Transfusion.* Oct 2009;49(10):2237–2240.
40. CDI Study Group. Community-directed interventions for priority health problems in Africa: results of a multicountry study. *Bulletin of the World Health Organization.* Jul 1 2010;88(7):509–518.
41. Onwujekwe O, Uzochukwu B, Ojukwu J, Dike N, Shu E. Feasibility of a community health worker strategy for providing near and appropriate treatment of malaria in southeast Nigeria: an analysis of activities, costs and outcomes. *Acta Tropica.* 2007;101(2):95–105.

42. Burns TL, Ferry BA, Malesker MA, Morrow LE, Bruckner AL, Lee DL. Improvement in appropriate utilization of recombinant human erythropoietin pre- and post-implementation of a required order form. *The Annals of Pharmacotherapy.* May 2010;44(5):832–837.

43. Smeets H, Hoes A, de Wit N. Effectiveness and costs of implementation strategies to reduce acid suppressive drug prescriptions: a systematic review. *BMC Health Services Research.* 2007;7(1):177.

44. Rotter T, Kugler J, Koch R, et al. A systematic review and meta-analysis of the effects of clinical pathways on length of stay, hospital costs and patient outcomes. *BMC Health Services Research.* 2008;8(1):265.

45. Dekker N, Hermens R, Elwyn G, et al. Improving calculation, interpretation and communication of familial colorectal cancer risk: protocol for a randomized controlled trial. *Implementation Science.* 5(1):6.

46. Vlemmix F, Rosman A, Fleuren M, et al. Implementation of the external cephalic version in breech delivery. Dutch national implementation study of external cephalic version. *BMC Pregnancy and Childbirth.* 2010;10(1):20.

47. McIntosh E. Economic evaluation of guideline implementation studies. In: Makela M, Thorsen T, eds. *Changing professional practice. Theory and practice of clinical guidelines implementation.* Copenhagen: Danish Institute for Health Services Research and Development; 1999:77–98.

48. Anderson DW, Bowland BJ, Cartwright WS, Bassin G. Service-level costing of drug abuse treatment. *Journal of Substance Abuse Treatment.* 1998;15(3):201–211.

49. Foster EM, Connor T. Public costs of better mental health services for children and adolescents. *Psychiatric Services.* Jan 2005;56(1):50–55.

50. Nabors LA, Leff SS, Mettrick JE. Assessing the costs of school-based mental health services. *Journal of School Health.* May 2001;71(5):199–200.

51. Cuffel BJ, Jeste DV, Halpain M, Pratt C, Tarke H, Patterson TL. Treatment costs and use of community mental health services for schizophrenia by age cohorts. *American Journal of Psychiatry.* Jul 1996;153(7):870–876.

52. Foster EM, Summerfelt WT, Saunders RC. The costs of mental health services under the Fort Bragg Demonstration. *Journal of Mental Health Administration.* Winter 1996;23(1):92–106.

53. Foster E, Johnson-Shelton D, Taylor T. Measuring time costs in interventions designed to reduce behavior problems among children and youth. *American Journal of Community Psychology.* Sep 2007;40(1/2):64–81.

54. McCrone P, Knapp M, Kennedy T, et al. Cost-effectiveness of cognitive behaviour therapy in addition to mebeverine for irritable bowel syndrome. *European Journal of Gastroenterology & Hepatology.* 2008;20(4):255–263.

55. Scheeres K, Wensing M, Bleijenberg G, Severens JL. Implementing cognitive behavior therapy for chronic fatigue syndrome in mental health care: a costs and outcomes analysis. *BMC Health Services Research.* 2008;8:175.

56. Foster EM, Olchowski AE, Webster-Stratton CH. Is stacking intervention components cost-effective? An analysis of the Incredible Years program. *Journal of the American Academy of Child and Adolescent Psychiatry.* 2007;46(11):1414–1424.

57. Byford S, Barrett B, Roberts C, et al. Cost-effectiveness of selective serotonin reuptake inhibitors and routine specialist care with and without cognitive behavioural therapy in adolescents with major depression. *The British Journal of Psychiatry.* Dec 1, 2007;191(6):521–527.

58. Drummond MF. *Methods for the economic evaluation of health care programmes.* 2nd ed. Oxford; New York: Oxford University Press; 1997.
59. Achenbach TM. *Manual for the Child Behavior Checklist/4–18 and 1991 Profile.* Burlington, VT: University of Vermont Department of Psychiatry; 1991.
60. Achenbach TM. *Manual for the Child Behavior Checklist/2–3 and 1992 Profile.* Burlington, VT: Department of Psychiatry; 1992.
61. Cohen JA, Mannarino AP, Deblinger E. *Treating trauma and traumatic grief in children and adolescents.* New York: Guilford Press; 2006.
62. Cohen JA, Mannarino AP, Deblinger E. *Child and parent trauma-focused cognitive behavioral therapy treatment manual.* Philadelphia: Drexel University College of Medicine; 2006.
63. Child Sexual Abuse Task Force and Research & Practice Core National Child Traumatic Stress Network. How to Implement Trauma-Focused Cognitive Behavioral Therapy. http://www.nctsnet.org/nctsn_assets/pdfs/TF-CBT_Implementation_Manual.pdf. Accessed 1/10/11.
64. Proctor EK, Knudsen KJ, Fedoravicius N, Hovmand P, Rosen A, Perron B. Implementation of evidence-based practice in community behavioral health: agency director perspectives. *Administration and Policy in Mental Health.* 2007;34(5): 479–488.
65. Deas TM, Jr. Health care value-based purchasing. *Gastrointestinal endoscopy clinics of North America.* Oct 2006;16(4):643–656.
66. Rosenthal MB, Dudley RA. Pay-for-performance: will the latest payment trend improve care? *JAMA.* Feb 21 2007;297(7):740–744.
67. Asada Y. A summary measure of health inequalities for a pay-for-population health performance system. *Preventing Chronic Disease.* http://www.cdc.gov/pcd/issues/2010/jul/09_0250.htm. Accessed 1/11/11.
68. Mason J, Freemantle N, Nazareth I, Eccles M, Haines A, Drummond M. When is it cost-effective to change the behavior of health professionals? *JAMA.* Dec 19, 2001;286(23):2988–2992.
69. Raghavan R. Using risk adjustment approaches in child welfare performance measurement: applications and insights from health and mental health settings. *Children and Youth Services Review.* Jan 2010;32(1):103–112.

6

Designing for the Dissemination of Environmental and Policy Initiatives and Programs for High-Risk Groups

■ NEVILLE OWEN, ANA GOODE,
BRIANNA FJELDSOE,
TAKEMI SUGIYAMA, AND
ELIZABETH EAKIN

■ INTRODUCTION

Epidemiologic, behavioral, and public health research has generated a plethora of findings with the potential to inform prevention in practice. There have been significant research advances: on understanding relationships of behavior with health outcomes; on developing measurement methods for use in public health research; on identifying the individual, social and environmental determinants of health behaviors; and, on a wide range of behavior change interventions that have been developed and tested systematically. However, the actual translation of this broad array of knowledge into effective policies and programs has been limited.[1]

It is now well accepted that major gaps exist between the body of research knowledge relevant to health promotion and disease prevention, and its numerous potential applications in policy and in practice. Research findings may be promulgated, but their uptake will not happen automatically. Designing explicitly for dissemination is required.

These translation gaps have been characterized severally. The metaphor of the "leaky pipeline"[2] is compelling: much that is important in maintaining the rigor and integrity of prevention efforts can leak away, as that knowledge moves from the research evidence base through the mechanisms of translation into the broadness of policy and the constraints of practical application. The "push-pull" metaphor[3] also characterizes the relevant challenges nicely: efforts at dissemination by researchers (the "push" element) can be limited in their momentum, or the initial momentum can rapidly decay; furthermore, the motivations and capacities of practitioners and policymakers (the "pull" element) to translate, adopt, and implement can be held back by the multiple limitations of systems for funding, administration, staffing, and implementation of programs. These models and related frameworks point to the need for an increased emphasis on designing for dissemination.[4,5] In practice, such models can guide initiatives through the relevant networks and partnerships required for successful dissemination.[6]

Using examples from the field of physical activity and health, this chapter illustrates: designing for the dissemination of population-based environmental and policy approaches; and, designing for the dissemination of broad-reach programs for groups with significant health disparities—adults living with chronic disease. These two approaches are complementary, reflecting Geoffrey Rose's[7,8] perspective on the *strategy of preventive medicine*: that overall health is improved by both population-wide and high-risk approaches. While the examples in this chapter focus mainly on physical activity, the principles may be applied to other health behaviors, and to other topics in public health.

■ POPULATION-BASED ENVIRONMENTAL AND POLICY APPROACHES TO IMPROVING HEALTH

Environmental and policy initiatives have the potential to be wide reaching, available broadly across the social spectrum, and sustainable. The broad strategic aim is to make healthy choices more-realistic choices within the context of people's everyday lives. As has been previously documented,[9] there have been remarkable successes in the dissemination of environmental and policy approaches, particularly in the field of tobacco control in countries like the United States and Australia, in reducing road traffic accidents, and in changing public attitudes and behaviors in relation to alcohol use. However, systematic approaches to dissemination of environmental and policy initiatives, through translating research knowledge and applying it in practical ways, present many challenges.

In this chapter the focus is on physical activity, which illustrates how designing for dissemination may be approached. As was the case during the early stages of tobacco control efforts (e.g., stop-smoking groups, self-help books), initiatives to increase participation in physical activity have focused on factors operating at the individual level (motivation, goal setting, confidence, incentives for change, social support, etc.). Such approaches have an important role to play in health improvement, and particularly so for high-risk groups. However, promoting individual responsibility for behavioral change through educational/motivational strategies alone is unlikely to influence population-wide physical activity levels.[10,11]

For physical activity, the role of environmental attributes is receiving increasing attention because the probability of individuals' decisions on whether or not to engage in physical activity can depend crucially on contextual opportunities and constraints. Widespread and sustainable behavioral changes are likely to be achieved by making participation in physical activity a more probable choice, through dissemination of the relevant environmental and policy initiatives.

Disseminating environmental and policy initiatives to change health behaviors requires both contextual and behavioral specificity,[12,13,14] focusing on the different "behavior settings" for dissemination.[14] For example, exercise for fitness or health purposes, carried out in health club facilities or gymnasia, may be determined by distinct individual, social, and environmental factors that dissemination will need to address. Similarly, the multiple levels of determinants for light-intensity workplace physical activity will operate in distinct ways, as will recreational- or health-related walking in natural environment settings, or physically active transport through walking and avoiding automobile use for short trips and errands.

In this perspective, physical activity may be conceived of as taking place in four particular domains: transportation, recreation, the workplace, and the home. These domains need to be addressed distinctly because they provide quite different dissemination settings, the relevant behaviors are likely to be influenced by different factors, and the engagement of different partners will be required for successful dissemination initiatives. The domain of active transport is discussed as a discrete "behavior setting" to illustrate issues related to designing for dissemination of environmental and policy initiatives to increase physical activity.

Dissemination of Environmental and Policy Initiatives to Increase Physical Activity

A key issue for public health is how to disseminate broadly, evidence-based initiatives that will increase the physical activity levels of populations, by decreasing dependency on automobiles and increasing the use of active transport modes (walking and biking). Active transport contributes to health because the alternatives to automobile use involve physically active options.[15] Furthermore, less automobile use will result in less sitting time, which is now known to have favorable effects on weight gain, metabolic health outcomes, and risk of major chronic diseases, additional to the risks associated with lack of physical activity.[16]

The rapidly increasing body of evidence in the public health benefits of active transport, combined with advocacy for environmental and policy initiatives to promote walking, has engaged multiple sectors beyond health.[15,17] Active transport initiatives are being implemented, advocacy and policy frameworks are being disseminated, and serious resources are being devoted to large-scale practical efforts in many developed countries. However, as is the case for other health behaviors, the systematic use of research evidence to inform the relevant detail of such dissemination lags behind the enthusiasm and the imperative for doing so.[18]

Neighborhood walkability is a composite construct based on population density, land use mix, and street connectivity, which was developed by urban planning and transportation researchers and is used in physical activity research. Neighborhood walkability indexes have been positively associated with physical activity in a number of studies.[13,19,20] The implications of this evidence are important for engaging policymakers and the other "gatekeepers" of dissemination, who are in the urban planning, transportation, and environmental-sustainability fields. However, the indexes used to define neighborhood walkability in physical activity research need to be translated into practical terms to inform policy and practice. Practically, the attributes of destinations and routes within neighborhoods that are likely to determine the relevant behavioral choices include:[21,22]

- The presence of destinations, such as retail outlets or entertainment venues in the local neighborhood, and the attributes of the routes by which they may be accessed can provide *instrumental cues* (relating to the feasibility and efficiency of walking or biking).

- Aesthetic attributes can provide *evaluative and affective cues* that may make active behavioral choices more or less attractive (in a negative way, poor neighborhood aesthetic attributes might foster residents' staying indoors to watch television, or driving an automobile, rather than spending time outdoors or walking or biking to destinations).
- Built-environment attributes can provide *normative cues* about behavioral choices that are expected of people (large parking lots and the absence of sidewalks around shopping centers, seeing few other people in the local neighborhood walking or using bicycles).
- Built-environment attributes may prompt people to anticipate the likely *positive or negative outcomes* of such behavioral choices. Such outcomes might include a greater variety of pleasant social interactions, or prolonged waiting to cross busy roads and exposure to exhaust fumes.

Practitioners and policymakers who are the gatekeepers for dissemination of environmental innovations for active transport need to know what the sometimes abstract constructs and research findings mean in concrete terms. Communication between researchers and practitioners must be clearly defined, must be targeted, and is best facilitated by supportive networks of locally driven, yet internationally connected organizations.

To this end, the Council on the Environment and Physical Activity (CEPA) of the International Society for Physical Activity and Health has been established. The purpose of CEPA is to build strong, evidence-based links from the research that is being supported through the International Physical Activity and the Environment Network (IPEN) study. IPEN investigators from multiple disciplines in multiple countries are conducting rigorous research on physical activity and the environment (*www.ipenproject.org*).

As a broad-based international dissemination strategy, the objective of CEPA is to encourage the use of research findings to advocate for the dissemination of evidence-based environmental and policy changes that will support and promote physical activity. The aims of CEPA are as follows:

1. To stimulate and support *interdisciplinary* research on physical activity and the environment internationally
2. To build capacity for using the best available methods, and encourage the use of common protocols and measures
3. To increase communication and collaboration among researchers in developing new measures, adapting measures for local contexts, and organizing networks focusing on specific population subgroups, geographic regions, and research questions
4. To encourage formation of interdisciplinary teams to conduct research that provides the evidence base for dissemination
5. To encourage teams from different countries to carry out joint and pooled analyses, with the aim of identifying unique environmental and cultural determinants of physical activity that may be more broadly disseminated
6. To support physical activity/environment researchers to become more effective advocates for disseminating evidence-based approaches to environmental and policy change

Success in the dissemination of environmental and policy initiatives to influence physical activity requires not only the relevant evidence, but also strong locally relevant engagement capacities and initiatives on the part of researchers. If CEPA ultimately is successful in building the relevant capacities and in strengthening communication and mutual support between researchers from multiple disciplines, there should be enhanced prospects for the broad international dissemination of environmental policy initiatives to promote physical activity. The elements of the strategy to support international dissemination and local initiatives that is encompassed by these six CEPA aims potentially may be applied to other health behavior and public health challenges.

■ DISSEMINATION TO GROUPS WITH SIGNIFICANT HEALTH DISPARITIES

For those with significant health disparities, defined here as adults at high risk of chronic disease, or who are living with chronic disease, appropriate health behavior change programs should be widely available, evidence-based, accessible, and capable of promoting changes that can be maintained. (For a thorough treatment of dissemination and implementation research in the broader array of populations with health disparities, see Chapter 22). For this to be an effective element of the overall strategy for preventive medicine described by Geoffrey Rose,[7,8] it requires the dissemination of such programs to large numbers of high-risk individuals, through approaches that can be delivered within health systems and services and by health professionals.

To develop the relevant interventions, practical intervention trials carried out in contexts that reflect the challenges of practice and the difficulties of implementation within complex systems are required.[23-25] There is a large and rapidly growing evidence base on health behavior interventions delivered via broad-reach modalities. These delivery mechanisms do not rely on face-to-face contact, such as the telephone, mobile telephone text messaging (SMS), the Internet (website and e-mail), and computer-tailored interventions (with the intervention delivered via print materials or on computer screens). Such interventions hold particular promise for evaluation in dissemination contexts (and for subsequent uptake into practice), as they have the potential to deliver evidence-based health behavior change interventions to large numbers of participants in an efficient and potentially cost-effective manner.[26]

Research documenting the effectiveness of broad-reach health behavior interventions has developed considerably in the past decade, such that there are now published reviews on interventions to influence physical activity and other health behaviors, for each of the above delivery modalities. However, in examining the evidence summarized in these reviews, it is clear that there has been limited attention to the maintenance of a behavioral change when interventions are delivered using such mass-reach modalities.

Evidence for Dissemination: Maintenance of Behavior Change Is Fundamental

In order for interventions to be adopted and institutionalized, evidence on the long-term effectiveness is crucial. Furthermore, evidence on the specific attributes of interventions related to maintenance of behavioral change is required. In the particular case of telephone-delivered interventions on physical activity and dietary change, the review by Eakin, Lawler, Owen, and Vandelanotte found significant end-of-intervention behavioral improvements in 20 of 26 studies included in the review, but only four of the eight studies that assessed outcomes following a subsequent period of no-intervention reported significant behavioral maintenance.[27] Thus, evidence that telephone-delivered interventions could produce lasting effects was found to be limited. In the case of interventions delivered via mobile telephone text messaging, the review by Fjeldsoe et al. found significant end-of-intervention behavioral improvements in 13 of 14 studies reviewed; however, none of the 14 studies assessed maintenance of behavior change beyond the end of intervention.[28]

For website-delivered physical activity interventions, the review by Vandelanotte et al. found significant end-of-treatment improvements in physical activity in 8 of the 15 studies reviewed; of the 5 studies in which maintenance of physical activity was examined, 3 reported a significant effect of the intervention on maintenance.[29] For computer-tailored interventions for physical activity and dietary change, the review by Kroeze et al. found significant intervention effects in 23 of 30 studies reviewed, but did not address the issue of maintenance of behavior change following the end of intervention delivery.[30]

Maintenance of intervention effects is a key issue for informing designing for dissemination, as the ultimate goal is to produce sustained improvements in behavior and related health outcomes. Health care decision makers thus need evidence on the duration and intensity of intervention delivery and related resources that are required to bring about such sustained changes. However, as is clear from the above summary of reviews of broad-reach intervention modalities, only limited attention has been paid to maintenance of behavioral change in the relevant research studies that must be relied upon to make the case for dissemination.

Recently, the evidence on maintenance of physical activity and dietary behavior change following interventions (delivered via both mediated and face-to-face modalities) was reviewed systematically.[31] The review defined maintenance of behavior change as a significant between-group difference at postintervention *and* at follow-up (at least three months after end of intervention), for one or more behavioral outcomes. The review found that maintenance outcomes were reported in 35% of the 157 intervention trials initially considered for review, suggesting that more research attention is needed on this issue. Of the 29 trials that met all inclusion criteria, 21 (72%) achieved maintenance as previously defined. Most importantly for informing designing for dissemination were the review findings on intervention characteristics common to trials achieving maintenance. Trials targeting women only were less likely to achieve maintenance, although the majority of these targeted women with chronic conditions, arguably a more challenging subgroup in terms of health behavior change.

Studies with higher attrition (>70%) and those employing pretrial behavioral screening (that is, excluding those who already were reaching a specific behavior threshold) were more likely to achieve maintenance. Interventions of longer duration (greater than six months), those using face-to-face contact, those employing more intervention strategies (more than six strategies used), and those using follow-up prompts (brief contact following a more intensive intervention phase) were also more likely to achieve maintenance. These findings indicate specific characteristics of interventions that may be important for facilitating maintenance of behavior change and need to be examined in practical behavioral trials.

■ CASE STUDY: PRACTICAL BEHAVIORAL TRIALS AS A BASIS FOR DISSEMINATION: *THE LOGAN HEALTHY LIVING PROGRAM*

The Logan Healthy Living Program (LHLP) was a cluster-randomized trial evaluating a 12-month telephone-delivered physical activity and dietary behavior intervention targeting Australian primary care patients with type 2 diabetes or hypertension from a low-income community.[32] The LHLP trial was a pragmatic trial designed explicitly to inform subsequent dissemination.[23,25] For more on pragmatic trials, see Chapter 4. In addition to documenting the primary behavioral outcomes of the trial,[33] key elements of the evidence base needed to inform dissemination were also examined. These included:

- cost-effectiveness analysis[34]
- data on intervention implementation that were systematically collected allowing for evaluation of dose–response outcomes[35]
- maintenance data six months following the end of the intervention[36]

In brief, the original LHLP trial, in which the primary outcomes were self-reported physical activity and dietary behavior, resulted in significant between-group improvements favoring the intervention group. This was the case for all dietary outcomes, including energy from total fat and saturated fat, vegetable intake, fruit intake, and grams of fiber; and, a significant within-group improvement was observed for both treatment and usual-care groups for moderate-to-vigorous physical activity.[33] Results were maintained at an 18-month follow-up, 6 months following the end of intervention.[36] The intervention was also shown to be cost effective, and a higher dose of intervention, particularly during the latter part of the intervention, was shown to be related to behavior change outcomes.[35]

As described below, the evidence generated in the LHLP trial, along with a systematic review of telephone-delivered interventions,[27] played a significant role in informing the dissemination of the LHLP intervention into community-based practice. To highlight the opportunities, practicalities, and compromises involved in the dissemination of the LHLP, an account of the adaptations and supportive factors that were necessary to facilitate adoption and implementation in a community setting is provided.[37]

Funding and Broader Contextual Opportunity

Resources for dissemination are crucial, particularly those related to the infrastructure and staffing necessary for program delivery. The ability to conduct the LHLP dissemination study was influenced in large part by the availability of dedicated state government funding to enable the implementation of locally relevant solutions to better manage and prevent chronic disease. One of the sites to receive funding was the Logan area in which the LHLP trial was conducted. As mandated by the initiative, this presented an opportunity to consider the dissemination of local, evidence-based programs targeted at the primary and secondary prevention of chronic disease within the Logan community.

Strong Credibility and Community Partnerships

The conduct of the LHLP research trial in the Logan community involved the development of a partnership with the South East Primary HealthCare Network (SPHN), a state-funded organization providing administrative, technical, and professional development support to local area primary care practices. This core partnership and other strong relationships in the Logan community were important to enhancing local trust in the trial, aiding recruitment and ultimately influencing dissemination: its successful translation from research to practice.

At the same time as Logan received funding, the LHLP trial was nearing completion, and the Principal Investigator of LHLP was invited to sit on the Steering Committee that oversaw the allocation of the program funding. That committee was charged with identifying evidence-based chronic disease self-management initiatives that could be undertaken in the community. The Principal Investigator advocated for uptake in the local community of the LIILP based on its consistency with the funding goals. Consequently, the LIILP was adopted by SPHN for delivery as part of the larger suite of programs offered under the Logan strategy. Central to its inclusion was the commitment of LHLP research staff to provide ongoing support for implementation, and to oversee its evaluation.

Measurement and Evaluation in the Program Dissemination Context

Documenting the dissemination context, the target group, and the relevant program content

The first adaptation concerned the target group of the intervention. To avoid duplication of existing chronic disease services, and given the increasing focus on overweight and obesity in primary care, SPHN resolved that the OHP should target physical activity, diet, and modest weight loss in overweight primary care patients *without* chronic disease. Due to these changes, new content around weight loss was incorporated into the intervention protocols and materials. The research team took the lead on these adaptations, which were based on a distillation of the evidence from previous reviews, were particularly concerned with program attributes that might enhance maintenance, and were developed in consultation with OHP program staff. Documenting precisely these changes and noting the relevant areas of difference compared to what was the case in the efficacy study context are crucial to developing systematic accounts of behavior change program dissemination.

Documenting Program Delivery

As the OHP was not being delivered in a research context, it was decided to allow more flexibility in program delivery, consistent with the norms of the clinical approach being used. Although maintaining the same call structure as the LHLP (a tapered call schedule over 12 months; weekly, fortnightly, then monthly phases), OHP telephone counselors had the discretion to tailor the frequency of calls according to individual participants' needs. Research staff assisted with the development of a database for participant and outcomes tracking.

Assessment of outcomes in the dissemination context

Like the LHLP, participant assessment in the OHP occurred at four time points (baseline, 4, 12, and 18 months) and was used to provide feedback to OHP program participants and for program evaluation. While LHLP participant assessments were completed by computer-assisted telephone interviewers blinded to study condition, OHP budgetary constraints meant that the telephone counselors also completed assessment calls. To address limitations concerning the potential biases engendered by the collection of self-report data by program staff delivering the intervention, the OHP also collected clinical objective measures, including physician-measured weight, waist circumference, and blood pressure, which were not collected in the LHLP trial.

The evaluation of this disseminated program required particular attention to the inevitable changes that take place in adapting the program from the efficacy study context. Several adaptations to the original LHLP, rebadged by SPHN as the Optimal Health Program (OHP), were necessary to ensure feasibility and program "fit" within the adopting organizational context, based largely on needs and availability of resources. Documenting the nature of such changes systematically is crucial to inform future efforts at designing for dissemination.

■ SUMMARY AND CONCLUSIONS

The perspective on designing for dissemination put forward in this chapter has dealt with two complementary and interrelated elements of Rose's[7,8] strategy of preventive medicine:

- primary-prevention through disseminating evidence-based environmental and policy initiatives to influence health risk behaviors in *populations and communities*
- dissemination of an evidence-based health behavior change program for those with *significant health disparities*

Table 6–1 identifies principles to guide the designing for the dissemination of evidence-based environmental and policy initiatives, and the implementation and evaluation of dissemination initiatives for evidence-based health behavior change programs.

This chapter has emphasized the need for research that is designed explicitly with dissemination in mind.[38] This was illustrated in relation to environmental and

TABLE 6-1. *Summary of Key Principles to Guide Designing for Dissemination of Environmental and Policy Initiatives and Broad-Reach Health Behavior Programs*

ENVIRONMENTAL AND POLICY INITIATIVES
- Emphasize environmental and policy initiatives to support broad dissemination
- Address multiple domains and levels of the determinants of health behaviors
- Build strong partnerships with influential instrumentalities outside of public health
- Develop advocacy networks to guide and support evidence-based dissemination

BROAD-REACH HEALTH BEHAVIOR PROGRAMS
- Partnerships with key stakeholders (funders and implementers)
  - Fit of program/intervention with organizational goals
  - Availability of ongoing resources to support sustained implementation (monetary and personnel)
  - On-the-ground constraints on program delivery
  - In-depth knowledge of target populations
- Rigorous study designs
  - Randomized designs where possible
  - Integration of outcomes important to informing funders and advancing science
  - Systematic tracking of resources needed for implementation and intervention
  - Maintaining program fidelity while being flexible and responsive

---

policy initiatives to influence physical activity. The crucial importance for dissemination of working with experts and gatekeepers in the transportation and urban planning was emphasized. The other element of this chapter, the broad-reach intervention dissemination case study of a health behavior change program, highlighted the need to maintain key elements of research quality in designing for dissemination: to the extent that is practically possible, a rigorous study design; the systematic tracking of implementation and related costs; and, the conduct of dose–response, maintenance, and cost-effectiveness analyses.

The examples on designing for dissemination presented in this chapter illustrate not only the exciting opportunities for real-world dissemination research, but also the resourcefulness and commitment required for success. Significant gaps remain to be bridged.[39] For public health researchers, the priorities are in the conduct of high-quality scientific investigation, and generally not in dissemination and communication of the findings and implications of their research. For policymakers and practitioners, the priorities are to act in practical ways on the policies and programs necessary for improving public health. The synthesis of relevant knowledge and the identification of evidence-based applications of research findings are generally not feasible within the constraints of policy formulation and delivery systems. Thus, many formidable challenges remain, and exciting opportunities exist for strengthening the knowledge bases, concepts, and systems needed in designing for dissemination.

SUGGESTED READINGS

Brownson RC, Haire-Joshu D, Luke DA. Shaping the context of health: a review of environmental and policy approaches in the prevention of chronic diseases. *Annu Rev Public Health*. 2006;27(1):341–370.

Describes broad-reach approaches in public health that can influence populations through changing important determinants of health-related behavioral choices.

Glasgow RE, Emmons KM. How can we increase translation of research into practice? Types of evidence needed. *Annu Rev Public Health*. 2007;28(1):413–433.

> *Describes the forms of evidence that can be gathered in the context of dissemination research, emphasizing types of evidence that can best inform translation into practice.*

Owen N, Glanz K, Sallis JF, Kelder S. Evidence-based approaches to dissemination and diffusion of physical activity interventions. *Am J Prev Med*. 2006;31(4)(suppl 1):35–44.

> *Describes examples of how broad-reach approaches to physical activity may be disseminated, drawing on dissemination models and approaches from other areas of public health.*

Goode A, Owen N, Reeves M, Eakin E. Translation from research to practice: community dissemination of a telephone-delivered physical activity and dietary behavior change intervention. *Am J Health Promot*. 2011;25(4):257-263.

> *Presents a case study of the process by which a telephone-delivered dietary-change and physical activity intervention previously tested in a controlled trial were implemented in a socially disadvantaged community.*

SELECTED WEBSITES AND TOOLS

Cancer Control P.L.A.N.E.T. <http://cancercontrolplanet.cancer.gov/index.html>. *Cancer Control P.L.A.N.E.T. acts as a portal to provide access to data and resources for designing, implementing, and evaluating evidence-based cancer control programs. The site provides five steps (with links) for developing a comprehensive cancer control plan or program.*

Designing for Dissemination Conference, 2002 <http://cancercontrol.cancer.gov/IS/pdfs/d4d_conf_sum_report.pdf> *Provides detailed reports on a conference sponsored by the U.S. National Cancer Institute, which focused on identifying and overcoming the barriers to research dissemination and on the adoption of evidence-based interventions. It provides the conference final report, plus access to presentations on the state of knowledge in disseminating cancer control initiatives, challenges in research translation, and action plans or designing for dissemination.*

RE-AIM (Reach, Effectiveness, Adoption, Implementation, Maintenance) <http://www.re-aim.org/> *RE-AIM is a framework designed to enhance the quality, efficiency, and public health impact of efforts to translate research into practice. Practical measurement tools, guidelines on application, and background readings are provided.*

Active Living Research (ALR) <http://www.activelivingresearch.org/> *ALR is an initiative supported by the Robert Wood Johnson Foundation, focused on the prevention of childhood obesity in low-income and high-risk groups. It describes how environment and policy research can be used to influence active living opportunities for children and families. The ALR website provides many useful links to accounts of research translation activities.*

■ REFERENCES

1. Glasgow RE, Emmons KM. How can we increase translation of research into practice? Types of evidence needed. *Annu Rev Public Health*. 2007;28(1):413–433.
2. Green LW, Ottoson JM, Garcia C, Hiatt RA. Diffusion theory, and knowledge dissemination, utilization, and integration in public health. *Annu Rev Public Health*. 2009;30(1):151–174.
3. Orleans CT. Increasing the demand for and use of effective smoking-cessation treatments reaping the full health benefits of tobacco-control science and policy gains—in our lifetime. *Am J Prev Med*. 2007;33(6)(suppl 1):S340-S348.

4. Glasgow RE, Goldstein MG, Ockene JK, Pronk NP. Translating what we have learned into practice: principles and hypotheses for interventions addressing multiple behaviors in primary care. *Am J Prev Med.* 2004;27(2)(suppl 1):88–101.

5. Wandersman A, Duffy J, Flaspohler P, et al. Bridging the gap between prevention research and practice: the interactive systems framework for dissemination and implementation. *Am J Community Psychol.* 2008;41(3–4):171–181.

6. Cameron R, Brown KS, Best JA. The dissemination of chronic disease prevention programs: linking science and practice. *Can J Public Health.* 1996;(87)(suppl 2): S50–S53.

7. Rose G. *The Strategy of Preventive Medicine.* Oxford, UK: Oxford University Press; 1992.

8. Rose G. Sick individuals and sick populations. *Int J Epidemiol.* 2001;30(3):427–432, 433–434.

9. Brownson RC, Haire-Joshu D, Luke DA. Shaping the context of health: a review of environmental and policy approaches in the prevention of chronic diseases. *Annu Rev Public Health.* 2006;27(1):341–370.

10. Glanz K, Owen N, Wold JA. Perspectives on behavioral sciences research for disease prevention and control in populations. *J Natl Inst Public Health.* 2009;58(1): 40–50.

11. Sallis JF, Owen N. *Physical Activity and Behavioral Medicine.* Thousand Oaks, CA: Sage; 1999.

12. Giles-Corti B, Timperio A, Bull F, Pikora T. Understanding physical activity environmental correlates: increased specificity for ecological models. *Exerc Sport Sci Rev.* 2005;33(4):175–181.

13. Owen N, Humpel N, Leslie E, Bauman A, Sallis JF. Understanding environmental influences on walking: review and research agenda. *Am J Prev Med.* 2004;27(1): 67–76.

14. Sallis JF, Owen N, Fisher EB. Ecological models of health behavior. In: Glanz K, Rimer BK, Viswanath K, eds. *Health Behavior and Health Education: Theory, Research, and Practice.* 4th ed. San Francisco, CA: Jossey-Bass; 2008:465–482.

15. Frank LD, Greenwald MJ, Winkelman S, Chapman J, Kavage S. Carbonless footprints: promoting health and climate stabilization through active transportation. *Prev Med.* 2010;(50)(suppl 1):S99–S105.

16. Owen N, Healy GN, Mathews CE, Dunstan DW. Too much sitting: the population-health science of sedentary behavior. *Exerc Sport Sci Rev.* 2010;38(3):105–113.

17. Handy SL, Boarnet MG, Ewing R, Killingsworth RE. How the built environment affects physical activity: views from urban planning. *Am J Prev Med.* 2002;23(2)(suppl 1):64–73.

18. Kerner J, Rimer B, Emmons K. Introduction to the special section on dissemination: dissemination research and research dissemination: how can we close the gap? *Health Psychol.* 2005;24(5):443–446.

19. Frank LD, Schmid TL, Sallis JF, Chapman J, Saelens BE. Linking objectively measured physical activity with objectively measured urban form: findings from SMARTRAQ. *Am J Prev Med.* 2005;28(2)(suppl 2):117–125.

20. Owen N, Cerin E, Leslie E, et al. Neighborhood walkability and the walking behavior of Australian adults. *Am J Prev Med.* 2007;33(5):387–395.

21. Owen N. Effects of the built environment on obesity. In: Bouchard C, Katzmarczyk P, eds. *Physical Activity and Obesity.* Champaign, IL: Human Kinetics; 2010: 199–202.

22. Sugiyama T, Neuhaus M, Owen N. Active transport, the built environment and human health. In: Rassia S, Pardalos P, eds. *Sustainable Environmental Design in Architecture: Impacts on Health*. London, UK: Springer. 2011;34–67.

23. Glasgow RE, Magid DJ, Beck A, Ritzwoller D, Estabrooks PA. Practical clinical trials for translating research to practice: design and measurement recommendations. *Med Care*. 2005;43(6):551–557.

24. Hooker S, Seavey W, Weidmer C, et al. The California active aging community grant program: translating science into practice to promote physical activity in older adults. *Ann Behav Med*. 2005;29(3):155–165.

25. Tunis SR, Stryer DB, Clancy CM. Practical clinical trials: increasing the value of clinical research for decision making in clinical and health policy. *JAMA*. 2003;290(12): 1624–1632.

26. Marcus BH, Dubbert PM, Forsyth LH, et al. Physical activity behavior change: issues in adoption and maintenance. *Health Psychol*. 2000;19(1)(suppl):32–41.

27. Eakin EG, Lawler SP, Owen N, Vandelanotte C. Telephone interventions for physical activity and dietary behavior change: a systematic review. *Am J Prev Med*. 2007;32(5): 419–434.

28. Fjeldsoe BS, Marshall AL, Miller YD. Behavior change interventions delivered by mobile telephone short-message service. *Am J Prev Med*. 2009;36(2):165–173.

29. Vandelanotte C, Spathonis K, Eakin E, Owen N. Website-delivered physical activity interventions: a review of the literature. *Am J Prev Med*. 2007;33(1):54–64.

30. Kroeze W, Werkman A, Brug J. A systematic review of randomized trials on the effectiveness of computer-tailored education on physical activity and dietary behaviors. *Ann Behav Med*. 2006;31(3):205–223.

31. Fjeldsoe B, Neuhaus M, Winkler E, Eakin E. Systematic review of maintenance of behavior change following physical activity and dietary interventions. *Health Psychol*. 2011;30(1):99–109.

32. Eakin EG, Reeves MM, Lawler SP, et al. The Logan Healthy Living Program: a cluster randomized trial of a telephone-delivered physical activity and dietary behavior intervention for primary care patients with type 2 diabetes or hypertension from a socially disadvantaged community—rationale, design and recruitment. *Contemp Clin Trials*. 2008;29(3):439–454.

33. Eakin E, Reeves M, Lawler S, et al. Telephone counselling for physical activity and diet in primary care. *Am J Prev Med*. 2009;36(2):142–149.

34. Graves N, Barnett A, Halton KA, et al. Cost-effectiveness of a telephone-delivered intervention for physical activity and diet. *PLoS ONE*. 2009;4(9):e7135.

35. Goode AD, Winkler EAH, Lawler SP, Reeves MM, Owen N, Eakin EG. Telephone-delivered physical activity and dietary intervention for type 2 diabetes and hypertension: does intervention dose influence outcomes? *Am J Health Promot*. 2011;25(4):43–47.

36. Eakin E, Reeves M, Winkler E, Lawler S, Owen N. Maintenance of physical activity and dietary change following a telephone-delivered intervention. *Health Psychol*. 2010;29(6):566–573.

37. Goode A, Owen N, Reeves M, Eakin E. Translation from research to practice: community dissemination of a telephone-delivered physical activity and dietary behavior change intervention. *Am J Health Promot*. 2011;25(4):257-263.

38. Klesges LM, Estabrooks PA, Dzewaltowski DA, Bull SS, Glasgow RE. Beginning with the application in mind: designing and planning health behavior change interventions to enhance dissemination. *Ann Behav Med.* 2005;29(2):66–75.
39. Cuijpers P, de Graaf I, Bohlmeijer E. Adapting and disseminating effective public health interventions in another country: towards a systematic approach. *Eur J Public Health.* 2005;15(2):166–169.

7

The Role of Organizational Processes in Dissemination and Implementation Research

■ GREGORY A. AARONS,
JONATHAN D. HOROWITZ,
LAUREN R. DLUGOSZ, AND
MARK G. EHRHART

■ INTRODUCTION

The science of dissemination and implementation (D&I) is a swiftly growing and broad field that commonly involves both outer (i.e., system) and inner (i.e., organization) contexts of health service systems and organizations at multiple levels.[1-4] While a broad view of organizational issues related to D&I at first glance implicates contextual factors as paramount, the inner workings of organizations, workforce trends, health care providers, and consumers also impact uptake and use of scientific discovery in practice.[5,6] This "topography" of D&I provides the backdrop for the proposed phases of the implementation process, including Exploration (consideration of whether to adopt or even consider an innovation), Adoption Decision/Preparation (preparing for implementation once the adoption decision is made), Active Implementation (enacting plans and working through emergent issues), and Sustainment (creating and supporting the structures and processes that will allow an implemented innovation to be maintained in a system or organization).[1,7] Considering D&I as a process with multiple phases has implications for how the various topographic levels (i.e., country, system, organization, provider, patient) may impact or be impacted by the D&I of evidence-based practices (EBPs) into routine care. Such bidirectional effects are key to conceptual models that recognize recipients of new technologies as not passive but as highly likely to react in various ways depending on characteristics of the context, the innovation to be implemented, and individual differences in health care providers and patients. It is becoming increasingly clear that organizational-level issues and factors are not only important but also are likely to have more impact on successful D&I of EBPs relative to individual-level factors.[8]

The bulk of health, mental health, public health, and social services are delivered within or through organizations. While the types of organizations are varied (e.g., for-profit, nonprofit, public) and range from large (e.g., Kaiser Permanente, Veterans Affairs Healthcare System, Los Angeles County Health Department) to small (e.g., single-program community-based nonprofits), there are a number of common organizational constructs or processes likely to be associated with successful D&I of health care innovations and EBPs.[2,4] Drawing from the business, management, and organizational literatures, this chapter focuses on several of the more common and well-researched organizational constructs and processes that may impact uptake and sustainment of EBPs in organizations. In particular, the chapter will focus on organizational culture, organizational climate, strategic climates, leadership, organizational readiness for change, attitudes toward EBP, organizational development, and organizational process improvement. Below, these factors are considered in relation to the questions and challenges of EBP implementation in health care, behavioral health, and social service settings.

As shown in Figure 7–1, each of the constructs addressed in this chapter may operate in ways that are unidirectional, are bidirectional, or more likely, have multiple determinants and influences that operate reciprocally. For example, state service and public health systems may be subject to gubernatorial influence, but local or state legislators may exert congruent or opposing influence as well.[9] Research has shown that how a given agency is positioned within a system may impact its influence in the service context.[10] Likewise, within a given public or private organization, the organization's culture can be determined through leadership, structures, and procedures within the organization.[11] From a "bottom-up" perspective, the

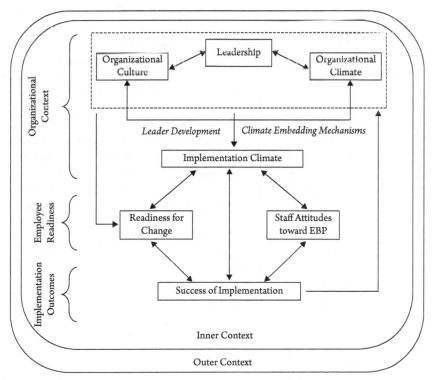

Figure 7–1. Multiple levels of organizational processes and implementation.

nature of the employees and their relationships, motives, and the influence of leaders at multiple levels can also help to shape the culture of an organization.[11,12] For instance, transformational leadership and leaders' relationships with subordinates and others in an organization are differentially important during active implementation compared with stable operations.[13,14] Thus, it is important to consider not only how organizational factors can impact the implementation process but also how implementation can impact organizational processes and functioning. For example, it may be that staff receptivity to EBP can impact the fidelity and integrity with which EBPs are delivered,[15,16] but the process of implementation in combination with the practice itself may impact the system or organization, its management, and its workforce.[17–19]

Another assumption deserving of consideration is that change in organizational processes or routines (such as implementing new interventions) takes time. Further, some changes take more time than others, as learning is frequently incremental and iterative.[20] For example, changing a relatively circumscribed aspect of organizational support for EBP could involve strategies such as making summaries of peer-reviewed literature available to staff and could be relatively low threshold, low cost, and quickly implemented. However, more complicated goals, such as improving the effectiveness or efficiency of safety in emergency medicine departments, may be slowed or facilitated by the organizational culture of the hospital or department in which change is to take place.[21] Thus, the type and size of the system or organization and the type and scope of the change target can impact the need for more or less protracted change strategies with the ultimate goal of incorporating evidence and EBP into usual care. Such changes may be fluid and require different time frames to become part of the ongoing organizational culture.[22] Also, as discussed below, developing a particular type of organizational culture or climate can require the use of a number of "embedding mechanisms" that emanate from leadership at multiple organizational levels.[11] Two types of organizational climate will be discussed, general organizational climate and more focused or "strategic" climates, both of which can be tailored to D&I activities. Finally, organizational readiness for change, organizational culture and climate change, and the tradition of organizational process improvement will be explored, particularly in regard to how they can be applied to health service improvement and EBP implementation.

One of the primary arguments of this chapter is that leaders within organizations must pay attention to the context in which the implementation takes place to increase the likelihood of implementation success and long-term sustainment.[23] Such attention must be consistent and goal directed and consider the outer context, the inner context, and the motivations and needs of people within the participating organizations.[1,2,4]

Our discussion of organizational issues in implementation will begin by focusing on two related but distinct concepts: organizational culture and organizational climate. Organizational culture and climate are sometimes confused for each other; one review found over 32 definitions of organizational climate and 54 definitions of organizational culture with some overlap between these constructs.[24] In what follows, the distinguishing features of these constructs are highlighted, with a specific emphasis on their role in the EBP implementation process.

■ ORGANIZATIONAL CULTURE

An organization's culture is essentially what makes that organization unique from all others, including the core values instilled in the organization by its founder(s) and the organization's history of how it has survived through successes and failures. It includes the values for the services or products provided as well as how individuals and groups within the organization treat and interact with one another. Our working definition of organizational culture for this chapter comes from Schein,[11] who described organizational culture as the "...pattern of shared basic assumptions that was learned by a group as it solved its problems of external adaptation and internal integration, and that has worked well enough to be considered valid and, therefore, to be taught to new members as the correct way to perceive, think, and feel in relation to those problems."[11(p.17)]

One way that scholars have discussed organizational culture is in terms of its layers or levels. Two examples are shown in Table 7–1. Frameworks along these lines specify outer layers that are more tangible and easily accessible (e.g., artifacts such as style of dress or the physical arrangement of space) but may have different meanings in different organizations. To truly understand these outer layers, Schein[25] and others have argued that one must gain a deeper understanding of the more deeply held, subjective, and less easily accessed values and assumptions that comprise inner layers.[11,26] Such basic, shared assumptions are so deeply ingrained in the organization that its members may not be able to readily articulate them; thus, scholars have argued that both qualitative and quantitative methods must be used to truly understand an organization's culture.[11,26]

Adding to the complexity of defining culture and its levels, scholars vary in their models of the specific components or dimensions of organizational culture. Table 7–2 lists six different ways in which scholars have conceptualized organizational culture and notes the reference(s) we cite for each approach. This is by no means an exhaustive list but is provided to give the reader a sense of some of the variability in conceptual models of organizational culture.

Part of the allure of the concept of organizational culture has been its connection to organizational performance. Its rise in popularity in the 1980s was linked

TABLE 7–1. *Layers of Organizational Culture*

Source	Number of Layers	Layers
Schein[25]	3	Underlying assumptions Espoused values Artifacts
Rousseau[26]	5	Fundamental assumptions Values Behavioral norms Patterns of behavior Artifacts

TABLE 7–2. *Dimensions of Organizational Culture as Defined in Different Models with Quantitative Assessments*

Source	# of Dimensions	Dimensions
Organizational Culture Inventory (Cooke & Rousseau)[27]	3	Constructive culture Passive/Defensive culture Aggressive/Defensive culture
Denison[28]; Denison & Neale[29]	4	Involvement Consistency Adaptability Mission
Organizational Culture Profile (Chatman[30]; O'Reilly et al.[31])	8	Attention to detail Outcome orientation Aggressiveness Emphasis on rewards Innovation Supportiveness Team orientation Decisiveness
Organizational Culture Profile (Ashkanasy et al.)[32]	10	Leadership Structure Innovation Job performance Planning Communication Environment Humanistic workplace Development of the individual Socialization on entry
Competing Values Framework (Cameron & Quinn)[33]	4	Clan Adhocracy Hierarchy Market
Organizational Social Context (Glisson[34]; Glisson et al.[35])	4	Proficiency Resistance Apathy Suppression

Note: There are two different conceptual models of culture both identified as the Organizational Culture Profile.

to books such as those authored by Deal and Kennedy[36] and Peters and Waterman[37] that influenced executives to attempt to change their culture in order to increase organizational effectiveness. Unfortunately, most of those efforts did not result in much success, as organizational culture is rather resistant to change, and, as such, some have even questioned the link between organizational culture and organizational performance.[38] While a few interventions designed to improve organizational culture in health care settings have been effective in improving clinical and organizational outcomes, including decreased infection rates in a hospital[39] and increased work satisfaction and organizational commitment in long-term care,[40] a recent review article was unable to identify a general, effective strategy for changing organizational culture.[41] Nevertheless, there is evidence to suggest that organizations with cultures that are more supportive of employees and that are adaptable to changes in the environment (e.g., EBP implementation) are more effective in general.[42,43]

▪ ORGANIZATIONAL CLIMATE

The popularity of the study of organizational culture among organizational research-ers throughout the 1980s and 90s was preceded by a time of high levels of interest in the construct of organizational climate from the late 1960s through the 1970s. The goal of the earliest research and writing on the topic of organizational climate was to describe the environment that emerged through the treatment of workers by their leaders. This, in turn, affected employee attitudes, motivations, and performance.[44,45] Over time, a number of differences emerged in how the organizational climate was conceptualized and studied, including in terms of level of analysis (individual vs. organizational unit), content (description vs. evaluation), focus (general vs. specific), and type of composition model (climate level vs. climate strength). Although a dis-cussion of individual perceptions of climate (also known as psychological climate) and climate strength (variability in climate perceptions) are outside the scope of this chapter, the content and focus of climate perceptions are particularly relevant. In response to early criticisms regarding overlap between the constructs of climate and job attitudes (e.g. job satisfaction),[46,47] some climate scholars have emphasized that climate involves employees' descriptions (but not evaluations) of the "events, prac-tices, and procedures and the kinds of behaviors that get rewarded, supported, and expected in a setting."[48(p.384)] Other climate researchers, particularly those who have studied climate in the context of mental health services, have emphasized climate as both perception of and affective response to employees' work environment.[34,49] In either case, it is important to note that climate is not merely defined by the pres-ence of practices and procedures in the work environment. Rather, it is the perceived meaning inferred by employees through management practices and procedures that ultimately defines the climate of the organization.[49,50]

In addition, the other important distinction for this chapter that emerged early in the history of the climate literature was between molar (or generic) climate and focused or "strategic" climate. The molar approach typically involves an attempt to measure climate at a broad level across multiple dimensions, such as role stress, autonomy, leadership support, and warmth.[51] These dimensions generally refer to the extent to which management provides a positive experience for employees at work, and thus has also been described as a climate for employee well-being.[50] In contrast, the focused climate approach involves employee perceptions of the prac-tices and procedures with regard to a specific criterion, whether it be a strategic outcome (e.g., climate for customer service, climate for safety) or an organizational process (e.g., ethics, fairness).[48] In other words, in contrast to molar climate that attempts to capture the general "feel" of the organization, the focused or strategic climate approach attempts to understand the extent to which employees perceive that management emphasizes a specific criterion of interest, whatever it may be. A relevant example is the notion of a climate for implementation of innovations in an organization,[52] discussed below as one type of strategic climate.

▪ IMPLEMENTATION CLIMATE

The strategic climate approach to organizational climate is highly relevant for research on D&I. Organizational culture and molar climate are important for successful implementation and for achieving successful clinical outcomes;[53,54] in fact, there is clear evidence that they are.[54,55] However, their role is important in laying the foundation for the development of an effective implementation climate. An implementation climate is defined as "...employees' shared perceptions of the importance of innovation implementation within the organization...[that] results from employees' shared experiences and observations of, and their information about and discussions about, their organization's implementation policies and practices."[56(p.813)] It is important to note that implementation climate is distinct from a climate for innovation, which involves the extent to which the organization encourages and supports the development of new ideas and technologies,[57,58] but does not capture how those ideas and technologies are actually implemented in the organization. However, climate for innovation may be associated with greater employee openness to adoption of EBP. Implementation climate focuses specifically on creating a fertile organizational context for putting a new innovation into practice. When management communicates the importance of the implementation of a new practice through its policies, procedures, and reward systems, employees are able to clearly understand that the leaders in the organization care about the implementation and use of the innovation, therefore enabling employees to better focus their energy and motivation for that goal. As a result, the overall implementation is more likely to succeed.[56]

There are many ways that leaders, managers, and supervisors can communicate the value of successful implementation. In the authors' own work on the implementation of EBPs in mental health agencies, a detailed measure of EBP implementation climate was developed to capture the variety of means through which management communicates the value of EBP for the organization. The measure was used as a framework for improving EBP implementation climate in the agencies that participated in the research project. In one agency, EBP guest speakers were brought in for staff, and educational materials such as manuals were made readily available. Another agency's chief executive officer attended a regular team meeting to recognize their efforts in EBP implementation. In all of the participating agencies, leaders made a concerted effort to recognize staff for successfully implementing EBP, including thanking staff via e-mail and recognizing positive client outcomes in staff meetings. All of these strategies communicated to staff members that management valued the successful implementation of EBP.

It is important to note that if management enacted only one of these strategies, implementation would not be as likely to be successful in contrast to an organization that strategically employed a number of these aspects of implementation climate. More importantly, if management contradicts itself, for instance by talking about the importance of EBP but not providing appropriate supports or incentives for its proper use, then a strong implementation climate will not result. Thus, it is the concerted convergence of targeted strategies to promote EBP uptake that creates a positive EBP implementation climate.[55] The role of leaders is crucial in creating and implementing such strategies during the EBP implementation process, and thus we now turn to the nexus of leadership, culture, and climate.

■ LEADERSHIP

Leadership is one organizational contextual factor that has come under extensive investigation[59] across a range of private,[60] military,[61] medical,[62] mental health,[63,64] and nonprofit[65] settings. Leadership is a critical and important factor in implementation of community initiatives.[66] Of the many theories of leadership (see Avolio et al.[67] for a review), one particularly useful and well-researched framework is the Full Range Leadership (FRL) model.[68–71] According to this model, leadership behaviors fall into three broad categories, with more specific dimensions within each. The first, *transformational* leadership, includes those behaviors in which a leader attends to and develops followers to higher levels of performance and potential (individualized consideration), engages followers in thinking about issues in new ways (intellectual stimulation), communicates an appealing vision for the future (inspirational motivation), and becomes a trusted role model for staff (idealized influence).[72] *Transactional* leadership, the second category in the FRL model, involves exchanges between leaders and followers in which leaders reinforce or reward followers for engaging in certain behaviors and meeting practical and/or aspirational goals (contingent reward) as well as monitoring and correcting performance (passive or active management by exception). The final general category in the FRL model, *passive or laissez-faire leadership* (i.e., nonleadership), refers to withdrawal behaviors on the part of the purported leader in which little exchange between the leader and follower is enacted. It is, however, not merely a nonimpactful or neutral set of behaviors but is thought to represent an actively destructive abdication of responsibility.[73] Obviously, this is considered to be an ineffective style of leadership.

The FRL model has been subject to a high degree of scrutiny in many countries and cultures, and in many different types of organizations, and has been the subject of at least five meta-analyses[71,74–77] that support its predictive validity. Specifically, transformational leadership is positively associated with follower job satisfaction,[78] job well-being, individual follower performance,[79] group performance,[60,61,80] and cohesive organizational culture,[81] as well as decreased turnover,[82] absenteeism,[83] risk of injury,[80] and employee burnout.[81,84] The contingent reward dimension of transactional leadership is also associated with group performance[85] and individual follower performance.[79] Passive leadership is associated with poor job satisfaction and poor efficiency,[86] higher workplace stress, psychological distress, increased risk of bullying at work,[73] and lower safety climate and conscientiousness.[87] These findings have been supported across a broad range of organizational settings[76,88] and cultures,[78,89] including health care organizations and behavioral health organizations.[81,83,84,90]

Several studies have shown that leaders can be trained to display more transformational leadership behaviors. One approach stemming from the FRL model that has come under extensive investigation is the Full Range Leadership Program (FRLP),[91] a training that consists of leadership feedback and a personal development plan that is used during an initial three-day workshop and a two-day workshop three months later.[92] Several studies have shown the FRLP to be effective in increasing staff ratings of transformational leadership[93,94] and other positive organizational outcomes such as staff productivity, attendance, and prosocial behavior.[93] Several adaptations of the FRLP have also been found effective in improving transformational leadership,[95–97] including a more targeted one-day leadership training.[98]

■ LEADERSHIP AND ORGANIZATIONAL CHANGE

In addition to the more general benefits of effective leadership in organizations, leadership is also important for facilitating change processes in organizations.[10,38] Positive and effective leadership in health care systems can help to create climates that support quality of care and implementation of EBPs. For example, Corrigan and colleagues[39] found a positive association between strong mental health program leadership and consumer satisfaction and quality of life. Stronger transformational leadership has been associated with positive work attitudes in both for-profit and nonprofit organizations,[40] and more positive leadership in human service organizations has been associated with staff members' higher organizational commitment.[41] Aarons and colleagues[42] found that organizational climate mediates the association of leadership on therapeutic alliance such that positive leadership is associated with positive organizational climate, which was in turn associated with more positive clinician ratings of working alliance. Aarons[99] also found that more positive leadership is associated with more positive staff attitudes toward adopting EBPs.[5]

Glisson and Durick[100] identified leadership as a positive predictor of organizational commitment within human service organizations. Corrigan and colleagues[101] found that mental health team members want their leaders to display a range of behaviors similar to those prescribed by the FRL model. In addition, transformational leadership has been positively associated with positive organizational culture and reduced burnout[81] in mental health service teams. Both transformational and transactional leadership were found to be positively associated with clinicians' receptivity toward the use of EBP[99] and, as noted above, to positively predict consumer satisfaction and quality of life. In contrast, laissez-faire leadership predicted poor organizational and consumer outcomes.[102]

As alluded to above, leadership is critical for embedding a strategic climate for implementation.[11] Climate embedding mechanisms can be used strategically as part of ongoing management responsibilities, including reaction to crises, allocation of resources, and monitoring staff behavior.[11] Leaders in health care settings can use embedding mechanisms to develop implementation climate in several ways, including effectively problem solving when crises occur during implementation, providing rewards to staff based on implementation progress and excellence, and regularly discussing the benefits of the innovation being implemented.

While there are many practical and ideological challenges in EBP implementation,[103] it is important to consider the role of leadership at multiple levels within health and social service organizations. Indeed, there are many commonalities across service sectors that must be considered for effective implementation to occur.[1,7] Strategies and policies often emerge from top management; however, it is important to consider leadership at all levels in an organization so that there is congruence of message, reinforcement, and direction that is accessible and palpable for staff at the front line of services.[12] The notion of high investment in "first-level" leadership provides a backdrop for strongly supporting staff during the implementation process. Indeed, it is first-level transformational leadership that is likely key to creating a team climate for implementation that can lead to more positive attitudes toward adopting EBP during active implementation.[14]

Despite the importance of strong leadership during EBP implementation, first-level leaders often lack the management and leadership skills as well as the power necessary to develop positive organizational and implementation climates and effectively implement EBPs. This represents a critical gap between workforce readiness for EBP and the need to implement the most effective services for health and mental health care. The authors are currently developing and testing just such an intervention to simultaneously improve FRL and a positive EBP implementation climate. While acceptability and feasibility data for this intervention are promising, further tailoring and large-scale testing are needed to validate such approaches to leadership development and improving organizational readiness and effectiveness in implementing EBPs.[104]

■ ORGANIZATIONAL READINESS FOR CHANGE

An often-discussed concern that requires further research and attention is the degree to which organizational readiness for change impacts implementation. As with culture and climate, organizational readiness for change is the subject of different definitions that focus on various aspects of organizations including structure, process, equipment and technology, and staff attitudes. For the purposes of this chapter, organizational readiness for change is defined as the extent to which organizational members are psychologically and behaviorally prepared to implement a new innovation, technology, or EBP. Organizational readiness is widely regarded as an essential antecedent to successful implementation of change in health care and social service organizations.[105-107] The concept of organizational readiness for change arose from Lewin's three-stage model of change, which advocates "unfreezing" the mind-set of an organization and creating the motivation to change.[108] Several scholars have supported the notion that when employees exhibit readiness to change, they expend greater effort during the process of implementation, are more invested in the change, and are more persistent in the face of obstacles to successfully implementing change.[109-112] In many cases, health care organizations implement changes that require collective behavioral changes throughout the organization or a specific team to achieve desired outcomes.[113] However, even simple changes can become complex when considering organizational dynamics combined with individual and collective agendas goals. For example, in a large health care organization, implementing something seemingly as simple as a clinical reminder for a patient to receive a test requires overcoming the differing perceptions, agendas, priorities, and values of a number of stakeholders,[114] any of whom could derail the implementation process.

There are several interpersonal and social dynamics to consider when discussing organizational readiness, as well as a number of theories that inform this issue. For example, social information processing asserts that members of a team look to one another for clues on issues such as change in an organization, and suggests that an individual's readiness to change may be shaped by the readiness of peers.[115] Social cognitive theory suggests that when organizational readiness for change is high, organizational members are more likely to initiate change and exert greater efforts and persistence for change.[116,117] Motivation theory adds that when organizational readiness for change is high, members will exhibit prosocial, change-related behaviors that exceed job requirements.[106,118] Based on these theories, researchers have explored mechanisms for creating readiness for change in organizations. Several key change beliefs that lead to organizational readiness for change have been identified,[106,119,120] which are outlined below. In addition, examples of how each of the key change beliefs can be applied during implementation are included based on a current study by the first author on a dynamic adaption process for implementing an EBP in several counties throughout California.[121] This implementation study involves an adaptation resource team (comprised of investigators, EBP developers and trainers, county administrators, agency representatives, and clinical supervisors) that works to increase participating counties' readiness for change before beginning implementation and for shepherding the implementation process and problem solving as issues and challenges arise during the implementation process.

- **Change valence** refers to whether employees think the change being implemented is beneficial or worthwhile for them personally.[106,120] In an effort to create change valence among organizational members, change agents should discuss with employees the positive results of the change (e.g., improved patient or client outcomes) as well as any negative consequences should the implementation fail (e.g., as possible layoffs).[122] One potential benefit for many health care workers is the ability to include certification in a new intervention or technology on their resume, thus becoming more competitive in the job market. In fact, in our experience with EBP implementation, service providers in one agency were eligible to remain employed in their agency during a large funding cut primarily because they had been trained in a specific EBP.
- **Change efficacy**, the degree to which employees think they are capable of implementing a change, is another key belief in creating organizational readiness for change. When deciding whether they are capable of implementing a new practice, employees consider the task demands, availability of resources, and current situational factors.[106] Change advocates should include employees in activities, such as planning meetings, in order to increase their collective confidence in their ability to implement and manage the change.[123] They should focus on communicating to employees that training and support will be available throughout the implementation process and through the Sustainment phase. Some agencies participating in the dynamic adaptation implementation project decreased their service providers' caseloads by about 50%, which allowed staff more time to prepare for using the new intervention with clients. However, it was also clear that these issues needed to be balanced by outer-context exigencies including productivity and workflow requirements.
- **Discrepancy** refers to an employee's belief that organizational change is needed due to a gap between the organization's current state and some

desired end state. Organizational change agents may use external contextual factors, such as changes in economic conditions or new competition in the field, in order to create discrepancy beliefs.[124] A counterintuitive strategy is that of creating and spreading dissatisfaction among employees so they will perceive the discrepancy indirectly and come to perceive a need for change.[125] Once employees perceive a discrepancy in their workplace, they are likely to be motivated to lessen the discrepancy. For example, if there is an unacceptable level of iatrogenic effects of hospitalization on patients, leaders may communicate directly with organizational members about why an EBP was selected for implementation (i.e., how the decision makers think it will improve the current organizational state) to decrease the perceived discrepancy in quality-of-care targets and actual quality of care. One of the counties participating in the dynamic adaptation implementation project will be including service providers that are currently successful in the community and satisfied in their roles. As such, there may be a belief that the change to an EBP is not needed. The researchers and change agents within the county are working with all stakeholders to demonstrate a discrepancy between usual care and the EBP and use the other key change beliefs in order to capitalize on the perception that a service quality gap exists.

• **Principal support** is the last key belief, in which formal leaders and opinion leaders in the organization are committed to the successful implementation of a given change. This is highly related to the previously discussed notion of creating a positive implementation climate through strategic leader behaviors. Opinion leaders can promote organizational change, such as the implementation of EBP,[126] through the mechanisms described above. However, it is also beneficial to include employees in change efforts, as this has been shown to also increase motivation for organizational change.[127] A leader's ability to recognize and address individual staff members' motivations and attitudes[99] may also facilitate buy-in to strategic objectives such as EBP adoption and implementation. In some cases, a key leader can impact an entire organization or county. For example, a system leader in one county involved in the dynamic adaptation implementation study believed in the importance of using EBP in the community and was invested in its proper implementation. This leader was able to create an infrastructure for effective implementation that included developing a practical referral process, having funding lines in place, and making staff available to begin providing EBP immediately after initial training. The leader was also available to quickly solve significant problems as they arose during implementation and sustainment.

Organizational readiness for change, including the four aspects of readiness for change discussed above, can lead to better staff buy-in and willingness to adopt organizational change. Together with the organizational characteristics of culture, climate, and leadership, organizational readiness for change sets the stage for the implementation of EBP and specifically impacts the most proximal predictor of implementation behaviors: staff attitudes toward EBP.

■ ATTITUDES TOWARD EVIDENCE-BASED PRACTICE

Staff and leader attitudes toward EBP are important aspects to consider when implementing manualized treatments in health care settings. Attitudes toward EBP can be predicted by a number of organizational characteristics including the culture and climate of an organization,[128] leadership,[63] and the level of organizational support for EBP that is provided by the organization.[55] In addition, organizational characteristics such as transformational leadership can create a climate for innovation that is associated with better uptake of innovation,[129] better workplace and patient outcomes,[130] and more positive provider attitudes toward EBP.[13] In addition, Dobbins[131] has suggested that attitudes toward the use of research or an organizational "research culture" is a key factor in employee attitudes toward change. As noted above, organizational climate can be closely linked to employee attitudes and behaviors. It is important to consider the role of attitudes along with other factors such as behavioral intentions,[132] provider self-efficacy[122] and motivations, incentives, and infrastructure to support effective provider behavior change.

Addressing the issues discussed above is critical when considering change efforts related to EBP implementation. There are, however, additional approaches that come from models of culture and climate change and quality improvement and have more to do with strategies for the process of organizational change. These approaches are described next.

■ ORGANIZATIONAL DEVELOPMENT AND CHANGE

Barriers to health care provision arise not only from insufficient resources and the culture and climate of organizations, but also from issues along classic quality dimensions of service delivery. Too often, health care services fail to be efficient, timely, well organized, evidence based, and client centered.[133] Thus, attempts have been made to improve health care and social services via process improvement approaches that are drawn from fields outside of health care, such as organizational development and engineering.[134]

Organizational Culture and Climate

A recent systematic review of organizational culture change in health care settings found only two examples of empirical studies.[41] There is, however, work on organizational change being conducted in allied health care settings. One example of an organizational intervention that specifically addresses organizational culture and climate change has been developed by Charles Glisson and colleagues. The organizational intervention, called ARC (Availability, Responsiveness and Continuity), uses trained change agents to support the implementation of innovative practices in social and mental health services for children.[3] One major component of the ARC model is improving service provider behaviors and attitudes, flexibility, and openness to service improvements such as EBP.[54] Change agents work to develop positive staff attitudes that may promote openness to change and the adoption of effective practices, and this approach could be utilized to designate a EBP as a solution to a previously perceived problem area for effective services in the organization,[34] which coincides with the discrepancy notion discussed in the previous section. Change agents might also develop and maintain interest in new practices by providing information about EBP, resolving problems in the implementation process, and facilitating communication regarding implementation.[34] The ARC model has been effective in improving organizational factors such as organizational climate and in decreasing staff turnover rates.[34,135] The model has also been associated with significantly improved client outcomes and better outcomes when implemented in conjunction with EBP, compared with implementation of EBP without the ARC model.[54]

Process Improvement

Process improvement approaches are business management strategies that aim to improve efficiency by improving specific organizational processes usually for explicit outcomes or targets.[136] These efforts originated in the manufacturing sector and became prominent with the advent of such approaches as Six Sigma[137] and Lean thinking.[138] Typically intended to reduce manufacturing defects and increase the speed of manufacturing production, process improvement strategies have also been applied to health care and social service delivery.[139]

The application of improvement strategies can be challenging due to the high degree of variability in service delivery processes across different types of organizations and because culture change within service organizations is particularly difficult.[140] Improvement efforts typically include an emphasis on the following basic principles: quality leadership, focus on process, continuous improvement, evidence-based decision making, and a systems approach to management.[133] According to the World Health Organization (WHO), process improvement is both a philosophy and a set of technical methods, which includes a systematic review of delivery processes, operations research, teamwork improvement, the use of data and measurement, and the use of benchmarking.[141] Process improvement frequently relies on Plan-Do-Study-Act (PDSA) cycles that allow organizations to experiment with, implement, measure, and evaluate incremental change (or lack thereof) in relatively short periods of time.[133,136,142] Health care–specific process improvement strategies include reduction of medical errors,[143,144] decreases in admission and other wait times,[145] dissemination of clinical practices and guidelines,[146,147] improvement of patient discharge processes,[148] and improvement in hiring practices.[141,149]

One example of a widespread process improvement effort is the Institute for Healthcare Improvement's (IHI) Breakthrough Series, which intends to help health care organizations make specific clinical and operational process improvements. This series has undertaken a number of initiatives, including improving perinatal care, improving outcomes for high-risk and critically ill patients, and improving flow through acute care settings (see IHI website for examples). In their Pain Management collaborative with the Veterans Administration Health Care Administration (VA), they attempted to improve pain management across 70 clinical teams in the VA system. They documented significant decreases in patient pain ratings, increases in pain care plans for patients, and increases in proportion of patients provided with pain care materials.[150]

Another type of process improvement is the VA system Quality Enhancement Research Initiative (QUERI).[151,152] There are nine different QUERIs, and each focuses on specific health or clinical care targets. For example, there are QUERI divisions to address chronic heart failure, diabetes, HIV/hepatitis, ischemic heart disease, mental health, polytrauma and blast-related injuries, spinal cord injury, stroke, and substance use disorders. The QUERI approach utilizes a six-step model focused on improving care through the implementation of new practices.[153] The six steps include identifying the disease or health care problem, identifying the best practices or EBPs to address the problem, defining existing practice patterns and outcomes across the hospital or service system, identifying and implementing an intervention or interventions to implement and/or promote best practices, using data to document that new practices improve outcomes, and documenting that outcomes are associated with improving the patient's quality of life.

Another example of process improvement comes from the WHO. In an attempt to improve the treatment of chronic conditions in developing nations, the WHO and the MacColl Institute for Healthcare Innovation undertook a collaborative effort called the Innovative Care for Chronic Conditions (ICCC) framework.[154] This effort aims to reorganize health care systems in order to provide integrated and coordinated care.

The Network for the Improvement of Addiction Treatment (NIATx), which helps addiction treatment centers implement process improvement strategies,[139,155] applies process improvement principles such as continuous improvement, meeting customer needs, reducing variation and error, and using PDSA cycles to make incremental improvements. In one investigation of 13 addiction treatment agencies that instituted their recommendations, they demonstrated reduced wait time to treatment entry, and significant improvements in retention in care.[139]

Despite the promises involved in the application of organizational improvement techniques to health care settings, several challenges remain. First, these initiatives may occur in systems that are facing other competing priorities and demands, including legislative mandates, health care regulations, organizational policies, and existing external and internal networks. Thus, strategies for implementing process improvement techniques should address these realities. For example, it may be difficult to obtain buy-in from physicians and other medical personnel to take part in quality improvement measures when clinical and administrative demands are present.[156] Also, it may be difficult to embed quality improvement initiatives on an ongoing basis or as part of the culture of the organizations. Optimally, process improvement will be integrated into the health care or social service system and not be seen as an external time-limited "program."[141] Finally, process improvement strategies may be expensive and time consuming, and require substantial commitment from stakeholders.

In sum, it is critical that organizations not only focus on the processes for implementing EBPs but also to take into account the context in which those processes take place. The danger is the perception that addressing organizational and contextual issues requires additional time, effort, and expense, and might not be worth the investment. While addressing organizational context can be challenging, it is imperative for effective and sustained EBP implementation. In order for patients and clients to benefit from care, the best interventions that science has to offer must be implemented; however, in order for the implementation to be successful, the organizational contexts that provide the fertile ground for EBPs to take root must be addressed.

■ CONCLUSIONS

Taken as a whole, both organizational characteristics and specific organizational strategies are important for the effective D&I of EBPs in health and allied health care settings, as well as mental health, alcohol/drug treatment, and social service settings. This chapter summarizes some of the most critical organizational factors and strategies likely to impact successful EBP implementation. While there are myriad approaches to supporting organizational development and change, this chapter focuses on issues supported by relevant scientific literatures, and those most germane to EBP implementation in health care and related settings.

Certain organizational factors are likely to be more or less important across the phases of implementation. For example, effective and committed leadership may be particularly important during Exploration and Adoption Decision/Preparation phases.[23] Various organizational factors may have the most impact for particular types of D&I efforts or those focused on the unique aspects of a particular context. For example, leadership may impact D&I progress and process in diverse implementation contexts.[66] Focusing on improving organizational climate for implementation may also be more or less important for a particular team or workgroup that is implementing an EBP within an organization. For example, a given team might be implementing an EBP while the rest of the organization is continuing stable operations. Conversely, if the entire organization is becoming more committed to and focused on the use of EBP, then more global organizational culture and climate change strategies may be appropriate.

With the realization that development of organizational cultures, climates, and contexts supportive of EBP implementation takes time and concerted effort, there is hope that EBP implementation can be effectively pursued in diverse service settings. Understanding organizational context and applying organizational development strategies can aid in the improvement of health and mental health care, as well as social services. In order for patients and clients to benefit from care, the best interventions that science has to offer must be implemented effectively. Organizational change can lead to improved implementation outcomes[157,158] and ultimately improved clinical outcomes.[54] These goals can be achieved if we can create the organizational contexts that support EBP implementation.

While the concepts and constructs discussed in this chapter appear at times to be quite abstract, it is important to remember that they are created and are maintained by the behaviors, decisions, policies, and procedures developed and supported by people in the organization. In the same vein, they can be changed by individuals, groups, and teams with the vision, determination, and persistence to shepherd the organizational changes needed to implement and sustain EBPs. Any given implementation has the potential to improve the care needed by individuals, groups, and populations. It starts with a vision of how health care can be improved, and this can be global in scope or relate to a specific disease, its treatment, and specific subpopulations. While there is evidence that EBPs tend to be robust across populations, it is important for organizations to make the changes necessary to deliver those interventions to the right people at the right time. This is done by people in organizations creating organizational contexts open to change and able to implement and sustain that change.

It is imperative that those responsible for the implementation of EBPs take action to first identify the organizational issues to address. Then effective organizational change strategies must be identified, utilized, and consistently applied in order to improve the culture and climate of the organization to more effectively implement effective health care innovations and practices. The promise of this course of action is improved care, improved health, and improved lives for those we serve.

■ ACKNOWLEDGMENTS

Preparation of this chapter was supported by NIMH grants R21MH082731 and R01MH072961 (PI: Aarons), P30MH074678 (PI: Landsverk), and by the Chadwick Center at Rady Children's Hospital San Diego.

SUGGESTED READINGS

Aarons GA, Horwitz S, Hurlburt M, Landsverk J. Advancing a conceptual model of evidence-based practice implementation in public service sectors. *Administration and Policy in Mental Health and Mental Health Services Research*. 2011;38:4–23.
> *Presents a multilevel, four-phase model of the implementation and sustainment process as applied to public sector services.*

Aarons GA, Sommerfeld DH, Walrath-Greene CM. Evidence-based practice implementation: The impact of public vs. private sector organization type on organizational support, provider attitudes, and adoption of evidence-based practice. *Implementation Science*. 2009;4:1–13.
> *Examines the impact of organization type and organizational support for EBP on providers' use of and attitudes toward EBP.*

Ashkanasy NM, Broadfoot LE, Falkus S. Questionnaire measures of organizational culture. In: Ashkanasy NM, Wilderom CPM, Peterson MF, eds. *Handbook of Organizational Culture and Climate*. Thousand Oaks, CA: Sage; 2000: 131–147.
> *Presents a measures of organizational culture based on the ten major dimensions found in their comprehensive review of the literature on organizational culture.*

Klein KJ, Sorra JS. The challenge of innovation implementation. *Academy of Management Review*. 1996;21:1055–1080.
> *Discusses implementation outcomes and presents a model in which implementation effectiveness is a function of organizational climate for implementation and fit of the innovation with users' values.*

Schein E. *Organizational Culture and Leadership*. 3rd ed. San Francisco: Jossey-Bass; 2004.
> *A comprehensive review of organizational culture and leadership.*

Schneider B. *Organizational climate and culture.* San Francisco: Jossey-Bass; 1990.
  A comprehensive review of organizational climate and culture.
Sobo EJ, Bowman C, Halloran J, Aarons G, Asch S, Gifford AL. Enhancing organizational change and improvement prospects: Lessons from an HIV testing intervention for veterans. *Human Organization.* 2008;67:443–453.
  Presents a case study to examine how the structures and processes of a complex health care organizations impact implementation of an innovation.
Weiner BJ, Amick H, Lee SD. Conceptualization and measurement of organizational readiness for change: A review of the literature in health services research and other fields. *Medical Care Research and Review.* 2008;65:379–436.
  A comprehensive review of organizational readiness for change based on research in numerous organizational contexts.

SELECTED WEBSITES AND TOOLS
Institute for Healthcare Improvement

http://www.ihi.org/ihi provides resources for process improvement in health care.

Veterans Affairs Healthcare System Quality Enhancement Research Initiative
http://www.queri.research.va.gov/describes VA QUERI program.

Mind Garden

http://www.mindgarden.com/translead.htm#prompt2 provides information on the Multifactor Leadership Questionnaire. The authorized measures of the Full Range Leadership model are available from Mindgarden for research and/or applied purposes.

■ REFERENCES

1. Aarons GA, Hurlburt M, Horwitz SM. Advancing a conceptual model of evidence-based practice implementation in child welfare. *Adm Policy Ment Health and Ment Health Serv Res.* 2011;38:4–23.
2. Damschroder L, Aron D, Keith R, Kirsh S, Alexander J, Lowery J. Fostering implementation of health services research findings into practice: A consolidated framework for advancing implementation science. *Implement Sci.* 2009;4:50.
3. Glisson C, Schoenwald S. The ARC organizational and community intervention strategy for implementing evidence-based children's mental health treatments. *Ment Health Serv Res.* 2005;7:243–259.
4. Greenhalgh T, Robert G, Macfarlane F, Bate P, Kyriakidou O. Diffusion of innovations in service organizations: Systematic review and recommendations. *Milbank Q.* 2004;82:581–629.
5. Bond G, Drake R, McHugo G, Rapp C, Whitley R. Strategies for improving fidelity in the national evidence-based practices project. *Res Soc Work Pract.* 2009;19:569.
6. Torrey WC, Drake RE, Dixon L, et al. Implementing evidence-based practices for persons with severe mental illnesses. *Psychiatr Serv.* 2001;52:45–50.
7. Mendel P, Meredith L, Schoenbaum M, Sherbourne C, Wells K. Interventions in organizational and community context: A framework for building evidence on dissemination and implementation in health services research. *Adm Policy Ment Health and Ment Health Serv Res.* 2008;35:21–37.

8. Jacobs JA, Dodson EA, Baker EA, Deshpande AD, Brownson RC. Barriers to evidence-based decision making in public health: A national survey of chronic disease practitioners. *Public Health Rep.* 2010;125:736–742.
9. Brudney JL, Hebert FT. State agencies and their environments: Examining the influence of important external actors. *J Polit.* 1987;49:186–206.
10. Provan KG, Huang K, Milward HB. The evolution of structural embeddedness and organizational social outcomes in a centrally governed health and human services network. *Publ Admin Res Theor.* 2009;19:873–893.
11. Schein E. *Organizational Culture and Leadership.* 3rd ed. San Francisco: Jossey-Bass; 2004.
12. Priestland A, Hanig R. Developing first-level leaders. *Harv Bus Rev.* 2005;83:112–120.
13. Aarons GA, Sommerfeld DH, Willging C. The soft underbelly of system change: The role of leadership and organizational climate in turnover during statewide behavioral health reform. *Psychological Services.* 2011:8:269–281.
14. Aarons GA, Sommerfeld DH. Transformational leadership, team climate for innovation, and staff attitudes toward adopting evidence-based practice. Paper presented at: Academy of Management, 2008, August; Anaheim, CA.
15. McLeod BD, Southam-Gerow MA, Weisz JR. Conceptual and methodological issues in treatment integrity measurement. *School Psych Rev.* 2009;38:541–546.
16. Taxman FS, Friedman PD. Fidelity and adherence at the transition point: Theoretically driven experiments. *J Exp Criminol.* 2009;5:219–226.
17. Aarons GA, Sommerfeld DH, Hecht DB, Silovsky JF, Chaffin MJ. The impact of evidence-based practice implementation and fidelity monitoring on staff turnover: Evidence for a protective effect. *J Consult Clin Psychol.* 2009;77:270–280.
18. Aarons GA, Fettes DL, Flores LE, Sommerfeld DH. Evidence-based practice implementation and staff emotional exhaustion in children's services. *Behav Res Ther.* 2009;47:954–960.
19. Palinkas LA, Aarons GA. A view from the top: Executive and management challenges in a statewide implementation of an evidence-based practice to reduce child neglect. *Int J Child Health Hum Dev.* 2009;2:47–55.
20. Sproull L. Organizational learning. In: Bird Schoonhoven C, Dobbin F, eds. *Standford's Organization Theory Renaissance, 1970-2000.* Vol 28. Bingley, UK: Emerald Group Publishing Limited; 2010:59–69.
21. Van Noord I, Bruijne MC, Twisk WR. The relationship between patient safety culture and the implementation of organizational patient safety defences at emergency departments. *Int J Qual Health Care.* 2010;22:162–169.
22. Nutley SM, Davies HTO. Making a reality of evidence-based practice: Some lessons from the diffusion of innovations. *Public Money Manage.* 2001;20:35–42.
23. Aarons GA, Hurlburt M, Horwitz S. Advancing a conceptual model of evidence-based practice implementation in public service sectors. *Adm Policy Ment Health and Ment Health Serv Res.* 2011;38:4–23.
24. Verbeke W, Volgering M, Hessels M. Exploring the conceptual expansion within the field of organizational behaviour: Organizational climate and organizational culture. *J Manage Stud.* 1998;35:303–330.
25. Schein EH. Organizational culture. *Am Psychol.* 1990;45:109–119.
26. Rousseau DM. Normative beliefs in fund-raising organizations: Linking culture to organizational performance and individual responses. *Group Organ Stud.* 1990;15:448–460.

27. Cooke RA, Rousseau DM. Behavioral norms and expectations: A quantitative approach to the assessment of organizational culture. *Group Organ Stud.* 1988;13:245–273.
28. Denison DR. *Corporate Culture and Organizational Effectiveness.* New York: Wiley; 1990.
29. Denison DR, Neale W. *Denison Organizational Culture Survey.* Ann Arbor, MI: Denison Consulting; 2000.
30. Chatman J. Matching people and organizations: Selection and socialization in public accounting firms. *Adm Sci Q.* 1991;36:459–484.
31. O'Reilly CA, Chatman J, Caldwell DF. People and organizational culture: A profile comparison approach to assessing person-organization fit. *Acad Manage J.* 1991;34: 487–516.
32. Ashkanasy NM, Broadfoot LE, Falkus S. Questionnaire measures of organizational culture. In: Ashkanasy NM, Wilderom CPM, Peterson MF, eds. *Handbook of Organizational Culture and Climate.* Thousand Oaks, CA: Sage; 2000:131–145.
33. Cameron KS, Quinn RE. *Diagnosing and Changing Organizational Culture: Based on the Competing Values Framework.* San Francisco: Jossey-Bass; 2006.
34. Glisson C. The organizational context of children's mental health services. *Clin Child Fam Psychol Rev.* 2002;5:233–253.
35. Glisson C, Landsverk J, Schoenwald S, et al. Assessing the organizational social context (OSC) of mental health services: Implications for research and practice. *Admin Policy Ment Health and Ment Health Serv Res Special Issue: Improving Mental Health Services.* Mar 2008;35:98–113.
36. Deal TW, Kennedy AA. *Corporate Cultures.* Reading, MA: Addison-Wesley; 1982.
37. Peters TJ, Waterman RH. *In Search of Excellence.* New York: Harper & Row; 1982.
38. Siehl C, Martin J. Organizational culture: The key to financial performance? In: Schneider B, ed. *Organizational Climate and Culture.* San Francisco: Jossey-Bass; 1990:241–281.
39. Larson EL, Early E, Cloonan P, Sugrue S, Parides M. An organizational climate intervention associated with increased handwashing and decreased nosocomial infections. *Behav Med.* 2000;26:14–22.
40. Kinjerski V, Skrypnek BJ. The promise of spirit at work: Increasing job satisfaction and organizational commitment and reducing turnover and absenteeism in long-term care. *J Gerontol Nurs.* 2008;34:17–25.
41. Parmelli E, Flodgren G, Beyer F, Baillie N, Schaafsma ME, Eccles MP. The effectiveness of strategies to change organisational culture to improve healthcare performance: A systematic review. *Implement Sci.* 2011;6.
42. Kotter JP, Heskett JL. *Corporate Culture and Performance.* New York: The Free Press; 1992.
43. Wilderom CPM, Glunk U, Maslowski R. Organizational culture as a predictor of organizational performance. In: Ashkanasy NM, Wilderom CPM, Peterson MF, eds. *Handbook of Organizational Culture and Climate.* Thousand Oaks, CA: Sage; 2000:193–209.
44. Lewin K, Lippitt R, White RK. Patterns of aggressive behavior in experimentally created "social climates." *J Soc Psychol.* 1939;10:271–299.
45. McGregor DM. *The Human Side of Enterprise.* New York: McGraw-Hill; 1960.
46. Guion RM. A note on organizational climate. *Organ Behav Hum Perform.* 1973;9: 120–125.
47. Johannesson RE. Some problems in the measurement of organizational climate. *Organ Behav Hum Perform.* 1973;10:118–144.

48. Schneider B. *Organizational Climate and Culture.* San Francisco: Jossey-Bass; 1990.
49. James LR, Choi CC, Ko C-HE, et al. Organizational and psychological climate: A review of theory and research. *Eur J Work Organ Psy.* 2008;17:5–32.
50. Schneider B, Ehrhart MG, Macey WA. Organizational climate research: Achievements and the road ahead. In: Ashkanasy NM, Wilderom CPM, Peterson MF, eds. *Handbook of Organizational Culture and Climate.* 2nd ed. Newbury Park, CA: Sage; 2011:29–49.
51. James LA, James LR. Integrating work environment perceptions: Explorations into the measurement of meaning. *J Appl Psychol.* 1989;74:739–751.
52. Klein KJ, Sorra JS. The challenge of innovation implementation. *Acad Manage Rev.* 1996;21:1055–1080.
53. Glisson C, Hemmelgarn A. The effects of organizational climate and interorganizational coordination on the quality and outcomes of children's service systems. *Child Abuse Negl.* 1998;22:401–421.
54. Glisson C, Schoenwald SK, Hemmelgarn A, et al. Randomized trial of MST and ARC in a two-level evidence-based treatment implementation strategy. *J Consult Clin Psychol.* 2010;78:537–550.
55. Aarons GA, Sommerfeld DH, Walrath-Greene CM. Evidence-based practice implementation: The impact of public vs. private sector organization type on organizational support, provider attitudes, and adoption of evidence-based practice. *Implement Sci.* 2009;4:1–13.
56. Klein KJ, Conn AB, Sorra JS. Implementing computerized technology: An organizational analysis. *J Appl Psychol.* 2001;86:811–824.
57. West MA, Wallace M. Innovation in health care teams. *Eur J Soc Psychol.* 1991;21: 303–315.
58. Siegel SM, Kaemmerer WF. Measuring the perceived support for innovation in organizations. *J Appl Psychol.* 1978;63:553–562.
59. Avolio BJ. Examining the Full Range Model of Leadership: Looking back to transform forward. In: Day DV, Zaccaro SJ, Halpin SM, eds. *Leader Development for Transforming Organizations.* Mahwah, NJ: Lawrence Erlbaum Associates, Inc.; 2004.
60. Howell JM, Avolio BJ. Transformational leadership, transactional leadership, locus of control, and support for innovation: Key predictors of consolidated-business-unit performance. *J Appl Psychol.* 1993;78:891–902.
61. Bass BM, Avolio BJ, Jung DI, Berson Y. Predicting unit performance by assessing transformational and transactional leadership. *J Appl Psychol.* 2003;88:207–218.
62. McDaniel C, Wolf GA. Transformational leadership in nursing service: A test of theory. *J Nurs Adm.* 1992;22:60–65.
63. Aarons GA, Palinkas LA. Implementation of evidence-based practice in child welfare: Service provider perspectives. *Adm Policy Ment Health and Ment Health Serv Res.* 2007;34:411–419.
64. Corrigan PW, Garman AN. Transformational and transactional leadership skills for mental health teams. *Community Ment Health J.* 1999;35:301–312.
65. Drucker PF. *Managing the Nonprofit Organization.* New York: HarperCollins Publishers, Inc; 1990.
66. Goodman RM. A construct for building the capacity of community-based initiatives in racial and ethnic communities: A qualitative cross-case analysis. *J Public Health Manag Pract.* 2009;15:E1–E8.

67. Avolio BJ, Walumbwa FO, Weber TJ. Leadership: Current theories, research, and future directions. *Annu Rev Psychol.* 2009;60:421–449.
68. Bass BM, Avolio BJ. *The Multifactor Leadership Questionnaire.* Palo Alto, CA: Consulting Psychologists Press; 1989.
69. Avolio BJ, Bass BM, Jung DI. Re-examining the components of transformational and transactional leadership using the Multifactor Leadership Questionnaire. *J Occup Organ Psychol.* 1999;72:441–462.
70. Jung D, Sosik JJ. Who are the spellbinders? Identifying personal attributes of charistmatic leaders. *J Leadersh Stud.* 2006;12:12–26.
71. Judge TA, Piccolo RF. Transformational and transactional leadership: A meta-analytic test of their relative validity. *J Appl Psychol.* 2004;89:755–768.
72. Bass BM, Avolio BJ. *Training full range leadership.* Menlo Park, CA: Mind Garden;1999.
73. Skogstad A, Einarsen S, Torsheim T, Aasland MS, Hetland H. The destructiveness of laissez-faire leadership behavior. *J Occup Health Psychol.* 2007;12:80–92.
74. DeGroot T, Kiker DS, Cross TC. A meta-analysis to review organizational outcomes related to charismatic leadership. *Can J Adm Sciences.* 2000;17:356–371.
75. Dumdum UR, Lowe KB, Avolio BJ. A meta-analysis of transformational and transactional leadership correlates of effectiveness and satisfaction: An update and extension. In: Avolio BJ, Yammarino FJ, eds. *Transformational and Charismatic Leadership: The Road Ahead.* Oxford: Elsevier Science; 2002.
76. Lowe KB, Kroeck KG, Sivasubramaniam N. Effectiveness correlates of transformational and transactional leadership: A meta-analytic review of the MLQ literature. *Leadersh Q.* 1996;7:385–425.
77. Gasper JM. *Transformational Leadership: An Integrative Review of the Literature.* Kalamazoo, MI: Western Michigan University; 1992.
78. Walumbwa FO, Orwa B, Wang P, Lawler JJ. Transformational leadership, organizational commitment, and job satisfaction: A comparative study of Kenyan and U.S. financial firms. *Hum Resour Manage Q.* 2005;16:235–256.
79. MacKenzie SB, Podsakoff PM, Rich GA. Transformational and transactional leadership and salesperson performance. *J Acad Mark Science.* 2001;29:115–134.
80. Zohar D. Modifying supervisory practices to improve subunit safety: A leadership-based intervention model. *J Appl Psychol.* 2002;87:156–163.
81. Corrigan PW, Diwan S, Campion J, Rashid F. Transformational leadership and the mental health team. *Adm Policy Ment Health.* 2002;30:97–108.
82. Griffith J. Relation of principal transformational leadership to school staff job satisfaction, staff turnover, and school performance. *J Educ Adm.* 2004;42:333–356.
83. Kuoppala J, Lamminpaa A, Liira J, Vainio H. Leadership, job well-being, and health effects—A systematic review and meta-analysis. *J Occup Environ Med.* 2008;50:904–915.
84. Constable JF, Russell DW. The effect of social support and the work environment upon burnout among nurses. *J Human Stress.* 1986;12:20–26.
85. Geyer ALJ, Steyrer JM. Transformational leadership and objective performance in banks. *Appl Psychol: Int Rev.* 1998;47:397–420.
86. Frischer J, Larsson K. Laissez-faire in research education—An inquiry into a Swedish doctoral program. *High Educ Policy.* 2000;13:131–155.
87. Kelloway EK, Mullen J, Francis L. Divergent effects of transformational and passive leadership on employee safety. *J Occup Health Psychol.* 2006;11:76–86.

88. Antonakis J, Avolio BJ, Sivasubramaniam N. Context and leadership: An examination of the nine-factor full-range leadership theory using the multifactor leadership questionnaire. *Leadersh Q.* 2003;14:261–295.

89. Koh WL, Steers RM, Terborg JR. The effects of transformational leadership on teacher attitudes and student performance in Singapore. *J Organ Behav.* 1995;16: 319–333.

90. Garman AN, Davis-Lenane D, Corrigan PW. Factor structure of the transformational leadership model in human service teams. *J Organ Behav.* 2003;24:803–812.

91. Avolio BJ, Bass BM. *The Full Range of Leadership Development: Basic and Advanced Manuals.* Binghamton, NY: Bass, Avolio, & Associates; 1991.

92. Bass BM, Riggio RE. The development of transformational leadership. *Transformational Leadership.* 2nd ed. Mahwah, NJ: Lawrence Erlbaum Associates, Inc.; 2006:142–166.

93. Crookall P. Management of inmate workshops: A field test of transformational and situational leadership. London, ON, Canada: University of Western Ontario; 1989.

94. Avolio BJ, Bass BM. *Evaluate the impact of transformational leadership training at individual, group, organizational and community levels.* (Final report to the W. K. Kellog Foundation). Binghamton, NY: Binghamton University;1994.

95. Dvir T, Eden D, Avolio BJ, Shamir B. Impact of transformational leadership on follower development and performance: A field experiment. *Acad Manage J.* 2002;45: 735–744.

96. Kelloway EK, Barling J, Helleur J. Enhancing transformational leadership: The role of training and feedback. *Leadership and Organization Development Journal.* 2000;21: 145–149.

97. Dettmann JR, Beehr T. Training transformational leadership: A field experiment in the non-profit sector. Paper presented at: Meeting of the Society for Industrial and Organizational Psychology, July 2004; Chicago.

98. Barling J, Weber TJ, Kelloway EK. Effects of transformational leadership training on attitudinal and financial outcomes: A field experiment. *J Appl Psychol.* 1996;81: 827–832.

99. Aarons GA. Transformational and transactional leadership: Association with attitudes toward evidence-based practice. *Psychiatr Serv.* 2006;57:1162–1169.

100. Glisson C, Durick M. Predictors of job satisfaction and organizational commitment in human service organizations. *Adm Sci Q.* 1988;33:61–81.

101. Corrigan PW, Garman AN, Lam C, Leary M. What mental health teams want in their leaders. *Adm Policy Ment Health.* 1998;26:111–123.

102. Corrigan PW, Lickey SE, Campion J, Rashid F. Mental health team leadership and consumers' satisfaction and quality of life. *Psychiatr Serv.* 2000;51:781–785.

103. Aarons GA, Wells RS, Zagursky K, Fettes DL, Palinkas LA. Implementing evidence-based practice in community mental health agencies: A multiple stakeholder analysis. *Am J Public Health.* 2009;99:2087–2095.

104. Aarons GA, Ehrhart MG, Horowitz JD. Leadership to facilitate evidence-based practice implementation in healthcare organizations. Paper presented at: Academy of Management Annual Meeting, August 2010; Montreal.

105. Lehman WE, Greener JM, Simpson DD. Assessing organizational readiness for change. *J Subst Abuse Treat.* 2002;22:197–209.

106. Weiner BJ. A theory of organizational readiness for change. *Implement Sci.* 2009;19:67.

107. Weiner BJ, Amick H, Lee SD. Conceptualization and measurement of organizational readiness for change: A review of the literature in health services research and other fields. *Med Care Res Rev.* 2008;65:379–436.

108. Lewin K. Frontiers in group dynamics: Concept, method and reality in social science; social eqilibria and social change. *Hum Relat.* 1947;1:5–41.

109. Armenakis AA, Harris SG. Crafting a change message to create transformational readiness. *J Organ Change Manage.* 2002;15:169–183.

110. Beckhard R, Harris RT. *Organizational Transitions: Managing Complex Change.* Reading, MA: Addison-Wesley; 1987.

111. Kimberly JR, Quinn RE. *Managing Organizational Transitions.* Homewood, IL: Irwin; 1984.

112. Kotter JP. *Leading Change.* Cambridge, MA: Harvard Business School Press; 1996.

113. Edmondson AC, Bohmer RM, Pisano GP. Disrupted routines: Team learning and new technology implementation in hospitals. *Adm Sci Q.* 2001;46:685–716.

114. Sobo EJ, Bowman C, Halloran J, Aarons G, Asch S, Gifford AL. Enhancing organizational change and improvement prospects: Lessons from an HIV testing intervention for veterans. *Hum Org.* 2008;67:443–453.

115. Griffin RW, Bateman TS, Wayne SJ, Head TC. Objective and social factors as determinants of task perceptions and responses: An integrated perspective and empirical investigation. *Acad Manage J.* 1987;30:501–523.

116. Bandura A. Social cognitive theory: An agentic perspective. *Annu Rev Psychol.* 2001;52:1–26.

117. Gist ME, Mitchell TR. Self-efficacy: A theoretical analysis of its determinants and malleability. *Acad Manage Rev.* 1992;17:183–211.

118. Herscovitch L, Meyer JP. Commitment to organizational change: Extension of a three-component model. *J Appl Psychol.* 2002;87:474–487.

119. Holt DT, Armenakis AA, Feild HS, Harris SG. Readiness for organizational change: The systematic development of a scale. *J Appl Behav Sci.* 2007;43:232–255.

120. Armenakis AA, Harris SG. Reflections: Our journey in organizational change research and practice. *J Change Manage.* 2009;9:127–142.

121. Aarons GA, Green AE. A dynamic adaptation approach towards implementation of evidence based practice. Paper presented at: The Quality of Behavioral Healthcare: A Drive for Change through Research, April, 2010; Clearwater Beach, FL.

122. Bandura A. Self-efficacy mechanism in human agency. *Am Psychol.* 1982;37:122–147.

123. Armenakis AA, Harris SG, Mossholder KW. Creating organizational readiness to change. *Hum Relat.* 1993;46:681–704.

124. Pettigrew AM. Context and action in the transformation of the firm. *J Manage Stud.* 1987;24:649–670.

125. Jex SM, Spector PE. The generalizability of social information processing to organizational settings: A summary of two field experiments. *Percept Mot Skills.* 1989;69:883–893.

126. Flodgren G, Parmelli E, Doumit G, Gattellari M, O'Brien MA, Grimshaw J, Eccles MP. Local opinion leaders: effects on professional practice and health care outcomes. *Cochrane Database of Systematic Reviews* 2011, Issue 8. Art. No.: CD000125. DOI:10.1002/14651858.CD000125.pub4.

127. Coch L, French JRP. Overcoming resistance to change. In: Burke WW, Lake DG, Paine JW, eds. *Organization Change: A Comprehensive Reader.* Hoboken, NJ: Jossey-Bass; 1965:341–363.

128. Aarons GA, Sawitzky AC. Organizational climate partially mediates the effect of culture on work attitudes and staff turnover in mental health services. *Adm Policy Ment Health and Ment Health Serv Res.* 2006;33:289–301.

129. Anderson NR, West MA. Measuring climate for work group innovation: Development and validation of the Team Climate Inventory. *J Organ Behav.* 1998;19:235–258.

130. Proudfoot J, Jayasinghe U, Holton C, et al. Team climate for innovation: What difference does it make in general practice? *Int J Qual Health Care.* 2007;19:164–169.

131. Dobbins M. Dissemination and use of research evidence for policy and practice: A framework for developing, implementing, and evaluating strategies. In: Rycroft-Malone J, Bucknall T, eds. *Models and Frameworks for Implementing Evidence-Based Practice: Linking Evidence to Action.* Oxford: Wiley-Blackwell; 2010:147–153.

132. Ajzen I, Fishbein M. The influence of attitudes on behavior. In: Albarracín D, Johnson BT, Zanna MP, eds. *The Handbook of Attitudes.* Mahwah, NJ: Lawrence Erlbaum Associates, Inc.; 2005:173–222.

133. Schneider A. How quality improvement in health care can help to achieve the Millennium Development Goals. *Bull World Health Organ.* 2006;84:259–260.

134. Ford JH, Green CA, Hoffman KA, et al. Process improvement needs in substance abuse treatment: Admissions walk-through results. *J Subst Abuse Treat.* 2007;33: 379–389.

135. Glisson C, Dukes D, Green P. The effects of the ARC organizational intervention on caseworker turnover, climate, and culture in children's service systems. *Child Abuse Negl.* 2006;30:849–854.

136. Evans AC, Rieckmann T, Fitzgerald MM, Gustafson DH. Teaching the NIATx model of process improvement as an evidence-based process. *J Teach Addict.* 2008;6:21–37.

137. Eckes G. *The Six Sigma Revolution: How General Electric and Others Turned Process into Profits.* New York: John Wiley & Sons; 2000.

138. George ML. *Lean Six Sigma for Service: How to Use Lean Speed & Six Sigma Quality to Improve Services and Transactions.* New York: McGraw-Hill; 2003.

139. McCarty D, Gustafson DH, Wisdom JP, et al. The network for the improvement of addiction treatment (NIATx): Enhancing access and retention. *Drug Alcohol Depend.* 2007;88:138–145.

140. Sehwail L, DeYong C. Six sigma in health care. *Leadersh Health Serv.* 2003;16:1–5.

141. Leatherman S, Ferris TG, Berwick D, Omaswa F, Crisp N. The role of quality improvement in strengthening health systems in developing countries. *Int J Qual Health Care.* 2010;22:237–243.

142. Ragsdale MA, Mueller J. Plan, do, study, act model to improve an orientation program. *J Nurs Care Qual.* 2005;20:268–272.

143. Leape LL, Berwick DM. Five years after *To Err Is Human*: What have we learned? *JAMA.* 2005;293:2384–2390.

144. Becher EC, Chassin MR. Improving quality, minimizing error: Making it happen. A five-point plan and why we need it. *Health Aff.* 2001;20:68–81.

145. Boe DT, Riley W, Parsons H. Improving service delivery in a county health department WIC clinic: An application of statistical process control techniques. *Am J Public Health.* 2009;99:1619–1625.

146. Rosenheck RA. Organizational process: A missing link between research and practice. *Psychiatr Serv.* 2001;52:1607–1612.

147. Pearson ML, Wu S, Schaefer J, et al. Assessing the implementation of the chronic care model in quality improvement collaboratives. *Health Serv Res.* 2005;40:978–996.

148. Kim CS, Spahlinger DA, Kin JM, Billi JE. Lean health care: What can hospitals learn from a world-class automaker? *J Hosp Med.* 2006;1:191–199.

149. De Koning H, Verver JPS, van den Heuvel J, Bisgaard S, Does RJMM. Lean six sigma in healthcare. *J Heathc Qual.* 2006;28:4–11.

150. Cleeland CS, Reyes-Gibby CC, Schall M, et al. Rapid improvement in pain management: The Veterans Health Administration and the Institute for Healthcare Improvement collaborative. *Clin J Pain.* 2003;19:298–305.

151. Demakis JG, McQueen L, Kizer KW, Feussner JR. Quality Enhancement Research Initiative (QUERI): A collaboration between research and clinical practice. *Medical Care.* 2000;38:17–25.

152. Rubenstein LV, Mittman BS, Yano EM, Mulrow CD. From understanding health care provider behavior to improving health care: The QUERI framework for quality improvement. *Med Care.* 2000;38:129–141.

153. Goetz MB, Bowman C, Hoang T, Anaya H, Osborn T, Gifford AL. Implementing and evaluating a regional strategy to improve testing rates in VA patients at risk for HIV, utilizing the QUERI process as a guiding framework: QUERI series. *Implement Sci.* 2008;3:16.

154. Epping-Jordan JE, Pruitt SD, Bengoa R. Improving the quality of health care for chronic conditions. *Qual Saf Health Care.* 2004;13:299–305.

155. McCarty D, Gustafson D, Capoccia VA, Cotter F. Improving care for the treatment of alcohol and drug disorders. *J Behav Health Serv Res.* 2009;36:52–60.

156. Kaluzny AD, McLaughlin CP, Kibbe DC. Continuous quality improvement in the clinical setting: Enhancing adoption. *Qual Manag Health Care.* 1992;1:37–44.

157. Dadich A. From bench to bedside: Methods that help clinicians use evidence-based practice. *Aust Psychol.* 2010;45:197–211.

158. Saldana L, Chamberlain P, Wang W, Brown CH. Predicting program start-up using the stages of implementation measure. *Adm Policy Ment Health and Ment Health Serv Res.* 2011.

8 Viewing Dissemination and Implementation Research through a Network Lens

■ DOUGLAS A. LUKE

■ INTRODUCTION

Dissemination and implementation (D&I) are complex social and organizational processes by which new scientific discoveries and advances can be translated and transferred to people, settings, and communities to affect and improve public health. Despite their complexity, D&I processes can be viewed as a type of information transmission. A new scientific discovery (or innovation) is a piece of information that needs to be transferred to a different part of society, which can put that information to use. It turns out that this type of information transmission has important structural and relational properties that can best be understood using a relatively new systems science tool: network analysis. The purpose of this chapter is to propose a network analytic model of D&I and illustrate how network analysis can be used both to study and shape D&I processes and outcomes. Understanding the D&I process more fully through network analysis can be an important domain of D&I research.

For an orienting example, consider the ride of Paul Revere, a part of American history that many of us learn about in primary school. On the evening of April 18th, 1775, Paul Revere and his compatriot William Dawes rode from Boston to Lexington, warning people of the mobilizing British forces. Paul Revere's ride is a classic dissemination problem: how to get new important information ("The British are Coming!") disseminated quickly, reliably, and broadly. Although lanterns were actually hung in Christ Church in Boston at the beginning of the ride, Revere and Dawes disseminated the information by riding and stopping at towns and farmhouses along the way to Lexington (Figure 8–1), "alarming" the patriots there, many of whom set off on horseback on their own to further spread the message. Thus, Paul Revere's ride was an early type of "phone tree" where a message could be spread quickly through a network of people. Figure 8–2 shows schematically how the Paul Revere dissemination network was structured, and illustrates the relational and structural nature of dissemination. For example, we can see that the success of Paul Revere's ride rests not only on how many towns Revere and Dawes could reach in one night, but also in how many patriots hear the message in each town, and how many of them spread the message further. More specifically, this example suggests that in order to understand dissemination, and design more effective dissemination processes and structures, it is important to be able to study and analyze the structural and relational aspects of dissemination networks. The rest of this chapter describes how network analysis can be used in this way to study D&I.

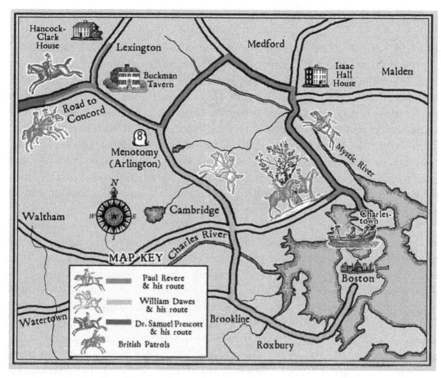

Figure 8–1. Map of Paul Revere's ride (www.paulreverehouse.org).

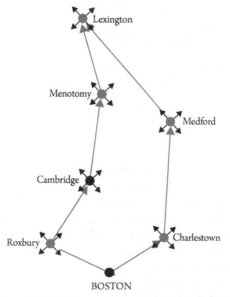

Figure 8–2. Network analytic depiction of Revere's and Dawes's ride.

■ NETWORK ANALYSIS FUNDAMENTALS

Network analysis is not just a set of quantitative techniques—it is a paradigmatic approach to the social and health sciences that embodies a fundamentally different view of social phenomena.[1] The unit of analysis in network science is a relationship between social objects, not an object or characteristic of an object. Relationships can be many things—friendship, money exchange, an e-mail transmission, disease transmission, and so on. Because of this shift in focus from the object to relationships among objects, network analysis is one of the most useful tools for studying context, environment, process, and social structure.[2] Network analysis has been used widely in public health and health sciences to study infectious disease transmission, social influences on health behavior, social support and social capital, organizational systems, and Diffusion of Innovations.[3]

To support the rest of this chapter, it is helpful to understand basic network analysis terminology. A network is made up of a set of nodes and ties that connect the nodes. A node can be almost any type of object—a person, organization, state, country, animal, computer, and so on. Similarly, a tie can represent almost any type of relationship. Nodes are also called actors, members, or vertexes. Ties are sometimes called links, arcs, or edges. Networks can include directed or nondirected relationships. A directed tie (usually indicated by an arrow in a network graph) shows what direction the relationship goes in. For example, money exchange is usually measured and analyzed as a directed tie. Money is given from one node and received by another node. Many other types of relationships are nondirected. For example, organizational collaboration is typically viewed as a nondirected relationship. Two organizations work together on a common project, and it does not make sense to think of the direction of that collaboration. Nondirected ties are usually indicated by straight lines (without arrowheads) in a network graphic. For those interested in more in-depth treatment of network data collection and analysis, see books by Wasserman & Faust, Valente, or de Nooy.[4-6]

■ CONNECTING DISSEMINATION AND IMPLEMENTATION THEORIES TO NETWORK THEORIES

Diffusion of Innovations

Probably the most important and influential theoretical framework relevant to D&I is the theory of Diffusion of Innovations[7] (see also Chapter 3).[8] Rogers defined Diffusion of Innovations as "the process by which an innovation is communicated through certain channels over time among the members of a social system." The early work on Diffusion of Innovations emphasized the types of members (Figure 8–3) as well as the cumulative adoption over time (Figure 8–4). Thus, early understanding of dissemination of scientific findings concentrated on the roles that different members of society played (e.g., innovators vs. opinion leaders) or the amount of time it took for an innovation to be disseminated and adopted in clinical or community practice.

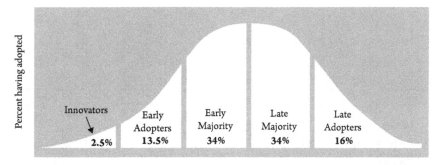

Figure 8–3. Distribution of role types according to time of adoption (based on Bohlen et al., 1962).[9]

However, this emphasis on types of persons involved in diffusion or the amount of time it takes for a discovery to be completely adopted begged the question about what processes drove diffusion in the first place. That is, what distinguishes early adopters from opinion leaders other than their simple temporal ordering in the diffusion process? This question did not start to get answered until Diffusion of Innovations theory started incorporating structural and relational aspects.[10]

This can be seen most clearly by actually looking at one of the well-known diffusion networks studied by social scientists: the adoption of new hybrid seed corn among Iowa farmers.[9,11] In this diagram (Figure 8–5), arrows connect the farmers and scientist, and the arrows point to the source of the information about the innovation. The diagram shows us that Farmer #1 was the innovator and the first to adopt the farm practice in 1948. However, most of the farmers did not learn about this new technology from him. Instead, it wasn't until after 1950 when Farmer #2 (the opinion leader) had adopted the new technology that the practice became more widespread. This network and geography map reveals that there is not just a temporal structure to the diffusion process, but also a relational structure. The opinion leader is much more densely connected to the rest of the diffusion network than the

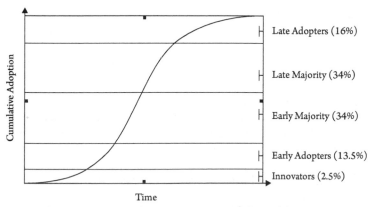

Figure 8–4. S-shaped diffusion of innovation curve (adapted from Rogers, 2003).[7]

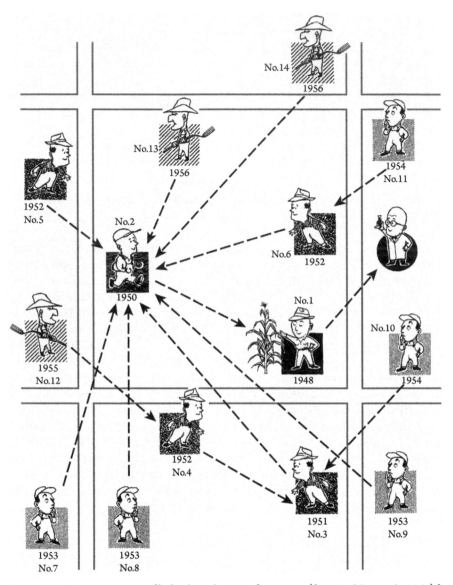

Figure 8–5. Dissemination of hybrid-seed corn information (from Bohlen et al., 1962).[9]

innovator is. That is, the pattern of informational ties can be used to understand the diffusion process. Consistent with U.S. federal definition and those described in Chapter 2 of this book, elsewhere in this chapter the broader term "dissemination" is used, which includes diffusion concepts.

Dissemination and Implementation Frameworks

Implementation science is a newly emerging discipline that focuses, in part, on the discovery and identification of social, organizational, and cultural factors affecting the uptake of evidence-based practices and policies.[12] Although the early developers of this field have recognized the importance of systems thinking and methods,[13] there has been a lack of explicit discussion or demonstration of the utility of network analysis methods for implementation science. However, close examination of new D&I science theoretical models makes it clear that network analysis could be a powerful tool.

For example, Proctor and colleagues have introduced an implementation research framework that groups outcomes into three categories: implementation outcomes, service outcomes, and client outcomes.[14] A number of the implementation outcomes, including penetration, acceptability, sustainability, and uptake, could be examined using network methodology. Tenkasi and Chesmore provide a good example of this in their study of implementation outcomes among 40 units of a multinational corporation.[15] They found that both between-unit and within-unit density of strong ties predicted change implementation cycle time (penetration) and change use (uptake).

The utility of network analysis for studying implementation is made more explicit in the theoretical framework proposed by Feldstein & Glasgow: the Practical, Robust Implementation and Sustainability Model (PRISM).[16] As suggested in Figure 8–6, when studying the implementation process of a new treatment or intervention, the social networks of both the organization members and patients are important tools for understanding predictors of adoption, implementation, and maintenance outcomes. In a successful empirical application of the PRISM model, Beck and colleagues further demonstrated the usefulness of network analysis.[17] Organizational

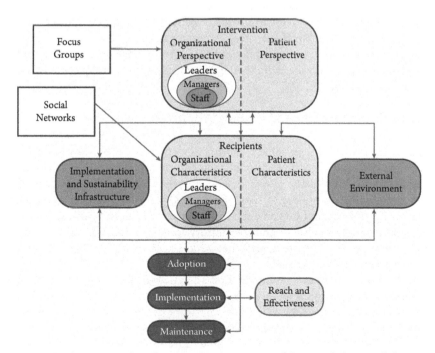

Figure 8–6. The Practical, Robust Implementation and Sustainability Model (PRISM) (adapted from Feldstein & Glasgow, 2008).[16]

advice-seeking patterns among clinicians and staff at two HMO sites were identified using network analysis. These network maps were then used to help drive the subsequent implementation of a new well-child care intervention.

Both of these examples utilize frameworks of implementation processes and outcomes. There have been fewer theoretical treatments of dissemination that highlight the role of network analysis. One exception is Wandersman and colleagues' Interactive Systems Framework for Dissemination and Implementation.[18] In their critical analysis of existing frameworks, they note that traditional models of dissemination tend to ignore the infrastructure and systems that support the dissemination processes. In arguing for a more dynamic and interactive model of D&I, they recognize the importance of network-related concepts such as social capital, community capacity, and collective efficacy.

Although network analysis has not been used widely in D&I science, this is likely to change as more researchers come to grips with the systems approach to studying dissemination and implementation processes and outcomes.

■ USING NETWORK ANALYSIS FOR DISSEMINATION AND IMPLEMENTATION RESEARCH

In the previous section, we have seen how a network theoretical framework can be useful for framing research questions about D&I processes and outcomes. This leads to scientific studies of D&I that collect and analyze data quite differently than in traditional social and health science research. The fundamental difference is the unit of analysis: traditional research poses questions about the attributes or characteristics of individual objects (i.e., people, organizations, etc.), whereas in network analysis the questions are about relationships among those objects. In the rest of this chapter, we will consider a number of network analysis techniques that are most useful for exploring D&I.

Network Description and Visualization

To provide a real-world example for the next two sections, data are shown from an ongoing evaluation of how state tobacco control programs use evidence-based guidelines such as CDC's *Best Practices for Comprehensive Tobacco Control Programs-2007*.[19] States are implementing new policies and practices based on these guidelines, and the successful implementation is supported by broad dissemination of these guidelines through state and community agencies.[20] A main goal of this evaluation was to assess the dissemination networks in each state to help CDC improve tobacco control D&I activities.

In D&I research or evaluation, the first analytic task is often to simply describe the basic dissemination structures or processes. For example, who is involved in the dissemination network? Who in this network has been actively involved with dissemination? How tightly connected is the dissemination network? How efficient is the network? All of these questions can be addressed with basic network analytic and visualization techniques.

For example, Figure 8–7 presents the *Best Practices* dissemination network for the Oregon state tobacco control program. Each node in the graphic is a critical agency or partner in the state program. Nodes are connected by a line if they have communicated with each other about CDC's *Best Practices* guidelines in the past year. The nodes are colored to indicate type of agency, and they are sized to reflect network prominence (see below.) This type of network graphic can reveal a lot about dissemination structures and processes. In this case we can quickly see that most of the Oregon partners have communicated about *Best Practices* with multiple other partners. There is one isolated agency (DHS MedAsst). The lead agency for the state program (TPEP) is highly interconnected. Contractors and grantees show a lower level of dissemination connections than other types of agencies such as advocacy groups.

Although network graphics such as this one can be constructed by hand for small networks, typically specialized network software such as Pajek or UCINet is used. Network software uses specialized visual display algorithms that can enhance the interpretability of the graphics—for example, by placing highly interconnected nodes in the center of the graph, placing disconnected nodes along the periphery, and minimizing crossing lines.[21]

In addition to network graphics, there are a number of useful basic network descriptive statistics that can be used to summarize important network properties. The two most useful of these are network density and diameter. Network *density* is a measure of the overall interconnectedness of the network. It is defined as the proportion of observed network ties to the total number of possible network ties.

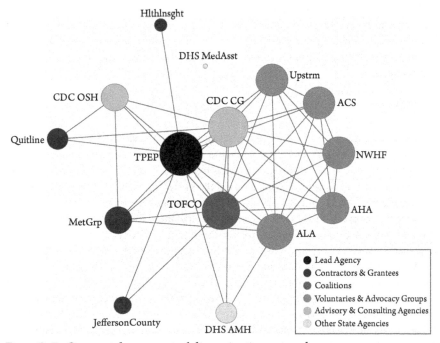

Figure 8–7. Oregon tobacco control dissemination network.

Oregon's dissemination network has 15 members, and there are 45 observed dissemination ties. For a nondirected network, the total number of possible ties is k*(k–1)/2, with k being the number of nodes. So the density of Oregon's network is 45/105, or 0.43. Density can range from 0 to 1, and as networks get larger, the density tends to get smaller. Experience suggests that the density of Oregon's dissemination network (0.43) indicates a highly interconnected network.

Network size, in and of itself, is often not a very interesting statistic. The network size can be driven by a number of factors totally unrelated to the relation of interest (here, dissemination), including geographic boundaries, funding patterns, legislative mandates, or even study design issues. Instead, we can look at a measure of network efficiency designed to tell us how easy it is to get from one part of the network to any other part. The network *diameter* is the longest path between all pairs of a connected network.[22] One of the major discoveries of network science is that even in very large networks (such as the Internet with millions of nodes), the network diameter can be quite small.[23] In fact, the "small-world" phenomenon is based on this property of large networks with small diameters.

For the Oregon network, the diameter is defined as infinity, because of the disconnected node (DHS MedAsst). That is, because this node is not connected to the rest of the network, we cannot go from one node to any other node in the network. If we drop this node and just consider the rest of the connected network, then we can calculate the diameter as 2. Because TPEP is connected to every other agency in the network, it only takes two steps or hops to reach another node from any starting node. The diameter of the Oregon network (more than the rough measure of its size) indicates that this is a highly interconnected network.

With network visualization, and measures of network density and diameter, we can summarize the basic characteristics of a dissemination network. This can help us understand whether an organizational or informational system is ready to support widespread and efficient dissemination of new programs, policies, and innovations.

Prominence

As we saw earlier, our current understanding of how Diffusion of Innovations works includes structural and relational elements. In particular, as Figure 8–7 suggests, particular members of a dissemination network may play specific roles in the dissemination process, and these roles are determined in part by how they are connected (or not connected) to others in the network. Network analysis provides a number of useful tools to assess the roles that individual members play in a network. Possibly the most popular and flexible of these tools is the set of network statistics designed to measure the *prominence* of individual network members.

A network member is seen as prominent in the network to the extent that she (or it) is visible to others in the network. The most commonly used class of prominence measures is *centrality*, where network members are central when those members have high involvement in many relations with other network members. Centrality can actually be measured in a number of different ways—Table 8–1 presents three different centrality statistics for the Oregon dissemination

TABLE 8-1. *Centrality Measures for Oregon Dissemination Network*

Agency	Centrality		
	Degree	Closeness*	Betweenness
TPEP	0.928	1.000	0.294
Metropolitan Group	0.357	0.619	0.003
American Lung Assoc.	0.643	0.765	0.033
Health InSight	0.071	0.520	0.000
Jefferson County Dept of Health	0.143	0.542	0.000
Tobacco Free Coalition	0.714	0.812	0.072
American Heart Assoc.	0.500	0.684	0.000
Upstream Public Health	0.500	0.684	0.000
American Cancer Society	0.500	0.684	0.000
Northwest Health Foundation	0.500	0.684	0.000
DHS-Addictions & Mental Health Div.	0.214	0.565	0.000
DHS-Medical Assistance	0.000	—	0.000
CDC-Office on Smoking and Health	0.357	0.619	0.007
CDC-Community Guide	0.786	0.867	0.096
Free & Clear	0.214	0.565	0.000
Overall Network Centralization	0.577	0.703	0.279

*Closeness centrality calculated after dropping the isolate: DHS-Medical Assistance.

network: *degree* centrality, *closeness* centrality, and *betweenness* centrality.[24] For all three measures, scores can range from 0 to 1, with numbers closer to 1 indicating greater centrality. Degree centrality is the easiest to understand—it is based on the number of direct connections (degree) that a network member has with other members. The lead agency, TPEP, has the highest overall degree (13), so it also has the highest degree centrality (0.93). Closeness centrality takes into account not just direct ties, but also indirect ties. A network member will have high closeness centrality if it lies close to all other members in the network. Closeness is measured by the smallest path that connects two nodes. For the Oregon network, closeness centrality can only be calculated after dropping the single isolate (DHS-Medical Assistance), because closeness is only defined for a connected network. TPEP has the highest possible closeness centrality because it is directly connected to every other network member. Health InSight, on the other hand, has the lowest closeness centrality because it has to go through TPEP to get to any other member of the network. Finally, betweenness centrality is another centrality measure that takes both direct and indirect ties into account. A node will have high betweenness if it sits in between many other shortest paths between network members. Betweenness is usually interpreted as control over the flow of information in a network.[25]

As Table 8-1 illustrates, these three measures of centrality give similar, but not identical information. What is the best measure to use? Each measure is based on a different aggregation of information about network ties (only direct ties considered vs. all ties) and network structure (distance vs. location). A researcher should use a measure of centrality that most closely matches the theoretical framework being used. For dissemination studies, if the focus were on identifying network members who are most responsible for driving the dissemination, then perhaps degree centrality would be most appropriate. If the interest were more in the flow of dissemination across an entire network, then betweenness centrality would be useful. Finally, if the researcher were more interested in dissemination efficiency (how quickly or easily the entire network can be reached with the information), then closeness centrality would be a good candidate.

Centrality measures are useful for identifying critical network members, such as TPEP in the Oregon dissemination network. TPEP's prominence makes sense given that it is the lead agency for the state's tobacco control program. Part of the Oregon analysis was to understand the impact of the CDC's Community Guide, which is a comprehensive systematic review of a whole range of public health interventions.[26] The centrality measures revealed that the Community Guide is playing an important role in the dissemination of Best Practices, which makes sense given the Community Guide's focus on evidence-based strategies.

Prominence measures can also be very useful for making comparisons across different networks or among different types of relationships in the same network. First, individual node-level centrality measures can be aggregated into network-level *centralization* indices. These are presented for the Oregon dissemination network at the bottom of Table 8–1. These numbers are actually measures of the variability of the node-level measures and also range from 0 to 1. Higher numbers indicate greater variability of centrality. This is usually interpreted as greater hierarchy in the communication structure. That being said, it is often difficult to interpret a single measure of centralization—instead, these numbers are more useful when making comparisons. For example, consider Figure 8–8, which compares the centralization

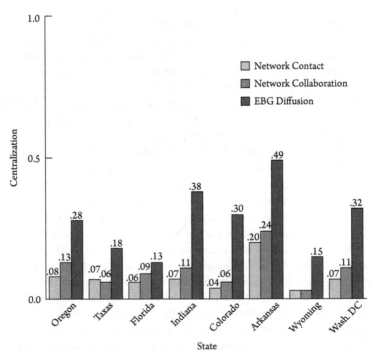

Figure 8–8. Betweenness centralization for eight tobacco control programs and three network relations.

of three types of network relations for eight different state tobacco control programs. Contact is simply how often two agencies talk to each other, collaboration is how extensively the two agencies work together on common projects, and EBG diffusion is whether the two agencies have talked to each other about CDC's *Best Practices* guidelines. The graphic shows a striking pattern: across all eight state programs, EBG diffusion shows much higher betweenness centralization than for contact or collaboration. This suggests that contact and collaboration are shared among state partners in comparable ways, but a small number of agencies are driving the *Best Practices* diffusion process in each state. This fits a staged communications model of Diffusion of Innovations, where interagency communication and collaboration must precede the more challenging task of broad dissemination of practice and policy innovations.

Analyzing Diffusion Processes

The previous two sections have shown that basic node-level and network-level statistics can provide information relevant to studies of D&I processes and structures. More advanced network analysis techniques are available that can help analyze or model more specific diffusion processes in social or organizational networks: main path analysis and threshold modeling.

Main path analysis

Diffusion occurs across time, and this time dimension can be taken into consideration with network analysis of diffusion processes. If we want to trace diffusion across a network, then we will be dealing with a network structure that has two important properties. First, the network will be directed; the ties between nodes will go *from* one actor *to* another actor. The Iowa farmers network (Figure 8–5) is an example of a directed network, while the Oregon tobacco control network is nondirected. Second, diffusion processes usually move in one direction over time; they do not double back. That is, once Farmer B learns about a new innovation from Farmer A, later on Farmer A will not learn about the same innovation again from Farmer B. This produces what are known as *acyclic* networks; these are networks without loops.[4]

Main path analysis was developed by Hummon and his colleagues and was used to trace the development of the theory of DNA.[27] Citations among scientific papers are a particular type of diffusion process, where scientists form the dissemination community. Main path analysis can be used to identify the most important path of information flow through a connected set of scientific papers. Figure 8–9 shows the main path through the DNA literature identified by Hummon (indicated by the thick black line). This main path includes Crick & Watson's famous 1953 paper describing the structure of DNA (node #27).

We can see how main path analysis works by turning back to the Iowa farm network as a simple diffusion process example. Although the Iowa farmers are not a citation network, this diffusion network meets the requirements for main path analysis: the network is directed, and acyclic (no loops). The main path in a

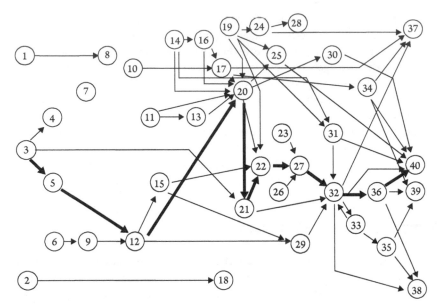

Figure 8–9. Main citation path of DNA research (reprinted from Hummon and Doreian, 1989).[27]

diffusion network is the set of links through which most of the information flows. The analysis works by first identifying sources and sinks. A source node is one that has no links coming into it, only links leaving it. That is, a source link is a place where information starts flowing in a network. A sink is the opposite: a node that only has links coming into it. A sink is therefore a final stopping place for information flow. Once sources and sinks are identified, the entire network is examined to see which ties account for the largest proportion of information flow from all sources to all sinks in a network. Figure 8–10 shows the results of the main path analysis for the Iowa farmers. (The arrows have been reversed to make the direction of the diffusion flow clearer.)

Along each diffusion link in the graph, the traversal weight is shown. The higher this number (up to 1) indicates, the higher proportion of information flow. The main path, identified by the thicker black line, is the path from a source node to a sink node with the highest traversal weights on its links. So, we can see here that the main path of diffusion in the farmers network starts with the scientist, flows through the most centrally connected farmer (#2), and ends with farmers #10 and #12. This type of network analysis can be very useful for larger, more complicated diffusion networks, as long as you have the appropriate data to allow for directed, acyclic networks.

Threshold models of diffusion

Another approach to understanding the structural and relational determinants of D&I is to more explicitly examine how network characteristics influence the

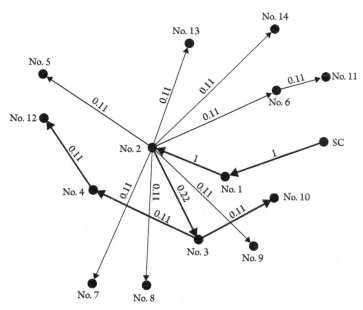

Figure 8–10. Main dissemination path of Iowa farmers.

likelihood of adoption (of some new idea, technology, behavior, or policy) over time. These are variously called contagion, threshold, or exposure models.[1,5] The central ideas of these models are that diffusion occurs over time, network characteristics influence the diffusion processes over time, and that there are thresholds that occur at specific points in time.[5] Many of these models examine the influence of network exposure. Exposure can be defined in a number of ways but is most simply seen as the proportion of an actor's social network that has already adopted the behavior of interest. The usual hypothesis is that as exposure increases over time, the likelihood of adoption for any actor in a network will also increase.

Much of the empirical work testing these threshold models in public health comes from Valente and his colleagues. For example, he has shown that exposure helps explain the diffusion of new family planning information among Korean families, but it did not predict diffusion of new medical technologies among doctors.[10] In a more recent example, an exposure model was used to explore how network ties influenced the ratification of the Framework Convention on Tobacco Control among 168 nations.[28] They were able to show that exposure to other countries who were members of GLOBALink (an online network of global tobacco control researchers) was significantly associated with ratification of the FCTC treaty (AOR = 2.92; 95% CI = 1.25, 6.78). Many of these threshold studies use longitudinal logistic regression or survival analysis. Although these models are fairly sophisticated in combining relational and attribute data, the models can be hard to refute and are fraught with concerns about nonindependence.[5] Newer statistical models of network processes and structure help avoid these technical problems, as described in the next section.

Statistical Modeling of Networks

Our previous examples of network analytic techniques have been primarily descriptive. They can be incredibly useful for exploring hypotheses about D&I processes, but they are limited in their ability to more formally test statistical hypotheses. Recent statistical and computational advances, however, now allow us to build and test statistical models of social networks.[29] These are new techniques that are just starting to be used in public health research.[30]

These statistical models are relational models—they work by predicting the likelihood that a network tie exists between two network members.[31] The attraction of these models for D&I research is threefold. *First*, and most important, the models allow for relational and actor predictors. This means that characteristics of the network member can be used in the model. So, for example, we can determine if participation in dissemination training results in a greater likelihood of dissemination activity. *Second*, despite the complexity of the underlying statistical computations, these models produce confidence intervals and p-values, which can be used to support traditional hypothesis testing. *Finally*, the models can use simulation techniques to provide goodness-of-fit tests, which are invaluable for model testing and model comparisons.

To see how this type of model can be used to test hypotheses about diffusion processes, consider Figure 8–11. This shows a main path citation network of 40 years of secondhand smoke research.[32] The dark blue nodes in the upper part of the graph are the basic science (i.e., epidemiology and biology) studies, and the lighter blue nodes at the bottom are the intervention, prevention, and policy studies. The red dashed lines were the only direct citations of the basic science literature from the policy and prevention literature. We had a hypothesis that there was a "discovery-to-delivery" diffusion gap in the secondhand smoke literature. The citation network suggests that this gap was real, that the secondhand smoke policy, prevention, and intervention studies were not directly citing the basic science upon which their interventions were based.

We used these new statistical network-modeling techniques to test this hypothesis. Table 8–2 summarizes the main modeling results. We found that secondhand smoke articles that were published in high-impact journals were more likely to be cited, regardless of type of study. However, we also found that there was little cross-citation between discovery and delivery research. In particular, a delivery article was 64.3% less likely (OR = 0.36, CI = 0.33–0.39) to cite a discovery article than a discovery article was to cite another discovery article. This statistical analysis supports a hypothesis of an important diffusion gap, that basic science information may not be quickly or easily disseminated to the practice community.

■ SUMMARY

One persistent challenge in the health and social sciences is the mismatch between theory and methods. Many important behavioral and organizational theories in public health embrace the importance of context, assume that behavior changes over time, and assume that these changes are dynamic in nature and have complex interrelationships with other dynamic systems. Yet, despite calls for increases in

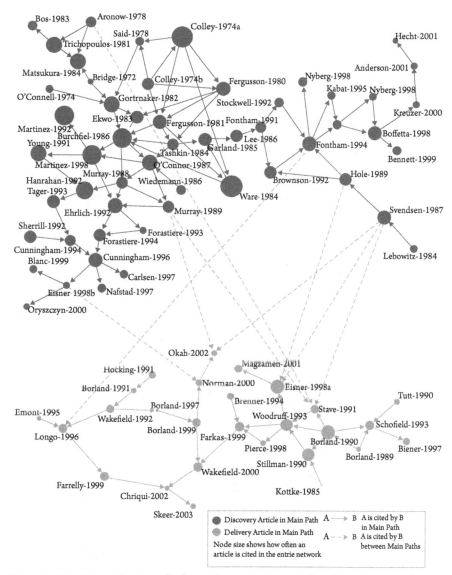

Figure 8–11. Dissemination of information among secondhand smoke research (adapted from Harris et al., 2009).[32]

multilevel and ecological approaches to public health science,[33] we still tend to use research methods and analytic techniques that ignore context, focus on single snap-shots in time, assume processes only operate at a single level of analysis, and are not dynamic.[2] Dissemination and implementation in public health is still in many ways an emerging discipline, but the important theoretical and conceptual frameworks guiding this new field all recognize that D&I are complex and dynamic social and organizational processes.

TABLE 8-2. *Likelihood of Citation Relation among Secondhand Smoke Studies (Adapted from Harris et al., 2009).*[32]

Coefficient	Model 1				Model 2			
	Logit	SE	OR	95% CI	Logit	SE	OR	95% CI
Edges/Arcs	−5.27	0.10	0.005	0.004–0.006	−5.14	0.10	0.006	0.005–0.007
Year Citation Patterns								
Cites articles by year (indegree)	−0.10	0.001	0.905	0.903–0.907	−0.10	0.001	0.905	0.903–0.907
Cited by year (outdegree)	0.04	0.002	1.041	1.037–1.045	0.04	0.002	1.041	1.037–1.045
Journal Citation Patterns								
Cites articles (indegree)								
Impact factor <3	Ref	—	—	—	Ref	—	—	—
Impact factor 3–5	0.79	0.03	1.259	1.187–1.335	0.80	0.03	2.226	2.098–2.360
Impact factor >5	1.58	0.03	4.855	4.578–5.149	1.61	0.03	5.003	4.717–5.306
Cited (outdegree)								
Impact factor <3	Ref	—	—	—	Ref	—	—	—
Impact factor 3–5	0.23	0.03	1.259	1.187–1.335	0.22	0.03	1.246	1.176–1.322
Impact factor >5	0.32	0.04	1.377	1.273–1.489	0.31	0.04	1.363	1.261–1.475
Subfield citation patterns								
Discovery cites discovery					Ref	—	—	—
Discovery cites delivery					−1.80	0.09	0.165	0.139–0.197
Delivery cites discovery					−1.03	0.04	0.357	0.330–0.386
Delivery cites delivery					1.47	0.04	4.349	4.021–4.704

As seen in this chapter, network analysis is a very useful tool for studying how new scientific discoveries and evidence-based policies and practices are disseminated to target audiences and implemented by communities, organizations, and governments. If appropriate network data are collected from these D&I activities, then a number of empirical possibilities open up. Network visualization can be used to map and describe the dissemination networks themselves. Network descriptive statistics such as density and diameter can be used to summarize and compare these networks. More specific network concepts such as prominence can be used to identify important elements or characteristics of the network. For example, network centrality and centralization can be used to identify important gaps or gatekeepers in a dissemination network. Specific theories of D&I process, such as Diffusion of Innovations, can be developed and tested using network methods. Finally, new statistical and computational abilities allow us for the first time to build and test statistical models of D&I network processes.

There is much that remains a mystery about how to build and sustain successful D&I in public health. However, it is clear that successful D&I happens in a social and organizational context (see Chapter 7)[34] and that the relationships among those persons and organizations can make or break the entire enterprise. Network analysis is uniquely suited to elucidating these relationships and thus is an important tool for future D&I research.

SUGGESTED READINGS

Goodreau S. Advances in exponential random graph (p') models applied to a large social network. *Social Networks.* 2007;29:231–248.

This article describes recent advances in statistical network analysis. The ability to apply exponential random graph models to large datasets offers many practical applications for drawing inferences and represents real progress in the field.

Luke DA. Getting the big picture in community science: Methods that capture context. *American Journal of Community Psychology.* 2005;35:185–200.

This article presents a review of empirical community psychology articles showing that social scientists utilize a narrow range of statistical tools that are not well suited to analyze contextual data and effects. The paper recommends a broader set of analytic approaches to understand the effects of context on health behavior, including multilevel modeling, geographic information systems, cluster analysis, and social network analysis.

Luke DA, Harris JK. Network analysis in public health: History, methods and applications. *Annual Review of Public Health.* 2007;28:69–93.

Luke and Harris describe the basics of network analysis and how its techniques are applied to public health problems. Historically, network analysis has been used in public health to examine the transmission of HIV and other STDs, the diffusion of innovations, and how social support and social capital impact public health outcomes.

Rogers EM. *Diffusion of Innovations.* 5th ed. New York: Free Press; 2003.

Rogers's classic text on how ideas and opinions diffuse over time through various communication channels and networks. Because many new ideas involve taking a risk, people seek out others who have already adopted it. As a result, the new idea is spread through social networks over a period of weeks, months, or years.

Valente TW. *Network Models of the Diffusion of Innovations*. Cresskill, NJ: Hampton Press; 1995.

Diffusion of innovations refers to the idea of certain concepts or opinions spreading rapidly throughout society. This process is dependent on the presence of social networks. Valente's text presents an examination of this process and methods for estimating how fast or slow diffusion occurs; to be used by students, researchers, and policymakers.

Valente TW. *Social Networks and Health: Models, Methods, and Applications*. New York: Oxford University Press; 2010.

Networks, by definition, focus on connections between individuals, organizations, or other units. Valente describes how social network models can be used to understand and even change a range of human health behaviors.

Wasserman S, Faust K. *Social Network Analysis: Methods and Applications*. New York: Cambridge University Press; 1994.

Wasserman and Faust's reference on social networks can be used as a comprehensive review or to recommend specific network analysis methods for researchers who have already gathered network data. The book is divided into six parts, providing a broad overview of social network's properties, types of network data, and statistical methods, accompanied by substantive examples.

SELECTED WEBSITES AND TOOLS

INSNA—International Network for Social Network Analysis <http://www.insna.org>. INSNA is the primary professional association for network analysis and network science. In addition to useful data and software resources, the INSNA website provides information on the main network analysis professional and scientific journals (*Connections* and *Social Networks*) as well as the annual international *Sunbelt Conference*.

Complexity and Social Networks Blog < http://www.iq.harvard.edu/blog/netgov/>. An interesting blog that covers a wide variety of network analysis and complexity science topics.

Pajek Wiki <http://pajek.imfm.si/doku.php?id=start>. Main support website for Pajek, a widely used free software package for network analysis.

Support website for *statnet* <http://csde.washington.edu/statnet/>. This website provides information on, background material for, and access to the *statnet* suite of packages for network analysis. The packages are written for the *R* statistical computing environment. Statistical modeling of networks can be done using procedures in *statnet*.

■ ACKNOWLEDGMENT

The author is grateful to Laura Brossart for her help in locating and editing the figures used in this chapter.

■ REFERENCES

1. Monge PR, Contractor N. *Theories of Communication Networks*. New York: Oxford University Press; 2003.
2. Luke DA. Getting the big picture in community science: Methods that capture context. *American Journal of Community Psychology*. 2005;35:185–200.

3. Luke DA, Harris JK. Network analysis in public health: History, methods and applications. *Annual Review of Public Health*. 2007;28:69–93.
4. Wasserman S, Faust K. *Social Network Analysis: Methods and Applications*. New York: Cambridge University Press; 1994.
5. Valente TW. *Social Networks and Health: Models, Methods, and Applications*. New York: Oxford University Press; 2010.
6. de Nooy W, Mrvar A, Batagelj V. *Exploratory Social Network Analysis with Pajek*. New York: Cambridge University Press; 2005.
7. Rogers EM. *Diffusion of Innovations*. 5th ed. New York: The Free Press; 2003.
8. Dearing JW, Kee KF. Historical roots of dissemination and implementation science. In: Brownson R, Colditz G, Proctor E, eds. *Dissemination and Implementation Research in Health: Translating Science to Practice*. New York: Oxford University Press; 2011.
9. Bohlen JM, Coughenour CM, Lionberger HF, Moe EO, Rogers EM. *Adopters of new farm ideas*. North Central Regional Extension Publication No. 13. East Lansing, MI: Michigan State University. 1962:3-12.
10. Valente TW. *Network Models of the Diffusion of Innovations*. Cresskill NJ: Hampton Press; 1995.
11. Ryan B. The diffusion of hybrid seed corn in two Iowa communities. *Rural Sociology*. 1943;8(1):15–24.
12. Bhattacharyya O, Reeves S, Zwarenstein M. What is implementation research?: Rationale, concepts, and practices. *Research on Social Work Practice*. 2009;18: 491–502.
13. Bammer G. Integration and implementation sciences: Building a new specialization. *Ecology and Society*. 2005;10. http://www.ecologyandsociety.org/vol10/iss2/art6/
14. Proctor EK, Landsverk J, Aarons G, Chambers D, Glisson C, Mittman, B. Implementation research in mental health services: An emerging science with conceptual, methodological, and training challenges. *Administration and Policy in Mental Health*. 2009;36:24–34.
15. Tenkasi RV, Chesmore MC. Social networks and planned organizational change: The impact of strong network ties on effective change implementation and use. *The Journal of Applied Behavioral Science*. 2003;39:281–300.
16. Feldstein AC, Glasgow RW. A Practical, Robust Implementation and Sustainability Model (PRISM) for integrating research findings into practice. *The Joint Commission Journal on Quality and Patient Safety*. 2008;34:228–243.
17. Beck A, Bergman D, Rahm AK, Dearing JW, Glasgow RE. Using implementation and dissemination concepts to spread 21st-century sell-child care at a health maintenance organization. *The Permanente Journal*. 2009;13(3):10–17.
18. Wandersman A, Duffy J, Flaspohler P, et al. Bridging the gap between prevention research and practice: The Interactive Systems Framework for Dissemination and Implementation. *American Journal of Community Psychology*. 2008;41:171–181.
19. US DHHS. *Best Practices for Comprehensive Tobacco Control Programs-2007*. Atlanta: CDC; 2007.
20. Mueller NB, Luke DA, Herbers SH, Montgomery TP. The *Best Practices*: Use of the guidelines by ten state tobacco control programs. *American Journal of Preventive Medicine*. 2006;31:300–306.
21. Batagelj V, Mrvar A. Pajek. Analysis and visualization of large networks. In: Junger M, Mutzel P, eds. *Graph Drawing Software*. Springer; 2003:77–104.

22. Kolaczyk ED. *Statistical Analysis of Network Data: Methods and Models.* New York: Springer; 2009.

23. Newman MEJ. The structure and function of complex networks. *SIAM Review.* 2003;45:167–256.

24. Freeman LC. Centrality in social networks: Conceptual clarification. *Social Networks.* 1979;1(3):215–239.

25. Freeman LC. A set of measures of centrality based on betweenness. *Sociometry.* 1977;40:35–41.

26. Zaza S, Briss PA, Harris KW, eds. *The Guide to Community Preventive Services: What Works to Promote Health?* New York: Oxford University Press; 2005.

27. Hummon NP, Doreian P. Connectivity in a citation network: The development of DNA theory. *Social Networks.* 1989;11:39–63.

28. Wipfli HL, Fujimoto K, Valente TW. Global tobacco control diffusion: The case of the Framework Convention on Tobacco Control. *American Journal of Public Health.* 2010;100:1260–1266.

29. O'Malley J, Marsden PV. The analysis of social networks. *Health Services and Outcomes Research Methodology.* 2008;8:222–269.

30. Luke DA, Harris JK, Shelton S, Allen P, Carothers BJ, Mueller NB. Systems analysis of collaboration in 5 national tobacco control networks. *American Journal of Public Health.* 2010;100:1290–1297. doi:10.2105/APH.2009.184358

31. Goodreau S. Advances in exponential random graph (p*) models applied to a large social network. *Social Networks.* 2007;29:231–248. doi:10.1016/j.socinet.2006.08.001

32. Harris JK, Luke DA, Zuckerman R, Shelton SC. Forty years of secondhand smoke research: The gap between discovery and delivery. *American Journal of Preventive Medicine.* 2009;36:538–548.

33. Office of Behavioral and Social Sciences Research. *Toward higher levels of analysis: Progress and promise in research on social and cultural dimensions of health.* NIH Publication No. 21–5020. 2001. Available online at: http://obssr.od.nih.gov/publications/books_and_projects/books_and_reports.aspx

34. Aarons GA, Horowitz J, Dlugosz L, Ehrhart M. (2011). The role of organizational processes in dissemination and implementation research. In: Brownson R, Colditz G, Proctor E, eds. *Dissemination and Implementation Research in Health: Translating Science to Practice.* New York: Oxford University Press; 2011.

9 Systems Thinking in Dissemination and Implementation Research

BEV J. HOLMES, DIANE T. FINEGOOD, BARBARA L. RILEY, AND ALLAN BEST

■ INTRODUCTION

Population and public health issues such as obesity and chronic disease are increasingly described as complex problems, deeply embedded within the fabric of society.[1] Similarly, health care systems are acknowledged to have greatly increased in complexity over the last 30 years.[2] This may seem obvious and not particularly new, especially to those who have been working in these fields for some time. However, despite the increasing recognition of their complex nature, public health issues continue to attract simple, independent, "one-off" solutions that are rarely adequate to result in significant change.[3]

It is perhaps not surprising that the common response to the public health issues that plague society is to eliminate, or at least reduce, their complexity. This chapter suggests that a more productive response, though, is to acknowledge complexity, and to design and study solutions that address it. In support of this view, the purpose of the chapter is to present systems thinking as an approach to intervene in and study health issues such as obesity and chronic disease—complex problems in the sense that they are unpredictable and influenced by many interacting and multilevel variables. First, the evolution of dissemination and implementation (D&I) health research is briefly reviewed, revealing an increasing recognition of complexity. This evolution parallels events in the field of knowledge translation, a term by which dissemination and implementation is more commonly known in Canada, where the authors live and work. The notion of "systems" is then introduced—what they are, and why an understanding of them is critical to improved health and health care through dissemination and implementation. Systems thinking is then described and its implications explored, with two in particular expanded on: the need to rethink cause and effect, and the importance of considering different levels of intervention. Obesity is presented as an example of an issue whose complexity demands a systems approach in order to address it meaningfully. The final section of the chapter demonstrates systems thinking in action, using the examples of two new Canadian projects, funded by the Canadian Partnership Against Cancer, based on such an approach: Youth Excel and The CAPTURE Project.

■ EVOLUTION OF DISSEMINATION AND IMPLEMENTATION IN HEALTH AND ITS RELATIONSHIP TO SYSTEMS THINKING

In Chapter 3, Dearing and Kee refer to the historically separate spheres of the state of the science (what researchers collectively know) and the state of the art (what practitioners collectively do). Relatively new to health research, D&I attempts to close the gap and as such is a growing priority for health-related funding agencies,[4] which are being pressured by governments to demonstrate the results of the research they support. Many such agencies were initially focused primarily on biomedical and clinical research, but are now also supporting health systems and population health research in an attempt to ensure that evidence from the laboratory and from clinical studies is translated into practice.

Of course, realizing this translation is no straightforward matter. The discourse of the trajectory—from basic to clinical to health system to population research—is deceptive, implying a linear progression from the generation of evidence to its implementation and ongoing use. Indeed, D&I has for the most part followed the linear processes of basic research and clinical research, where progressive, replicable steps are seen to lead to results. Crowley and colleagues illustrate this linear thinking with a model that represents the dominant view behind biomedical research and has driven the design of much D&I.[5] Such models describe a one-way process in which researchers produce new knowledge, which gets disseminated to end users, and then incorporated into practice and policy.

In their historical overview of D&I science, however, Dearing and Kee dispel the idea that D&I is a series of steps to ensure that information is moved from one source to another. The traditional notion of an intervention as predesigned and ready to implement is increasingly inaccurate, they claim, replaced by a view in which such innovations are coproduced by researchers and research users.

A parallel evolution in thinking can be traced in the field of knowledge translation (KT—also called knowledge transfer, knowledge exchange, research utilization, and more recently, knowledge mobilization), a term used to describe knowledge- to-action approaches in Canada. Historically, knowledge was seen as a product, generalizable across contexts, whose use depended on effective packaging. The emphasis on information technologies perpetuated the myth that knowledge is the same as data, and that transferring it effectively depends on sophisticated computer systems.[6] Many models were based on a fundamental belief that knowledge is created and tested by academic researchers, taught to students by instructors, adopted and diffused by consultants, and practiced by practitioners.[7]

Although the reliance on linear models is still evident,[8] growing evidence from D&I and KT activity is demonstrating that attempts to control multiple contexts during the process of implementation are fraught with theoretical and methodological challenges. Acknowledging these challenges, models such as the PARiHS framework (Promoting Action on Research Implementation in Health Services)[8] engage with the complexities of moving evidence into practice. The framework sees successful implementation as a function of the nature and type of evidence, the qualities of the context in which the evidence is being introduced, and the way the process is facilitated. Brown and McCormack use the PARiHS model to explore factors that influence the use of evidence in practice related to acute pain services.[9] They argue that pain management practices could be improved through a systematic, rigorous, and multidimensional approach, using the PARiHS framework as a guide. Wright et al. use the framework to determine the contextual indicators that enable or hinder continence care and management in rehabilitation settings for older people.[10] Their study led to the development of a tool to enable practitioners to assess the context within which continence care is provided.

In other examples, Wandersman and colleagues present an interactive systems framework as a heuristic for understanding systems, functions, and relationships relevant to the D&I process.[11] They argue that traditional research-to-practice models focus almost exclusively on the separate functions that take place as part of D&I, rather than the infrastructure or systems that support and carry out the functions. Damschroder and colleagues combine 19 research-to-practice theories to develop a consolidated framework for implementation research.[12] The framework is offered as a pragmatic structure for approaching complex, interacting, multilevel and transient states of constructs in the real world. Ward and colleagues review 28 knowledge transfer models to identify five common components (problem iden-tification and communication, knowledge/research development and selection, analysis of context, knowledge transfer activities or interventions, and knowledge/ research utilization), and from them construct a conceptual framework of the knowledge-to-action process.[13] Their framework demonstrates that these five com-ponents comprise a complex, multidirectional (rather than linear) set of interac-tions. They can occur simultaneously or in any given order as well as occur more than once during the knowledge transfer process.

The above examples are only a few among an increasing number that strive to acknowledge the complexity in health care and population health settings. They rep-resent a promising shift in the conceptualization of D&I—a shift that appreciates that the transfer of knowledge is not a one-way process, and that there are many fac-tors at play in how research and practice inform each other. Despite this shift, still lacking is a conceptualization of these factors at play as part of an overarching system whose dynamic whole is different from the structural properties of its subparts.[8] This conceptualization is at the heart of systems thinking, discussed next.

■ SYSTEMS THINKING

Systems and Their Attributes

Mandel notes the difficulty in defining a system and suggests it is easier to explain what a system *does* than what it *is*: a system unites elements into a meaningful rela-tionship that acts as a whole.[14] A system can be understood only as this integrated whole, since it is not constituted only by the sum of its components, but also by the relationships among these components.[15]

Systems can be thought of as simple, complicated, or complex.[16,17] Simple and complicated systems are predictable and can be understood if taken apart and ana-lyzed. Complex systems are not predictable and therefore cannot be understood through reductionism; however, it is possible to achieve a level of understanding of a complex system by studying how it operates. Table 9–1 describes some of the differences between simple or complicated systems and complex systems.

As the table suggests, not all systems are complex, even in health settings. For example, clinical reminder systems for physicians—which have been found to

TABLE 9-1. *Differences between Simple or Complicated and Complex Systems (Adapted from Finegood[17])*

Simple or Complicated Systems	Complex Systems
Homogeneous: identical/indistinguishable structural elements	**Heterogeneous**: large number of structural variations
Linear: a relationship with constant proportions	**Nonlinear**: cause does not produce a proportional effect.
Deterministic: same result always occurs for a given set of circumstances; predictable	**Stochastic**: an element of randomness leads to a degree of uncertainty about the outcome.
Static: nothing changes over time	**Dynamic**: changes over time; past has an impact on the future.
Independent: subsystems are not influenced or controlled by other parts of the system.	**Interdependent**: subsystems are interconnected or interwoven, not just interacting,
No feedback: open chain of cause and effect	**Feedback**: a closed chain of causal connections
No adaptation or self-organization	**Adaptation and self-organization**: ability of a system to structure itself, to create new structure, to learn, or diversify
No connection between levels or subsystems	**Emergence**: collective behavior that cannot be simply inferred from the behavior of components

increase the use of guideline-based care in general practice[18]—could be considered simple, consisting as they do of basic issues of technique and terminology that, once mastered, contain a very high assurance of success.[19] Complicated systems demand more coordination and more specialized expertise than simple ones; in this sense, a medical surgery can be viewed as complicated. The assumptions underlying rational planning, however, which could greatly enhance clinical reminder and surgical systems, do not apply in complex systems, with their features as described in the above table. Complex systems, unlike simple or complicated ones, are ultimately unknowable, given their many dynamic and interacting variables. Such is the case with most population and public health problems in the 21st century: they are too complex to "know," and therefore to "solve" through rational planning. The situation creates a profound challenge for D&I, requiring a paradigm shift and attendant new ways of doing business.[6] This shift is encompassed in the concept of systems thinking.

Systems Thinking and Its Implications

Given their nature as described above, complex problems in society require intervention at many different levels and the engagement of actors and organizations across levels ranging from the home, school, and work environments to communities, regions, and entire countries.[17] This multilevel, multiactor view is at the heart of systems thinking, a process of understanding how things influence one another other within a whole.

The systems view may sound deceptively similar to the well-known social-ecological approaches to health promotion and disease prevention.[20,21] While social-ecological models have usefully reinforced the need for multiple levels of influence and multiple strategies (e.g., education, policy, media), they have been less effective in focusing attention on the interrelationships within and across levels and how interventions need to take these relationships into account in their design and implementation.

Systems thinking addresses these limitations—but in the process implies the need to reconceptualize a number of factors related to D&I. Best and Holmes[6] outline three: what is meant by "evidence" and what kinds of evidence will be useful to improve health from a systems point of view, what is the most effective type of leadership to facilitate systems change, and how we can use networks to bring about improvements to health (see Chapter 8 on networks).

A further implication is the need to reconceptualize boundaries: If a systems perspective suggests that everything is directly or indirectly connected with everything else, decisions must be made about the "cutoff point" within which interventions will be studied; the values inherent in making such decisions must also be acknowledged.[22] Evaluation is another critical area of reflection, with huge implications for systems thinking. From a traditional scientific point of view, randomization is ideal; systems thinking, on the other hand, implies a need to learn from natural experiments and case studies. To build a body of more practice-based evidence,[23] evaluation systems are needed that both support continuous learning at the application level and pool practice-based evidence across contexts. This idea underpins a further implication: the need to rethink the current division of research and practice in population and public health. Ideally, these would not be seen as separate activities undertaken by separate groups of people (researchers and practitioners) but would be conceptualized as an overall approach to linking the generation and use of evidence.

Yet another implication stems from systems thinking's rejecting the conception of intervention as "flawlessly preplanned change based on accurate predictions of the consequences of action."[22, p.77] This being the case, how can the likely effects of actions or inaction be forecasted? Recognizing that the causes of and solutions to complex health issues defy simple calculations, researchers are using systems dynamics modeling to anticipate potential outcomes and effects of policies and programs in dynamic and complex environments.[24–26] These and other implications indicate the extent of the shift that systems thinking demands. Two further implications explored in more detail below are the need to re-examine the notion of causation, and the importance of intervention levels.

Rethinking causation

A reductionist approach to research generates knowledge and understanding of phenomena by breaking them down and studying their elements in terms of cause and effect.[27] It is an approach that demands seeing causal factors as being either independent of other factors or dependent on variables that were observed or changed in an experimental setting.[17] The approach works in many areas of science, where a notion of causation is based on regularities in natural phenomena. In an example given by Wagner,[28] if the activity of an enzyme in a metabolic pathway is increased, the rate at which substances are metabolized in this pathway is likely to increase; that is, changes in enzyme activity cause changes in metabolic rates. However, as Wagner goes on to explain, such causality can be meaningfully defined only for systems with similarly linear interactions among their variables. Assuming a linear cause-and-effect relationship becomes problematic in many settings, providing as it does only a limited and short-term perspective for understanding how things really work.

Despite some recognition that a reductionist approach to complex problems is likely to fail, many people persist in believing that the scientific method, including controlled experiments, testing of rival hypotheses, and replication of results, is the best way to solve problems, even if they are complex. Many still believe that the solutions must be based on the root of the problem.[29] Wagner[28] attributes this persistence to the fact that causation is a notion fundamental to human cognition, and suggests that

> in the social sciences, the linearity of causal models is often due to a lack of insight into functional relations among the variables of a model. This lack of insight probably exists for good reasons, such as the inability to do experiments, and methodological difficulties in collecting even observational data. Given this lack of insight, the most parsimonious assumption about a system is that it is in equilibrium, and that the interactions among its state variables and parameters in equilibrium are linear. (p. 98)

Robinson and Sirard[30] argue that this problem-oriented approach or reductionism is responsible for leaving many of the most important applied research questions unanswered, and for slowing efforts to improve individual and population health. They recommend a complementary, solution-oriented paradigm that emphasizes experimental research to identify the contributors to improved health, and suggest that this subtle conceptual shift has significant implications for the types of research performed and for making the results more relevant to policy and practice.

Rethinking levels of intervention

It is well known that with many public health and health systems issues, one or even multiple interventions in any one area (for example, at the level of the individual) are insufficient to create sustainable change. This understanding provides a rationale for the use of social ecological models and a comprehensive (multilevel, multistrategy) approach to address health issues (e.g., tobacco use, obesity).[31,32] In the case of social-ecological models, multilevel refers to multiple levels within a social-ecological system, including: individual, interpersonal, family, organizational, interorganizational/network, community, and societal levels. Systems thinking expands our view of multilevel.

As Meadows noted, to resolve complex problems, action is needed at a variety of levels.[33] A leading systems thinker in environmental and social analysis, Meadows described twelve leverage points or places to intervene in a complex system, from

TABLE 9-2. *Levels of a System*

Level	Explanation
Paradigm	The system's "mindset," the deepest held, often unspoken beliefs about the way the system works. Goals, rules, and structures that govern the system arise out of the paradigm. Actions and ideas at this level propose to either shift or reinforce the existing paradigm. Intervention at this level is very difficult.
Goals	Targets that need to be achieved for the paradigm to shift. Actions at this level focus or change the aim of the system.
System structure	Elements that make up the system as a whole, including the subsystems, actors, and interconnections among these elements. The structure conforms to the system's goals and paradigms. Actions at this level can change the system structure by changing linkages within the system or incorporating new types of structural elements.
Feedback and delays	Feedback allows the system to regulate itself by providing information about the outcome of different actions back to the source of the actions. Feedback occurs when actions by one element of the system affect the flows into or out of that same element. Actions at this level attempt to create new, or increase the gain around existing, feedback loops. Adding new feedback loops or changing feedback delays can restructure the system.
Structural elements	The smaller subsystems, actors, and physical elements of the system, connected through feedback loops and information flows. Actions at this level affect specific subsystems, actors, or elements of the system.

the paradigm (the highest level and the hardest to change, but the level at which there would be most impact) through the goals and rules of the system (important tools for system change), through system-level structures (for example, information flows) to subsystems that give rise to the system as a whole (the lowest level, at which changes can be effective, but whose impact tends to be local). Malhi and colleagues used Meadows's ideas to develop a five-level framework (Table 9-2) to sort qualitative data on systems change related to obesity (discussed further in the next section):[34]

Studying various levels of a system, one quickly realizes that no public health problem, despite how local it may seem, occurs on one level but rather involves a range of levels. The importance of intervention levels as well as the need for new perspectives on causality can be demonstrated briefly with the issue of obesity in the section below.

A systems view on the challenge of obesity

Obesity is increasingly recognized as a complex population health issue that must be viewed from a systems perspective. For example, the Institute of Medicine's L.E.A.D. (**L**ocate, **E**valuate, **A**ssemble Evidence and Inform **D**ecisions) Framework for Obesity Prevention Decision Making acknowledges the large number of contextual factors relevant to the development of obesity and encourages solutions that take these factors, the interactions among them, and the multiple system levels into consideration.[35]

Theory aimed at understanding what has become known as the obesity epidemic has evolved over the last few decades.[17] Initially obesity was conceived of as a result of energy imbalance; a later physiological model suggested it is the result of aberrant homeostatic control.[36] As discussed above, more recently, behaviors related to physical activity and eating—among the determinants of obesity—are framed by social and ecological models that recognize that such behaviors are developed and shaped in social and physical environments.[37,38] It is recognized that interventions aimed at improving physical activity and eating behaviors, when conducted in isolation of environmental and policy interventions, have limited success.

Although social-ecological models acknowledge the problem of obesity as complicated, they do not tend to convey it as *complex*—that is, possessing the characteristics noted in Table 9–1: being heterogeneous, nonlinear, stochastic, interdependent, generating feedback, self-organizing, and involving emergence. Figure 9–1 demonstrates the broad causal factors contributing to obesity and maps their interactions. The figure's complexity makes it a challenge to understand—but at the same time establishes obesity very clearly as a problem that reductionist approaches will fail to solve. It is clear that attributing obesity to specific, isolated causes will not be helpful. It is also clear that interventions must be implemented at a number of different levels and involve actors from multiple sectors—the food industry, media, marketing, transportation, urban planning, health care, public health, education, and the public.

Of course, it is one thing to understand problems as complex, and quite another to take action toward resolving them. Finegood acknowledges that the dozens of recommendations to address the problems of obesity also make it difficult to grasp the full picture of what needs to be done.[17] She and her colleagues used the five-level framework discussed in the previous section to systematically sort recommendations to address childhood obesity.[34] The intervention-level framework enables a consideration of (a) the issue at hand in its entirety, and (b) a range of actions toward resolving the issue, both at each level and overall. In a preliminary application of the framework to sort recommendations for resolving the issue of childhood obesity, they found that most actions put forward as suggestions to address obesity were at the level of structural elements, which demonstrates a strong tendency to make recommendations only where there is an obvious evidence base—in other words, where a cause and effect relationship can be inferred. Although these evidence-based actions are considered the gold standard, interventions at the structural elements level are usually the least effective in creating complex system change.[34]

In sum, a systems view of obesity reinforces the need to think differently about D&I. We need to go beyond the search for linear, cause-and-effect relationships and applying these "evidence-based" actions. Instead, we need to consider leverage points for influencing change within a complex system, which take into account properties of a system, such as feedback and delays, system structures, goals, and paradigms.

■ SYSTEMS THINKING IN ACTION

This section illustrates systems thinking in action in two projects funded by the Canadian Partnership Against Cancer (CPAC). Youth Excel is building a

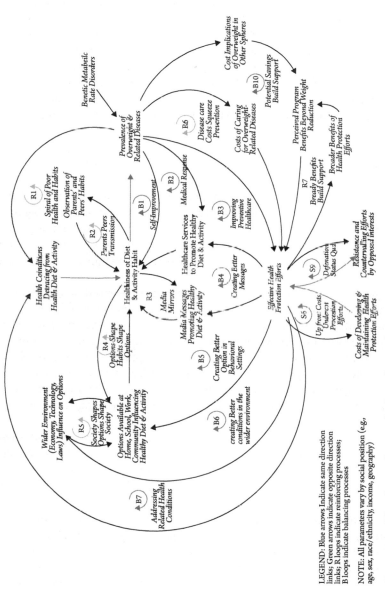

LEGEND: Blue arrows indicate same direction
links; Green arrows indicate opposite direction
links; R loops indicate reinforcing processes;
B loops indicate balancing processes

NOTE: All parameters vary by social position (e.g.,
age, sex, race/ethnicity, income, geography)

Figure 9–1. The obesity "system": a broad causal map.

multisectoral, multijurisdictional "learning system" as a vehicle for D&I that integrates evidence and action and can guide and redirect prevention efforts in a rapidly evolving social environment. The CAPTURE Project focuses on improving the use of "real-world" evidence to provide both a feedback loop to the D&I research agenda and to strengthen the use of evidence in practice. Both Youth Excel and The CAPTURE Project are focusing their attention on the systems for capturing and using practice-based evidence. Youth Excel is supporting a specific community of practice around youth health and preventing chronic disease, and The CAPTURE Project is building a platform and the capacity to support multiple projects where learning about effective dissemination and implementation depends on shared measurement. By addressing gaps in the systems that support the collection of practice-based evidence, Youth Excel and CAPTURE hope to help decision makers learn what works in which contexts and for whom.

Youth Excel

Youth Excel (*Youth* Health Collaborative: *Excel*erating Evidence-informed Action) was awarded under a CPAC funding program known as Coalitions Linking Action and Science for Prevention (CLASP). CPAC's goals for CLASP represent goals for D&I: to integrate science, policy, and practice to optimize prevention efforts, and to catalyze cross-provincial/territorial partnerships to improve individual and population health.[40]

Youth Excel's vision and approach are anchored in systems thinking about what is required to link evidence and action in the field of population and public health. The best available evidence must inform action, and such evidence must be continually generated to improve prevention policies and programs on an ongoing basis.[41,42] These imperatives require leaders in policy, practice, and research fields to work together to jointly plan, conduct, and act on relevant evidence. Youth Excel is implementing this approach; it is a multisector, multiprovince initiative that brings together national and provincial organizations from health and education sectors who share a goal to optimize youth health.

The Youth Excel initiative is timely, given the challenge at hand. Canada's youth are at risk for serious health issues due to tobacco use, unhealthy eating, and physical inactivity.[43] Unhealthy behaviors that are highly prevalent in youth tend to persist into adulthood,[44] perpetuating a complex cycle of health problems that defy attempts to discover which cause(s) leads to which effect(s).

The emerging approach in Canada assumes that changes in environments will be centrally important in reducing risk and promoting youth health. Moreover, the approach assumes that it is unlikely that any one policy or program will solve the problem. Rather, a mix of interventions will be required to create physical, social, and policy environments that promote healthy behavior patterns and discourage unhealthy patterns.[32] These assumptions have implications for evidence and approaches to D&I. Piecemeal, time-limited research projects are insufficient. What is needed is a system for ongoing learning within and across jurisdictions about what works, for whom, and under what circumstances.[3,45] Foundational assets for such a learning system include data systems and networks to provide and enable use of pertinent evidence. Building these foundational assets is at the core of Youth Excel. Youth Excel is a team of teams that link researchers, policy, and practice leaders, initially in seven provinces; the pan-Canadian Joint Consortium for School Health; and the Propel Centre for Population Health Impact (which serves as the Youth Excel secretariat).

Consistent with developing a youth health learning system, Youth Excel aims to establish and act on shared priorities for (a) moving evidence to action, and (b) deriving evidence from action. To advance this aim, Youth Excel is developing minimal datasets of indicators in the areas of tobacco use and physical activity (as initial priorities), with the scope encompassing both individual- and school-level variables. The product will be standard measures to optimize the ability to do comparative youth health studies across Canadian jurisdictions as innovative policies and programs are introduced (e.g., new physical and health curricula, provincial wellness strategies). Over time, additional components of a youth health learning system will be built, including a pan-Canadian database and an expanded network of colleagues who collaborate in developing a data feedback system, and in using it to support D&I through impact-oriented surveillance, evaluation, research, and planning.

The CAPTURE Project

Current models for generating the evidence on which program managers and policymakers base their decisions clearly fall short of filling the gap in practice-based evidence.[23] Academic research frequently addresses questions about whether an intervention is efficacious or effective, but rarely determines how it can be adapted to different populations or settings and how long effects are likely to be sustained (see Chapter 15). Program evaluation can give decision makers information about outputs and about some outcomes, but given the complexity of most challenges and the limited size of most interventions, it is hard to tell what is contributing to real change.

A systems approach to learning about the importance of context is to share measurement. Kramer and colleagues examined a handful of innovative organizations that had developed Web-based systems for reporting the performance, measuring the outcomes, and coordinating the efforts of hundreds or even thousands of social enterprises within their field.[46] They identified three types of breakthroughs in shared measurement: shared measurement platforms, comparative performance systems, and adaptive learning systems that improve knowledge, efficiency, and impact.

Developed to enable such shared measurement, CAPTURE (CAnadian Platform To increase Usage of Real-world Evidence) was funded by the Canadian Partnership Against Cancer. The CAPTURE vision is that we have effective primary prevention in Canada because we learn from what we do. The project includes a Web-based platform to support organizations and individuals in various functions including program and evaluation planning, reporting on progress, sharing and reflecting on the results of interventions, and connecting with others who are working with similar populations or implementing the same intervention.

During the first phase of CAPTURE's development, more than 500 chronic disease prevention informants, including public health practitioners, evaluators, public health decision makers, and public health and intervention researchers, were engaged in a series of consultations using a variety of methods, including concept mapping (a Web-based process in which participants brainstorm, sort, and rate topic-related statements, which are then represented visually in the form of a map); an expert panel meeting; stakeholder workshops, key informant interviews, and focus groups; Web surveys; and usability testing.

Through these consultations, CAPTURE learned about the needs and opportunities to make changes in the systems that support evaluation for learning, including that:

- program managers and policymakers want to be able to compare outcomes across program type;
- there is nowhere to learn how to adapt efficacious programs into different contexts or to identify the elements essential to making an efficacious intervention effective in a specific context;
- people have difficulty connecting with others working on similar issues;
- there is nowhere to share the results of evaluations or to learn how others implemented programs;
- setting up evaluation systems is expensive and time consuming; and
- data analysis is difficult for most practitioners.

By using a systems thinking lens and focusing on gaps in the system, rather than by trying to directly fill the gaps in the evidence base, CAPTURE will help to address the needs identified during the consultation phase. With this support for the collection of practice-based evidence, over time the CAPTURE databases will become a resource to learn what worked in specific populations and in particular geographic regions, whether an intervention is feasible to implement and acceptable to particular populations, what resources are required, and what barriers need to be overcome to implement an intervention.

■ CONCLUSION

Increasingly, the literature highlights the benefits of systems thinking in approaching D&I.[47,48] This chapter aimed to contribute to and further this literature by drawing attention to some of the implications inherent in adopting a systems view, in particular of causation and of leverage points for change in a complex system. We argue that the quest for solutions to complex health and social problems cannot be underpinned by reductionist science. Instead, it can be guided by a multilevel framework for complex solutions that identifies places to intervene in a complex system. As illustrated by Youth Excel and the CAPTURE project, systems-oriented D&I requires greater attention to foundational assets and infrastructure (e.g., data systems, common measures, networks) that enable learning in real time and continuous improvement of policies and programs operating in complex and dynamic environments.

SUGGESTED READINGS

Best A, Holmes BJ. Systems thinking, knowledge and action: Towards better models and methods. *Evidence and Policy.* 2010;6(2):145–159.

Best & Holmes examine models of systems thinking and their impact on translating knowledge into action (KTA). They identify four aspects of the KTA model—evidence and knowledge, leadership, networks, and communications—and its potential uses for changing research, policy, and practice.

Finegood D. The complex systems science of obesity. In: Cawley J, ed. *The Social Science of Obesity.* Oxford University Press; 2011.

This chapter considers obesity as a complex problem and illustrates the various characteristics that make obesity complex. It considers the usual responses to complexity and solutions appropriate for complex problems. Two frameworks for intervention are also presented.

Flood R. The relationship of 'systems thinking' to action research. *Systemic Practice and Action Research.* 2010;23(4):269–284.

Flood examines the relationship between action research and systems thinking and describes two lines of thought—systems thinking and systemic thinking—that consider action research in different lights. Systemic thinking is reported to have greater relevance as a foundation for action research.

Meadows, DH. *Thinking in Systems: A primer.* White River Junction, VT: Chelsea Green Publishing; 2008.

Published posthumously, this succinct primer describes a shift in systems thinking that can be applied to local and international contexts alike. Meadows asserts that understanding the relationship between structure and behavior can produce a new, improved way of thinking about systems.

Institute of Medicine. *Bridging the Evidence Gap in Obesity Prevention: A Framework to Inform Decision Making.* Washington, DC: Institute of Medicine of The National Academies; 2010.

Presents the Institute of Medicine's (IOM) framework for assisting researchers and policymakers with decision making about obesity prevention policies and programs. To write the report, the IOM organized a committee to answer two questions: How can current evidence about obesity prevention be identified, evaluated, and compiled to best inform decision making? How can additional, high-quality evidence be developed that is relevant to decision making about obesity prevention?

Rittel H, Webber M. Dilemmas in a general theory of planning. *Policy Sciences.* 1973;4: 155–169.

The search for the scientific bases of many societal problems is bound to fail, say Rittel and Webber, because these are "wicked" problems in the sense that they are difficult to define and locate. The authors describe 10 properties of such problems to which attention must be paid in the identification of actions towards their resolution.

Sterman J. Learning from evidence in a complex world. *American Journal of Public Health.* 2006;96:505–514.

Using evidence-based practices should result in more effective policies and practices, but too often policies intended to promote health do just the opposite. Sterman uses principles of systems thinking and simulation modeling to help researchers and policymakers better understand existing evidence and how to create real, positive changes in public health.

Wandersman A, Duffy J, Flaspohler P, et al. Bridging the gap between prevention research and practice: The interactive systems framework for dissemination and implementation. *Am J Community Psychol.* 2008;41(3–4):171–181

Wandersman et al. describe the gap between research and practice and the need for new approaches to close this gap. Their design, the Interactive Systems Framework for Dissemination and Implementation (ISF), can be used by a wide variety of stakeholders to recognize the various needs and resources of different systems.

Ward, V, House, A, Hamer, S. Developing a framework for transferring knowledge into action: A thematic analysis of the literature. *J Health Serv Res Policy.* 2009;14: 156–164.

Ward et al. thematically analyze 28 knowledge transfer (KT) models and based on these themes develop a conceptual framework for translating knowledge into action. The framework provides a foundation for gathering evidence about the effectiveness of KT interventions.

SELECTED WEBSITES

The CAPTURE Project <http://www.thecaptureproject.ca>

Keeps track of advances in the development of the program planning and evaluation platform, which will be available at www.thecaptureplatform.ca.

Youth Excel <www.propel.uwaterloo.ca/youthexcel>

Provides an overview of Youth Excel, updates on specific initiatives, and access to products and learning opportunities.

■ REFERENCES

1. Kreuter MW, De Rosa C, Howze EH, Baldwin GT. Understanding wicked problems: A key to advancing environmental health promotion. *Health Education & Behavior.* 2004;31:441–454.
2. Plsek P, Greenhalgh T. Complexity science: The challenge of complexity in health care. *British Medical Journal.* 2001;323(7313):625–628.
3. Bar-Yam Y. *Making Things Work: Solving Complex Problems in a Complex World.* Cambridge, MA: NECSI - Knowledge Press; 2004.
4. Rabin BA, Brownson RC, Haire-Joshu D, Kreuter MW, Weaver NL. A glossary for dissemination and implementation research in health. *Journal of Public Health Management and Practice.* 2008;14(2):117–123.
5. Crowley WF, Sherwood L, Salber P. Clinical research in the United States at a crossroads: Proposal for a novel public-private partnership to establish a national clinical research enterprise. *JAMA.* 2004;291(9):1120–1126.
6. Best A, Holmes BJ. Systems thinking, knowledge and action: Towards better models and methods. *Evidence and Policy.* 2010;6(2):145–159.
7. Van de Ven A, Johnson P. Knowledge for theory and practice. *Academy of Management Review.* 2006;31(4):808–821.
8. Kitson A, Rycroft-Malone J, Gill H, McCormack B, Seers K, Titchen A. Evaluating the successful implementation of evidence into practice using the PARiHS framework: Theoretical and practical challenges. *Implementation Science.* 2008;3:1.

9. Brown D, McCormack B. Developing postoperative pain management: Utilising the Promoting Action on Research Implementation in Health Services (PARIHS) Framework. *Worldviews of Evidence-Based Nursing.* 2005;2(3):131–141.

10. Wright J, McCormack B, Coffey A, McCarthy G. Evaluating the context within which continence care is provided in rehabilitation units for older people. *International Journal of Older People Nursing.* 2007;2:9–19.

11. Wandersman A, Duffy J, Flaspohler P et al. Bridging the gap between prevention research and practice: The interactive systems framework for dissemination and implementation. *American Journal of Community Psychology.* 2008;41:171–181.

12. Damschroder L, Aron DC, Keith RE, Kirsch SR, Alexander JA, Lowery JC. Fostering implementation of health services research findings into practice: A consolidated framework for advancing implementation science. *Implementation Science.* 2009;4:50.

13. Ward V, House A, Hamer S. Developing a framework for transferring knowledge into action: A thematic analysis of the literature. *Journal of Health Services Research and Policy.* 2009;14:156–164.

14. Mandel T. ed. (2000). The General System In: International Society for the Systems Sciences (2000). Accessed January 14, 2012 http://www.isss.org/members/papers/sysround.htm.

15. Cilliers P. *Complexity and Postmodernism: Understanding Complex Systems.* New York: Routledge. 1998.

16. Westley F, Zimmerman B, Patton MQ. *Getting to Maybe: How the World Is Changed.* Toronto: Vintage ; 2007.

17. Finegood D. The complex systems science of obesity. In: Cawley J, ed. *The Social Science of Obesity.* New York: Oxford University Press; 2011:208–236.

18. Nease DE Jr, Green LA. ClinfoTracker: A generalizable prompting tool for primary care. *Journal of the American Board of Family Practice.* 2003;16(2):115–123.

19. Glouberman S, Zimmerman B. Complicated and complex systems: What would successful reform of Medicare look like? Discussion paper number 8. Commission on the Future of Health Care in Canada; Ottawa. 2002.

20. McLeroy KR, Bibeau D, Steckler A, Glanz K. An ecological perspective on health promotion programs. *Health Education Quarterly.* 1988;15:351–177.

21. Stokols D, Allen J, Bellingham RL. The social ecology of health promotion: Implications for research and practice. *American Journal of Health Promotion.* 1996; 10(4):247–251.

22. Midgely G. Science as systemic intervention: Some implications of systems thinking and complexity for the philosophy of science. *Systemic Practice and Action Research.* 2003;16(2):77–97.

23. Green LW. Public health asks of systems science: To advance our evidence-based practice, can you help us get more practice-based evidence? *American Journal of Public Health.* 2006;96:406–409.

24. Glied S, Tilipman N. Simulation modelling of health care policy. *Annual Review of Public Health.* 2010;31:439–455.

25. Homer J, Milstein B, Wile K et al. Simulating and evaluating local interventions to improve cardiovascular health. *Public Health Research, Practice, and Policy.* 2010;7(1). http://www.cdc.gov/pcd/issues/2010/jan/08_0231.htm

26. Milstein B, Homer J, Hirsch G. Analyzing national health reform strategies with a dynamic simulation model. *American Journal of Public Health.* 2010;100(5):811–819.

27. Flood R. The relationship of 'systems thinking' to action research. *Systemic Practice and Action Research*. 2010;23(4):269–284.
28. Wagner A. Causality in complex systems. *Biology and Philosophy*. 1999;14:83–101.
29. Rittel H, Webber M. Dilemmas in a general theory of planning. *Policy Sciences*. 1973;4:155–169.
30. Robinson TN, Sirard JR. Preventing childhood obesity. A solution oriented research paradigm. *American Journal of Preventive Medicine*. 2005;28:192–201.
31. National Cancer Institute. *ASSIST: Shaping the Future of Tobacco Prevention and Control*. Tobacco Control Monograph 16. Bethesda, MD: U.S. Department of Health and Human Services, National Institutes of Health, National Cancer Institute. NIH Pub. No. 05–5645. May 2005.
32. Kumanyika S. Obesity prevention concepts and frameworks. In: Kumanyika S, Brownson R, eds. *Handbook of Obesity Prevention: A Resource for Health Professionals*. 2007:85–114.
33. Meadows DH. (1999). Leverage points: Places to intervene in a system. http://www.sustainer.org/pubs/Leverage_Points.pdf. Accessed June 15, 2010.
34. Malhi L, Karanfil O, Merth T, Acheson M, Palmer A, Finegood DT. Places to intervene to make complex food systems more healthy, green, fair and affordable. *Journal of Hunger and Environmental Nutrition*. 2009;4(3&4):466–476.
35. Institute of Medicine. *Bridging the Evidence Gap in Obesity Prevention: A Framework to Inform Decision Making*. Washington, DC: Institute of Medicine of The National Academies. 2010.
36. Bray GA, Bouchard C, James WPT, eds. *Handbook of Obesity*. New York: Marcel Dekker, Inc. 1998.
37. Doak CM, Visscher TL, Renders CM, Seidell JC. The prevention of overweight and obesity in children and adolescents: A review of interventions and programmes. *Obesity Review*. 2006;7(1):111–136.
38. Kumanyika S, Jeffery RW, Morabia A, Ritenbaugh C, Antipatis V, Public health approaches to the prevention of obesity (PHAPO) working group of the international obesity task force (IOTF). Obesity prevention: The case for action. *International Journal of Obesity and Related Metabolic Disorders: Journal of the International Association for the Study of Obesity*. 2002;26(3);425–436.
39. Milstein B, Homer J. System dynamics simulation in support of obesity prevention decision making. [Workshop]. Irvine, CA: Institute of Medicine. March 16, 2009.
40. Riley BL, Manske S, Cameron R. Youth Excel: Towards a Pan-Canadian platform linking evidence and action for prevention. *Cancer*. 2011;117(10 Suppl):2281-2288.
41. Cameron R, Riley B, Campbell S, Manske S, Lamers-Bellio K. The imperative of strategic alignment across organizations: The experience of the Centre for Behavioural Research and Program Evaluation. *Canadian Journal of Public Health*. 2009;100(1): 127–I30.
42. Speller V, Wimbush E, Morgan A. Evidence-based health promotion practice: How to make it work? *Promotion & Education*. 2005;12(suppl 1):15–20.
43. World Cancer Research Fund/American Institute for Cancer Research. *Food, Nutrition, Physical Activity, and the Prevention of Cancer: A Global Perspective*. Washington, DC: AICR; 2007.
44. Sallis J, Simons-Morton B, Stone E et al. Determinants of physical activity and interventions in youth. *Medicine & Science in Sport and Exercise*. 1992;24(suppl 2) S248–S257.
45. Sterman J. Learning from evidence in a complex world. *American Journal of Public Health*. 2006;96:505–514.

46. Kramer M, Parkhurst M, Vaidyanathan L. *Breakthroughs in shared measurement and social impact.* FSG Social Impact Advisors. 2009. http://www.hewlett.org/uploads/files/Breakthroughs_in_Shared_Measurement_complete.pdf

47. Best A, Hiatt RA, Norman CD. Knowledge integration: Conceptualizing communications in cancer control systems. *Patient Education and Counseling.* 2008;71:319–327.

48. Best A, Terpstra JL, Moor G, Riley B, Norman CD, Glasgow RE. Building knowledge integration systems for evidence-informed decisions. *Journal of Health Organization and Management.* 2009;23(6):627–641.

10 Participatory Approaches for Study Design and Analysis in Dissemination and Implementation Research

■ MEREDITH MINKLER AND
ALICIA L. SALVATORE

■ INTRODUCTION

The importance of community and other stakeholder participation for improving the quality and relevance of research has long been acknowledged.[1-4] With the growing interest in closing the "chasm"[5] between research and practice and more effectively eliminating health disparities, the potential benefits of participatory approaches for dissemination and implementation of research findings are increasingly being be considered. In particular, Community-Based Participatory Research (CBPR), with its commitment to action as part of the research process, holds great potential not only for improving the relevance of research to communities and stakeholders but also for ensuring that research results are effectively disseminated and translated into programs and policies to promote health. This partnership orientation to research has become recognized as an important means through which the distance between research and action might be more effectively bridged.[6] Indeed, as Horowitz and her colleagues point out, "CBPR may be the ultimate form of translational research…moving discoveries bidirectionally from bench to bedside to el barrio (the community) to organizations and policy makers."[7] Although CBPR is not possible or applicable in all research contexts, when it is appropriate, much value can be added to the research process and subsequent dissemination and implementation of findings through high-level community and other stakeholder participation. As discussed below, the level of community engagement in research takes place along a continuum, from limited consultation on specific aspects of the study, through high-level co-collaboration at every step in the process.

For readers unfamiliar with CBPR, this chapter seeks to demonstrate the value added from community participation to the research process itself. It also shows how CBPR methods are useful in the dissemination and implementation (D&I) of research findings and some of the lessons from CBPR for D&I research. There is a large and growing literature on CBPR that cannot be covered in a single chapter, so entry points into this body of writing are provided. After briefly describing a continuum of such participation, the discussion is focused, in particular, on CBPR. Challenges that can play out in participatory research are discussed, followed by a more detailed examination of the specific ways in which a CBPR approach can enhance the D&I of research findings through collaborative design, analysis, dissemination, and research translation. A case study of a community-university-health department CBPR project, in which both authors were involved, that endeavored to study and improve the health and working conditions of restaurant workers in San Francisco's Chinatown District is presented. Then, some of the methods used to involve all partners in study design, data analysis, and translation of findings into action, as well as some of the benefits of doing so, are discussed. Finally, key lessons learned, through this and other CBPR efforts, are shared, and their implications for improving the breadth and effectiveness of the critical dissemination and implementation phases of research are summarized.

Continuum of Participation in Research

Community and other stakeholder participation in research can be seen as occurring along a continuum, with benefits accruing at each stage, and the most substantial value added often occurring at the farthest end of the continuum. Over two decades ago, Biggs developed a continuum of community involvement in research, which remains frequently cited in the field.[8] He described the levels of participation as (1) *contractual*, in which community and other stakeholders simply take part in researchers' studies; (2) *consultative*, in which they are asked their opinions as interventions and other research instruments are designed and implemented; (3) *collaborative*, in which researchers and community and other stakeholders work together on projects designed, initiated, and managed by researchers; and (4) *collegiate*, in which all partners work as colleagues with different skills to offer, and there is mutual learning, and local control over the research process.

The second, third, and fourth levels in Biggs's model each can be seen as adding successively greater potential value to research processes and outcomes. Consultation with community and other stakeholders, for example, can result in higher recruitment rates and lower attrition, as well as fewer cultural and linguistic barriers, which in turn can increase the accuracy of data reporting and the appropriateness and effectiveness of interventions.[9-11] Investigator-initiated and managed studies that emphasize true collaboration with community and other stakeholders can increase still further the relevance and efficacy of research, resulting in greater community buy-in and trust, interventions that are better tailored to the study population, and enhanced efficacy in data collection, interpretation, and dissemination.[11] Finally, research that is truly collaborative in nature ensures that the research topic itself comes from, or is of substantial importance to, the community, and that the research process includes high levels participation throughout, including dissemination and use of study findings to help address the problem under study.[3,11,12]

Community-Based Participatory Research (CBPR) involves the most intensive form of community and stakeholder participation and typically takes place at the collaborative level. In this chapter, CBPR is used as an umbrella term for an orientation to research that goes by many names (among them participatory action research, community-partnered research, mutual inquiry and participatory research) and that have in common a commitment to combining research, participation, education, and action.[2,12] When feasible and appropriate, CBPR may be particularly well suited to translational research aimed at studying and addressing health disparities. This orientation to research adds value at each stage of the research process—from identification of the problem and of community assets to study design, analysis, and the dissemination and use of research findings. Although it also presents substantial challenges, including the time- and labor-intensive nature of the work, this orientation to research has achieved growing attention both in North America and internationally.

CBPR Definition and Principles

Community-Based Participatory Research is concisely defined by Green and his colleagues (1994) as "systematic inquiry, with the participation of those affected by the issue being studied, for the purposes of education and taking action or effecting change."[1] Building on this definition, as well as earlier work by Israel et al.,[3] the Kellogg Community Health Scholars Program[13] crafted a definition that situates CBPR within the context of efforts to study and address health disparities.[3,13] In its words, CBPR is "A collaborative process that equitably involves all partners in the research process and recognizes the unique strengths that each brings. CBPR begins with a research topic of importance to the community with the aim of combining knowledge and action for social change to improve community health and eliminate health disparities."[13]

The research dimension of CBPR can involve a wide range of qualitative and quantitative methods. Developing and administering community surveys or focus groups; conducting walkability assessments or air monitoring; using Geographic Information Systems (GIS) mapping; conducting secondary data analysis; and using randomized controlled trials (RCTs) to assess intervention effectiveness all have been used by as part of CBPR efforts.[10,11,14] Regardless of the particular research methods used, however, what is unique about this orientation to research is the *way* in which the research is conceptualized and conducted,[4] the heavy accent placed on genuine community and stakeholder engagement throughout the process, and the use of findings to help bring about change.

CBPR Principles

Eleven principles of CBPR (Table 10–1), described below, help to further articulate how CBPR differs from more traditional "top-down" approaches to research and is consistent with translational research that is indeed "community based," rather than merely "community placed." Israel and her community and academic colleagues[3,15] developed nine guiding principles of CBPR that are widely used to inform and guide the process of CBPR. Two other principles, added subsequently by Minkler and Wallerstein,[12] are also critical to this work. Although translational research partnerships wishing to utilize CBPR should adapt these principles (or develop new ones), as appropriate, given their own unique contexts, these eleven principles may be helpful in providing initial guidance.

TABLE 10-1. *CBPR Principles*

---

1. Recognizes community as a unit of identity, whether community is defined in geographic, racial/ethnic or other terms.
2. Builds on strengths and resources within the community
3. Facilitates a collaborative, equitable partnership in all phases of research, involving an empowering and power-sharing process that attends to social inequalities.
4. Fosters colearning and capacity-building among all partners
5. Integrates and achieves a balance between knowledge generation and intervention for the mutual benefit of all partners.
6. Focuses on the local relevance of public health problems and on ecological perspectives that attend to the multiple determinants of health.
7. Involves systems development using a cyclical and iterative process
8. Disseminates results to all partners and involves them in the wider dissemination of results
9. Involves a long-term process and commitment to sustainability
10. Openly address issues of race, ethnicity, racism, and other social divides, and embody "cultural humility"[16], recognizing that while no one can be truly "competent" in another's culture, we can demonstrate a commitment to self-reflection and critique, working to redress power imbalances and to develop authentic partnerships.
11. Work to assure research rigor and validity but also "broaden the bandwidth and validity"[17] to insure that the research question is valid (coming from, or being of importance to the community) and that different "ways of knowing," including community lay knowledge, are valued alongside more traditional scientific sources of knowledge.[17]

Source: Israel et al., 1998[3] and 2005[15]; Minkler and Wallerstein, 2008[12].

Following these principles may help strengthen the quality of data and the statistical power of analysis. Yet as Green and Glasgow[18] point out (see Chapter 15), although CBPR improves one facet of external validity—its relevance to "end users" of findings in a particular community—CBPR may make it less relevant to other communities. The more we make a study locally relevant, tailoring it to a particular population or community group, the more we make it ungeneralizable beyond that setting and population.[18] Such research remains important and relevant to others, however, in that it was made more applicable to typical circumstances, rather than settings that are "artificially constructed and controlled" for academic purposes.[18]

We turn now to the more specific ways in which CBPR may add value to community-based translational research.

Benefits of CBPR for Improving D&I Research Quality and Relevance

A CBPR orientation to inquiry has the potential to strengthen research quality at each step of the process, many of which have direct relevance for study design and analysis as well as the dissemination and implementation of findings. Although there are fewer examples of CBPR in D&I research specifically, the strengths of CBPR, highlighted below, are increasingly being pointed to as a way to remedy the "lack of "fit" between an intervention/research design on the one hand and, on the other hand, the realities inherent to target and practice settings, and the information needed by policymakers. Such mismatch often leads to "low adoption and implementation."[18]

CBPR can help ensure the relevance of the research topic. When "bench-to-bedside" or "bench-to-curbside" translational research is not seen by patients or communities as holding relevance for their lives and contexts, even the most elegant of research designs may fail to achieve their intended effects. Although the far end of the CBPR continuum involves communities or other stakeholders in identifying the topic to be studied, engaging such partners early in the process can help to ensure that even investigator-driven research is locally relevant and likely to yield useful results. Stanford University's Chronic Disease Self-Management Program has been tested through numerous peer-reviewed RCTs,[19-21] yet whether this program would have relevance to Native Americans, who are believed to have the nation's highest rates of diabetes,[22] was open to question. Working closely with a Community Advisory Board of Native Americans with diabetes in Santa Clara County, California, Jernigan and her colleagues determined that the program did have relevance but would need to be adapted, for example, in beginning each weekly session with a blessing and smudging ceremony, increasing session length to allow time for story-telling, and incorporating the image of a dream catcher into the program's visual of the symptom cycle.[23] With these changes, and led by Native American peer educators, the pilot program had a 100% retention rate, with significant changes seen in a variety of disease symptoms and self-management behaviors. Based on this success, the program was adapted for dissemination over the Internet[24]— a medium widely used by Native Americans across the United States since a major, cross-tribal newspaper is most easily accessed online.

CBPR can enhance the quality, validity, sensitivity, and practicality of research instruments by involving the local knowledge of community members. Surveys and other research instruments that lack cultural sensitivity or that appear naive or ill suited to the community being studied can reinforce feelings of disconnection and sometimes even be hurtful or insulting. Community insights into how to rephrase questions, or what type of research instrument may be best suited to a given community (e.g., focus groups versus in-depth interviews) can improve recruitment and retention[9-12] and, as Cargo and Mercer[11] point out, help in "reducing measurement error from survey and interview questions that are not culturally aligned." In the Healthy Homes Project in Seattle–Kings County, Washington, Community Health Workers administering a standard baseline survey to assess exposure to indoor asthma triggers noted that, despite earlier pretesting, questions about whether residents smoked at home were not sensitive enough to pick up whether or not *others* were smoking inside the house, and survey modifications resulted. As the study's epidemiologists pointed out, "Any loss in the ability to make 'pure' baseline and exit comparisons may have been outweighed by the higher quality of the exit data" as a result of community partner input.[25] The integration of different types of information and knowledge, through CBPR's inclusion of local knowledge and multiple stakeholder perspectives, is particularly relevant to D&I research, which, as Glasgow and Emmons (2007) and Green (2001) point out, has largely employed "...a limited and researcher-centered perspective as to what constitute 'evidence.' "[6,26]

CBPR can enhance the likelihood of overcoming the distrust of research by communities that traditionally have been the "subjects" of such research by bringing together partners with different skills, knowledge, and expertise to address complex problems. Deloria[27] coined the term "helicopter research" in reference to the fact that in "Indian country," outside researchers often enter to collect their data and then leave, offering nothing in return to local community members. Although such an approach has been noted—and criticized—by many communities, it is particularly problematic with respect to marginalized groups and populations for whom decades and sometimes centuries of oppression, including unethical research, at the hands of the dominant population have engendered deep distrust.[12,28]

By increasing the relevance of research interventions, CBPR can increase the likelihood of success. When community input is earnestly sought and valued, interventions may deviate from what the outside researchers originally had in mind.[29] Yet such changes may have positive effects for relevance and adaptation, improving external validity in the process.[28] Furthermore, participation of community members, including practitioners and policymakers, can enhance the probability of an intervention's adoption, "closing the gap between discovery and delivery."[18] Community Partners in Care, an RCT to improve the relevance of quality improvement approaches to depression care among African Americans, was planned using a community-partnered participatory research approach[30] and is now being implemented in Los Angeles, California, following these same participatory research principles and practices.[31] The inclusion of multiple stakeholders, among them a wide network of agencies, policymakers, and the arts community (since community partners felt the arts would provide culturally appropriate avenues for opening discussion about the stigma of depression), led to a robust community engagement model whose efficacy compared to more traditional resources for services models and is in the final stages of testing.[31]

CBPR can improve data analysis and interpretation by enhancing our understanding of the meaning of study findings through the contribution of lay knowledge. Although community members often have neither the time for nor the interest in being engaged in hands-on data analysis,[12,15,32] their help in reviewing and interpreting preliminary findings may add important nuance and deeper understandings of study results.

CBPR can improve the potential for disseminating findings to diverse audiences and translating evidence-based research into sustainable changes in programs, practices, and policies. Publication of CBPR translational research studies in peer-reviewed journals is critical, particularly since to date, the number of such publications that present their methodological approaches in detail and can demonstrate significant health outcomes, remains small.[11,33] Community and other stakeholder partners, however, can identify additional dissemination channels (e.g., ethnic media and relevant community events) as well as strategies to more effectively reach key community members and decision makers with the findings. A number of CBPR projects also have created workbooks or replication manuals to assist other partnerships interested in adapting and utilizing their approaches, and many of these, along with myriad other resources, are now available online through the Community Tool Box (http://ctb.ku.edu) and Community-Campus Partnerships for Health (www.ccph.info). The combination of community engagement and relevant scientific research further can pack substantial political punch, helping to effect policy and systems-level changes conducive to more health-promoting environments.[34] A successful CBPR effort in a low-resource San Francisco neighborhood with little access to fresh fruits and vegetables not only led to the creation of a local "Good Neighbor

Program" offering incentives to local stores that agreed to stock more fresh fruits and vegetables, but it also played a key role in helping secure the passage of legislation for a statewide demonstration program to help replicate this approach in other communities.[34–36] Although no funding was allocated after the measure was signed into law, a subsequent amendment for a public-private partnership will enable the program to be taken to scale.

Ethical and Methodological Challenges

Although CBPR can indeed help enhance the quality and relevance of translational research, including making substantial contributions to research design and analysis, this approach also raises difficult ethical and methodological challenges that merit attention.[12,14,29] Community and other stakeholders may make recommendations that would weaken the rigor of study instruments (e.g., altering validated scales) or propose changes in study design that may weaken the science, for example, when community members object to an RCT or staggered design that may be needed to prove whether an intervention had an effect. To avoid such difficulties, many partnerships now begin by developing memorandums of understanding (MOUs) and/or holding colearning workshops where the meaning of terms like *validity* and *research rigor* are explored from both academic and community perspectives, and decisions are made ahead of time about how difficult issues will be handled. Partnerships further have benefited by the development of tools, such as Mercer et al.'s[37] reliability-tested guidelines for assessing partnership process and progress along multiple dimensions, and tools developed by Israel and her colleagues,[38,39] which also have been widely adapted and used.

When trained community members are engaged in conducting interviews or administering surveys, perceptions of bias also may be raised. In communities characterized by high levels of distrust borne of years of discriminatory treatment, however, as in some rural parts of the Southern United States, involving outside researchers in face-to-face data gathering may be unrealistic, especially initially. Creative ways of dealing with such problems, such as having residents of neighboring communities accompany and introduce university researchers in data collection activities (e.g., door-to-door surveys) may help in building trust and increasing participation rates.[40]

In the data interpretation and dissemination phases of translational research, ethical and methodological challenges also may arise if community partners are perceived as having an "axe to grind" that could lead them to present findings selectively to further their community's best interests. Additionally, if data emerge that could cast the community in an unfavorable light,[41] thorny questions of community ownership and decision-making processes may ensue. As in other stages of the research process, colearning sessions and trainings on the importance of accurately collecting, analyzing, and reporting findings, as well as frank discussions of community and outside researcher roles and responsibilities in this regard, are critical. At the same time, instruments such as Flicker et al.'s[41] recommendations for Institutional Review Boards reviewing participatory research may be useful to CBPR partnerships in asking hard questions up front, including, for example, "What will be done if findings emerge that are unflattering to the community?" As noted earlier, process appraisal instruments that CBPR partnerships can use throughout the research process[37-39] and careful MOUs between partners can aid in preventing or openly confronting such challenges when they arise. Several ethical and methodological challenges and how they were dealt with are highlighted in the case study that follows.

■ CBPR CASE EXAMPLE: THE SAN FRANCISCO CHINATOWN RESTAURANT WORKER STUDY

The Chinatown Restaurant Worker Study is an ongoing CBPR effort to examine and address the health and working conditions of restaurant workers in San Francisco's Chinatown. Nationwide, workers in the restaurant industry face high rates of injury and other challenges such as low wages and few benefits, limited opportunities for upward mobility or wage increases, and other types of occupational injustice.[42-44] Studying the relationships between restaurant work and worker health is particularly important for immigrant workers who comprise a large portion of this workforce and who may experience disproportionately greater rates of illness and injury due to immigration concerns, language barriers, and lack of awareness of U.S. workplace regulations.[42] Given that restaurants are the largest employer of Chinese immigrants,[45] one of the largest and most rapidly growing immigrant populations in the United States research and intervention efforts with Chinese restaurant workers are critical. San Francisco's Chinatown, home to almost 5,000 people and more than 100 restaurants, offered an important setting in which to study and address the working conditions and health of this important community.

Building on strong mutual interest in promoting the health and welfare of Chinatown restaurant workers, a partnership was developed in 2007 comprised of a community-based organization (the Chinese Progressive Association [CPA]), two universities (the University of California, Berkeley School of Public Health, including UC Berkeley's Labor Occupational Health Program [LOHP], and the University of California San Francisco School of Medicine), and a local health department (the San Francisco Department of Public Health's Occupational and Environmental Health Section). Many of the partners had worked previously together on other CBPR projects, and the project coordinator (a university partner) was a founding member of CPA and a former resident of Chinatown. These existing relationships greatly facilitated the establishment of the partnership as well as initial trust between partners.

The community-university-health department collaborative aimed to follow CBPR principles[3,12] and included an ongoing participatory evaluation of partnership process and effectiveness.[46] A 12-member Steering Committee, comprised of representatives from each partner organization, was formed to serve as the project's primary coordinating and decision-making body. A six-member Restaurant Worker Leadership Group (RWLG) was established with the goal of facilitating in-depth participation from restaurant workers throughout all phases of the project.

A CBPR grant from the National Institute for Occupational Safety and Health (NIOSH) supported partnership development, an ecologic study of Chinatown restaurant worker health and safety, described in more detail below, a participatory evaluation of the partnership, and some dissemination activities. In keeping with its CBPR orientation, the Chinatown project kept the "final" phases of CBPR—dissemination and translation of findings into action—at the forefront of planning from the study's onset. For example, the team sought additional funding early in project from a large philanthropic organization, The California Endowment, which supports and encourages CBPR and policy-level intervention. This additional funding enabled the partnership to more broadly disseminate study findings and translate research findings into programs and policies to promote worker health. The community partner's long history and success in organizing and advocacy made CPA well suited to lead these expanded dissemination and translational activities, and it served as the lead agency on the California Endowment grant.

Participation in Study Design

Partners' collaboration in study design began during grant writing and intensified once study funds, the Steering Committee, and the RWLG were all in place. Consistent with partners' values and CBPR principles and recognizing the multi-level nature of factors influencing restaurant worker health, the Chinatown study employed an ecologic design. The study was comprised of a community-based cross-sectional survey of Chinatown restaurant workers, conducted by trained worker partners. It also included standardized observations of hazards to workers in Chinatown restaurants conducted by health department staff during food safety inspections. All partners, including RWLG members, actively participated in working groups to develop data collection protocols and study instruments. Involving all partners in study development required significant time and commitment from all partners. In addition, considerable resources were needed for critical services such as translation of documents into Chinese and English and simultaneous interpretation into Cantonese or English at project team meetings.

To more effectively involve RWLG members, Chinatown restaurant workers with no prior research experience, an eight-week training was held at the beginning of the study on topics such as workplace health and safety, workers' rights, research goals, and research-related topics such as confidentiality, informed consent, and survey administration. After the initial training, the RWLG met biweekly to provide feedback on study instruments, develop a recruitment plan for the worker survey, and prepare to pilot-test the survey instrument. Interactive activities such as risk mapping,[47-49] neighborhood mapping, and mock food inspections in a simulated kitchen were used to enhance workers' participation.

The instruments developed by the collaborative are described below with some examples of how the involvement of diverse partners improved their quality, and thereby enhanced their application and outcomes.

Worker Survey

A standardized questionnaire was developed to measure Chinatown restaurant workers' health and work experiences. A draft instrument, created with inputs from all partners, was reviewed and revised by the RWLG and then finalized after piloting with 15 restaurant workers. The participation of CPA in the development of the questionnaire resulted in many additions to the original draft created by university partners. These included questions designed to learn more about the broader context of workers' lives (e.g., wages, housing, health and social service utilization, and workers' civic engagement). The RWLG's participation in survey development resulted in some important wording additions to standardized scales (e.g., explaining such idioms as "butterflies in my stomach"), as well as new questions to document previously ignored hardships in their work environments such as harassment, violence, and wage and tip theft.[46]

Procedures for survey recruitment and administration similarly were collaboratively developed by all partners. The participation of CPA and the RWLG, in particular, was critical for anticipating possible risks to participants (e.g., worker retaliation) and developing a protocol that assuaged participants' fears and safeguarded their identities. Members of the RWLG and 17 additional community members who were hired as surveyors went through intensive training in informed consent and study procedures prior to their involvement in recruiting participants and administering the survey.

Restaurant Observations

A 13-item observational survey, the Restaurant Worker Safety Checklist, was developed to collect restaurant-level information about the presence of required labor law postings, occupational hazards, and safety measures, equipment, and behaviors during regularly scheduled food service inspections. The health department partner, SFDPH, took the lead on the development of the checklist, with additional inputs from community and academic partners and health department food inspection staff. RWLG members' recommendations resulted in important improvements to the final tool. As they pointed out, for example, the checklist should not only assess whether posters detailing Occupational Safety and Health Administration's (OSHA) regulations and San Francisco's wage ordinance were present but also whether Chinese language versions were posted. Further, the checklist should not just assess whether first aid kits were visible but document whether they were fully stocked (82% of restaurants did not have fully stocked kits).[46]

SFDPH was solely responsible for the administration of the checklist. However, community and university partners shadowed health department staff during checklist piloting. This enhanced partners' understanding of the types of challenges present in restaurants that affect both data collection and worker health.

Participation in Data Analysis and Interpretation

The collaborative was successful in exceeding research targets. Surveys were completed with 433 restaurant workers, and observational data using the Restaurant Worker Safety Checklist were collected by health department staff in 98% of Chinatown restaurants that were open for business at the time of data collection (n = 106 of 108 possible restaurants). Once data were collected, the partnership followed an agreed-upon process for preparing and analyzing the findings. This process included all partners and was designed to build upon partners' existing skills and expertise (e.g., data analysis and knowledge of local context) as well as codevelop and enhance additional skills necessary for improved interpretation of study results (e.g., "outsiders'" understanding of local culture and context and RWLG members' knowledge of how to read data tables).

University partners took the lead in preparing and analyzing the survey data, and health department partners did so for the observational restaurant-level data. During the analysis period, preliminary results were routinely shared with all partners through e-mail communications and presentations at Steering Committee, RWLG, and other project meetings. A critical component of the analysis phases of the study was the ongoing involvement of restaurant workers in data interpretation. Six monthly data interpretation workshops were held with the RWLG members at CPA's office in Chinatown. These workshops, conducted in Chinese by CPA staff and the project coordinator with additional support from other university and health department partners, employed hands-on learning to teach RWLG members to speak "data language" and to facilitate their participation in the interpretation of checklist and survey findings.

RWLG members provided many insights into the data not originally apparent to other partners. For example, when considering findings indicating that cooks wore long-sleeved shirts or cook jackets in only 10% of restaurant observations conducted,[50] RWLG members suggested that, in addition to the high kitchen temperatures, this was likely due to Chinese male cooks' viewing of burns and cuts as "badges of honor."[46] Similarly, RWLG members helped identify and provide context for some survey findings that they believed to be overreported due to workers' fears of employer retaliation or misinterpretation. For example, the RWLG doubted that 58% of restaurant worker respondents actually received paid sick days, as reported, explaining, "When people ask for a day off, they work another day later ... workers often understand this [having to make up a day for taking a sick day] as sick leave." Similarly, the RWLG explained that many of the statistics related to health, such general health status (SF-36) and work-related injuries, were likely underestimated due to the fact that many workers would only report major problems "like cancer." One member summed up this phenomenon, saying that Chinese workers think that "unless you're *really* sick, you're healthy." RWLG members felt that the same phenomenon resulted in an underreporting of abusive treatment at work such as being yelled at (reported by 42%). RWLG felt that those responding in the affirmative were probably only those for whom the "yelling had made them cry," explaining that they are constantly being yelled at by their supervisors.

The in-depth participation of all partners in data analysis and interpretation resulted in all partners, including restaurant workers themselves, having a detailed knowledge of study findings. This greatly enhanced equitable and high-level involvement in dissemination of study results as well as the use of data in the creation of translational strategies, discussed below.

Community and stakeholder participation in disseminating and translating results into programs and policies

In contrast to the research phase of the study, in which the researchers, in many ways, took the lead on guiding activities, the community and health department partners are leading in the "final phase" of the Chinatown CBPR effort. The partnership's dissemination plan includes sharing study findings through both scientific and lay/ethic media as well as targeted meetings with restaurant workers, restaurant owners, and key policy and decision makers. Recognizing that diverse purposes and audiences would require different types of communications, the partnership created several different reports to share findings: (1) a report of worker survey findings authored by university partners;[51] (2) a report of restaurant observation findings written by health department partners;[50] and (3) a comprehensive, visually appealing, and action-oriented report authored by CPA[52] that draws from the two previous reports to lay out a vision for improving working conditions for a healthy Chinatown. The collaborative's dissemination activities, like other CBPR efforts,[53,54] are guided by agreements regarding publication and presentation established early in the study. These guidelines emphasize coownership of data and coauthorship. To date, all partners have participated in presenting study findings and have served as coauthors on the peer-reviewed papers published to date.[46,55]

Multiple efforts are currently underway to translate study finding into sustainable improvements for Chinatown restaurant workers. As a result of the significant lack of labor law posting documented in this study (e.g., only 15% of observed restaurants had posted workers' compensation in English and 8% in Chinese; just 24% had the city's sick leave regulation posted in English and 23% in Chinese), and the results of a subsequent study to examine compliance with labor law posting in restaurants within and beyond Chinatown, SFDPH began requiring proof of workers' compensation insurance coverage for all new and change-of-business health permits. The health department is also taking additional steps to assess citywide compliance with these policies. For example, as a result of study findings that 50% of Chinatown restaurant workers did not receive minimum wage, 52% reported not receiving paid sick leave, 40% didn't received mandated work breaks, and 97% did not receive the city's required health care coverage, SFDPH sent formal letters to regulatory bodies such as the local Office of Labor Standards Enforcement (OSLE) to share study findings and request collaboration in improving enforcement of these laws. As a result, OLSE and SFDPH are exploring mechanisms to improve violator identification and enforcement.[55] Additionally, the health department has obtained new funding with study partner LOHP to explore feasible ways to involve food safety inspectors (who have legal access to restaurant environments) in the promotion of workers' health.

CPA is leading a number of efforts to implement or support action interventions based on study findings. Educational activities with restaurant workers, which began early in the project with the RWLG, have been scaled up in number and scope, to reflect study findings. Efforts to educate workers are a result of our finding that 64% of workers surveyed did not receive any mandated health and safety training at work, and documentation, through the study, of wage theft and many other regulatory violations. Ongoing educational efforts include Worker Teas held monthly at CPA, educational exchanges with other workers and worker rights groups around San Francisco and nationally (e.g., at a large workers' Social Forum), and others. Since no study of this magnitude had previously been conducted with Chinese restaurant workers in the United States, and since restaurants remain the largest employer of immigrant

Chinese workers throughout the nation study findings have been cited by worker centers and other organizations in New York, Los Angeles, and other major cities.

Additionally, in consultation with project partners and other stakeholders, and based in part on study findings, CPA has developed a key set of recommend actions to improve the health and well-being of Chinatown restaurant workers. These include: (1) convening community stakeholder roundtables to develop solutions for creating healthy jobs and a healthier community; (2) strengthening government enforcement of labor, health, and safety laws; and (3) significantly increasing investments in healthy economic development and responsible employment practices in Chinatown. Along with these general recommendations, CPA has drawn up a number of municipal policy actions. The above-mentioned report authored by CPA details these recommendations and the associated policy agenda.[52] The report was launched in September 2010, with many project partners and close to 170 community members, neighborhood organization representatives, media personnel and policymakers in attendance. With the launch, which received widespread media coverage in local newspapers, television and radio programs, as well as on line, CPA initiated a Low Wage Worker Bill of Rights organizing campaign to create support for policy change. At a kickoff event on the steps of the City Hall in Spring 2011, CPA and its partner organization, the Progressive Workers Alliance, introduced a multipronged policy approach to preventing or redressing wage theft and related violations, as well as improving worker education and protection for employer retaliation. When speaking on the bill he cosponsored, a prominent local Supervisor remarked, "I am proud to be introducing local legislation that is drawn from action-based research and bottom-up grassroots organizing that will help strengthen labor law enforcement in San Francisco and give workers a meaningful voice in stopping wage theft in our city." The event, attended by many community, academic, and health department partners from the study, as well as policymakers and others, was captured on several nightly news programs, and in a prominent story in the leading local newspaper the next day. It also was widely covered in the ethnic media locally and beyond.

Parallel dissemination activities underway by members of the partnership include efforts by the Labor Occupational Health Program and the San Francisco Department of Health to investigate the potential for disseminating the Restaurant Worker Checklist to other health departments within California and nationally. The sharing of the final report of restaurant observation findings and the project's observational checklist tool through the SFDPH's website (http://www.sfphes. org/publications/Restaurant_Health_Safety_Checklist.pdf), as well as an article about the check list in *Public Health Reports*,[55] a journal that is received by many health departments and public health practitioners around the nation, also are expected to help facilitate the dissemination process.

■ **LESSONS LEARNED AND IMPLICATIONS FOR DISSEMINATION AND IMPLEMENTATION RESEARCH**

The Chinatown Restaurant Worker Project described above in many ways exemplifies the potential value of CBPR for improving the relevance of research and enhancing the dissemination and implementation of findings through collaborative design, analysis, dissemination, and research translation. Drawing on this and other participatory research case studies, as well as the now substantial body of literature in the field of CBPR, we present key lessons learned and their implications for research dissemination and implementation.

Through the codevelopment of research priorities and design with community and other stakeholders, CBPR can help ensure that the research is relevant to the community, potentially helping improve its external validity.[56] Further, such cogeneration of research topic and study design can enhance buy-in and shared commitment on the part of all partners in moving from research to action. In the Chinatown CBPR study and numerous others,[11,12,15,25,57] the participation of community partners in the design of research instruments resulted in the generation of new survey items and improved data-gathering tools that in turn proved critical to a fuller understanding of the topic under investigation—and the design of subsequent research-based action.

Inclusion of multiple stakeholders, including but not limited to a strong community partner, also is advised. As illustrated in the Chinatown case study, having as a partner a local health department can be important for gaining entrée into the community and to environments (i.e., worksites) that otherwise would likely be "off limits." Further, including as partners one or more policymakers, and/or having a strong policy mentor, may be critical for those partnerships wishing to help affect broader, systems-level change. In West Oakland, California, a CBPR partnership to study and address the large number of diesel trucks driving through and idling in a low-income portside community, profited early on by including a local city council member as a policy mentor and active partner. By holding monthly meetings in the councilor's office, where study findings were discussed and a proposed new truck route ordinance designed, the partnership was able to get many disparate stakeholders to the table, and several subsequent policy wins followed in part as a result.[58]

The special benefits of a participatory approach for dissemination of study findings through diverse channels and to multiple audiences also should be underscored. Publication of study methods and findings in respected peer-reviewed journals is, of course, critical, both for extending the study's reach and underscoring its scientific merit. Yet as Canadian scholar Dennis Raphel is fond of asking, "If an article is published in *Social Science and Medicine* but nobody reads it, does it exist?" A prolific scholar himself, Raphel's message is not to *avoid* publishing, but rather to insure that we do not stop there. Many CBPR partnerships, including the Chinatown study, have a special subcommittee that helps to ensure the wide dissemination of findings through a diversified strategy. Proposed journal articles and abstracts for presentations at professional meetings, typically with community partner coauthors, are reviewed by these committees. But attention also is focused on effective use of the mass media (including local language newspapers), presentations at community forums, development of policy briefs based on study findings, and other nonacademic means of disseminating findings to promote education and action. The involvement of multiple stakeholders, especially those "in" the community, increases the capacity to disseminate findings in a meaningful and culturally appropriate way.

Furthermore, as in the Chinatown project, the inclusion of a health department may enhance the partnerships' ability to speak the "language" of, and have greater success in engaging, regulators and policymakers in organizational- and policy-level interventions to address research findings. As an inherently collaborative and colearning process, CBPR enhances the expertise and capacity of all partners for culturally appropriate research and prevention that addresses contextual factors. While university partners bring research expertise to the table, the inclusion of community and health department partners, who often are more skilled in organizing and policy advocacy than their academic counterparts, can be critical for ensuring that findings are translated more broadly into innovative actions to address social, economic, and political determinants of health. Such actions may be more likely to result in sustainable and long-term impacts than more traditional health and public health interventions.[34,59]

Ethical and methodological challenges will almost invariably emerge in the course of a CBPR effort—a fact that underscores the importance of preparing, in advance via MOUs or less formal mechanisms, as well as encouraging ongoing dialogue around tough issues such as funding and workload equity. Although as noted above, useful instruments have been developed to help guide such discussions,[37–39,41] the unique composition and needs of each partnership suggest the utility of tailoring such tools, or devising new ones, to best serve a particular partnership.

Among the most challenging aspects of CBPR, with special relevance to D&I research, is that this orientation to research requires a long-term commitment from all partners. In addition to the added time involved in front-end partnership building and maintenance (e.g., involving numerous steering committee and advisory board meetings, community meetings, retreats, etc.), the translation and action phases of such work may often not take place until after the funded research period. In a Harlem, New York–based CBPR effort to promote the successful community reintegration of former substance-abusing inmates, several key policy victories were achieved only well after the project's federal support had ended. Had the Harlem Community and Academic Partnership members not continued to work together, the impressive policy changes to which they contributed, including legislation mandating discharge planning services, help finding housing and drug treatment services, and reinstatement of Medicaid coverage immediately upon release from prison or jail, might never have been achieved.[57,60] Complicated issues take time to understand and address, and rarely align neatly with academic or community partner timetables.

Successful translation and use of CBPR findings also may require obtaining additional funding, including some from nongovernmental and other sources that can constrict or preclude advocacy on behalf of relevant legislation. In the Chinatown case study, substantial supplemental funding from a large and progressive foundation committed to policy-level change, with the community partner as the lead agency, proved particularly suited for translating study finding into policy-level interventions. Yet philanthropic organizations differ in their support for policy-related activities, and CBPR partnerships whose goals include action on the legislative level should determine in advance whether and to what extent their funding source(s) will support and/or even allow such activity.

■ SUMMARY

An inherently action-focused research orientation, CBPR is particularly well suited to D&I research. As suggested in this chapter, although CBPR is not relevant in all or even most research contexts, when there is goodness-of-fit between this orientation to research and a proposed study, significant value can be added to both the processes and outcomes of the research. Prominent among the latter are enhanced dissemination and implementation of findings through the authentic engagement of community partners and other stakeholders throughout. In our discussion of CBPR, and our use of the Chinatown Restaurant Worker Study to illustrate its principles in action, we have highlighted many of the benefits CBPR can offer to research and its dissemination and implementation. Drawing on this and other CBPR case studies and literature, we also have suggested a number of implications that CBPR holds for dissemination and implementation research and bridging the gap between research and practice.

In concluding, we would like to emphasize an additional and important strength that CBPR offers for reducing health disparities (as discussed in Chapter 22). When conducted in accordance with its key tenets and principles, CBPR can be an important paradigm for promoting not only health equity in the sense of distributive justice, but also the "procedural justice"[61] necessary for real change to take place, and be sustained over time. Procedural justice has been described as involving "equitable processes through which low-income communities of color, rural residents, and other marginalized groups can have a seat at the table—and stay at the table—having a real voice in decision making affecting their lives."[34] In the words of one RWLG member from the Chinatown study, involvement in a CBPR study and its subsequent translational efforts can yield "courage to confront problems in [our] community." Through reciprocal capacity building of community, university, and other partners; its establishment of "structures for participation"; and its provision, especially for underrepresented communities, of a "place" for their voices to be heard and a way to make change,[33] CBPR can be a potent mechanism for addressing some of the social and other inequalities at the heart of many health disparities.

SUGGESTED READINGS

Cargo M, Mercer SL. The value and challenges of participatory research: strengthening its practice. *Annu Rev Public Health*. 2008;29:325–350.

This thorough and sophisticated article on CBPR in the health field provides a critical review of the literature, followed by an "integrative practice framework" highlighting key domains including values and drivers (such as knowledge transfer and self-determination), partnership processes, and the interpretation and application of research outcomes.

Israel BA, Schulz AJ, Parker EA, Becker AB. Review of community-based research: assessing partnership approaches to improve public health. *Annu Rev Public Health*. 1998;19:173–202.

The single most cited paper in CBPR in the health field. This paper introduces CBPR, its core principles, as well as some of the challenges entailed in their implementation. In addition to providing a review of the literature, this work uses early lessons of the Detroit Community-Academic Research Center to explicate CBPR principles and their implementation.

Israel BA, Eng E, Schultz A, Parker E. *Methods in Community-Based Participatory Research for Health.* San Francisco, CA: Jossey-Bass;2005.

> *Edited by four leaders in the field, this book provides an introduction to a wide range of methods in CBPR, including topics such as partnership development and maintenance; community assessment and diagnosis; definition of issues, documentation of partnership processes, and the interpretation, dissemination, and application of research findings. Its 17 chapters and 16 appendixes include many tools and examples from the Detroit Community-Academic Research Center and elsewhere to illustrate the methodological approaches and other topics under consideration.*

Minkler M, Wallerstein N. *Community-Based Participatory Research for Health: From Process to Outcomes.* 2nd ed. San Francisco, CA: Jossey-Bass;2008.

> *The first major volume on CBPR in the health field in the United States, this coedited text, now in its second edition, includes 21 chapters and 12 appendixes covering a wide range of theoretical, methodological, ethical, and practical issues in CBPR, with a special emphasis on policy and other health-related outcomes. Key topics include the theoretical and practice roots of CBPR, issues of power and trust in working cross-culturally, ethical and methodological challenges, participatory evaluation, and CBPR and policy. Numerous case studies and practical tools are included, for example, reliability-tested guidelines for appraising participatory research and guidelines for institutional review boards (IRBs).*

O'Fallon L, Dearry A. Community-based participatory research as a tool to advance environmental health sciences. *Environ Health Perspect.* 2002;110(Suppl 2): S155–159.

> *Although specifically focused on CBPR as it relates to environmental health and environmental justice, this seminal article provides a thoughtful laying out of the ways in which community engagement strengthens research processes and outcomes, as well as the challenges inherent in this approach. Several case studies from environmental health are used to illustrate the issues raised, and the article remains widely cited in public health and other disciplines.*

SELECTED WEBSITES AND TOOLS

The Community Tool Box (http://ctb.ku.edu). Created by the Work Group for Community Health and Development at the University of Kansas, and over 6,000 pages in length, this well-organized website offers numerous tools for participatory community assessment and evaluation, as well as other aspects of CBPR and related approaches.

Community-Campus Partnerships for Health (www.ccph.info). This site is a portal to a wide array of resources for partnerships undertaking CBPR, including sample memoranda of understanding, tools for collaborative asset and risk mapping, research dissemination, and articles and workbooks on the translation of findings into policy and practice change.

■ REFERENCES

1. Green L, George M, Daniel M, et al. *Study of participatory research in health promotion.* Ottawa: The Royal Society of Canada;1994.
2. Hall B. From margins to center: The development and purpose of participatory action research. *Am Sociol.* 1992;23(4):15–28.
3. Israel BA, Schulz AJ, Parker EA, Becker AB. Review of community-based research: assessing partnership approaches to improve public health. *Annu Rev Public Health.* 1998;19:173–202.

4. Cornwall A, Jewkes R. What is participatory research? *Soc Sci Med*. Dec 1995;41(12): 1667–1676.
5. Am. IMCQHC. *Crossing the Quality Chasm: A New Health System for the 21st Century*. Washington, DC: Natl. Acad. Press;2001.
6. Glasgow RE, Emmons KM. How can we increase translation of research into practice? Types of evidence needed. *Annu Rev Public Health*. 2007;28:413–433.
7. Horowitz CR, Robinson M, Seifer S. Community-based participatory research from the margin to the mainstream: are researchers prepared? *Circulation*. 2009;119: 2633–2642.
8. Biggs SD. *Resource-Poor Farmer Participation in Research: A Synthesis of Experiences from Nine National Agricultural Research Systems*. The Hague, Netherlands: ISNAR;1989.
9. Kaplan SA, Dillman KN, Calman N, Billings J. Opening doors and building capacity: employing a community-based approach to surveying. *J Urban Heatlh*. 2004;81: 291–300.
10. O'Fallon L, Dearry A. Community-based participatory research as a tool to advance environmental health sciences. *Environ Health Perspect*. 2002;110(Suppl 2): S155–159.
11. Cargo M, Mercer SL. The value and challenges of participatory research: strengthening its practice. *Annu Rev Public Health*. 2008;29:325–350.
12. Minkler M, Wallerstein N. *Community-Based Participatory Research for Health: From Process to Outcomes*. 2nd ed. San Francisco, CA: Jossey-Bass; 2008.
13. W.K. Kellogg Foundation Community Health Scholars Program. Stories of Impact [brochure]. Ann Arbor, MI: University of Michigan, School of Public Health, Community Health Scholars Program, National Program Office; 2001.
14. Minkler M. Community based research partnerships: Challenges and Opportunities. *J Urban Health*. 2005;82(2):3–12.
15. Israel BA, Eng E, Schultz A, Parker E. *Methods in Community-Based Participatory Research for Health*. San Francisco, CA: Jossey-Bass; 2005.
16. Tervalon M, Murray-Garcia J. Cultural humility versus cultural competence: a critical distinction in defining physician training outcomes in multicultural education. *J Health Care Poor Underserved*. May 1998;9(2):117–125.
17. Reason P, Bradbury H. *Handbook of Action research: Participative Inquiry and Practice (Concise ed.)*. Thousand Oaks, CA: Sage; 2008.
18. Schillinger D. An introduction to effectiveness, dissemination and implementation research. In: P. Fleisher and E. Goldstein, eds. *UCSF Clinical and Translational Science Institute (CTSI Resource Manuals and Guides to Community-Engaged Research, P. Fleisher, ed.)*: Published by Clinical Translational Science Institute Community Engagement Program, University of California San Francisco; 2010. Accessed December 19, 2010. http://accelerate.ucsf.edu/files/CE/edi_introguide.pdf
19. Lorig KR, Ritter P, Stewart AL, et al. Chronic disease self-management program: 2-year health status and health care utilization outcomes. *Med Care*. Nov 2001;39(11): 1217–1223.
20. Lorig KR, Sobel DS, Ritter PL, Laurent D, Hobbs M. Effect of a self-management program on patients with chronic disease. *Eff Clin Pract*. Nov–Dec 2001;4(6):256–262.
21. Lorig KR, Sobel DS, Stewart AL, et al. Evidence suggesting that a chronic disease self-management program can improve health status while reducing hospitalization: a randomized trial. *Med Care*. Jan 1999;37(1):5–14.

22. Galloway JM. Cardiovascular health among American Indians and Alaska Natives: successes, challenges, and potentials. *Am J Prev Med.* Dec 2005;29(5 Suppl 1):11–17.

23. Jernigan VB. Community-based participatory research with Native American communities: the Chronic Disease Self-Management Program. *Health Promot Pract.* 2010;11(6):888–899.

24. Jernigan VB, Lorig K. The Internet Diabetes Self-Management Workshop for American Indians and Alaska Natives. *Health Promot Pract.* 2011;12(2):261–70.

25. Kreiger J, Allen C, Roberts J, Ross L, Takaro T. What's with the wheezing? Methods used by the Seattle-King County Healthy Homes Project to assess exposure to indoor asthma triggers. In: Israel BA, Eng E, Schultz A, Parker E, eds. *Methods in Community-Based Participatory Research for Health.* Vol. 230–250. San Francisco, CA: Jossey-Bass; 2005.

26. Green L. From research to "best practices" in other settings and populations. *Am. J. Health Behav.* 2001;25:165–178.

27. Deloria V, Jr. Commentary: research, redskins, and reality. *Am Indian Q.* 1991;15(4): 457–468.

28. Green LW, Mercer SL. Can public health researchers and agencies reconcile the push from funding bodies and the pull from communities? *Am J Public Health.* 2001;9(12):1926–1929.

29. Buchanan D, Miller F, Wallerstein N. Ethical issues in community-based participatory research: balancing rigorous research with community participation in community intervention studies. *Progr Community Health Partnersh.* 2007;1.2:153–160.

30. Jones D, Franklin C, Butler BT, Williams P, Wells KB, Rodriguez MA. The Building Wellness project: a case history of partnership, power sharing, and compromise. *Ethn Dis.* Winter 2006;16(1 Suppl 1):S54–66.

31. Bowen C, Jones L, Dixon EL, Miranda J, Wells K. Using a community partnered participatory research approach to implement a randomized controlled trial: planning community partners in care *J Health Care Poor Underserved.* 2009;21(780–795).

32. Cashman SB, Adeky S, Allen A, et al. Analyzing and interpreting data with communities. In: Minkler M, Wallerstein N, eds. *Community-Based Participatory Research for Health: From Process to Outcome.* Second ed. San Francisco, CA: Jossey-Bass; 2008:285–301.

33. Viswanathan M, Ammerman A, Eng E, et al. *Community-Based Participatory Research: Assessing the Evidence. Summary, Evidence Report/Technology Assessment No. 99.* Rockville, MD: Agency for Healthcare Research and Quality;2004.

34. Minkler M. Linking science and policy through community-based participatory research to eliminate health disparities. *Am J Public Health.* 2010;100(Suppl 1): S81–87.

35. Hennessey Lavery S, Smith ML, Esparza AA, Hrushow A, Moore M, Reed DF. The community action model: a community-driven model designed to address disparities in health. *Am J Public Health.* Apr 2005;95(4):611–616.

36. Vasquez VB, Lanza D, Hennessey-Lavery S, Facente S, Halpin HA, Minkler M. Addressing food security through public policy action in a community-based participatory research partnership. *Health Promot Pract.* Oct 2007;8(4):342–349.

37. Mercer SL, Green LW, Cargo M, et al. Reliability-tested guidelines for assessing participatory research projects. In: Minkler M, Wallerstein N, eds. *Community-Based Participatory Research for Health from Process to Outcome.* San Franciso, CA: Jossey-Bass; 2008:408–418.

38. Israel BA, Lantz PM, McGranaghan RJ, Kerr D, Guzman JR. Detroit Community-Academic Urban Research Center In-Depth, Semistructured Interview Protocol for Board Evaluation, 1996–2002. In: Israel BA, Eng E, Schultz A, Parker E, eds. *Methods in Community-Based Participatory Research for Health*. San Francisco, CA: Jossey-Bass; 2005:425–429.

39. Israel BA, Lantz PM, McGranaghan RJ, Kerr D, Guzman JR. Detroit Community-Academic Urban Research Center Closed-Ended Survey Questionnaire for Board Evaluation, 1997–2002. In: Israel BA, Eng E, Schultz A, Parker E, eds. *Methods in Community-Based Participatory Research for Health*. San Francisco, CA: Jossey-Bass; 2005:430–433.

40. Farquhar S, Wing S. Methodological and ethical considerations in community-driven environmental justice research: two case studies from rural North Carolina. In: Minkler M, Wallerstein N, eds. *Community-Based Participatory Reserach: From Process to Outcome*. Second ed. San Francisco, CA: Jossey-Bass; 2008: 263–280.

41. Flicker S, Travers R, Guta A, McDonald S, Meagher A. Ethical dilemmas in community-based participatory research: recommendations for institutional review boards. *J Urban Health*. Jul 2007;84(4):478–493.

42. Restaurant Opportunities Center of New York (ROC-NY). *Behind the Kitchen Door: Pervasive Inequality in New York's Thriving Restaurant Industry*. New York: Restaurant Opportunities Center of New York and the New York City Restaurant Industry Coalition; 2005.

43. United ROC. *A Summary of Restaurant Industry Summaries in New York, Chicago, Metro Detroit, New Orleans, and Maine: National Executive Summary*. New York, Chicago, Detroit, New Orleans, Portland: Restaurant Opportunities Center United; 2010.

44. Webster T. Occupational hazards in eating and drinking places. *Compensation and Working Conditions*. 2001;2001(Summer):27–33.

45. U.S. Census Bureau (2000). *Summary File 3: P49; Sex by Industry for the Employed Civilian Population over 16+ Years*. http://factfinder.census.gov/.

46. Minkler M, Tau Lee P, Tom A, et al. Using community-based participatory research to design and initiate a study on immigrant worker health and safety in San Francisco's Chinatown restaurants. American J Ind Med. 2010;53(4):361–371.

47. Mujica J. Coloring the hazards: risk maps research and education to fight health hazards. *Am J Ind Med*. 1992;22(5):767–770.

48. Brown MP. Worker risk mapping: an education-for-action approach. *New Solut*. 1995;5:22–30.

49. Brown MP. Risk mapping as a tool for community-based participatory research and organizing. In: Minkler M, Wallerstein N, eds. *Community-Based Participatory Research for Health*. San Francisco, CA: Jossey-Bass; 2008.

50. San Francisco Department of Public Health. *Health and Safety in San Francisco's Chinatown Restaurants: Findings from an Observational Survey*. San Francisco, CA: San Francisco Department of Public Health; 2009.

51. Salvatore AL, Krause N. *Health and Working Conditions of Restaurant Workers in San Francisco's Chinatown: Report of Survey Findings*. UC Berkeley and UC San Francisco; 2010.

52. Chinese Progressive Association. *Check Please!: Health and Working Conditions in San Francisco Chinatown Restaurants*. San Francisco, CA; 2010.

53. Wing S, Horton RA, Muhammad N, Grant GR, Mansoureh T, Thu K. Integrating epidemiology, education, and organizing for environmental justice: community health effects of industrial hog operations. *Am J Public Health.* 2008;98(8):1390–1397.

54. Parker E, Israel B, Robins T, et al. Evaluation of community action against asthma: a community health worker intervention to improve children's asthma-related health by reducing household environmental triggers for asthma. *Health Education and Behavior.* 2008;35(3):376–395.

55. Gaydos M, Bhatia R, Morales A, et al. Promoting health equity and safety in San Francisco's Chinatown restaurants: findings and lessons learned from a pilot observational survey. *Public Health Rep.* 2011;126(suppl 3):62–69.

56. Green LW, Glasgow RE. Evaluating the relevance, generalization, and applicability of research: issues in external validation and translation methodology. *Eval Health Prof.* Mar 2006;29(1):126–153.

57. Minkler M, Breckwich Vásquez V, et al. *Promoting Healthy Public Policy Through Community-Based Participatory Research: Ten Case Studies.* Oakland, CA: PolicyLink; 2008.

58. Gonzalez P, Minkler M, Gordon M, et al. Community-Based-Participatory Research and Policy Advocacy to Reduce Diesel Exposure in West Oakland, California. *Am J Public Health.* May 9, 2011. [Epub ahead of print.]

59. Morello-Frosch R, Pastor MJ, Sadd J, Porras C, Prichard M. Citizens, science and data judo: leveraging secondary data analysis to build a community-academic collaborative for environmental justice in Southern California. In: Israel BA, Eng E, Schultz A, Parker E, eds. *Methods in Community-Based Participatory Research for Health.* San Francisco, CA: Jossey-Bass; 2005:371–393.

60. Minkler M, Freudenberg N. From community-based participatory research to policy change. In: Fitzgerald H, Burack C, Seifer S, eds. *Handbook for Engaged Scholarship: Contemporary Landscapes, Future Directions Vol. 1: Institutional Change.* East Lansing, MI. Michigan State University; 2010:275–294.

61. Kuehn R. A taxonomy of environmental justice. *Environmental Law Reporter.* 2000;30(10681–10703).

11 Enhancing Dissemination through Marketing and Distribution Systems: A Vision for Public Health

■ MATTHEW W. KREUTER,
CHRISTOPHER M. CASEY,
AND JAY M. BERNHARDT

■ INTRODUCTION

The long lag time between discovery of new knowledge and its application in public health and clinical settings is well documented[1] and described in numerous other chapters in this book. Along this evidence-to-practice cycle, there is no shortage of evidence-based approaches and empirically supported programs to enhance the public's health,[2,3] but there are few *systems* in place to bring these discoveries to the attention of practitioners and into use in practice settings. In business, the process of taking a product or service from the point of development to the point of use by consumers is carried out by a *marketing and distribution system*.[4] In previous work, we have argued that marketing and distribution responsibilities are largely unassigned, underemphasized, and/or underfunded for disseminating effective public health programs, and without them widespread adoption of evidence-based approaches is unlikely.[5] This chapter builds on our earlier work by proposing three specific components of a marketing and distribution system for evidence-based public health practices, and describing how the potential benefits of such a system could be evaluated through dissemination research.

■ A CASE STUDY

In the late 1990s, a team of public health researchers in St. Louis, Mo., created the ABC Immunization Calendar. It was a simple computer software program designed to help community health centers boost low rates of immunization among babies and toddlers. The program used information from new parents and a digital photograph of their baby to create personalized monthly calendars that were given to the family during their baby's first two years of life. The calendars provided health and developmental information matched to the baby's age and reminders of the baby's next appointment in the vaccination series. Each time the parent and baby returned for a required vaccination, the program would take a new picture of the baby and print more months of the calendar (to cover the period leading to the next vaccination).

The program was well received in a pilot study[6] and increased child vaccination rates from 65% to 82% in an efficacy trial.[7] Based on these results, the research team obtained dissemination grant funding and adapted the program for widespread use.[8] A survey was conducted among potential user organizations to determine what computer platform and operating systems they were using. The ABC software was then reprogrammed to maximize compatibility with existing infrastructure. A user's guide was developed to help organizations install and use the program. An implementation guide was developed to help organizations decide how to integrate the program into their standard procedures and implement it. A promotional brochure with sample calendars and published articles was created and distributed at national meetings and to any person or organization that expressed interest. Training was provided, and some computer equipment was made available on loan. These efforts led to four Federally Qualified Health Centers (FQHCs) in the St. Louis area adopting the ABC Immunization Calendar. The program was delivered to thousands of families, and some centers used the program for many years.

Was the ABC Immunization Calendar a dissemination success? The research team adhered closely to conventional wisdom about translating public health science into practice. The intervention was tested for feasibility, acceptability, and efficacy in real-world settings. When positive results were found, the research team identified potential adopters, learned about their practice settings, and adapted the program accordingly. They created instruction manuals to help adopters use the software and to customize an implementation plan for their organization. They provided training and technical assistance. Local organizations adopted and used the program. But there are 7,500 FQHCs in the United States, reaching 17 million Americans. The ABC Immunization Calendar was adopted by four of them. In the grand scheme of things, the program's impact on the public's health was negligible.

Why didn't a program that's fast, easy, cheap, and effective find a home in more FQHCs? What should the research team have done differently to maximize its adoption and use? This story illustrates the limitations of current approaches to disseminating evidence-based programs and the need for marketing and distribution systems to support those efforts. For example, it's not the case that 7,496 FQHCs rejected the ABC Immunization Calendar. Rather, they *never even heard of it*. And if they had heard of it and wanted to adopt it, how would they obtain a copy? Could a small, university-based research team duplicate and distribute software and instruction manuals to hundreds or thousands of potential adopters? Could such a team also provide timely training and technical assistance to a mass of users? Are they trained to do this? Would they know how to set up such an operation? Would they *want* to do it? Would their university reward them for spending time on this? Thus, even well-intentioned, dissemination-minded researchers trying to do the right thing and following recommendations that are nearly universally accepted today will run up against demands that they are not trained to understand or address, they lack the capacity to carry out, and are not viewed as central to the mission of the organizations where they work.

■ A MARKETING AND DISTRIBUTION PERSPECTIVE

Marketing and distribution systems are designed to bring products and services from their point of development to their point of use. This typically occurs through a system of interconnected organizations or intermediaries.[4] Collectively, these intermediaries identify potential users, promote the product to them, provide them with easy access to the product through convenient (and usually local) channels, allow them to see and use the product before acquiring it, help them acquire it, and support the product after purchase if the buyer has questions or problems.[9] Without such systems, every "producer" would have to interact directly with every potential customer or user to promote, distribute, and support a product or program. As illustrated by the previous case example, such interaction would be impractical and inefficient, and in business practice it is rare.

In understanding how a marketing and distribution system might improve dissemination of evidence-based interventions into public health practice, three key characteristics of the business model stand out. First, there is specialization of labor. It is not expected that the person (or organization) that developed a product will be the same one that manufactures it, distributes it, promotes it, sells it, services it, and supports the users that buy it. Second, each of these responsibilities is assigned. It is the primary responsibility of someone (or some organization) to assure that its part of distribution chain is fulfilled. It is someone's job. If it's not carried out, they don't get paid. Finally, all parts of the process are integrated. Even when carried out by different individuals (or organizations), these efforts are highly coordinated. In public health, most steps in the marketing and distribution process are unassigned, underemphasized, and underfunded. If they are undertaken at all, it is usually only as one of many responsibilities of someone who may lack the training or resources to do it well. And rarely are there financial or other tangible incentives for distributing or adopting evidence-based public health programs and services.

■ A SYSTEM FOR PUBLIC HEALTH

In the remainder of this chapter, we propose and discuss three parts of a marketing and distribution system that could help bring more evidence-based interventions into public health practice. These are: (1) user review panels, (2) design and marketing teams, and (3) dissemination field agents. After each is described, we present a model system that would incorporate all three in an integrated fashion.

User Review Panels

On the popular TV show *American Idol*, aspiring singers compete to earn a recording contract. To identify contestants for the program, auditions are held in cities across the country. Tens of thousands of hopeful contestants wait hours to sing before a panel of judges comprised of professionals from the music industry. Only a dozen or so are chosen to be finalists and invited to appear on the TV program. Once on the program, these contestants perform and are critiqued by celebrity judges. Each week the TV audience votes for their favorite performer. The contestant that receives the fewest votes is eliminated from the competition. This continues until there is only one contestant remaining, the winner. *American Idol* then invests heavily in developing, marketing, and promoting the music and career of this singer.

American Idol's process and format illustrates key differences between expert reviews and user reviews. Selecting the most talented 12–18 singers from 10,000+ aspirants is done by *expert review*. The judges evaluate auditioning singers based on a range of criteria they believe predicts success. This is not unlike the process of systematic evidence reviews in public health, wherein teams of scholars (i.e., experts) evaluate the strength of scientific findings for different types of interventions. Those with strong and consistent supporting evidence are "selected" and recommended for use in practice. On *American Idol*, expert reviews are also provided after each song performed by a contestant. These critiques provide voters in the TV audience with some additional information on which they might base their decisions. But the viewing audience ultimately determines who wins and loses. This is *user review*. Members of the voting audience are "users" because they will be the ones who purchase (or don't) the music recorded by the winner. In essence, their votes reflect market demand for one singer versus another.

On *American Idol*, it's striking how often this market demand diverges from expert critiques. Why is that? One explanation is that not all viewers value the same things as music experts. Assuming that all of the finalists have a very high level of talent (and therefore a high likelihood of career success), it makes sense to leave this decision to market demand. We can apply the same logic to the process of disseminating evidence-based public health programs and strategies. When expert review has provided a menu of proven strategies and programs, adopters and users (i.e., the market) will determine which, if any, meet their own unique needs and preferences. Knowing this, and in the absence of high-cost, in-depth marketing research on intermediaries and end users, we should consider how to integrate formal user review processes into dissemination efforts.

We start with two assumptions: (1) not all evidence-based interventions will work equally well in real-world practice settings; and (2) there are insufficient resources to develop every successful (i.e., empirically supported) prototype into a program or policy for active dissemination to adopters. Thus, a primary goal of user review panels in public health dissemination would be to identify those evidence-based programs and approaches that adopters really want and believe can be implemented in their types of organizations. In other words, identify programs and approaches likely to be in high demand by different market segments. Just like the winner of *American Idol*, this subset of evidence-based interventions would then receive priority treatment and resources to be developed, adapted, and promoted for wider use. Programs and approaches not selected for focused development and marketing could still be adopted and used, but would not benefit from the same attention and resources.

Depending on the nature and type of evidence-based interventions being considered (and therefore, the types of organizations likely to adopt a particular program or approach), user review panels might include representatives from community-based organizations, schools, local health departments, city planners, policymakers, state and local health departments, Federally Qualified Health Centers, health care systems, primary care providers, health foundations, and other organizations. These panels would review types of evidence-based based interventions (e.g., client reminder systems) as well as specific programs within each type. They could rate each on criteria like ease of use, organizational fit, implementation burden, acceptability to clients or patients, and feasibility, as well as classic predictors of adoption such as relative advantage and trialability as described by Rogers (2003).[10] Interventions rated as most promising by a user review panel would be turned over to a Design and Marketing Team to prepare them for widespread use and active promotion.

Design and Marketing Teams

At a 2002 *Designing for Dissemination* conference of invited researchers, practitioners, and intermediaries from across the United States, researchers were consistently the least likely to believe that translation and dissemination of research findings were their responsibility, felt unprepared in the science of dissemination and communication, and expressed concerns that their interests and strengths were in areas other than translational work.[11] Researchers' interests and skills in translational science have likely increased in the decade since this meeting, but formal training in disciplines related to the design, marketing, and distribution of public health programs and services is still uncommon for scientists. In addition, there are few, if any, incentives—financial or otherwise—for researchers to actively disseminate their evidence-based public health programs.

As noted in Chapter 15 in this book and elsewhere,[12] greater attention to external validity during research design, analysis, and dissemination can help researchers and practitioners to design programs that have higher translational potential. While we agree that greater understanding of these steps would enhance the translational efforts of scientists, we will argue that design and marketing functions are sufficiently important and complex and they require specialized expertise and dedicated personnel.

Although the details may vary case by case, there is a general sequence of actions that design and marketing teams carry out to make a promising product—like an evidence-based intervention—ready for the market. *Market research* is used to learn as much as possible about organizations that might adopt the intervention. What are their goals? How would this intervention help them achieve those goals? How would they use the intervention? How would it be integrated within their current client flow, operations, systems, and processes? Who within the organization would make the decision whether or not to adopt the intervention? Who would be responsible for implementing it? What are their concerns about the intervention? What would they change about the intervention?

Responses to questions like these would inform a wide range of design and distribution functions. For example, products routinely undergo *adaptation* or *reformulation* to maximize their appeal to potential users. If market research shows that potential adopters of a particular public health intervention are excited about feature X or concerned about feature Y, a smart design team would adapt the intervention accordingly. Also, it is often the case that the version of a program used in research under controlled conditions is not yet ready for use in practice settings. Knowing how, by whom, and for what purposes it will be used will help a design team reshape and package the program for use in specific nonresearch settings.

Using *audience segmentation*, a design team can distinguish between different subgroups of users and create targeted marketing and distribution strategies for each. Audience segments might be defined by organization type (e.g., schools, public health departments, Federally Qualified Health Centers), populations served, intended use of the intervention, or any combination of these and other characteristics. What's important is that the characteristics shared within each subgroup, or segment, lead to distinct, actionable strategies for promoting and distributing the evidence-based intervention. For example, different message strategies (e.g., "cost-effective" vs. "clients love it"), messengers (e.g., trusted peers vs. trade associations), and channels (e.g., conferences vs. online communities) might be indicated for different segments.

A design and marketing team would not only create the dissemination strategy but would execute it as well. This would include many critical operational functions, including building partnerships, establishing a distribution system, providing training, technical assistance and user support services, coordinating and evaluating the overall process, and creating tangible incentives and rewards for adoption. These and other operational functions of a marketing and distribution system have been described in our previous work.[5] The question is not *whether* these functions are needed to more effectively disseminate evidence-based public health interventions, but rather *who* will perform them.[9] For the most part, they are currently unassigned. We believe it is unrealistic to expect public health researchers to possess the skills and have the time that would be needed to do these tasks well. A dedicated public health Design and Marketing Team would have both.

Dissemination Field Agents

What do real estate agents, travel agents, and talent agents have in common? Each has specialized expertise and provides assistance with complex tasks that are often unfamiliar to those who use their services. They do this through direct contact—in person, by phone, and/or electronically—with their clients. These interactions are usually goal directed: buying or selling a house, planning a trip, negotiating a contract.

In public health, a corps of Dissemination Field Agents could operate in a similar fashion, as a kind of evidence-based public health sales force. These specialists would have extensive knowledge of evidence-based interventions and expertise in how to adapt and implement the interventions in different settings and for different populations. They would work closely and proactively with organizations to help them understand and choose from available strategies. They could provide detailed information about specific evidence-based programs, approaches, or policies across health topics and practice settings. If an organization decided to try an intervention, Dissemination Field Agents would help them prepare and succeed by providing training and ongoing technical assistance to adapt, implement, and evaluate the evidence-based program, practice, or policy they chose. These Field Agents would have similar training and functions as the knowledge brokers described in Chapter 2.

Elements of this approach have shown promise. New York City's Public Health Detailing Program aims to help primary care providers improve patient care related to key public health challenges like vaccination, cancer screening, obesity, and HIV testing.[13,14] Program representatives—*agents*, in our terminology—work in three communities with a high burden of poor health. They meet with doctors, physician assistants, nurse practitioners, and administrators to promote clinical preventive services and chronic disease management, and to distribute "detailing action kits" that include evidence summaries, patient education materials, other small media, referral forms, chart stickers, community resource guides, and lists of service providers. Other public health efforts like this, modeled after physician detailing by pharmaceutical representatives, have been around for at least 40 years,[15] though mostly on a local level.

Nationally, the National Cancer Institute's Cancer Information Service (CIS) created the Partnership Program to help put cancer control science into practice to eliminate health disparities.[16] The CIS hired and trained 45 partnership coordinators in 35 states. These staff developed relationships with local, regional, and national organizations for the purposes of sharing information and networking, jointly developing cancer control projects using evidence-based approaches in minority and medically underserved populations, and increasing the capacity of partners to move science into practice. With its national scope, emphasis on translating science into practice, and coordination under a single administrative unit (CIS), elements of the Partnership Program could be followed in establishing a corps of Dissemination Field Agents. However, despite a promising start and numerous successes, the Program was short lived and has been replaced by NCI's National Outreach Network.[17]

■ AN INTEGRATED APPROACH

How would these three recommendations—*User Review Panels, Design and Marketing Teams, and Dissemination Field Agents*—come together in a coordinated marketing and distribution system to bring more evidence-based interventions into public health practice? Here's one vision. Imagine a new administrative unit within one of the nation's public health agencies being charged with accelerating the translation of science to practice. A first step would be to identify the universe of evidence-based approaches and practices. This is easier today than it ever has been, with a growing number of inventories of effective programs as well as systematic evidence reviews like The Community Guide.[18]

User Review Panels would be charged with narrowing this pool of eligible interventions to a smaller set that addresses genuine user demand in ways that are highly appealing to potential adopters. Because the scope of this task would be great, it may be necessary to impose some initial restrictions, like focusing on evidence-based approaches that address leading causes of death and disease or setting up separate panels for specific practice settings and/or health problems. These user reviews would necessarily be ongoing but would provide periodic priority rankings of which evidence-based interventions were in greatest demand. A major collateral benefit of this process would be that its results, when shared, could redirect the efforts of public health scientists to better meet the needs of practice organizations and even suggest specific partnerships for practice-based research.

These priority rankings would set the agenda for a *Design and Marketing Team*. Starting with the highest priority interventions, the team would work closely with developers and potential adopters to: (1) define specific target audiences most likely to adopt each program, (2) make the programs ready for use in practice by these targeted adopters, and (3) develop strategies to effectively promote the program to these groups. Over time, the number of programs would grow. The result of these efforts would be an ever-expanding menu of evidence-based, high-demand, practice-ready programs. As user demand shifts (e.g., for emerging public health challenges), the items on the menu would expand accordingly.

This "menu" would establish the parameters of activity for a corps of *Dissemination Field Agents*. Initially, agents would execute the plans of the Design and Marketing Team. They would seek out organizations identified as potential adopters and share with them the menu of programs designed for their unique practice setting. They would aim to establish positive relationships with organizations, ideally viewed as trusted and competent sources of information about evidence-based public health and prevention programs. When organizations express interest in one or more menu item, agents would shift their focus to providing technical assistance and support for implementation. One of the great advantages of having a field corps is that its members will quickly gain first-hand knowledge of the strengths and limitations of programs in different settings, and the challenges and solutions related to implementation. This invaluable information would inform ongoing and iterative activities of the Design and Marketing Team via a formal feedback loop. It would also create a network of agents that could help each other (and each other's clients) by sharing their experiences.

Figure 11–1 illustrates how User Review Panels, Design and Marketing Teams, and Dissemination Field Agents might be linked in an integrated approach to disseminating evidence-based public health programs.

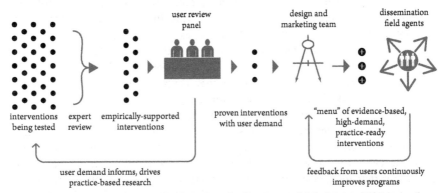

Figure 11–1. Integrating User Review Panels, Design and Marketing Teams, and Dissemination Field Agents in a new system for moving evidence-based programs into public health practice.

▪ CONCLUSION

We realize that this vision likely raises more questions than it answers. Who would build and operate such a system? Who would pay for it? Would researchers who have developed and evaluated public health interventions cooperate in sharing their programs and products? What tangible incentives can be created at each step of the process to encourage dissemination and adoption? What would constitute success for such an effort, and how would we measure it? All are important questions and worthy of thoughtful answers that match their complexity. Doing so is beyond the scope of this chapter, but ongoing in our work. We hope the ideas presented here will stimulate others' thinking about systems and infrastructure to enhance dissemination, and welcome critiques, refinement, and additions to our proposed model.

SUGGESTED READINGS

Kreuter MW, Bernhardt J. Reframing the dissemination challenge: A marketing and distribution perspective. *American Journal of Public Health.* 2009;99(12):2123–2127.

    Critiques current approaches to disseminating evidence-based public health programs and explains how and why a marketing and distribution system would enhance these efforts.

Kotler P. Marketing Management. Upper Saddle River, NJ: Prentice Hall; 2000.

    A useful introduction from an author with extensive experience in health and social marketing.

Larson K, Levy J, Rome MG, Matte TD, Silver LD, Frieden TR (2006). Public Health Detailing: A strategy to improve the delivery of clinical preventive services in New York City. *Public Health Reports.* 121(3):228–234.

    Describes application of an "agent" model intervention to facilitate implementation of public health practices in primary care settings.

SELECTED WEBSITES AND TOOLS

Cancer Control P.L.A.N.E.T. <http://cancercontrolplanet.cancer.gov/index.html>. Cancer Control P.L.A.N.E.T. acts as a portal to provide access to data and resources for designing, implementing, and evaluating evidence-based cancer control programs. The site provides five steps (with links) for developing a comprehensive cancer control plan or program.

Diffusion of Effective Behavioral Interventions < http://www.effectiveinterventions.org/en/home.aspx> provides an inventory of effective HIV and STD prevention and control programs, as well as information on how to use them.

▪ ACKNOWLEDGMENTS

Preparation of this chapter was funded in part by a grant from the National Cancer Institute's Center of Excellence in Cancer Communication Research Program (P50-CA095815) and by Cooperative Agreement Number (U48-DP001903) from the Centers for Disease Control and Prevention, Prevention Research Centers Program.

■ REFERENCES

1. Green L, Ottoson J, Garcia C, Hiatt R. Diffusion theory and knowledge dissemination, utilization and integration. *Annual Review of Public Health.* 2009;30:151–174.
2. Zaza S, Briss P, Harris K, eds. *The guide to community preventive services: What works to promote health?* New York: Oxford University Press; 2005.
3. The Cochrane Collaboration. http://www.cochrane.org/. Accessed August 28, 2010.
4. Coughlan A, Anderson E, Stern L, El-Ansary A. *Marketing channels.* Upper Saddle River, NJ: Pearson Prentice Hall; 2006.
5. Kreuter M, Bernhardt J. Reframing the dissemination challenge: A marketing and distribution perspective. *American Journal of Public Health.* 2009;99(12): 2123–2127.
6. Kreuter M, Vehige E, McGuire A. Using computer-tailored calendars to promote childhood immunization. *Public Health Reports.* 1996;111(2):176–178.
7. Kreuter M, Caburnay C, Chen J, Donlin M. Effectiveness of individually tailored calendars in promoting childhood immunization in urban public health centers. *American Journal of Public Health.* January 2004;94(1):122–127.
8. Caburnay C, Kreuter M, Donlin M. Disseminating effective health promotion programs from prevention research to community organizations. *Journal of Public Health Management & Practice.* March 2001;7(2):81–89.
9. Kotler P. *Marketing Management.* Upper Saddle River, NJ: Prentice Hall; 2000.
10. Rogers E. *Diffusion of Innovations.* 551 ed. New York: Free Press; 2003.
11. National Cancer Institute. *Conference Summary Report, Designing for Dissemination,* September 19–20, Washington, DC: Author; 2002.
12. Klesges L, Estabrooks P, Dzewaltowski D, Bull S, Glasgow R. Beginning with the application in mind: Designing and planning health behavior change interventions to enhance dissemination. *Annals of Behavioral Medicine.* 2005;29:S66–S75.
13. Larson K, Levy J, Rome M, Matte T, Silver L, Frieden T. Public Health Detailing: A strategy to improve the delivery of clinical preventive services in New York City. *Public Health Reports.* 2006;121(3):228–234.
14. New York City Department of Health and Mental Hygiene. Public Health Detailing Program. Available at http://www.nyc.gov/html/doh/html/csi/csi-detailing.shtml; accessed on December 27, 2010.
15. Butler B, Godfrey Erskine E. Public health detailing: Selling ideas to the private practitioner in his office. *American Journal of Public Health.* 1970;60(10):1996–2002.
16. LaPorta M, Hagood H, Kornfeld J, Treimann J. Partnerships as a means of reaching special populations: Evaluating the NCI's CIS Partnership Program. *Journal of Cancer Education.* 2007;22:S35–S40.
17. Robinson B. NCI plans to expand outreach through community-based research programs. *NCI Cancer Bulletin.* 2009;6(16):9.
18. Task Force on Community Preventive Services. *The Guide to Community Preventive Services: What Works to Promote Health?* New York: Oxford University Press; 2005.

Section THREE
Design and Analysis

12 Design and Analysis in Dissemination and Implementation Research

■ JOHN LANDSVERK,
C. HENDRICKS BROWN,
PATRICIA CHAMBERLAIN,
LAWRENCE PALINKAS,
MITSUNORI OGIHARA,
SARA CZAJA,
JEREMY D. GOLDHABER-FIEBERT,
JENNIFER A. ROLLS REUTZ,
AND SARAH MCCUE HORWITZ

■ INTRODUCTION

Dissemination and implementation research has evolved into an emerging field, implementation science, as exemplified by the launching of the journal *Implementation Science* in 2006, and the annual Dissemination and Implementation conferences, initiated in 2007 and sponsored by the Office of Behavioral and Social Science (OBSSR) in collaboration with other institutes and centers at the NIH. Not surprisingly, progress in this emerging science is uneven, with a greater volume of empirical studies mounted in the physical health care field than in the fields of mental health or social services, due largely to medicine's early focus on quality of care and, more recently, on comparative effectiveness. The Cochrane Collaboration (www.cochrane.org) has been an important resource for evaluating the evidence base for clinical interventions in medicine and, since 1994, has developed systematic reviews of studies of implementation strategies for health care settings through the Effective Practice and Organization of Care Group (EPOC, www.epoc.cochrane.org). However, despite these important scientific efforts, there remains a lack of consensus on methodological approaches to the study of dissemination and implementation processes and especially tests of implementation strategies.[1] To begin to address these deficiencies, this chapter reviews design issues for dissemination and implementation research and also presents an overview of some of the analytic approaches to dissemination and implementation research, recognizing that this analytic work is still at an early stage of development. Finally, the chapter presents a case study of research that crosses three of four recognized dissemination and implementation phases and illustrates a number of design and analysis issues.

Focus of Dissemination and Implementation Research

A useful organizing heuristic is to conceptualize dissemination and implementation studies (D&I) in relation to two other stages of research, efficacy and effectiveness. Nicely captured in the 2009 National Research Council and Institute of Medicine report on *Preventing Mental, Emotional, and Behavioral Disorders Among Young People*[2] (shown in Figure 12–1) and adapted from that report, dissemination and implementation (D&I) studies are the last stage of research in the science to practice continuum, preceded by efficacy and effectiveness studies that are distinct from and address different questions from D&I studies. The figure also demonstrates that distinct phases (albeit somewhat overlapping) exist within the D&I stage, characterized as Exploration, Adoption/Preparation, Implementation, and Sustainment similar to those proposed by Aarons, Hurlburt, and Horwitz.[3] These phases correspond to fundamentally different research questions from efficacy and effectiveness studies. In particular, the Exploration phase focuses on identifying or enlarging the set of organizations or communities that express interest in using or making available a particular intervention, strategy, or program. We may be interested in the sheer number of settings that express interest through a passive dissemination process, or we may want to identify whether some communities, say those serving high proportions

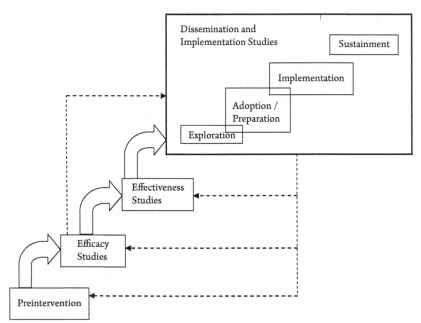

Figure 12–1. Stages of research and phases of dissemination and implementation. Adapted from "Figure 11–1. Stages of research in prevention research cycle" in Chapter 11 of: Implementation and Dissemination of Prevention Programs (2009) in National Research Council and Institute of Medicine. *Preventing Mental, Emotional, and Behavioral Disorders among Young People.* Washington DC: The National Academies Press, p. 326.

of minority or poor populations, are differentially interested in using a certain program.[4] In the Adoption phase, we are interested in factors related to the formal decision to implement, or strategies to increase, adoption of an intervention or program; the next phase is Implementation (or Implementation Fidelity), which involves strategies for improving program fidelity in the field; and finally Sustainment (and moving to scale), involving strategies to maintain delivery of the intervention or extend its use in communities or organizations. We can summarize the distinct emphasis of D&I research as follows : in contrast... to the traditional research questions of efficacy research, which routinely examines overall impact in a relatively homogeneous target population and of effectiveness research, which routinely asks who benefits and for how long in more realistic settings, dissemination and implementation research questions focus primarily on whether different strategies for informing communities or delivery of an intervention increase the speed of implementation, the quality of program delivery, or the degree of access or penetration of the intervention. We view these characteristics of speed, quality, and degree as leading to measurable quantities that can be used to monitor the implementation process. Implementation success would generally be measured by attainment of certain milestones, such as a decision that a community or organization adopts a program, certification that an agency has been credentialed, and other appropriate milestones. We also consider the three dimensions of the timing, quality, and quantity of milestone attainment as critical to evaluating implementation studies, and we view dissemination and implementation research as centrally concerned with answering these questions regarding improvement in one or more of these dimensions (see the case study for illustration of these dimensions). Consequently, the study designs, assessment instruments, analytical strategies, and analytic tools for D&I research all need to relate to speed, quality, or quantity. Given the very different purposes of efficacy, effectiveness, and D&I research as well as different purposes for phases within the D&I stage, it is likely that they may require different research designs or different emphases in the classic research design tension between internal and external validity. While specific research questions regarding dissemination and implementation research may most efficiently be addressed by a unique research design, there may remain questions about effectiveness of newly implemented strategies that are worth answering anew. Indeed, two papers have argued that it is possible to combine several different designs into one overall study so that efficacy, effectiveness, and implementation research questions can be addressed within a single study.[5,6]

We note that this research model typology is also reflected in the NIH Roadmap initiative for reengineering the clinical research enterprise currently driving the translational research initiative at the NIH.[7-9] The Roadmap initiative has identified three types of research leading to improvements in the public health of our nation, namely, basic research that informs the development of clinical interventions (e.g., biochemistry, neurosciences), treatment development that crafts the interventions and tests them in carefully controlled efficacy trials, and what has come to be known as service system and implementation research, where treatments and interventions are brought into and tested in usual-care settings.[10] Based on this tripartite division, the Roadmap further identified two translation steps that would be critical for moving from the findings of basic science to improvements in the quality of health care delivered in community clinical and other delivery settings. The first translation step brings together interdisciplinary teams that integrate the science work being done in the basic sciences and treatment development science, such as translating neuroscience and basic behavior research findings into new treatments. The focus of the second translation phase is to translate evidence-based treatments into service delivery settings and sectors in local communities, and it is this second step that we would identify as the D&I research enterprise.

Translation Steps and Randomized Designs

Historically, basic science and treatment research as partners in the first translation step have relied heavily on what has come to be known as the "gold standard" of designs: namely, the randomized controlled trial (RCT), involving randomization at the person level. In the efficacy phase, the primary aim is to determine whether an intervention has impact on its intended target. A great deal of methods development has been devoted to the use of randomized controlled trials to evaluate program efficacy for medical[11] and behavioral research.[12] While effectiveness research also has played an important role in the science-to-practice continuum, we are still in the process of defining rules for such basic terms as "intent-to-treat" analysis for these more complex longitudinal designs that often include multiple levels in the analysis.[13] In one of the few comprehensive discussions of the distinction between efficacy and effectiveness trials, Flay in 1986[14] noted that "whereas efficacy trials are concerned with testing whether a treatment or procedure does more good than harm when delivered under optimum conditions, effectiveness trials are concerned with testing whether a treatment does more good than harm when delivered via a real-world program."[14] Pertinent to this design discussion, Flay also introduced the concept of "implementation effectiveness" trials and indicates such trials "can be uncontrolled in the sense that variations in program delivery are not controlled, or they can be controlled experiments in which different approaches to the delivery or dissemination of an efficacious technology are tested."[14]

It is not accidental that Flay's language on implementation and dissemination includes a discussion of random assignment to different approaches for delivery. Flay's perspective then was that randomized trials could be used for such research. This perspective, however, is not universally accepted. This issue of control groups or comparison conditions and use of randomized trials for studies about translating research to practice has been recently discussed by Glasgow and colleagues around the concept of practical clinical trials[15] with a recommendation that such translation requires as much if not more attention to external validity as to internal validity. While the authors acknowledge that RCT designs provide the highest level of evidence, they argue that "in many clinical and community settings, and especially in studies with underserved populations and low resource settings, randomization may not be feasible or acceptable"[15] and propose alternatives to the randomized design such as "interrupted time series," "multiple baseline across settings" or "regression discontinuity" designs. Brown and colleagues have argued that the gap between some of these designs and true RCTs can be diminished by incorporating randomization across time and place instead of person-level randomization.[5,13,16]

The use of classic RCT designs in the second translation step has been even more vigorously and provocatively addressed by Berwick, the well-known leader of the Institute for Healthcare Improvement (IHI). In a recent *JAMA* commentary, he argues that there is an unhappy tension between "2 great streams of endeavor with little prospect for merging into a framework for conjoint action: improving clinical evidence and improving the process of care."[17] He proposes resolving this tension with a radical research design position (based in epistemology), namely, that the randomized clinical trial design—so important in evidence-based medicine—is not useful for studying health care improvement in complex social and organizational environments. Asserting the need for essentially new evaluation methods, he points to Pawson and Tilley's[18] position that the study of social change in complex systems requires a wider range of scientific methodologies in order to capture change mechanisms within social and organizational contexts. Berwick extends this argument, suggesting that "many assessment techniques developed in engineering and used in quality improvement—i.e., statistical process control, time series analysis, simulations, and factorial experiments—have more power to inform about mechanisms and context than do RCTs, as do ethnography, anthropology, and other qualitative methods."[17]

In summary, a robust debate ongoing for D&I efforts focuses on whether randomized designs, found so useful for efficacy and effectiveness research, can or should be applied to D&I research. If they do have a place in D&I research, for what questions are they most useful? Even if one rejected Berwick's conclusion that randomized designs are not useful for testing improvement in complex environments, it is useful to address Berwick's challenge to search nontraditional sources for alternative designs in the third stage of research, namely (D&I). The next section reviews the major issues in designs for D&I research, with a particular focus on randomization and alternatives to randomized designs and also discusses the emerging development of hybrid, adaptive, and staging designs as well as mixed-methods designs. This is followed by a section that discusses power calculations in multilevel implementation designs and the use of analytic strategies such as mediation and moderation. Although little work in the use of mediation and moderation analyses in D&I research exists to date, the section lays out the need for this approach if we are to better understand the mechanisms and limitations of implementation strategies. Finally, the chapter addresses a rapidly emerging set of tools for dissemination and implementation research under the label of system science and then concludes with a case example of a rigorous and complex study in California of the impact of two implementation strategies for a 40-county rollout of the robust evidence-based intervention "Multidimensional Treatment Foster Care".

■ DESIGNS IN DISSEMINATION AND IMPLEMENTATION RESEARCH

Designs in Current D&I Research

We begin by briefly reviewing what is known about types of designs used in published D&I research, using the extensive work of the Cochrane Collaborative Effective Practice and Organization of Care Review Group (EPOC) in conducting systematic reviews of studies testing implementation strategies, primarily in medical care, as well as a recent structured review of implementation research designs focused on mental health care in child mental health and child welfare settings.[19]

At the time of the review for this chapter, EPOC characterized study designs in four major categories in their Data Collection Checklist (http://epoc.cochrane. org/sites/epoc.cochrane.org/files/uploads/datacollectionchecklist.pdf):

Randomized controlled trial (RCT), that is, a trial in which the participants (or other units) were definitely assigned prospectively to one or two (or more) alternative forms of health care using a process of random allocation (e.g., random number generation, coin flips).

Controlled clinical trial (CCT) may be a trial in which participants (or other units) were: a) definitely assigned prospectively to one or two (or more) alternative forms of intervention using a quasi-random allocation method (e.g., alternation, date of birth, patient identifier) or; b) possibly assigned prospectively to one or two (or more) alternative forms of intervention using a process of random or quasi-random allocation.

Controlled before-and-after study (CBA), that is, involvement of intervention and control groups other than by random process, and inclusion of baseline period of assessment of main outcomes. There are three minimum criteria for inclusion of CBAs: (a) *Contemporaneous data collection*: Pre- and postintervention periods for study and control sites are the same. If it is not clear in the paper (e.g., dates of collection are not mentioned in the text), the paper should be discussed with the investigators before data extraction is undertaken. (b) *Appropriate choice of control site:* studies using second site as controls; if study and control sites are comparable with respect to site characteristics, level of care and setting of care. If not clear from paper whether study and control sites are comparable, the paper should be discussed with the investigators before data extraction is undertaken. (c) *Minimum number of sites:* a minimum of two intervention sites and two control sites.

Interrupted time series (ITS), that is, a change in trend attributable to the intervention. There are two minimum criteria for inclusion of ITS designs: (a) a clearly defined point in time when the intervention occurred; (b) at least three data points before and three after the intervention.

As of June 30, 2010, 66 systematic reviews and 26 protocols of reviews in progress were posted on the Cochrane Collaborative website by the EPOC review group, including 49 reviews of specific types of interventions, 34 of interventions to improve specific types of practice, and 9 broad reviews or protocols. This suggests that the EPOC reviews constitute a useful repository of information regarding implementation strategies and the use of a fuller range of design options, some of which may be transferable to nonmedical care service systems. In many of these reviews, the proportion of studies that meet the design requirements, for some comparison or control condition for inclusion into EPOC reviews, is often quite small, as many publications in the literature are still merely descriptive in nature or have weak designs without comparison or control conditions to answer critical research questions.[20] An examination of the 1,053 studies included in the 66 EPOC systematic reviews shows that RCT designs constitute 75% of the designs reviewed, with 2.1% classified as CCT, 9.4% as CBA, 10.2% as ITS, and 3.3% as other (usually a combination of design types). The EPOC reviews demonstrate the dominance of randomized studies in medical care D&I research where comparison or control conditions are employed, and also suggest that the vast majority of the literature in this field is descriptive and provides little in the way of generalized knowledge compared with the much smaller number with some degree of design.

This emphasis on randomized designs in implementation research is supported by a recent paper that used EPOC design categories to review types of designs published on D&I research in non–medical care service systems, namely child welfare and child mental health.[19] Using standardized search strategies and the categories established by the EPOC review group, nine relevant studies were identified, all involving randomization, eight at a single level and one at two levels (treatment intervention vs. control, and intervention strategy vs. control).

From these two sources of extant D&I research, randomized designs constitute the majority of implementation studies that met the criteria of some kind of control or comparison condition. We also note that approximately 1 in 10 studies reviewed by EPOC used an interrupted time series design as an alternative to randomization. This is one of the four alternatives to randomization reviewed by Glasgow and colleagues.[15]

The observed dominance of RCT designs in D&I research supports the benefits of such designs for addressing common threats to interpretation of study findings. However, it is well to consider the nature of threats to the integrity of a randomized trial for dissemination and implementation research before further reviewing a range of design options for D&I research.

Often, one emphasizes characteristics of well-conducted research studies or trials in order to guide researchers into conducting studies that will lead to accurate scientific inferences. While this is helpful, we believe this is too optimistic a perspective, since research needs more than an overly optimistic "glass half-full" attitude to make appropriate conclusions. Indeed, a study can do many things right but fail in just one way and thereby put all its inferences at risk. The critical scientific paradigm for assigning observed differences by condition to an implementation's effect is that the only systematic factor that differs by intervention condition is the assigned intervention. For example, an implementation trial can carry out an appropriate randomization of communities to one of two implementation conditions, use valid and reliable measures, and conduct statistical analyses that correctly take into account intraclass clustering within communities. But if community leaders in one arm of the trial are more likely to refuse to be interviewed or drop out more frequently, this effect on the quality of the inferences can never be compensated by other good parts of the study. To reduce the potential for such imbalance, and to hold an implementation design in place, requires a strong and active partnership between communities, institutions, and researchers.[21,22] Below, we list some of the factors that are known to affect the quality of inferences[23] with special attention to implementation and dissemination research.

Random assignment is the obvious choice for insuring that implementation condition is fairly distributed (sometimes with blocking into similar communities followed by random assignment within these block). While some have suggested that random assignment is not appropriate for implementation research, our review indicates that there have been a sizeable number of such randomized implementation trials conducted, and they do have an important place in this research agenda. The usual alternative is a comparative study where one or more select communities apply a specified implementation procedure while other communities, often selected afterward, are used as comparison. The problem with this design is that it hopelessly confounds two factors: the implementation itself as well as community readiness, since only those communities that are "ready" are prepared to implement. One can never distinguish whether the differences in communities are due to one of these factors or both. An alternative design is a "rollout" design[5] where communities that express their willingness are randomized to the timing of implementation. Such a dynamic wait-listed design[16,24] has been used in the comparison of two implementation strategies for an evidence-based intervention for foster care to be described later in the case study.[4,25,26]

A second major threat to an implementation trial is a failure to use valid and reliable measures to assess implementation outcomes. Because the implementation process is inherently multilevel, it is critical to assess impact across the appropriate levels. One potential flaw can occur if one only measures the distal outcome on a target population that is served, since these may not be comparable across intervention conditions. For example, suppose an implementation strategy is designed to increase the number of youth who receive an evidence-based program. If we compare findings from those youth in communities randomized to the new implementation strategy to those using implementation as usual, it is quite possible for systematic differences to occur between those target youth who are exposed to different interventions. There is no mechanism to guarantee that those who receive the intervention are equivalent, and it may be that the expansion of service delivery brings in more or less challenging populations that are served. Analytic strategies that use propensity scores to adjust for differences at the nonrandomized level could be considered.[27,28] There is ordinarily no need to adjust for covariates at the higher level where randomization occurs because randomization preserves balance.

While there are enormous benefits to randomization, the multilevel nature of D&I research creates issues for typical randomization at the individual-level designs. Figure 12–2 shows a classic multilevel structure with four levels that Shortell[29] has suggested for change in assessing performance improvement in organizations. While randomization can and is being done at levels higher than the individual, there is an issue in having sufficient power as one moves to higher levels with diminishing units to be used in a randomized design (see later section on calculation of power in multilevel designs). Since power is so critical to the use of randomized designs, it is reasonable to consider quasi-experimental designs without randomization for D&I research. This clearly is the thrust of Glasgow and colleagues[15] in their 2005 article on practical designs. Another useful source for the alternative designs and the trade-offs between randomized and nonrandomized designs is the *Handbook of Practical Program Evaluation*,[30] edited by Wholey, Hatry, and Newcomer, especially the contrasting chapters on "Quasi-Experimentation"[31] by Reichardt and Mark, and the chapter on "Using Randomized Experiments"[32] by St Pierre. We note that Reichardt and Mark describe four prototypical quasi-experimental study designs: (1) before–after, (2) interrupted time series, (3) nonequivalent group, and

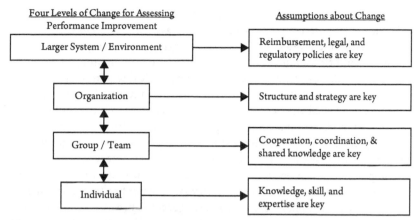

Figure 12–2. Four levels of change and assumptions about change. From Shortell, 2004.[29]

(4) regression–discontinuity designs. Their rendering of alternative designs is quite comparable to the EPOC classification of designs in implementation research and to the discussion of alternative designs by Glasgow and colleagues.[15]

We would also point to important recent studies that have compared the results between randomized experiments and observational studies. These have included both examples of strong divergence between observational studies and experimental studies, such as found in studies of hormone replacement therapy[33] as well as examples where the results were remarkably consistent. Notable is the paper published in 2000 by Concato et al.[34] that examined meta-analyses of randomized controlled trials and meta-analyses of either cohort or case-control studies on the same intervention. Across interventions addressing five very different medical conditions, the authors found remarkable similarity in the results in the two types of designs, which are perceived to be quite different in the hierarchy of evidence. The authors concluded that "The results of well-designed observational studies (with either a cohort or a case-control design) do not systematically overestimate the magnitude of the effects of treatment as compared to those in randomized, controlled trials on the same topic" (p. 1887). A later study published in 2008 by Cook et al.[35] came to the same conclusion when comparing the results from randomized experiments and regression discontinuity designs. In both papers, the authors argued that the quality of the observational studies had to be high to be comparable to the results in randomized designs. This line of research informs the emerging field of implementation science by suggesting that observational studies may also be seriously considered.

Rethinking Randomized Designs

An alternative approach to problems with the use of traditional RCT designs, so important in efficacy and effectiveness research stages, is to rethink how randomized designs can be adapted to meet the special needs of research across the four phases of the D&I stage. The next section discusses some of this rethinking, by considering nontraditional ways of using random assignment in D&I research.

Random assignment provides a method for making fair comparisons between intervention conditions, but the standard procedure for assigning individuals as well as organizations or communities often is impractical to administer, unacceptable to stakeholders, or irrelevant to the major research question.[36] In this section we describe nontraditional ways of using random assignment that can still be used to address important dissemination and implementation questions. One fundamental way of using random assignment involves the timing of delivery of an intervention. Often communities are uncomfortable withholding an intervention completely from a subpopulation, especially if the intervention is preventive in nature, holds little apparent risk of being iatrogenic, or addresses a major health problem in a community. In such a situation, researchers may suggest the use of a wait-listed design, which allows half the units to receive the intervention first, followed by the second set receiving it later. Communities are often more comfortable with this design compared with one involving a traditional control condition, and such a design can be used to address whether proximal impact on implementation targets (e.g., program adoption, fidelity, and reach into a target population) occurs. However, such standard wait-listed designs are inherently inefficient because the data from the second half of the study when the wait-listed group receives the intervention is weak or of negligible use in answering questions on implementation and dissemination.

An alternative design is a dynamic wait-listed design[16] or equivalently a stepped-wedge design.[37,38] These designs randomly assign units, which may be schools[16,24] or larger settings such as counties,[13,25,26] to different times of training. Starting with a small number of units assigned at the first time point, eventually all of the units receive training. Because the timing of training is random and there is before-training and after-training data on most if not all the units, we can track whether intended changes occur both across time and across condition. This type of design has been used to evaluate the effectiveness of a youth suicide prevention program[24] and also to test two implementation strategies for an evidence-based program in foster care.[25,26] There are three appealing features about this dynamic wait-listed design compared with traditional wait-listed designs. First, the statistical power is substantially greater for the dynamic design in answering many relevant research questions.[16] Second, it is often not practical to train a large number of communities in an intervention all at once, and the dynamic feature nicely focuses on a small manageable number who can receive the training attention that they need. Third, the use of multiple times for assignment provides more robustness of the design in terms of influence by exogenous factors, such as economic downturns, that could otherwise destroy any chance to make inferences if its timing occurred at the most critical time in the assignment to training.

We recommend that a dynamic wait-listed design be considered when an implementation study is being "rolled out" into a set of communities as part of a federal, statewide, or local policy change.[5,16,24] Such "rollout" trials could be of high utility in implementation research. As an example of an appropriate use of such a trial, consider examining the following typical strategy for improving the quality and effectiveness of services by improving the training of mental health counselors.

There are four levels that we need to pay attention to: the level of the client who receives services, the therapist who delivers the services, the supervisor whose job it is to improve service delivery within a mental health agency, and the agency itself. We consider an implementation strategy that changes the supervision practices of therapists within agencies. A first question is what level of randomization should be used to provide maximum utility to understanding whether a new supervision strategy is effective relative to that now being used. We can consider randomizing at any and all four levels from the client to the agency, but many of these levels will not be very useful. A key step is to identify what the most salient "level of intervention" being examined is; here we are fundamentally interested in how the use of a new supervision program will affect outcomes downstream, and therefore the key level of intervention is at the supervisor level; this is the first level where we would expect behavior to change. An empirically validated rule is the following: whenever possible one should randomize at the level of intervention, since randomization at lower levels (e.g., therapist) would contort supervisors from using new techniques to train therapists in the standard condition, and randomization at higher levels (e.g., agency) will generally result in major reductions in power.[39] If we do randomize at the level of the supervisor within an agency, then the agency is considered a "blocking factor." Blocking is a well-known way of reducing variability and thereby increasing power. In a rollout design, we would randomly determine the order and timing of training of supervisors and, consequently, their transmission of new behaviors to their supervisee therapists and, in turn, their own clients.

To assess impact in this trial design, we would likely want to measure behaviors of the supervising process (supervisor–therapist interactions), as well as of the therapeutic session itself (therapist–client), and perhaps at the level of the client target behavior as well. All three of these measures would normally be assessed over time. Thus, the design in this study would typically involve multiple observation/coding times for supervisors before and after they were trained to deliver a different type of supervision, multiple observation/coding times for their respective therapists, and multiple observation times for different clients across time. Three levels of analysis could be done, with the first examining changes in supervisor behavior across time before and after training, the second involving therapist–client behavior, also coded in terms of how therapist behavior with clients related to the timing of the supervisory training they received, and third, the behavior of the clients themselves. To connect these three analyses, we would conduct mediation analyses, which are presented later in this chapter.

The "sample size" for such a trial would then be given by the number of agencies, number of supervisors in each agency, the distribution of the number of therapists who receive supervision within these agencies, and finally the number of clients served by each therapist. Characteristics of timing include when supervisors in each agency receive training, the number of observation points in each supervision, the number of observation points for each therapist in interacting with a client, and the baseline and follow-up times for assessing client behavior. To make sure that there is sufficient power in this design to answer all three questions of impact on supervisor behavior, on therapist behavior, and on client behavior, as well as on mediational pathways, we would need to carry out a sophisticated study of how statistical power relates to these sample sizes and timing. While there are programs that allow one to compute power in multilevel designs,[40,41] to date the calculations for dynamic wait-listed designs are generally only available to do by simulation (see next section on power calculations).

Special Issues in Design and Analysis of D&I Research

Power and sample size calculations

The simpler tables that exist for calculating statistical power and sample size are typically not appropriate for implementation studies because of the multilevel or clustering and longitudinal nature of the data. Two online tools are often useful for these calculations, the Optimal Design (OD) system available through the W.T. Grant Foundation, and the RMASS program developed by the Center for Health Statistics at the University of Chicago. Websites for both are listed in the appendix to this chapter.

Randomization at single versus multiple levels in D&I research

Designs that involve multiple levels of random assignment or allocation are often useful in increasing the precision of inferences. For example, to examine sustain-ability of a classroom-based intervention, we randomized first-grade teachers and classrooms within schools to the timing of training. This was the primary unit of intervention for this study. To compare early versus later training in this class-room-based intervention design, we would essentially rely on the average differences within schools for classrooms that had early versus late training. However, we knew that because schools ordinarily assign students with like ability in the same classrooms, called ability tracking, classrooms within schools would typically not be well matched. Therefore, a design that tried to compare outcomes for the one or two early trained teachers in each school with those who were trained later would have to introduce a large heterogeneity in classrooms unless children were matched into similar classrooms within schools. We, in fact, did this by random assignment of all children to classrooms as they were enrolled in the school,[42] and this design greatly increased the statistical power over a design that did not have balanced classrooms.[39,43] Such designs that use random assignment of groups at one level and random allocation of individuals into these groups can provide substantial improvement in power.

An alternative way to use randomization is to randomize units at two levels to different types of interventions. For example, a system-level intervention can be tested by random assignment of agencies to different intervention strategies, say to business as usual versus a new system for monitoring fidelity and providing correc-tives. A client-based intervention can be tested against standard practice by ran-domly assigning clients to these conditions within each agency. Such a two-level intervention design is known as a "split plot" and is commonly used in industrial experiments[44] but is suitable for implementation trials as well. It can be used to com-pare overall effect of the implementation strategy, overall effects of the client-based intervention, and their interaction. An example of such a design for implementation studies is given by Chambers.[45]

Pilot studies and estimating effect size

In developing a new implementation strategy, it is often very sensible to conduct a small-scale study to examine feasibility and assess sources of variation to determine the size one would need to have a fully powered study. While this is a useful approach, we want to convey some caution, especially with the estimation of effect sizes from a pilot study. As pointed out by Kraemer,[46] the precision of an effect size estimate from a pilot study is much lower than that in a fully powered study, and consequently, considerable uncertainty in power introduced with this estimated effect size from the pilot study is entered into power calculation programs. It is possible to use these pilot studies to get some useful information about the magnitude of different sources of variance,[5] but the intended magnitude of the effect that one is aiming to achieve should best be determined by clinical relevance, rather than the estimated value obtained from the pilot study.

Analyzing for mechanisms through mediation

A major task for D&I method development is to determine new mediation analysis methods for implementation modeling. There will be many challenging causality questions, particularly around how to best handle protocol deviations in implementation trials. One of these challenges will be to deal with the possibility of differential attrition in intervention agents in the intervention arms. For example, teachers who are successfully trained in an EBP such as the Good Behavior Game (GBG) that promotes improved classroom behavior may be less frustrated with teaching and less likely to leave the profession.[47] Such attrition differences can become manifest in a longitudinal comparison of teachers who have been trained in this intervention versus those not trained[6] and may be one explanation of persistent intervention effects.

This work also needs to incorporate innovative developments in causal inference for mediation models, that is, principal stratification (PS).[48-60] Traditional PS causal modeling characterizes subgroups that are responders to an intervention as well as nonresponders[48,51,53] and can assess the magnitude and extent of different impacts that these subgroups experience. PS techniques are also closely connected to latent variable modeling and mediation analysis,[61-66] and these latent variable approaches can be used for evaluating intervention impact and examining rates of differential response across intervention conditions.[67] There is, however, a need to extend these methods to take into account repeated measures over time and multilevel modeling. As one example, Brown and colleagues[68] have proposed developing two-level PSs to account for different strata of intervention agents' (e.g., teachers') responses to training. Like traditional PSs, teachers could be classified into always-successful managers of their classroom whether or not they received intervention training, always unsuccessful even if given training, and responders to the training. Also like PS, in implementation trials we cannot know any teacher's classification exactly, since we can only observe his or her response to the training or no-training condition. However, causal inferences for outcomes of *youth*, who are exposed to these teachers, are indeed possible in randomized trials. We have identified a class of such two-level PS models using the Georgia Gatekeeper Trial[69] and are developing and testing several approaches in implementation research.

Finally, work needs to consider application of existing methods for multistage follow-up[13,68] to evaluate the effect of prevention programs on severe levels of drug abuse, an area that has not received sufficient attention in the literature in many evaluations. These applications for new trials will involve epidemiologic assessment of the strength of antecedent risk factors, that is, multiple drug use in adolescence, on later severe abuse. While the method is straightforward, it will require complex calculations to take into account unknown levels of differential attrition and any direct effects from program to drug abuse that do not involve drug use.

Mixed-Methods Designs in D&I Research

Mixed-methods designs focus on collecting, analyzing, and merging both quantitative and qualitative data into one or more studies. The central premise of these designs is that the use of quantitative and qualitative approaches in combination provides a better understanding of research issues than either approach alone.[70] In such designs, qualitative methods are used to explore and obtain depth of understanding as to the reasons for success or failure to implement evidence-based practice or to identify strategies for facilitating implementation. Complementarily, quantitative methods are used to test and confirm hypotheses based on an existing conceptual model and obtain breadth of understanding of predictors of successful implementation.[71] Numerous typologies and guidelines for the adoption of mixed-methods designs exist. Teddlie and Tashakkori[71] identified 40 different types of mixed-methods designs in their review of the literature, and Cresswell and Plano Clark[70] highlighted 12 different typologies. These typologies represent mixed-methods research in the fields of nursing, evaluation, public health, primary care, education, and the social and behavioral sciences, and outline the structure, function, and process of using mixed methods.

In implementation research, quantitative and qualitative methods are used either simultaneously or sequentially. Moreover, one method is usually but not always perceived as being dominant or primary, and the other is subordinate or secondary. A review of published studies of dissemination and implementation found that most involved the simultaneous use of quantitative and qualitative methods, and most used quantitative methods as the primary or dominant method and qualitative methods as the secondary or subordinate method.[72] A little less than half of the studies used a balanced approach in which quantitative and qualitative methods were used simultaneously and given equal weight. For instance, Whitley and colleagues[73] documented the process of implementation of an illness management and recovery program for people with severe mental illness in community mental health settings using qualitative data to assess perceived barriers and facilitators of implementation and quantitative data to assess implementation performance based on assessments of fidelity to the practice model, with no overriding priority assigned to either aim. Some studies gave equal weight to qualitative and quantitative data for the purpose of evaluating fidelity and implementation barriers/facilitators even though the collection of qualitative data to assess implementation was viewed as secondary to the overall goal of evaluating the effectiveness of an intervention.[74–76]

In implementation research, mixed methods have been used to achieve one or more of five different functions.[72] First, qualitative and quantitative methods may be used sequentially or simultaneously to answer the same question. This is known as convergence. There are two specific forms of convergence: triangulation and transformation. Triangulation involves the use of one type of data to validate or confirm conclusions reached from analysis of the other type of data. Transformation involves the sequential quantification of qualitative data—for example, concept mapping[77]—or the use of qualitative techniques to transform quantitative data.[70] Second, quantitative and qualitative methods may be used to answer related questions for the purpose of evaluation or elaboration. This is known as complementarity. In evaluative designs, quantitative data were used to evaluate outcomes while qualitative data were used to evaluate process. In elaborative designs, qualitative methods were used to provide depth of understanding and quantitative methods are used to provide breadth of understanding. This includes studies that present descriptive quantitative data on subjects, and studies that used qualitative data to focus on beliefs and perspectives. Third, one method may be used in sequence to answer questions raised by the other method. This is known as expansion or explanation. Fourth, qualitative methods may be used to answer questions that will enable use of the other method to answer other questions. This is known as development. In implementation research, there are three distinct forms of development: instrument development, conceptual development, and intervention development or adaptation. Finally, there is the sequential use of one method to identify a sample of participants for use of the other method. This is known as sampling.

The process of integrating quantitative and qualitative data occurs in three forms: merging the data, connecting the data, and embedding the data.[70] In implementation research, merging the data occurs when qualitative and quantitative data are brought together in the analysis phase to answer the same question through triangulation or related questions through complementarity.[72] Connecting the data occurs when the analysis of one dataset leads to (and thereby connects to) the need for the other dataset, such as when quantitative results lead to the subsequent collection and analysis of qualitative data (i.e., expansion) or when qualitative results are used to build to the subsequent collection and analysis of quantitative data, (e.g., development). Embedding the data occurs when qualitative studies of treatment or implementation process or context were embedded within larger quantitative studies of treatment or implementation outcome for the purpose of complementarity, convergence, or expansion.

There are several reasons for using mixed-methods designs in intervention research. One might use quantitative methods to measure intervention and/or implementation outcomes and qualitative methods to understand process. Qualitative inquiry is highly appropriate for studying process because (1) depicting process requires detailed descriptions of how people engage with one another; (2) the experience of process typically varies for different people, so their experiences need to be captured in their own words; (3) process is fluid and dynamic, so it can't be fairly summarized on a single rating scale at one point in time; and (4) participants' perceptions are a key process consideration.[78]

A second reason for using mixed-methods designs is to conduct both exploratory and confirmatory research. In mixed-methods designs, qualitative methods are used to explore a phenomenon and generate a conceptual model along with testable hypotheses, while quantitative methods are used to confirm the validity of the model by testing the hypotheses.[71] This combined focus is also consistent with the call by funding agencies[79] and others[1] to develop new conceptual models and to develop new measures to test these models.

Mixed methods can also be used to examine both intervention content and context. Many studies use mixed methods to examine the context of implementation of a specific intervention.[73, 80–82] Unlike efficacy studies where context can be controlled, implementation research occurs in real-world settings distinguished by their complexity and variation in context.[19] Qualitative methods are especially suited to understanding context.[83] In contrast, quantitative methods are used to measure aspects of the content of the intervention in addition to the intervention's outcomes.

Mixed methods may also be used to incorporate the perspective of potential consumers of evidence-based practices (both practitioners and clients).[1] Use of qualitative methods gives voice to these stakeholders[84] and allows partners an opportunity to express their own perspectives, values, and opinions.[85]

Finally, mixed methods may be used to compensate for one set of methods by the use of another set of methods. For instance, convergence or triangulation of quantitative and qualitative data was an explicit feature of the mixed-methods study of the implementation of SafeCare® in Oklahoma by Aarons and Palinkas[86,87] because of limited statistical power in quantitative analyses that were nested in teams of services providers, a common problem of implementation research.[1,19]

■ SYSTEM SCIENCE APPROACHES IN IMPLEMENTATION RESEARCH

The term *system science* refers to a transdisciplinary approach to understanding how interactions between elementary units produce complex patterns. System science methods, using the NIH/OBSSR definition, take into account the "complexity, dynamic nature, and emergent phenomena" and typically uses social network analysis, agent-based modeling, and systems dynamics as well as other tools such as decision analysis and systems engineering (see Chapter 9). We view these system science methods as critical to moving implementation research forward as a science for the following reasons. First, implementation is inherently interactional, across multilevels within systems and between as well as across systems, and only when different systems function together can we expect implementation to succeed. The system science methods we discuss directly deal with interactions, in contrast to, say, traditional statistical modeling involving standard regression modeling—which assumes complete independence- or multilevel growth modeling—which allows correlation across persons and time but does not explicitly model these processes.

Second, implementation process data, which are essential in research to monitor progress, are heavily dependent on interactions between actors, as exemplified in the development of community–researcher partnerships.[21,22] Third, implementation process data also are essential for communities, organizations, and service systems themselves to provide monitoring and feedback for quality improvement. Most of today's research-level implementation process data are very expensive for these systems to collect. Consequently, we need to develop cost-effective ways to assemble quality implementation process data, conduct analyses on these data, and integrate this into a monitoring and feedback system. We fully anticipate that such systems can be built by automating these steps as much as possible. Systems science methods will need to be used for all these purposes. Below, we describe important system science methods that are available and then provide brief illustrations of how they can be used in implementation.

System Dynamics Method (SDM) is a method for understanding systems and how they change what was originally developed by Forrester at MIT[88] coming out of his field of industrial dynamics. Hovmand and his colleagues at the Washington University Social System Design Lab, a vibrant current organization in the field of system dynamics, describe it as a "method for understanding, designing, and managing change... (which) models the various relationships between elements of a particular system and how these relationships influence the behavior of the system over time."[89] Hovmand has also developed a creative approach to system dynamics methodology (http://gwbweb.wustl.edu/research/systemdynamics/Pages/SystemDynamicsDefinition.aspx) by incorporating a highly articulated use of participatory group model building as a multiple stakeholder qualitative approach to understanding system processes and more fully uncovering the assumptions driving the graphic models with feedback mechanisms or loops with causal relationships typically expressed in quantitative parameters.

An excellent example that illustrates how system dynamics modeling can be applied to implementation research is Hovmand and Gillespie's NSF funded study on the "Impact of implementing evidence based practices on organizational performance." This research project employed system dynamics modeling with human service agencies in St. Louis that were involved in adopting and implementing evidence-based practices.[91] Hovmand and Gillespie developed a conceptual framework represented as a system dynamics simulation model based on several sources of information, including extant literature, theory from organizational science, and key informant interviews with mental health services administrators and clinical directors. "Results from the simulations show how gains in performance depended on organizations' initial inertia and initial efficiency and that only the most efficient organizations may see benefits in organizational performance from implementing EBP."[91]

Agent-Based Modeling (ABM) refers to computational methods that simulate the actions or interactions between units or between units and their environments. ABMs are used to model and compare outcomes of implementation strategies that are too difficult to evaluate any other way. Unlike system dynamics methods, ABM is built from the "bottom-up" as opposed to a "top-down" approach. Consequently, it can be used to model the dynamics of individuals and groups as they freely or restrictively interact with one another within defined environments. ABMs have been used to improve our understanding of social interactions,[92-98] including applications as complex as the growth and death of civilizations as they interact with finite environments, the spread of infectious diseases, and social interactions around illegal drug use. An agent-based model is an interacting set of objects, each having attributes and a set of rules for change and interaction. Agents can represent individuals, groups of individuals, social networks, or other definable objects. For implementation, we would often include facilitator and trainers or coaches as agents. Simulation studies of agent-based models are then used to track microlevel and macrolevel behavior over time as each agent[99] behaves autonomously and interacts with other agents or its environment. Agent-based models allow for heterogeneity across agents to reflect, say, varying levels of fidelity among facilitators. They also allow nonlinear effects. For example, increasing the amount of training that a facilitator receives may enhance fidelity up to a point; a facilitator may actively resist too much training with fidelity degrading accordingly. Although interactions are often simple and local, they can result in complex, emergent patterns. An important approach is to use "evidence-based" ABM simulations.[100] These use "pattern-oriented modeling,"[101] indicating that any ABM must at a minimum reproduce macrolevel measurable behavior. To examine the "pattern" or fit of ABMs, one would match predicted macrolevel behavior to observed quantities (e.g. predicted and observed distributions of waiting times to adoption). This pattern-oriented modeling is similar to the testing of the goodness of fit of latent growth models using observable quantities.[102] Once the model has been validated, it can be extended across time to predict outcomes under different circumstances or rules.[98]

Social network analysis (SNA) involves techniques to examine the social relationships between individuals, or across groups, organizations, and institutions. Social network analysis is a set of theories and techniques used to understand how social relationships (e.g., friendship, advice seeking, reputation) influence behaviors.[103-107] These methods quantify a person's position within a social hierarchy and characterize people's social influences such as the percent of their colleagues who have adopted an evidence-based program.[108-111] The basic elements as represented by *nodes* (e.g., individuals, agencies) and *edges.* Each edge identifies the existence and directionality of a relationship between two nodes.

Social networks influence behavior through several theoretical mechanisms. Networks transfer behavior change information, influence perception of social norms, and provide how-to knowledge. [108,110] Network data are used extensively in interorganizational research and functioning as they describe the cohesiveness, integration, or fragmentation of work.[112-114] Network maps also indicate where to intervene to improve network performance.[115,116] Social network analysis is relevant to studying the relationship between practitioners and scientists as they form collaborative partnerships around implementation. Valente et al. recently evaluated a Community-Based Participatory Research (CBPR) initiative and showed that the intervention increased bidirectional linkages between Community-Based Organizations (CBOs) and from CBOs to universities but not from university researchers to CBOs.[117] *Dynamic* social networks refers to changes that occur in these networks over time. Dynamic SNA is used to trace the adoption, uptake, and dissemination of interventions as well as to propose new network implementation strategies.

Networks can be used to design and implement behavior change programs in schools and communities.[118,119] In a randomized trial, Valente and colleagues[120] tested a school smoking prevention program led by network-selected leaders.[120-122] This showed that network-based groups were more effective than were groups created randomly.

Systems engineering refers to the processes of identifying and manipulating the properties of a system as a whole rather than by its component parts. Systems engineering is both a discipline and process to guide the development, implementation, and evaluation of complex systems.[123] A system is an aggregation of components structurally organized to accomplish a set of goals or objectives. All systems have the following characteristics: a structure, interacting components, inputs and outputs, goals, and objectives. Systems are dynamic in that each system component has an effect on the other components.[124]

System optimization requires design consideration of all components of a system, in contrast to a more traditional reductionist approach focusing on individual components. Attempts to design a system without considering the dynamic physical and social environments where the system operates will degrade system performance. For example, if a school-based prevention program competes for time against instruction, output would be low. *Task analysis* (TA) is one systems engineering tool we will use to characterize the implementation process and necessary resource and skill requirements. It was successfully applied to describe 15 complex intervention programs in the Resources for Alzheimer's Caregiver Health (REACH) program conducted by Schultz and colleagues.[125] Another system engineering tool is the *Analytic Hierarchy Process* (AHP).[126] This can be used to capture decision making within systems. By focusing on the decision process and establishing priorities, the Analytic Hierarchy Process can identify critical attributes of an intervention and areas where an intervention might be modified or adapted.[127]

It is not well known that strategies for implementation vary dramatically. We have been struck by the vastly different approaches that have been used in different implementation strategies. To compare these alternatives, a full characterization of different strategies is required, and that requires the use of a standard procedure for eliciting intended implementation strategies as well as identifying where inefficiencies and other problems exist. The use of task analysis and the analytic hierarchical process and related techniques provides the ability to develop an ordering of priorities in decision making to distinguish different implementation models in theory and practice.

Intelligent Data Analysis refers to advanced computational methods to automate the generation of meaning from text, video, or audio signals. These techniques can be used to reduce large amounts of process data on implementation that come in digitized form. We point out that most implementation process data that are typically collected in agencies, such as number of people attending meetings or self-ratings of fidelity, are only crude indicators of the implementation process. However, there are other sources of information on the implementation process that are rarely codified but can be converted to analyzable data. Notably, these include audio and videotaped training as well as program delivery sessions. Such information is highly useful for supervision, but often just a small portion of this information is ever used. Automated signal processing and feature extraction of videotapes are possible using intelligent data analysis, and the outcomes of such methods would help to identify specific ways to improve facilitator fidelity.

As one illustration of the use of intelligent data analysis, we point to the availability of contact logs, process notes, e-mail, and other communications to monitor implementation. Automated generation of meaning from text is one important tool to convert information that generally requires time-consuming human judgment. If we were able to automate the process of transferring such information into meaningful data on the implementation process, it would result in a major savings in costs for agencies and service providers. The transfer of text to meaningful terms involves intelligent data analysis. Similar to psychometrics, computer science research has used latent variables via the Hidden Markov Model (HMM) to derive meaning from text information. In HMM, there is a time-dependent process governed by state changes and its associate state-dependent distribution that produce observations at each step (e.g., in speech a syllable is a state and the sound is the observation). In HMM the goal is to estimate the number of states, the state transition matrix, and the state-dependent distributions of observations.[128] A more advanced Latent Semantic Indexing method models elicit meanings behind texts[129,130] and has been used extensively in research, including our own,[131,132] to classify and categorize documents (i.e., automatic groupings). A general assumption is that the documents come from a set of unknown categories and the words and phrases appearing in the documents are produced by category-dependent distributions. Given a set of observed data, these methods construct matrices that explain document generation and word/phrase generation using iterative optimization and/or matrix decomposition. We note that completely automated systems for converting text to meaning are not likely to succeed by themselves. However, intelligent data analysis provides not only a best classification based on similarity to correctly classified text information, but also a probability assessment of this correct classification. Thus, we can discriminate between text that is clearly classified and text that may be incorrectly classified. By screening this text, we can concentrate the high-cost human interaction on those messages that have uncertain classification, greatly limiting the cost involved in producing valid implementation process data.

Decision analysis with microsimulation modeling (DA) is the final method presented with an implementation research example. This method is often combined with an economic analysis because in support of an overall decision analysis, cost-effectiveness analyses or benefit-analyses explicitly acknowledge the reality of budget constraints and other limited resources, identifying those interventions that can feasibly maximize the decision makers' objectives. Such analyses often employ computer-based models that simulate the long-term, systemic impact of each specified alternative and compare them to provide recommendations about the best action(s) to take. It is important to note that such analyses provide their greatest value when they are employed in an iterative fashion, allowing policymakers to consider a variety of what-if scenarios and to evaluate multiple decisions holistically.

Decision analyses have been used successfully to consider complex decisions involving health conditions with long time courses and multiple outcomes. Such analyses have considered the prevention and management of HIV/AIDS, cardiovascular disease, diabetes, and HPV and cervical cancer.[133–138] For example, they have informed policy recommendations for HIV/AIDS prevention. Relying in part on model-based cost-effectiveness analyses, the Institute of Medicine recommended a shift from funding programs based on high AIDS prevalence to targeting prevention efforts to subgroups at high risk of infection (e.g., needle exchange for injection drug users).[139]

These tools of decision science are also well suited to supporting human service policymakers (such as child welfare directors and managers) as they confront the challenges of complex, real-world operations.[140] Such analyses can identify policies and interventions that are most likely to achieve a set of desired objectives given current uncertainties. In the context of ongoing child welfare operations, evidence-based interventions' superior effectiveness must be considered with respect to how well they enhance safety, permanence, and well-being and to any additional resources required to implement and maintain them at levels ensuring effectiveness. As decision makers contemplate these interventions, they require actionable information to overcome uncertainty as to whether the long-term benefits and averted costs of evidence-based interventions justify the investment.

With over 1 million children served by the U.S. child welfare system at a cost of $20 billion annually, the use of evidence-based interventions has the potential to improve the health and well-being of a large, vulnerable population in a more cost-effective manner. However, substantial investments may be required to incorporate such interventions into child welfare agencies requiring evidence to support these decisions as they weigh the various trade-offs.[141]

An excellent illustration of the use of decision analysis is provided by Goldhaber-Fiebert and colleagues[142] presented at the NIH supported Dissemination and Implementation conference in March, 2011. The authors used a computer-based microsimulation model to evaluate the effect of implementing one such evidence-based foster parent training intervention: KEEP (Keeping Foster Parents Trained and Supported).[143] The microsimulation computed policy-relevant outcomes such as increased rates of adoption and reunification (positive exits) along with improved foster care placement stability (e.g., reduced lateral foster placement changes and reduced negative exits to group care, etc.) resulting from the application of KEEP. The microsimulation incorporated data on children in foster care from randomized controlled trials of KEEP[144,145] as well as large, population-representative longitudinal studies (e.g., National Survey of Child and Adolescent Well-Being [NSCAW-1]), using multivariate Cox proportional hazard models and bootstrapping to provide estimates of the rates of foster care placement change, the main covariates that determine these rates, and their associated uncertainty.

The detailed microsimulation developed for this analysis simulated large cohorts of individual children whose characteristics matched those of the actual foster care populations within the U.S. child welfare system. The model then followed these "simulated individuals" on their paths through the system, tracking their placement changes and allowing past experiences to influence their future risks of placement change and exit. This approach permitted the consideration of the rich, complex effects of each individual's experience in the system over time, identifying cumulative benefits to KEEP, emphasizing higher-risk groups of children who may differentially benefit from the application of the intervention, and gauging the heterogeneous mediating effects that different state child welfare systems could have on KEEP. The paper demonstrated decision-analytic methods to employ existing data to project policy-relevant child welfare outcomes related to permanence and stability. Decision-analytic microsimulation modeling is a feasible and useful methodology to inform challenging child welfare policy decisions and can be extended to consider multiple evidence-based interventions and outcomes.

■ CASE STUDY: COMMUNITY DEVELOPMENT TEAMS TO SCALE-UP MTFC IN CALIFORNIA

Background: Each year, 87,000 children and adolescents are placed in group, residential, and institutional care settings in the United States (http://www.childwelfare.gov/pubs/factsheets/foster.cfm) with over 15,000 in California. While there is some quasi-experimental evidence to support positive short-term effects for highly structured and individualized group care models such as Teaching Family Homes,[146] the majority of studies have linked placement in group and residential care with increased odds of an array of negative outcomes such as association with delinquent peers,[147] delinquency,[148] isolation from family, and lowered odds of reunification.[149] Group home placements are also expensive, consuming 43% of the substitute care dollars in California in 2001. Multidimensional Treatment Foster Care (MTFC) was developed as an alternative to group and residential care for children and adolescents with severe emotional, behavioral, and mental health problems being placed through juvenile justice and child welfare systems. In MTFC, the children/teens are placed singly in a highly trained and supported community foster home where they and their family (biological, adoptive) receive intensive clinical services. A series of randomized trials have shown significantly better outcomes for participants in MTFC versus group care,[150,151] leading MTFC to be designated as a top-tier evidence-based model by multiple scientific advisory boards and organizations.[152-155] MTFC has been implemented in over 90 agencies in the United States and Europe since 2001; however, these agencies likely do not reflect typical publicly funded service systems; they are early innovators.[156] In fact, it is estimated that 90% of public systems do not implement evidence-based practice models. It is these non-early-adopting agencies that are the focus of this case study.

Context

The California Institute of Mental Health (CIMH) originated the Community Development Team (CDT) model[157] to increase the number of California counties that successfully adopt, implement, and sustain evidence-based practices. CDTs operate through several well-specified mechanisms including multicounty team meetings, expert local consultation, peer-to-peer exchanges, and regular multicounty conference calls. Forty California counties who were non-early-adopters of

MTFC were invited to participate in an NIMH-funded randomized trial to scale up MTFC in California, and all agreed to be part of this trial. After matching counties on demographic characteristics (e.g., size, percent minority, poverty, previous use of mental health funding) into three cohorts of 12–14 counties, a two-step randomization process was used. Counties were first randomized to condition (CDT or individualized or standard "as usual" implementation). Then they were randomized again to one of three time frames for implementation start date that spanned across three years. Randomization to start date allowed us to manage issues related to implementation capacity as training all counties at once was impossible. The random assignment of counties to cohort also increased protection against the influence of exogenous factors.[16]

Measurement and Analytic Framework

A primary research question relates to whether participation in the CDT condition improves the adoption, implementation, fidelity/adherence, and sustainability of MTFC. Secondarily, contextual and organizational factors are hypothesized to mediate the association between experimental condition and implementation outcomes. For example, as a result of participating in the CDTs, counties are expected to make better progress due to more positive attitudes toward the MTFC model and supportive organizational climates. However, regardless of experimental condition, those counties with higher scores on the hypothesized mediators are expected to achieve better implementation outcomes.

One of the main implementation outcomes to be examined is how long it takes for a county to place their first child in an MTFC home, an event that comes after the decision by multiple social service systems in the county to adopt MTFC, the selection and training of agency workers to support MTFC, and the selection and training of a foster parent in MTFC. We use survival analysis techniques, including Cox regression modeling,[158] to compare the time it takes for placement for CDT and standard-setting counties. Survival analysis is well suited for these data as cohorts will vary in the amount of time that they have been involved in the study, thereby creating an outcome measure that is right censored. Survival analyses will use the entire time period available for each cohort (4.5 years for Cohort 1; 2.5 years for Cohort 2; and 1.5 years for Cohort 3). By modeling how the hazard rate depends on intervention status and other covariates, a formal test can be conducted to assess the CDT intervention impact. An unusual feature in this study is that the outcomes for counties in the CDT groups could be correlated because they work together in a peer-to-peer setting. In contrast, those counties assigned to the standard implementation condition are expected to have outcomes that are independent. To account for how this clustering effect in the CDT group affects the standard error and testing of the intervention, the Generalized Estimating Equation (GEE) sandwich-type variance estimator will be used to adjust for nonindependence in Cox regression modeling, using techniques similar to those employed previously in schizophrenia studies where family factors caused clustering.[159–161] These methods correct for nonindependence; test statistics can be based on exact tests where the distribution under the null is simulated and critical values are thereby obtained.

In addition to the time to first placement, implementation progress is measured using a Stages of Implementation Completion (SIC) scale developed for this trial that includes both time-based and quality indicators of completion of each of eight implementation stages: (1) Engagement, (2) Feasibility, (3) Readiness Planning, (4) Staff Hired/Trained, (5) Fidelity Monitoring System in Place, (6) Services and Consultation Begins, (7) Adherence and Competence Tracked and Feedback, and (8) Certification/Licensure. Activities are specified at each stage and measured using dates of accomplishment and quality ratings. Progression through each stage involves unique (although sometimes overlapping) groups of constituents. For example, leaders of child welfare, mental health, and juvenile justice systems first explore the possibility of implementation (Stage 1), and access the feasibility/fit of the model for their local circumstances (Stage 2). If the determination to proceed is made, system leaders are likely to step back from the process and involve others who will be directly involved in the active implementation and in the planning (Stage 3). During active implementation when staff are hired and trained (Stage 4) and fidelity monitoring is set up (Stage 5), intervention and agency staff are the primary agents involved, not the system leadership. Therefore, the SIC is populated by data from a variety of agents at the various stages. Quality-of-participation ratings are made within several of the SIC stages.[25,162] Interestingly, this real-world implementation instrument reflects, quite closely, the theoretical model developed by Aarons et al.[3] and adds considerable support for the importance of different factors at various stages of the implementation process.

In addition to the SIC time to completion and quality-of-completion ratings, qualitative measures aimed at adding to the understanding of what factors influence decision makers to adopt evidence-based models are being examined. Palinkas found that the social networks of system leaders played a key role in their decision to adopt during the exploration stage. Network size and density (the number of reported links divided by the maximum number of possible links) was not associated with the size of the county but was significantly associated with stage of participation; individuals in counties that were considering participation in the Cal-40 study had larger and more dense networks than individuals in counties that had already made a decision to participate or not participate.[163] For those who had agreed to participate or were considering participation, information about MTFC and the Cal-40 study was obtained from presentations given by CIMH representatives at state or regional meetings, direct contact by CIMH with county agency directors, direct contact by other agency directors within the county, or staff within the agency. In addition, how leaders interpret and make use of evidence is being examined, including what sources of information they find credible, where they obtain information, and what types of evidence they see as relevant. The findings from the qualitative measures will enhance and extend the SIC outcomes by providing insights into specific mechanisms that drive decisions to adopt/not adopt.

Preliminary Findings

The trial is still underway. Of the 40 non-early-adopting California counties invited to participate, none declined, and 39 consented to at least consider implementing

MTFC. No counties objected to the randomization to condition, but several noted that the time frame to which they were assigned did not fit their circumstances.[26] Counties with more children placed in care and those that had more positive organizational climates consented to participate more quickly.[4] The study has recently been extended to include 11 additional Ohio counties that are not early adopters of MTFC. Recruitment, enrollment, and randomization methods used in Ohio mirrored those used in California. In Ohio, the CDT intervention is being implemented by the Center for Innovative Practices at Kent State University under the direction of CIMH consultants.

SUGGESTED READINGS

Berwick D. The science of improvement. *JAMA*. 2008;299(10):1182.

This article describes four recommended changes in the use of health care evidence that would speed along health care and practice improvements: (1) use a range of scientific methodologies, considering both mechanisms and contexts; (2) reconsider thresholds for action on evidence, making incremental changes; (3) reconsider concepts of trust and bias; and (4) engage both academics and patient caregivers with respect.

Brown CH, Wyman PA, Guo J, Peña J. Dynamic wait-listed designs for randomized trials: new designs for prevention of youth suicide. *Clin Trials*. 2006;3(3):259–271.

This article describes a modification to the traditional wait-listed design, in which random assignment occurs multiple times during a trial, thus enabling subjects to receive the intervention. Still, these designs can only be used to assess short-term impact, and there is no control group left as a comparison.

Brown CH, Ten Have TR, Jo B, et al. Adaptive designs for randomized trials in public health. *Annu Rev Public Health*. 2009;30:1–25.

Suggests adaptations to the traditional randomized trial. In this article, "adaptive design" refers to a trial in which characteristics of the study, such as assignment to an intervention or control group, change during the data collection process.

Flay B. Efficacy and effectiveness trials (and other phases of research) in the development of health promotion programs. *Prev Med*. 1986;15(5):451–474.

This early work from Flay provides a useful overview of the concepts of efficacy and effectiveness. While the science of translational research has evolved considerably over the past three decades, many of the principles from Flay's article remain highly relevant.

Glasgow R, Magid D, Beck A, Ritzwoller D, Estabrooks PA. Practical clinical trials for translating research to practice: design and measurement recommendations. *Med Care*. 2005;43(6):551.

Building on the influential work of Tunis et al.[164] on practical clinical trials (PCTs), this article provides examples of conducting PCTs with enhanced external validity, without sacrificing internal validity. The authors suggest that in order to reduce the gap between academia and real-world practice, it is necessary to increase the relevance of PCTs for appropriate audiences.

Landsverk J, Brown C, Rolls Reutz J, Palinkas L, Horwitz S. Design elements in implementation research: a structured review of child welfare and child mental health studies. *Admin Policy Ment Health and Ment Health Serv Res*. 2011:1–10.

This paper discusses the need for the development of methodological approaches to the study of implementation processes and tests of implementation strategies through a structured review of nine studies. The authors present limitations of randomized designs and potential design alternatives to consider.

Palinkas L, Aarons G, Horwitz S, Chamberlain P, Hurlburt M, Landsverk J. Mixed method designs in implementation research. *Admin Policy Ment Health and Ment Health Serv Res.* 2011:1–10.

This paper examines mixed-methods designs in implementation research over a five-year period and offers suggestions for their use. The authors found that design complexity was associated with context, number of objectives, and implementation phase.

Pierre RG. Using randomized experiments. In: Wholey J, Hatry H, Newcomer K, eds. *Handbook of Practical Program Evaluation.* San Francisco, CA: Jossey-Bass Inc.; 2004: 150–175.

In this chapter, Pierre considers the recent push to use randomized experiments for obtaining evidence. He offers recommendations for using and designing randomized experiments, as well as how they should be executed and evaluated.

Reichardt C, Mark M. Quasi-experimentation. In: Wholey J, Hatry H, Newcomer K, eds. *Handbook of Practical Program Evaluation.* San Francisco, CA: Jossey-Bass Inc.; 2004: 126–149.

In this chapter, Reichardt and Mark consider four quasi-experimental designs: before–after, interrupted time series, nonequivalent group, and regression discontinuity. They describe the strengths and weaknesses of each design, as well as threats to validity.

West SG, Duan N, Pequegnat W, et al. Alternatives to the randomized controlled trial. *Am J Public Health.* 2008;98(8):1359–1366.

The authors consider alternatives to the randomized controlled trial that also allow for drawing causal inferences. They describe the strengths and weaknesses of each design, including threats to validity and the strategies that can be used to diminish those threats.

SELECTED WEBSITES AND TOOLS

http://www.wtgrantfoundation.org/resources/consultation-service-and-optimal-design
Optimal Design is a software package, developed by Stephen Raudenbush and colleagues,[165] which helps researchers determine sample size, statistical power, and optimal allocation of resources for multilevel and longitudinal studies. This includes group-randomized trials, also called setting-level experiments. Version 3.0 was released in October 2011. The software, a description of the updates from the previous version, and a manual containing software documentation are available for download.

http://www.healthstats.org/rmass/
The **RMASS** program computes sample size for three-level mixed-effects linear regression models for the analysis of clustered longitudinal data. Three-level designs are used in many areas, but in particular, multicenter randomized longitudinal clinical trials in medical or health-related research. In this case, Level 1 represents measurement occasion, Level 2 represents subject, and Level 3 represents center. The model allows for random effects of the time trends at both the subject level and the center level. The sample size determinations in this program are based on the requirements for a test of treatment by time interaction(s) for designs based on either subject-level- or cluster-level randomization. The approach is general with respect to sampling proportions and number of groups, and it allows for differential attrition rates over time.

http://epoc.cochrane.org/
The **Cochrane Effective Practice and Organization of Care (EPOC) Group** is a review group of The Cochrane Collaboration—an international network of people helping health care providers, policymakers, patients, their advocates, and carers make well-informed decisions about human health care by preparing and publishing systematic reviews (SRs). The research focus of the EPOC Group is interventions designed to improve the delivery, practice, and organization of health care services. The EPOC editorial base is located in Ottawa, Canada with satellite centers in Norway, Australia, and England.

▪ ACKNOWLEDGMENTS

Support for this chapter was provided by the following grant funded by the National Institute of Mental Health and the National Institute on Drug Abuse: P30 MH074678, DA019984, MH040859, DA024370, P30 MH068579, MH080916 and P30 DA027828.

▪ REFERENCES

1. Proctor E, Landsverk J, Aarons G, Chambers D, Glisson C, Mittman B. Implementation research in mental health services: an emerging science with conceptual, methodological, and training challenges. *Administration and Policy in Mental Health and Mental Health Services Research.* 2009;36(1):24–34.
2. National Research Council and Institute of Medicine. Division of Behavioral and Social Sciences and Education, Board on Children, Youth, and Families, Committee on the Prevention of Mental Disorders and Substance Abuse Among Children, Youth, and Young Adults: Research Advances and Promising Interventions, O'Connell ME, Boat T, and Warner KE, eds. *Preventing mental, emotional, and behavioral disorders among young people: Progress and possibilities.* Washington, DC: National Academy Press; 2009.
3. Aarons GA, Hurlburt M, Horwitz SM. Advancing a conceptual model of evidence-based practice implementation in public service sectors. *Administration and Policy in Mental Health and Mental Health Services Research.* 2011;38(1):4–23.
4. Wang W, Saldana L, Brown CH, Chamberlain P. Factors that influenced county system leaders to implement an evidence-based program: a baseline survey within a randomized controlled trial. *Implementation Science.* 2010;5(1):72.
5. Brown CH, Ten Have TR, Jo B, et al. Adaptive designs for randomized trials in public health. *Annual Review of Public Health.* 2009;30:1–25.
6. Poduska J, Kellam S, Brown C, et al. Study protocol for a group randomized controlled trial of a classroom-based intervention aimed at preventing early risk factors for drug abuse: integrating effectiveness and implementation research. *Implementation Science.* 2009;4(1):56.
7. Zerhouni E. The NIH roadmap. *Science (Washington).* 2003;302(5642):63–72.
8. Zerhouni E. Translational and clinical science—time for a new vision. *New England Journal of Medicine.* 2005;353(15):1621.
9. Culliton B. Extracting knowledge from science: a conversation with Elias Zerhouni. *Health Affairs.* 2006;25(3):w94.
10. Westfall J, Mold J, Fagnan L. Practice-based research— "Blue Highways" on the NIH roadmap. *JAMA.* 2007;297(4):403.

11. Friedman LM, Furberg C, DeMets DL. *Fundamentals of clinical trials.* 3rd ed. New York: Springer; 1998.

12. Torgerson D, Torgerson C. *Designing and running randomised trials in health and the social sciences.* Basingstoke, UK: Palgrave Macmillan; 2008.

13. Brown CH, Wang W, Kellam SG, et al. Methods for testing theory and evaluating impact in randomized field trials: intent-to-treat analyses for integrating the perspectives of person, place, and time. *Drug and Alcohol Dependence.* Jun 2008;95(Suppl 1):S74–S104; Supplementary data associated with this article can be found, in the online version, at doi:110.1016/j.drugalcdep.2008.1001.1005

14. Flay B. Efficacy and effectiveness trials (and other phases of research) in the development of health promotion programs. *Preventive Medicine.* 1986;15(5):451–474.

15. Glasgow R, Magid D, Beck A, Ritzwoller D, Estabrooks P. Practical clinical trials for translating research to practice: design and measurement recommendations. *Medical Care.* 2005;43(6):551.

16. Brown CH, Wyman PA, Guo J, Peña J. Dynamic wait-listed designs for randomized trials: new designs for prevention of youth suicide. *Clinical Trials.* 2006;3(3): 259–271.

17. Berwick D. The science of improvement. *JAMA.* 2008;299(10):1182.

18. Pawson R, Tilley N. *Realistic evaluation.* London: Sage Publications Ltd; 1997.

19. Landsverk J, Brown C, Rolls Reutz J, Palinkas L, Horwitz S. Design elements in implementation research: a structured review of child welfare and child mental health studies. *Administration and Policy in Mental Health and Mental Health Services Research.* 2011:1–10.

20. Evensen A, Sanson-Fisher R, D'Este C, Fitzgerald M. Trends in publications regarding evidence-practice gaps: a literature review. *Implementation Science.* 2010 2010;5(1):11.

21. Brown CH, Kellam SG, Kaupert S, et al. Partnerships for the design, conduct, and analysis of effectiveness, and implementation research: experiences of the prevention science and methodology group. *Administration and Policy in Mental Health.* Accepted for publication.

22. Chamberlain P, Marsenich L, Sosna T, Roberts R, Jones H, Price JM. Three collaborative models for scaling up evidence-based practices. *Admininstration and Policy in Mental Health and Mental Health Services Research.* Published online April 12, 2011. DOI: 10.1007/s10488-011-0349-9.

23. Brown CH, Berndt D, Brinales JM, Zong X, Bhagwat D. Evaluating the evidence of effectiveness for preventive interventions: using a registry system to influence policy through science. *Addictive Behaviors.* Nov–Dec 2000;25(6):955–964.

24. Brown CH, Wyman PA, Brinales JM, Gibbons RD. The role of randomized trials in testing interventions for the prevention of youth suicide. *International Review of Psychiatry.* Dec 2007;19(6):617–631.

25. Chamberlain P, Saldana L, Brown CH, Leve LD. Implementation of multidimensional treatment foster care in California: A randomized trial of an evidence-based practice. In: Roberts-DeGennaro M, Fogel S, eds. *Empirically supported interventions for community and organizational change.* Chicago: Lyceum Books, Inc.; 2010.

26. Chamberlain P, Brown C, Saldana L, et al. Engaging and recruiting counties in an experiment on implementing evidence-based practice in California. *Administration and Policy in Mental Health and Mental Health Research.* 2008;35:250–260.

27. Marcus SM, Gibbons RD. Estimating the efficacy of receiving treatment in randomized clinical trials with noncompliance. *Health Services & Outcomes Research Methodology.* Dec 2001;2(3-4):247-257.
28. Stuart EA, Green KM. Using full matching to estimate causal effects in nonexperimental studies: examining the relationship between adolescent marijuana use and adult outcomes. *Developmental Psychology.* Mar 2008;44(2):395-406.
29. Shortell SM. Increasing value: a research agenda for addressing the managerial and organizational challenges facing health care delivery in the United States. *Medical Care Research and Review.* 2004;61:12-30S.
30. Wholey J, Hatry H, Newcomer K. *Handbook of practical program evaluation.* San Francisco: Jossey-Bass Inc. Pub; 2004.
31. Reichardt C, Mark M. Quasi-experimentation. In: Wholey J, Hatry H, Newcomer K., eds. *Handbook of practical program evaluation.* San Francisco: Jossey-Bass Inc. Pub; 2004:126-149.
32. Pierre R. Using randomized experiments. In: Wholey J, Hatry H, Newcomer K., eds. *Handbook of practical program evaluation.* San Francisco: Jossey-Bass Inc. Pub; 2004:150-175.
33. Barrett-Connor E, Grady D, Stefanick M. The rise and fall of menopausal hormone therapy. *Annual Review of Public Health.* 2004;26:115-140.
34. Concato J, Shah N, Horwitz R. Randomized, controlled trials, observational studies, and the hierarchy of research designs. *The New England Journal of Medicine.* 2000; 342(25):1887.
35. Cook T, Shadish W, Wong V. Three conditions under which experiments and observational studies produce comparable causal estimates: new findings from within-study comparisons. *Journal of Policy Analysis and Management.* 2008;27(4):724-750.
36. West SG, Duan N, Pequegnat W, et al. Alternatives to the randomized controlled trial. *American Journal of Public Health.* August 1, 2008;98(8):1359-1366.
37. Brown CA, Lilford RJ. The stepped wedge trial design: a systematic review. *BMC Medical Research Methodology.* 2006;6:54.
38. Bonell CP, Hargreaves J, Cousens S, et al. Alternatives to randomisation in the evaluation of public health interventions: design challenges and solutions. *Journal of Epidemiology and Community Health.* 2009.
39. Brown CH, Liao J. Principles for designing randomized preventive trials in mental health: an emerging developmental epidemiology paradigm. *American Journal of Community Psychology.* 1999;27(5):673-710.
40. Raudenbush SW, Liu X. Statistical power and optimal design for multisite randomized trials. *Psychological Methods.* Jun 2000;5(2):199-213.
41. Bhaumik DK, Roy A, Aryal S, et al. Sample size determination for studies with repeated continuous outcomes. *Psychiatric Annals.* 2008;38(12):765-771.
42. Brown CH, Kellam SG, Ialongo N, Poduska J, Ford C. Prevention of aggressive behavior through middle school using a first grade classroom-based intervention. In: Tsuang MT, Lyons MJ, Stone WS, eds. *Towards prevention and early intervention of major mental and substance abuse disorders.* Arlington, VA: American Psychiatric Publishing, Inc.; 2007:347-370.
43. Kellam SG, Brown CH, Poduska JM, et al. Effects of a universal classroom behavior management program in first and second grades on young adult behavioral, psychiatric, and social outcomes. *Drug and Alcohol Dependence.* Jun 2008;95(Suppl 1):S5-S28;

supplementary data associated with this article can be found in the online version, at doi:10.1016/j.drugalcdep.2008.1001.1004.

44. Jones B, Nachtsheim CJ. Split-plot design: what, why, and how. *Journal of Quality Technology.* 2009;41(4):340–361.

45. Chambers DA. Advancing the science of implementation: a workshop summary. *Administration and Policy in Mental Health and Mental Health Services Research.* 2008;35(1–2):3–10.

46. Kraemer HC, Mintz J, Noda A, Tinklenberg J, Yesavage JA. Caution regarding the use of pilot studies to guide power calculations for study proposals. *Archives of General Psychiatry.* May 2006;63(5):484–489.

47. Kellam SG, Ling X, Merisca R, Brown CH, Ialongo N. The effect of the level of aggression in the first grade classroom on the course and malleability of aggressive behavior into middle school. *Development & Psychopathology.* Spr 1998;10(2):165–185.

48. Frangakis CE, Rubin DB. Principal stratification in causal inference. *Biometrics.* 2002;58:21–29.

49. Greenland S, Lanes S, Jara M. Estimating effects from randomized trials with discontinuations: the need for intent to treat design and G-estimation. *Clinical Trials.* 2007;5:5–13.

50. Robins JM, Greenland S. Identifiability and exchangeability for direct and indirect effects. *Epidemiology.* 1992;3:143–155.

51. Barnard J, Frangakis CE, Hill JL, Rubin DB. Principal stratification approach to broken randomized experiments: a case study of school choice vouchers in New York City/Comment/Rejoinder. *Journal of the American Statistical Association.* 2003; 98(462):299–323.

52. Frangakis C, Brookmeyer R, Varadhan R, Safaiean M. *Methodology for evaluating a partially controlled longitudinal treatment using principal stratification, with application to a needle exchange program.* Baltimore, MD: 2002. NEP-06–02.

53. Frangakis CE, Brookmeyer RS, Varadham R, Safaeian M, Vlahov D, Strathdee SA. Methodology for evaluating a partially controlled longitudinal treatment using principal stratification, with application to a needle exchange program. *Journal of the American Statistical Association.* 2004;99(465):239–250.

54. Barnard J, Frangakis CE, Hill J, Rubin DB. School choice in NY city: A Bayesian analysis of an imperfect randomized experiment. In: Gatsonis C, Kass RE, Carlin BP, et al., eds. *Case studies in Bayesian statistics.* Vol V. New York: Springer; 2002:3–98.

55. Muthén BO, Jo B, Brown CH. Comment on the Barnard, Frangakis, Hill & Rubin article, Principal stratification approach to broken randomized experiments: a case study of school choice vouchers in New York City. *Journal of the American Statistical Association.* Jun 2003;98(462):311–314.

56. Frangakis CE, Rubin DB, Frangakis CE, Rubin DB. Principal stratification in causal inference. *Biometrics.* Mar 2002;58(1):21–29.

57. Frangakis CE, Varadham R. Systematizing the evaluation of partially controlled studies using principal stratification: from theory to practice *Statistica Sinica.* 2004;14:945–947.

58. Jin H, Rubin DB. Principal stratification for causal inference with extended partial compliance. *Journal of the American Statistical Association.* 2008;103(481):101–111.

59. Rubin DB. Direct and indirect causal effects via potential outcomes. *Scandinavian Journal of Statistics.* Jun 2004;31(2):161–170.

60. Angrist JD, Imbens GW, Rubin DB. Identification of causal effects using instrumental variables. *Journal of the American Statistical Association.* 1996;91(434):444–455.
61. Asparouhov T, Muthén BO. Multilevel mixture models. In: Hancock GR, Samuelsen KM, eds. *Advances in latent variable mixture models.* Charlotte, NC: Information Age Publishing, Inc.; 2008:27–51.
62. Muthen B. Latent variable mixture modeling. In: Marcoulides GA, Schumacker RE, eds. *Advanced structural equational modelling: New developments and techniques.* Mahwah, NJ: Lawrence Earlbaum Associates; 2001:1–33.
63. Muthen B. Second-generation structural equation modeling with a combination of categorical and continuous latent variables. In: Collins LM, Sayer AG, eds. *New methods for the analysis of change, Decade of behavior.* Washington, DC: American Psychological Association, 2001:291–322.
64. Muthen B. Statistical and substantive checking in growth mixture modeling. *Psychological Methods.* 2003;8(3):369–377.
65. Muthen B. Latent variable modeling of longitudinal and multilevel data. *Soiological Methodology.* 2005;27:453–480.
66. Muthén B. Latent variable modeling of longitudinal and multilevel data. *Sociological Methodology.* 1997;27:453–480.
67. Muthén B, Brown CH. Estimating drug effects in the presence of placebo response: causal inference using growth mixture modeling. *Statistics in Medicine.* 2009;28(27): 3363–3395.
68. Brown CH, Indurkhya A, Kellam SG. Power calculations for data missing by design with application to a follow-up study of exposure and attention. *Journal of the American Statistical Association.* 2000;95:383–395.
69. Guo J. *Extending the Principal Stratification Methods to Multi-Level Randomized Trials* [Doctoral Dissertation]. Tampa, FL: Epidemiology and Biostatistics, University of South Florida; 2010.
70. Creswell JW, Plano Clark VL. *Designing and conducting mixed methods research.* Thousand Oaks, CA: Sage Publications, Inc; 2007.
71. Teddlie C, Tashakkori A. Major issues and controversies in the use of mixed methods in the social and behavioral sciences. In: Tashakkori A, Teddlie C, eds. *Handbook of mixed methods in the social and behavioral sciences.* Thousand Oaks, CA: Sage; 2003:3–50.
72. Palinkas L, Aarons G, Horwitz S, Chamberlain P, Hurlburt M, Landsverk J. Mixed method designs in implementation research. *Administration and Policy in Mental Health and Mental Health Services Research.* 2011;38(1):44–53.
73. Whitley R, Gingerich S, Lutz W, Mueser K. Implementing the illness management and recovery program in community mental health settings: facilitators and barriers. *Psychiatric Services.* 2009;60(2):202.
74. Marshall T, Rapp C, Becker D, Bond G. Key factors for implementing supported employment. *Psychiatric Services.* 2008;59(8):886.
75. Marty D, Rapp C, McHugo G, Whitley R. Factors influencing consumer outcome monitoring in implementation of evidence-based practices: results from the National EBP Implementation Project. *Administration and Policy in Mental Health and Mental Health Services Research.* 2008;35(3):204–211.
76. Rapp C, Etzel-Wise D, Marty D, et al. Barriers to evidence-based practice implementation: results of a qualitative study. *Community Mental Health Journal.* 2009;46(2): 112–118.

77. Trochim WMK. An introduction to concept mapping for planning and evaluation. *Evaluation and Program Planning.* 1989;12(1):1–16.
78. Patton MQ. *Qualitative evaluation and research methods (3rd Ed).* Thousand Oaks, CA: Sage; 2002.
79. Chambers D. Advancing the science of implementation: a workshop summary. *Administration and Policy in Mental Health and Mental Health Services Research.* 2008;35(1):3–10.
80. Henke R, Chou A, Chanin J, Zides A, Scholle S. Physician attitude toward depression care interventions: implications for implementation of quality improvement initiatives. *Implementation Science.* 2008;3(1):40.
81. Sharkey S, Maciver S, Cameron D, Reynolds W, Lauder W, Veitch T. An exploration of factors affecting the implementation of a randomized controlled trial of a transitional discharge model for people with a serious mental illness. *Journal of Psychiatric and Mental Health Nursing.* 2005;12(1):51–56.
82. Slade M, Gask L, Leese M, et al. Failure to improve appropriateness of referrals to adult community mental health services—lessons from a multi-site cluster randomized controlled trial. *Family Practice.* 2008;25(3):181.
83. Bernard H, ed. *Research methods in anthropology.* 3rd ed. Newbury Park, CA: Sage; 1994.
84. Sofaer S. Qualitative methods: what are they and why use them? *Health Services Research.* 1999;34(5):1101–1118.
85. Palinkas L, Aarons G, Chorpita B, Hoagwood K, Landsverk J, Weisz J. Cultural exchange and the implementation of evidence-based practices. *Research on Social Work Practice.* 2009;19(5):602.
86. Aarons GA, Palinkas LA. Implementation of evidence-based practice in child welfare: service provider perspectives. *Administration and Policy in Mental Health.* Jul 2007;34(4):411–419.
87. Palinkas L, Aarons G. A view from the top: executive and management challenges in a statewide implementation of an evidence-based practice to reduce child neglect. *International Journal of Child Health and Human Development.* 2009;2(1):47–55.
88. Forrester JW. System dynamics and the lessons of 35 years. In: De Greene KB, ed. *The systemic basis of policy making in the 1990s.* Cambridge, MA: MIT Press, 1991:199–240.
89. George Warren Brown School of Social Work Social System Design Lab. "What is System Dynamics?". Accessed 2/3/2011. http://gwbweb.wustl.edu/research/systemdynamics/Pages/SystemDynamicsDefinition.aspx
90. Proctor EK, Knudsen KJ, Fedoravicius N, Hovmand P, Rosen A, Perron B. Implementation of evidence-based practice in community behavioral health: agency director perspectives. *Administration and Policy in Mental Health and Mental Health Services Research.* 2007;34(5):479–488.
91. Hovmand PS, Gillespie DF. Implementation of evidence-based practice and organizational performance. *The Journal of Behavioral Health Services and Research.* 2010;37(1):79–94.
92. Epstein JM, Axtell R. *Growing artificial societies.* Cambridge, MA: MIT Press; 1996.
93. Epstein JM. *Nonlinear dynamics, mathematical biology, and social science.* Boston, MA: Addison-Wesley; 1997.
94. Miller JH, Page SE. *Complex adaptive systems: An introduction to computational models of social life.* Princeton, NJ: Princeton University Press; 2007.

95. Heath B, Hill R, Ciarallo F. A survey of agent-based modeling practices (January 1998 to July 2008). *Journal of Artificial Societies and Social Simulation.* Oct 2009;12(4):A143–A177.

96. Sun R, ed. *Cognitive and multi-agent interaction: From cognitive modeling to social simulation.* New York: Cambridge University Press; 2006.

97. Epstein JM. *Generative social science: Studies in agent-based computational modeling.* Princeton, NJ: Princeton University Press; 2007.

98. Epstein JM. Why model? *Journal of Artificial Societies and Social Simulation.* 2008;11(4):12.

99. Anderies JM, ed. *The transition from local to global dynamics: A proposed framework for agent-based thinking in social-ecological systems.* Northhampton, MA: Edward Elgar; 2002.

100. Alam SJ, Meyer R, Ziervogel G, Moss S. The impact of HIV/AIDS in the context of socioeconomic stressors: an evidence-driven approach. *Journal of Artificial Societies and Social Simulation.* 2007;10(4):7.

101. Grimm V, Revilla E, Berger U, et al. Pattern-oriented modeling of agent-based complex systems: lessons from ecology. *Science.* Nov 11 2005;310(5750): 987–991.

102. Wang C-P, Brown CH, Bandeen-Roche K, Jaccard J. Residual diagnostics for growth mixture models: examining the impact of a preventive intervention on multiple trajectories of aggressive behavior. *Journal of the American Statistical Association.* 2005;100(471):1054–1076.

103. Borgatti SP, Everett MG, Freeman LC. *Ucinet for Windows: Software for social network analysis.* Lexington, KY: Analytic Technologies; 2005.

104. Monge PR, Contractor NS. *Theories of communication networks.* New York: Oxford University Press; 2002.

105. Scott J. *Network analysis: A handbook.* 2nd ed. Newbury Park, CA: Sage; 2000.

106. Wasserman S, Faust K. *Social networks analysis: Methods and applications.* Cambridge, UK: Cambridge University Press; 1994.

107. Valente TW, Mouttapa M, Gallaher M. Social network analysis for understanding substance abuse: a transdisciplinary perspective. *Substance Use & Misuse.* 2004; 39:1685–1712.

108. Burt R. Social contagion and innovation: cohesion versus structural equivalence. *American Journal of Sociology.* 1987;92:1287–1335.

109. Marsden MG, Treacy S, Stewart D. Reduced injection risk and sexual risk behaviours after drug misuse treatment: results from the National Treatment Outcome Research Study. *AIDS Care.* 2002;14(1):77–93.

110. Valente TW. *Network models of the diffusion of innovations.* Cresskill, NJ: Hampton Press; 1995.

111. Valente TW. *Models and methods for innovation diffusion.* Cambridge, UK: Cambridge University Press; 2005.

112. Knoke D, Kuklinski JH. *Network analysis.* Thousand Oaks, CA: Sage; 1982.

113. Kwait J, Valente TW, Celentano DD. Interorganizational relationships among HIV/AIDS service organizations in Baltimore: a network analysis. *Journal of Urban Health.* 2001;78:468–487.

114. Brass DJ, Galaskiewicz J, Greve HR, Tsui W. Taking stock of networks and organizations: a multilevel perspective. *Academy of Management Journal.* 2004;47: 795–799.

115. Valente TW, Chou CP, Pentz MA. Community coalition networks as systems: effects of network change on adoption of evidence-based prevention. *American Journal of Public Health.* 2007;97:880–886.
116. Valente TW, Fosados R. Diffusion of innovations and network segmentation: the part played by people in the promotion of health. *Journal of Sexually Transmitted Diseases.* 2006;33:S23–S31.
117. Valente TW, Fujimoto K, Palmer P, et al. A network assessment of community-based participatory research: linking communities and universities to reduce cancer disparities. *American Journal of Public Health.* 2010;100(7):1319–1325.
118. Lomas J, Enkin M, Anderson GM, Hanna WJ, Vayda E, Singer J. Opinion leaders vs. audit feedback to implement practice guidelines: delivery after previous cesarean section. *Journal of American Medical Association.* 1991;265:2202–2207.
119. Valente TW, Pumpuang P. Identifying opinion leaders to promote behavior change. *Health Education & Behavior.* 2007;34:881–896.
120. Valente TW, Hoffman BR, Ritt-Olson A, Lichtman K, Johnson CA. The effects of a social network method for group assignment strategies on peer led tobacco prevention programs in schools. *American Journal of Public Health.* 2003;93:1837–1843.
121. Buller D, Buller MK, Larkey L, et al. Implementing a 5-a-day peer health educator program for public sector labor and trades employees. *Health Education & Behavior.* 2000;27(2):232–240.
122. Valente TW, Sussman S, Unger J, Ritt-Olson A, Okamoto J, Stacy A. Peer acceleration: effects of a network tailored substance abuse prevention program among high risk adolescents. *Addiction.* 2007;102:1804–1815.
123. Kossisakoff A, Sweet WN. *Systems engineering principles and practice.* Hoboken, NJ: John Wiley & Sons Inc.; 2003.
124. Czaja SJ, Nair SN. Human factors engineering and systems design. In: Salvendy G, ed. *Handbook of human factors and ergonomics.* 3rd ed. Hoboken, NJ: John Wiley & Sons Inc; 2006:32–49.
125. Schulz R, Belle SH, Czaja SJ, Gitlin LN, Wisniewski SR, Ory MG. Introduction to the special section on Resources for Enhancing Alzheimer's Caregiver Health (REACH). *Psychology and Aging.* 2003;18(3):357–360.
126. Saaty TL. The Analytic Hierarchy Process in conflict management. *International Journal of Conflict Management.* 1990;1(1):47–68.
127. Czaja SJ, Schulz R, Lee CC, Belle SH. A methodology for describing and decomposing complex psychosocial and behavioral interventions. *Psychology and Aging.* 2003;18(3):385–395.
128. Rabiner LR. A tutorial on hidden Markov models and selected applications in speech recognition. *Proceedings of the IEEE.* 1989;77(2):257–286.
129. Deerwester S, Dumais ST, Furnas GW, Landauer TK, Harshman R. Indexing by latent semantic analysis. *Journal of the American Society for Information Science.* 1990;41(6):391–407.
130. Hofmann T. Probabilistic latent semantic indexing. *SIGIR '99: Proceedings of the 22nd annual international ACM SIGIR conference on research and development in information retrieval.* Berkeley, CA: ACM; 1999:50–57.
131. Li T, Zhu S, Ogihara M. Hierarchical document classification using automatically generated hierarchy. *Journal of Intelligent Information Systems.* 2007;29(2):211–230.
132. Li T, Zhu S, Ogihara M. Text categorization via generalized discriminant analysis. *Information Processing & Management.* 2008;44(5):1684–1697.

133. Frazier AL, Colditz GA, Fuchs CS, Kuntz KM. Cost-effectiveness of screening for colorectal cancer in the general population. *JAMA.* 2000;284(15):1954.
134. Gaspoz JM, Coxson PG, Goldman PA, et al. Cost effectiveness of aspirin, clopidogrel, or both for secondary prevention of coronary heart disease. *New England Journal of Medicine.* 2002;346(23):1800.
135. Goldhaber-Fiebert JD, Stout NK, Salomon JA, Kuntz KM, Goldie SJ. Cost-effectiveness of cervical cancer screening with human papillomavirus DNA testing and HPV-16, 18 vaccination. *Journal of the National Cancer Institute.* 2008; 100(5):308.
136. CDC Diabetes Cost-effectiveness Group. Cost-effectiveness of intensive glycemic control, intensified hypertension control, and serum cholesterol level reduction for type 2 diabetes. *JAMA.* 2002;287(19):2542–2551.
137. Sanders GD, Bayoumi AM, Sundaram V, et al. Cost-effectiveness of screening for HIV in the era of highly active antiretroviral therapy. *New England Journal of Medicine.* 2005;352(6):570.
138. Tosteson ANA, Stout NK, Fryback DG, et al. Cost-effectiveness of digital mammography breast cancer screening. *Annals of Internal Medicine.* 2008;148(1):1.
139. Ruiz MS. *No time to lose: Getting more from HIV prevention.* Washington, DC: National Academies Press; 2001.
140. Gold MR, Siegel JE, Russell LB, Weinstein MC, eds. *Cost-effectiveness in health and medicine.* New York: Oxford University Press; 1996.
141. Goldhaber-Fiebert JD, Snowden LR, Wulczyn F, Landsverk J, Horwitz SM. Economic evaluation research in the context of child welfare policy: a structured literature review and recommendations. *Child Abuse and Neglect.* 2011;35(9): 722–740.
142. Goldhaber-Fiebert, JD. "Evaluating Child Welfare Policies with Decision-analytic Simulation Models." Paper presented at the 4th Annual NIH Conference on the Science of Dissemination and Implementation: Policy and Practice, Bethesda, Maryland, March 21–22, 2011.
143. Price JM, Chamberlain P, Landsverk J, Reid J. KEEP foster parent training intervention: model description and effectiveness. *Child & Family Social Work.* 2009;14(2):233–242.
144. Price J, Chamberlain P, Landsverk J, Reid J, Leve L, Laurent H. Effects of a foster parent training intervention on placement changes of children in foster care. *Child Maltreatment.* 2008;13(1):64.
145. Chamberlain P, Price J, Reid J, Landsverk J. Cascading implementation of a foster and kinship parent intervention. *Child Welfare.* 2008;87(5):27.
146. Larzelere RE, Daly DL, Davis JL, Chmelka MB, Handwerk ML. Outcome evaluation of Girls and Boys Town's Family Home Program. *Education & Treatment of Children.* 2004;27(2):130–150.
147. Dodge KA, Sherrill MR. Deviant peer group effects in youth mental health interventions. In: Dodge K, Dishion T, Lansford J, eds. *Deviant peer influences in programs for youth.* New York: Guilford Press; 2006:97–121.
148. Ryan J, Marshall J, Herz D, Hernandez P. Juvenile delinquency in child welfare: investigating group home effects. *Children and Youth Services Review.* 2008;30(9): 1088–1099.
149. Wulczyn F, Orlebeke B, Melamid E. Measuring contract agency performance with administrative data. *Child Welfare.* 2000 Sep–Oct 2000;79(5):457–474.

150. Chamberlain P, Leve L, DeGarmo D. Multidimensional treatment foster care for girls in the juvenile justice system: 2-year follow-up of a randomized clinical trial. *Journal of Consulting and Clinical Psychology.* 2007;75(1):187.

151. Eddy J, Bridges Whaley R, Chamberlain P. The prevention of violent behavior by chronic and serious male juvenile offenders. *Journal of Emotional and Behavioral Disorders.* 2004;12(1):2.

152. U.S. Department of Education, Office of Special Educational Research and Improvement, Office of Reform Assistance and Dissemination. *Safe, Disciplined, and Drug-Free Schools Programs.* Washington, DC: 2001.

153. U.S. Department of Health and Human Services, ed. *Youth Violence: A Report of the Surgeon General.* Rockville, MD: U.S. Department of Health and Human Services, Centers for Disease Control and Prevention, National Center for Injury Prevention and Control; Substance Abuse and Mental Health Services Administration, Center for Mental Health Services; and National Institutes of Health, National Institute of Mental Health; 2001.

154. U.S. Department of Health and Human Services, ed. *Mental Health: A Report of the Surgeon General.* Rockville, MD: U.S. Department of Health and Human Services, Substance Abuse and Mental Health Services Administration, Center for Mental Health Services, National Institutes of Health, National Institute of Mental Health; 1999.

155. Aos S, Phipps P, Barnoski R, Leib R, eds. *The comparative costs and benefits of programs to reduce crime, 4.0.* Olympia, WA: Washington State Institute for Public Policy; 1999.

156. Rogers E. *Diffusion of innovations.* New York: Free Press; 1995.

157. Sosna T, Marsenich L. *Community Development Team Model: Supporting the model adherent implementation of programs and practices.* Sacramento, CA: California Institute for Mental Health; 2006.

158. Kalbfleisch JD, Prentice RL. *The statistical analysis of failure time data.* 2nd ed. New York: Wiley; 2002.

159. Liang K-Y, Zeger SL. Longitudinal data analysis using generalized estimating equations. *Biometrika.* 1986;73(1):13–22.

160. Zeger SL, Liang KY, Albert PS. Models for longitudinal data: a generalized estimating equation approach. [erratum appears in *Biometrics* 1989 Mar;45(1):347]. *Biometrics.* Dec 1988;44(4):1049–1060.

161. Pulver AE, Liang K-y, Brown C, et al. Risk factors in schizophrenia: season of birth, gender, and familial risk. *British Journal of Psychiatry.* 1992;160:65–71.

162. Chamberlain P, Brown CH. Observational measure of implementation progress: the stages of implementation completion (SIC). Submitted for publication.

163. Palinkas L, Fuentes D, Holloway I, Wu Q, Chamberlain P. Social Networks and Implementation of Evidence-Based Practices in Public Youth-Serving Systems. *Sunbelt XXX, International Network for Social Network Analysis Conference.* Vol Riva del Garda, Italy: 2010.

164. Tunis, SR., Stryer, DB., and Clancy, CM. Practical Clinical Trials Increasing the Value of Clinical Research for Decision Making in Clinical and Health Policy. *JAMA.* 2003;290(12):1624–1632.

165. Raudenbush, S.W., Spybrook, J., Congdon, R., Liu, X., Martinez, A. (2011). Optimal Design Plus Empirical Evidence (Version 3.0)

13 Measurement Issues in Dissemination and Implementation Research

■ ENOLA K. PROCTOR
AND ROSS C. BROWNSON

■ INTRODUCTION

The dissemination and implementation (D&I) of evidence-based programs and interventions are increasingly understood to be crucial to improving the public's health.[1] Yet research progress in D&I is currently hampered by underdeveloped concepts and measurement tools. Citing a critical need to create a repertoire of appropriate metrics with which to evaluate D&I research efforts,[2] the planning committee for the 2010 Third Annual NIH Conference on the Science of D&I chose a theme of "methods and measurement." This chapter addresses measurement challenges on four key fronts: measuring D&I processes, measuring outcomes of D&I, measuring stakeholder perspectives on these processes and outcomes, and measuring the incremental impact of successful D&I to public health outcomes. Chapter 5 on the economics of D&I addresses an additional measurement challenge—capturing the incremental costs of implementation.

The chapter follows the definitions of D&I offered by Rabin and colleagues[3]: dissemination is an active approach of spreading evidence-based interventions to target audiences via determined channels using planned strategies. Implementation is the process of putting to use, or integrating, evidence-based interventions within a specific setting. The language of D&I is highly varied, as these processes also may be described as diffusion or translation.[3]

The constructs for measurement derive from conceptual models of D&I. The framework of D&I reflected in Figure 13–1 makes a number of key distinctions that carry implications for conceptualizing and measuring implementation processes. First, the model distinguishes between the evidence-based prevention program, treatment, or policy being introduced and the *dissemination strategies* for spreading information about them and *implementation strategies* for putting those programs into place in usual settings of prevention or care. Second, these implementation strategies are different from their *outcomes,* which in turn need to be distinguished according to their several types. *Dissemination and implementation outcomes* serve as intermediate outcomes, or the proximal effects that are presumed to contribute to more distal outcomes, such as changes in service systems, in consumer health, behavior change, and larger population health. Service system outcomes reflect the six quality improvement aims set out in the Crossing the Quality Chasm reports:

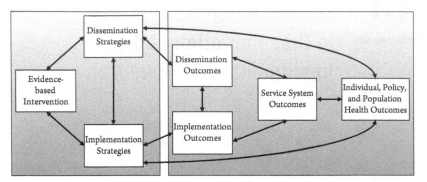

Figure 13–1. A framework for dissemination and implementation.

the extent to which services are safe, effective, patient centered, timely, efficient, and equitable.[4,5] D&I outcomes along with service system outcomes are viewed as contributing to individual and population health outcomes.[6]

The objectives of this chapter are to advance the concept of "dissemination and implementation outcomes" distinct from service system and health outcomes. The chapter proposes several concepts that comprise D&I outcomes and discusses challenges and opportunities in their measurement. Conceptualizing and measuring D&I outcomes will advance understanding of D&I processes and their empirical study.

The current literature reflects a wide array of terms that are used when discussing D&I processes, terms that are often used inconsistently. Moreover, when these constructs have been studied, they are measured in different ways—ranging from qualitative, quantitative survey, and record archival.[7,8] but often without any reporting of their measurement properties or rigor. Grimshaw et al.[9] report that meta-analyses of the effectiveness of implementation strategies has been thwarted by lack of detailed information about outcomes, use of widely varying constructs, reliance on dichotomous rather than continuous measures, and unit of analysis errors.[7] Clearly the progress of D&I science requires the development of reliable and valid measures of outcomes. Reliable and valid measures of D&I outcomes will enable empirical testing of the success of efforts to disseminate and implement new interventions, and pave the way for comparative effectiveness research on D&I strategies.

■ MEASURING DISSEMINATION AND IMPLEMENTATION STRATEGIES

Fortunately for our nation's public health, basic, clinical, and population research has generated a growing supply of evidence-based interventions, programs, and services. Recognizing their heterogeneity across such fields as obesity, cancer, violence control, substance abuse, and mental health, this chapter will refer to these collectively as evidence-based interventions (EBIs). Unfortunately, knowledge of how to effectively disseminate and implement these EBIs has not kept pace. In other words, our supply of the "what" (to be implemented) significantly outstrips our supply of the "how" (evidence-based D&I strategies). This evidence on how an intervention can be "scaled up" and the contextual conditions for implementation has been described as Type 3 evidence (which builds on Type 1 etiologic evidence and Type 2 intervention effectiveness evidence).[10,11] As noted in Chapter 15, studies to date have tended to overemphasize internal validity (e.g., well-controlled efficacy trials) while giving sparse attention to external validity (e.g., the translation of science to the various circumstances of practice).[12,13] The D&I evidence that can be found is largely descriptive, often reflecting observations of naturalistic spread or change in usual care. Failure to deliver effective services, programs, and policies has been attributed largely to our lack of knowing how to best implement and sustain change.[14] The NIH Program Announcement for Dissemination and Implementation research calls for better understanding of the "…mechanisms and approaches to package and convey the evidence-based information necessary to improve public health and clinical care services…similarly with respect to implementation strategies:…"[15(pg6)]

D&I Strategies: Definition and Measurement Challenges

Building on definitions in Chapter 2 of this book and following the definitions provided by the National Institutes of Health Program Announcement on Dissemination and Implementation Research, the chapter uses the term *dissemination strategy* to refer to "the targeted distribution of information and intervention materials to a specific public health or clinical practice audience." The term *implementation strategy* refers to the systematic intervention processes undertaken to adopt and integrate evidence-based health interventions; impact organizational structure, climate, and culture; and change practice patterns within specific settings, thus enabling the implementation of effective clinical interventions. This definition is consistent with the use of the term *implementation strategies* in the NIH PAR-10-0380. The term *D&I processes* is more inclusive, comprising (1) implementation strategies, (2) the naturally unfolding events that result in the dissemination of information or the way new prevention programs, services, and treatments are put into place, and (3) the various changes—often iterative, unintended, and nonlinear in addition to the planned and desired outcomes. The most basic level of measurement is determining a categorical or nominal definition. Mittman and colleagues wrote one of the earliest articles about strategies for implementing clinical practice guidelines.[16] However, the literature is just now providing category typologies for D&I strategies. Such work is critical in order to distinguish one strategy from another.

Dissemination strategies have been described as targeted approaches to make potential adopters aware of an innovation and encouraged to adopt it.[17] Although dissemination has often been approached in unsystematic and uncoordinated ways,[1] the literature increasingly specifies dissemination strategies for delivering information about evidence-based health programs and policies. Dissemination processes have been characterized as involving a "push–pull capacity,"[18] in that the potential adopter must be receptive (pull) concurrent with systematic "push" efforts. Dissemination strategies have been grossly distinguished as either passive or active[1] information diffusion, although the literature increasingly emphasizes the importance of active processes. Passive approaches include mass mailings, publication of information including practice guidelines, and untargeted presentations to heterogeneous groups.[18] Active dissemination strategies include hands-on technical assistance, replication guides, point-of-decision prompts for use, and mass media campaigns.[18] A commonly used active dissemination strategy is some kind of training (e.g., train the trainer, certificate training, work[19] described a staff development workshop that was developed for the dissemination of a physical education program to schools across the United States. The training workshop was described as a hands-on experience where participants were actively engaged in the lessons, physical skills, and activities that they will teach.

The AHRQ reviewed 31 published dissemination strategies in the areas of smoking cessation, healthy diet, mammography, cervical cancer screening, and cancer pain control. The poor quality of research limited the evidence about which strategies were most effective. However, it was clear that active approaches such as media campaigns are likely to be more effective than passive mailings.[20] More recently, Rabin et al.[3] systematically reviewed D&I research on community-based cancer prevention and listed D&I strategies. Although they did not distinguish dissemination strategies from implementation strategies, they list the following strategies that correspond to common understandings of dissemination strategies: conveying programs through media and interpersonal channels and Web sites; providing written materials; written reports and publications (e.g., of guidelines), holding workshops and training sessions; making phone calls and convening teleconferences; using train-the-trainer methods; and providing technical support.

Implementation strategies also have been grossly dichotomized as "top down" or "bottom up," although an increasing number of articles report listings and typologies of implementation strategies. Magnabosco[21] empirically identified 106 discrete state-level implementation activities in state public mental health systems and categorized these into five types: state infrastructure building and commitment, stakeholder relationship building and communications, financing, continuous quality management, and service delivery practices and training. Leeman and colleagues identified 14 different implementation strategies and also grouped them into five (different) categories: Increasing Coordination, Raising Awareness, Persuasion via Interpersonal Channels, Persuasion via Reinforcing Beliefs, and Increasing Behavioral Control. The EPOC effort of the Cochrane Collaboration identified four types of implementation strategies: professional, financial, organizational, and regulatory. And the Agency for Health Research and Quality (AHRQ) also distinguished five categories of implementation strategies, highly similar to those of EPOC: Provider, Information Systems, Financial, Organizational, and Patient Education and Reminder.

While these taxonomies are useful for signaling the level (policy, organizational, provider, patient) at which the strategies are directed, they often contain different elements within categories. The "professional" or "provider" strategy types often contain such specific implementation strategies as audit and feedback; educational materials, meetings, or outreach visits; and local consensus building. Licensure falls within the regulatory category.

The heterogeneity within categories likely reflects this field's early state of measurement. Most strategies are "bundled" or "packaged" approaches, likely because we don't know which specific components are effective, and in what way. Most implementation strategies are behavioral, educational, and psychosocial interventions rather than technological, making them challenging to specify and measure. Advancing the clarity of definition, classification, and operationalization of implementation processes is a high priority. Michie et al.[22] note that our current knowledge of implementation is thwarted by lack of theoretical understanding of the processes involved,[23] and declare an "imperative that there be a consensual, common language"[23] to describe strategies. As these processes become more clearly defined, their primary mechanisms of change and targeted "leverage points" should also be specified. Research on implementation strategies needs to subject specific components to more granular testing, yielding strategies that are more parsimonious, "leaner," and more cost effective. These discrete strategy components can then be used in more targeted ways. Once effective mechanisms are discerned, empirical study should be directed to testing whether components can be blended or bundled, and targeted to particular purposes and contexts.

■ DISSEMINATION AND IMPLEMENTATION OUTCOMES

Dissemination outcomes are defined here as the effects of dissemination strategies, that is, the consequences of targeted distribution of information and intervention materials to a specific public health or clinical practice audience. Similarly, implementation outcomes are defined as the effects of deliberate and purposive actions to implement new interventions. D&I outcomes are proximal reflections of their respective processes and thus serve as intermediate outcomes in larger efforts to improve the service system, and ultimately individual or population health.[7] Kottke and Isham[24] addressed the many conceptual and methodological challenges inherent in measuring population health outcomes. Distinguishing D&I effectiveness from program or intervention effectiveness is critical. When efforts to transport new programs, or the information about them, from laboratory settings to community health and mental health venues fail—as they often do—we must be able to determine if failure occurred because the intervention was ineffective in the new setting (intervention failure), or if a good intervention was conveyed and deployed incorrectly (dissemination/implementation failure). As with D&I strategies, the conceptualization and measurement of D&I outcomes is also at an early stage, leaving the field without clear directions for conceptualizing and evaluating success.

Table 13–1 shows a taxonomy of D&I outcomes. For each outcome, the table nominates a level of analysis, identifies the theoretical basis to the construct from literature, shows different terms that are used for the construct in the literature, suggests the point or stage within D&I processes at which the outcome may be most salient, and lists the types of existing measures for the construct that our search identified. The outcomes listed in Table 13–1 are only examples and probably the more obvious ones, and many other concepts will emerge from chapters in this book. Many of the D&I outcomes can be inferred or measured in terms of expressed attitudes and opinions, intentions, or reported or observed behaviors.

TABLE 13–1. *Taxonomy of Dissemination and Implementation (D&I) Outcomes*

Dissemination and Implementation Outcome	Level of Analysis	Theoretical Basis	Other Terms in the Literature	Salience by D & I Stage	Example Method of Measurement
Acceptability	Individual	Diffusion theory: complexity and relative advantage	Satisfaction with the innovation; System readiness	Early for adoption; Ongoing for penetration; Late for sustainability	Survey; Key informant interviews; Administrative data
Reach	Individual	RE-AIM	Participation	Early	Surveys; Administrative data
Adoption	Individual; Organization; Policy	Diffusion theory: trialability, observability; RE-AIM	Uptake; Utilization; Intention to try; Use of the innovation; Knowledge transfer	Early to mid	Surveys; Observation; Key informant interviews; Focus groups; Administrative data
Appropriateness	Individual; Organization; Policy	Diffusion theory: compatibility	Perceived fit; Relevance; Compatibility; Suitability; Usefulness; Practicability	Early (prior to adoption)	Surveys; Key informant interviews; Focus groups
Feasibility	Individual; Organization; Policy	Diffusion theory: compatibility, trialability, observability	Actual fit or utility; Suitability; Practicability; Community readiness	Early (during adoption)	Surveys; Administrative data
Fidelity	Individual	RE-AIM: part of implementation	Delivered as intended; Adherence; Integrity; Quality of program delivery	Early to mid	Observation; Checklists; Content analyses; Self-report; Administrative data
Cost	Individual; Organization; Policy	RE-AIM; TCU Program Change Model: costs and resources	Marginal cost; Cost effectiveness; Cost benefit; Economic evaluation	Early for adoption and feasibility; Mid for penetration; Late for sustainability	Administrative data
Penetration	Organization; Policy	RE-AIM necessary for reach	Spread; Access to services; Level of utilization	Mid to late	Surveys; Case studies; Key informant interviews
Sustainability	Organization; Policy	Diffusion theory: confirmation; RE-AIM: maintenance	Maintenance; Institutionalization; Continuation; Sustained use; Standard of practice or care	Late	Surveys; Case studies; Record and policy reviews; Key informant interviews

Dissemination Outcomes

The literature on dissemination outcomes is sparse and scattered, reflecting no conceptual typology or list of dissemination outcomes and tools for their measurement. Rabin and colleagues reported that nearly half of all published reports of dissemination research in cancer fail to report any outcomes.[3] However several constructs reflecting potential outcomes are mentioned in articles that discuss dissemination approaches, the most frequent of which is *change in attitude/behavior*.[3] Other commonly referenced, desired effects (outcomes) of dissemination include *awareness, receipt, acceptance,* and *use of information*.[18] Dingfelder & Mandell's[17] definition of dissemination strategies reflects such dissemination outcomes as *awareness of an innovation* and an *inclination to use* the innovation. The RE-AIM framework's (elaborated in Chapter 16) constructs of *reach, adoption, implementation,* and *maintenance* are sometimes referenced as outcomes, although Rabin et al.[25] present them as mediators of the extent and speed of dissemination. Clearly, *reach* may reflect the breadth with which health information spreads, and thus serves as a key dissemination outcome.

Implementation Outcomes

The literature reflects at least eight conceptually distinct implementation outcomes—*acceptability, adoption, appropriateness, feasibility, fidelity, implementation cost, penetration,* and *sustainability*.[7,8] Proctor and colleagues[8] developed a taxonomy of implementation outcomes, offered conceptual definitions, and addressed their measurement challenges (Table 13–1). *Acceptability* is the perception among implementation stakeholders that a given intervention or innovation is agreeable, palatable, or satisfactory. The referent of the implementation outcome "acceptability" (or the *"what" is acceptable*) may be a specific intervention, practice, technology, or service within a particular setting of care. Acceptability should be assessed based on the stakeholder's knowledge of or direct experience with various dimensions of the intervention to be implemented, such as its content, complexity, or comfort. Acceptability may be measured from the perspective of various stakeholders, such as administrators, payers, providers, and consumers, and rated acceptability is likely to be dynamic, changing with experience. Thus, ratings of acceptability may be different when taken, for example, preimplementation and later throughout various stages of implementation.

Adoption is the intention, initial decision, or action to try or employ an innovation or evidence-based practice.[25,26] Adoption also may be referred to as "uptake." Adoption could be measured from the perspective of provider or organization. *Appropriateness* is the perceived fit, relevance, or compatibility of the innovation or evidence-based practice for a given practice setting, provider, or consumer; and/or perceived fit of the innovation to address a particular issue or problem. "Appropriateness" is conceptually similar to "acceptability," and the literature reflects overlapping and sometimes inconsistent terms when discussing these constructs. However, an evidence-based intervention may be perceived as appropriate but not acceptable, and vice versa. For example, an intervention might be considered a good fit for treating a given condition, but its features (for example, rigid protocol) may render it unacceptable to the provider. The construct "appropriateness" may capture "pushback" to implementation efforts, as when providers feel a new program is a "stretch" from the mission of the health care setting or is not consistent with their skills, role, or job expectations. These perceptions may be function of the organization's culture or climate.[27]

Incremental implementation cost is the additional expense of implementing an evidence-based intervention. Chapter 5 on economic aspects of D&I provides a fuller exposition of this outcome and details the ways in which implementation costs vary. Direct measures of implementation cost are essential for studies comparing the costs of implementing alternative interventions and of various implementation strategies.

Feasibility is the extent to which a new program or policy can be successfully used or carried out within a given agency, in a particular setting, or in a certain population.[27] Typically, the concept of feasibility is invoked retrospectively as a potential explanation of an initiative's success or failure, as reflected in poor recruitment, retention, or participation rates. While feasibility is related to appropriateness, the two constructs are conceptually distinct. For example, a program may be appropriate for a service setting—in that it is compatible with the setting's mission or service mandate—but may not be feasible due to resource or training requirements. Fidelity is the most common implementation outcome, defined as the degree to which an intervention was implemented as it was prescribed in the original protocol or as it was intended by the program developers.[25,29] Fidelity is typically measured by comparing the original evidence-based intervention and the disseminated/implemented intervention in terms of (1) adherence to the program protocol, (2) dose or amount of program delivered, and (3) quality of program delivery. The literature identifies five implementation fidelity dimensions including adherence, quality of delivery, program component differentiation, exposure to the intervention, and participant responsiveness or involvement.[30,31]

Penetration is defined as the integration of a practice within a service setting and its subsystems[31] and is similar to Rabin et al.'s[25] notion of niche saturation. Stiles et al.[32] apply the concept of service penetration to service recipients (the number of eligible persons who use a service, divided by the total number of persons eligible for the service). Penetration also can be calculated in terms of the number of providers who deliver a given intervention divided by the total number of providers trained in or expected to deliver the service. From a service system perspective, the construct is also similar to "reach" in the RE-AIM framework.[33] Sustainability is the extent to which a newly implemented intervention is maintained or institutionalized within a service setting's ongoing, stable operations. The literature reflects quite varied uses of the term "sustainability."[25,34–37] Rabin et al.[25] emphasize the integration of a given program within an organization's culture through policies and practices, and distinguish three stages that determine institutionalization: (1) passage (a single event such as transition from temporary to permanent funding), (2) cycle or routine (i.e., repetitive reinforcement of the importance of the evidence-based intervention through including it into organizational or community procedures and behaviors, such as the annual budget and evaluation criteria), and (3) niche saturation (the extent to which an evidence-based intervention is integrated into all subsystems of an organization). Thus, the outcomes of "penetration" and "sustainability" may be related conceptually and empirically, in that higher penetration may contribute to long-term sustainability.

■ CONCEPTUAL AND METHODOLOGIC CHALLENGES

Conceptualizing and measuring implementation outcomes will advance understanding of implementation processes, enhance efficiency in implementation research, and pave the way for studies of the comparative effectiveness of implementation strategies. Advancing the nominal and operational measurement of D&I outcomes requires work on several fronts. First, accurate measurement of D&I outcomes requires more consistent nominal definition, including the use of consistent terminology. Studies often use different labels for what appear to be the same construct, or use one term for the outcome's label or nominal definition but a different term for operationalizing or measuring the same construct. While language inconsistency is typical in most still-developing fields, implementation research may be particularly susceptible to this problem. No single discipline is "home" to dissemination/implementation research. Studies are conducted across a broad range of disciplines, published in a scattered set of journals, and consequently, are rarely cross-referenced. The field now has only the beginnings of a common language to characterize D&I outcomes, a situation that thwarts its conceptual and empirical advancement. A taxonomy of D&I outcomes can organize the key variables and frame research questions required to advance implementation science. Their measurement and empirical test can help specify the mechanisms and causal relationships within D&I processes and advance a base of empirical evidence about successful D&I

The literature reflects a wide array of approaches for measuring implementation outcomes, ranging from qualitative, quantitative survey, and record archival.[7,8] Much measurement has been "homegrown," with virtually no work on the psychometric properties or measurement rigor. Grimshaw et al.[9] report that meta-analyses of the effectiveness of implementation strategies has been thwarted by lack of detailed information about outcomes, use of widely varying constructs, reliance on dichotomous rather than continuous measures, and unit of analysis errors.[7] Clearly the progress of D&I science requires the development of reliable and valid measures of outcomes. Reliable and valid measures of implementation outcomes will enable empirical testing of the success of efforts to implement new treatments, and pave the way for comparative effectiveness research on implementation strategies. Several key issues are highlighted below.

Level of Analysis for Outcomes

Dissemination of health information and the implementation of new preventive practices involve change at multiple levels, ranging from the individual (health consumer, provider) to the organization, to the community and in policy.[7,38] Some outcomes, such as attitude change and acceptance, may most appropriately be assessed at the individual level while others, such as spread or penetration, may be more appropriate for aggregate analysis, such as at the level of the organization. Currently, very few studies reporting D&I outcomes specify the level at which measurement was taken.

Construct Validity

Construct validity is the degree to which a measure "behaves" in a way consistent with theoretical hypotheses[39] and is predictive of some external attribute (e.g., rate of smoking). Qualitative data, reflecting language used by various stakeholders as they think and talk about D&I processes, is important for validating outcome constructs. Through in-depth interviews, stakeholders' cognitive representations and mental models of outcomes can be analyzed through such methods as cultural domain analysis (CDA).[40,41]

Criterion-Related Validity

Criterion-related validity (sometimes considered a subset of construct validity) is the degree to which a measure is predictive of some "gold standard" measure of the same attribute.[39] Assessment of criterion validity is common in many areas of medical and public health research. For example, to gauge the accuracy of self-reported smoking behavior one might compare self-reported data with biochemical measures of cotinine (a nicotine breakdown product). However, in most areas of D&I research the gold standard does not exist. Similarly, to assess accuracy of staff self-report of use of a new intervention, records might be audited for evidence of the intervention's delivery and supervisors might be queried. Currently, neither dissemination research nor implementation research adequately discusses or explores the validity of outcome measurement.

Salience of D&I Outcomes to Stakeholders

Any effort to change care involves a range of stakeholders, including the intervention developers who design and test the intervention effectiveness, policymakers who design and pay for service, administrators who shape program direction, providers and supervisors, patients/clients/consumers and their family members, and community members interested in health care. The success of efforts to implement evidence-based intervention may rest on their congruence with the preferences and priorities of those who shape, deliver, and participate in care. D&I outcomes may be differentially salient to various stakeholders, just as the salience of clinical outcomes varies across stakeholders.[42] For example, implementation cost may be most important to policymakers and program directors, feasibility may be most important to direct service providers, and fidelity may be most important to intervention developers. To ensure applicability of implementation outcomes across a range of health care settings and to maximize their external validity (described in detail in Chapter 15), all stakeholder groups and priorities should be represented in this research, as discussed below.

Salience of Implementation Outcomes by Point in the Implementation Process

Changing health care by disseminating and implementing new interventions is a process. Chamberlain has identified 10 steps for the implementation of an evidence-based intervention, Multidimensional Treatment Foster Care (MTFC), beginning with consideration of adopting MTFC and concluding when a service site meets certification criteria for delivering the intervention.[43] D&I outcomes are likely to differ in importance across phase. For example, feasibility may be most important once organizations and providers try new interventions. Later, it may be a "moot point," once the intervention—initially considered novel or unknown—has become part of normal routine. The literature suggests that studies usually capture measures of fidelity prior to, or during, initial implementation, while adoption is often assessed at 6,[44] 12,[45,46] or 18 months[47] after initial implementation. But most studies fail to specify a time frame or are inconsistent in choice of a time point in the implementation process for measuring outcomes. Research is needed to explore these issues, particularly longitudinal studies that measure multiple D&I outcomes.

Modeling Interrelationships among D&I Outcomes

The literature has only begun to address the ways in which D&I outcomes are interrelated.[7,8] Dingfelder and Mandell's model[17] positions dissemination as a contributor to successful implementation outcome. Yet dissemination outcomes are likely interrelated in dynamic and complex ways, as are implementation outcomes.[48–51] Moreover, their indicators are likely to reflect change throughout the adoption and implementation of change. For example, the perceived appropriateness, feasibility, and implementation cost associated with an intervention will likely bear upon ratings of the intervention's acceptability. Acceptability, in turn, will likely affect adoption, penetration, and sustainability. Similarly, consistent with Rogers's Diffusion of Innovations theory, the ability to adopt or adapt an innovation for local use may increase its acceptability.[52]

Important work remains to model these interrelationships, and this work will likely inform definitions and thus shape our language about D&I processes. For example, if two outcomes that we now define as distinct concepts are shown through research to always occur together, the empirical evidence would suggest that the concepts are really the same thing and should be combined. Similarly, if two of the outcomes are shown to have different empirical patterns, evidence would confirm their conceptual distinction.

Using Implementation Outcomes to Model Success

Success in D&I is probably a function of a "portfolio" of factors, including the effectiveness of the intervention itself and the skillful use of D&I strategies.[7,8] For example, implementation strategies could be employed to increase provider acceptance, improve penetration, reduce implementation costs, and achieve sustainability of the intervention being implemented. It is important to conceptually and empirically address how various implementation and dissemination outcomes contribute to success. For example, an evidence-based intervention may be highly effective, but it may be largely unknown to potential adopters; this poor dissemination outcome (low awareness) would likely undermine the likelihood of its implementation. This scenario may be modeled as follows:

$$Implementation\ success = f\ of\ effectiveness\ (= high) + awareness\ (= low)$$

As another example, a program may be only mildly acceptable to key stakeholders because it is seen as too costly to sustain. The overall potential success of implementation in this case might be modeled as follows:

$$Implementation\ success = f\ of\ effectiveness\ (= high) + acceptability\ (moderate)$$
$$cost\ (high) + sustainability\ (low)$$

In a third situation, a given intervention might be only moderately effective but highly acceptable to stakeholders because current care is poor, the intervention is inexpensive, and current training protocols ensure high penetration through providers. This intervention's potential might be modeled in the following equation:

$$Implementation\ success = f\ of\ intervention\ effectiveness\ (moderate) +$$
$$acceptability\ (high) + potential\ to\ improve$$
$$care\ (high) + penetration\ (high)$$

These examples suggest that successful change in public health and health delivery can be understood and modeled using the concepts of D&I outcomes, thereby making decisions about what to implement more explicit and transparent.

Measuring Stakeholder Perspectives

Successful D&I of evidence-based interventions depend largely on the fit of evidence-based interventions with the preferences and priorities of those who shape, deliver, and participate in care. Several groups of D&I stakeholders can be distinguished. Community members may include: (1) *health care consumers* who comprise the primary beneficiaries in the successful D&I of evidence-based health services and (2) the *whole population* in a community that benefits from dissemination of a population-level public health intervention (e.g., water fluoridation). Many dissemination efforts target health consumers directly, as in marketing campaigns designed to increase consumer demand for a particular program, drug, or service. *Families* comprise another group of D&I stakeholders, often sharing consumer desires for quality care and similarly affected by successful D&I. Service recipients and family members bring different perspectives to the evaluation of health care,[53] underscoring the importance of systematically assessing their perspectives on D&I of evidence-based health care.

Intervention developers constitute a third group of stakeholders. Many engage in D&I efforts, fueled by a desire that their interventions be used in real-world care. For example, many intervention developers (including nurse in-home visitation program developers) have launched their own implementation "shops," many of which are proprietary, as elaborated in Chapter 18. Many provide direct training, supervision, and consultation. Those who develop health policies, such as smoking bans, launch advertising campaigns, as do pharmaceutical firms, who also provide academic detailing aimed at changing provider prescribing behavior. Another set of stakeholders, *public health and health care advocates*, engage in similar efforts. Intervention developers and/or their marketing enterprises highly value the implementation outcomes of penetration, fidelity, and sustainability.

Many if not most D&I efforts target the *frontline practitioners* who deliver health care and prevention services or *agency administrators*, through organizational implementation strategies. Health care providers themselves can serve important dissemination roles. For example, Kerner et al.[1] suggest that primary care physicians, dentists, and community health workers have high potential for exposing the broader public to evidence-based health promotion and disease prevention. Personnel in public health agencies have an obligation to survey the evidence carefully and decide when the science base is sufficient for widespread dissemination. Finally, *policymakers* at the local, regional, state, national, and international levels are an important audience for D&I efforts. These individuals are often faced with macrolevel decisions on how to allocate the public resources for which they have been elected stewards. This often raises important dissemination issues related to balancing individual and social good or deciding on costs for implementing evidence-based policies.

Advancing methods to capture stakeholder perspectives is essential for D&I research.[54,55] A federal report, the "Road Ahead Report," calls for assessing the perspectives of multiple stakeholders, in order to improve the sustainability of empirically supported interventions in real-world care.[56]

Shumway has investigated the use of time trade-off, rating scale, paired comparison, and more simple ranking methods for preference assessment in research funded by the NIMH and industry. Her applications of these established methods with varied groups, including patients, patients' families, clinicians, policymakers, and members of the general public, show that stakeholders often differ markedly in their preferences for outcomes.[57–59]

A variety of established quantitative approaches for stakeholder preference assessment derive from medical decision making and health services research (standard gamble and time trade-off), psychophysics and psychology (category rating and magnitude estimation), marketing (conjoint analysis), cognitive anthropology (cultural domain analysis and cultural consensus analysis), and sorting and ranking approaches common to multiple disciplines. Research is needed to test these methods for assessing the feasibility, acceptability, and validity of stakeholder perspectives using, for example, cognitive interviewing techniques such as "think aloud"[57] and quantitative measures of method performance. The Sawtooth Software "Conjoint Value Analysis" Web System software can be used for conjoint analysis. ANTHROPAC 4.98,[60] a menu-driven DOS program, can be used to conduct metric and nonmetric multidimensional scaling and cluster analyses in exploratory analyses of stakeholder preference domains.

■ SUMMARY

The National Institutes of Health, the Agency for Healthcare Research and Quality (AHRQ), the CDC, and a number of private foundations have expressed the need for advancing the science of D&I. Internationally, interest in D&I research is present in many countries including the UK Centre for Reviews and Dissemination, the UK Medical Research Council, and the Canadian Institutes of Health Research. Improving health care requires not only effective programs and interventions, but also effective strategies to move them into community-based settings of care. But before discrete strategies can be tested for effectiveness, comparative effectives, or cost effectiveness, they must be identified and defined in such a way that enables their control, manipulation, and measurement. Measurement is underdeveloped for many aspects of population health, reflecting the historic emphasis on acute care.[24] A variety of tools are needed to capture health care access and quality, and no measurement issues are more pressing than those for D&I science.

SUGGESTED READINGS

Dusenbury L, Brannigan R, Falco M, & Hansen WB. A review of research on fidelity of implementation: implications for drug abuse prevention in school settings. *Health Educ Res.* 2003;18(2):237–256.

This article reviews the state of research on a key implementation outcome, fidelity. Of the implementation outcomes identified and discussed in this chapter, fidelity is that most frequently addressed in implementation trials and the one with the most advanced measurement work.

Glasgow RE, Vogt TM, Boles SM. Evaluating the public health impact of health promotion interventions: the RE-AIM framework. *Am J Public Health.* 1999;89(9):1322–1327.

In this seminal article, Glasgow et al. evaluate public health interventions using the RE-AIM framework. The model's five dimensions (Reach, Efficacy, Adoption, Implementation, and Maintenance) act together to determine a particular program's public health impact. The article also summarizes the model's strengths and limitations and suggests that failure to evaluate on all five dimensions can result in wasted resources.

Proctor E, Silmere H, Raghavan R, et al. Outcomes for implementation research: conceptual distinctions, measurement challenges, and research agenda. *Adm Policy Ment Health.* 2011;38:65–76.

Proctor et al. offer a groundbreaking summary of issues in the design and evaluation of implementation research, setting out a model that defines steps in the process and discussing a model for quantifying the benefits of program implementation. The ability to measure implementation outcomes leads to better understanding of the implementation process and improves efficiency.

Proctor EK, Landsverk J, Aarons G, Chambers D, Glisson C, & Mittman B. Implementation research in mental health services: an emerging science with conceptual, methodological, and training challenges. *Adm Policy Ment Health.* 2009;36(1):24–34.

The conceptual framework proposed in this article by Proctor et al. identifies the key components in implementaiton science—an evidence-based intervention or quality improvement to be implemented, an implementation strategy for putting the EBI into place in a new setting or health care context, and three types of outcomes that are conceptually related: *implementation outcomes, service system outcomes, and health outcomes. Proctor et al. address the training needs for the D&I field and offer a research agenda for advancing the field.*

Rabin BA, Brownson RC, Kerner JF, & Glasgow RE. Methodologic challenges in disseminating evidence-based intervention to promote physical activity. *Am J Prev Med.* 2006;31(4S):S24–S34.

This article addresses several of the methodological gaps in dissemination research. Through use of two scenarios (one at the population level and one at the clinical level), the authors illustrate a number of key approaches (i.e., issues of design, measures of outcomes and external validity, the balance between fidelity and adaptation to local settings, and the review and funding of dissemination science).

Rabin BA, Glasgow RE, Kerner JF, Klump MP, Brownson RC. Dissemination and implementation research on community-based cancer prevention: a systematic review. *Am J Prev Med.* 2010;38(4):443–456.

A systematic review of recent dissemination and implementation research of evidence-based interventions in smoking, healthy diet, physical activity, and sun protection. This review highlights, among other recommendations, the need for studies that cover a broader range of populations and settings, more consistent terminology use, more practice-based evidence, and measures with higher validity and reliability.

SELECTED WEBSITES AND TOOLS

Cancer Control P.L.A.N.E.T. <http://cancercontrolplanet.cancer.gov/index.html> Cancer Control P.L.A.N.E.T. acts as a portal to provide access to data and resources for designing, implementing, and evaluating evidence-based cancer control programs. The site provides five steps (with links) for developing a comprehensive cancer control plan or program.

CDC BRFSS <http://www.cdc.gov/brfss/> The BRFSS, an ongoing data collection program conducted in all states, the District of Columbia, and three U.S. territories, and the world's largest telephone survey, tracks health risks in the United States. Information from the survey is used to improve the health of the American people. The CDC has developed a standard core questionnaire so that data can be compared across various strata.

CDC WONDER <http://wonder.cdc.gov> CDC WONDER is an easy-to-use system that provides a single point of access to a wide variety of CDC reports, guidelines, and numeric public health data. It can be valuable in public health research, decision making, priority setting, program evaluation, and resource allocation.

National Center for Health Statistics <http://www.cdc.gov/nchs/> National Center for Health Statistics is the principal vital and health statistics agency for the U.S. government. NCHS data systems include information on vital events as well as information on health status, lifestyle, and exposure to unhealthy influences; the onset and diagnosis of illness and disability; and the use of health care. NCHS has two major types of data systems: systems based on populations, containing data collected through personal interviews or examinations (e.g., National Health Interview Survey and National Health and Nutrition Examination Survey), and systems based on records, containing data collected from vital and medical records. These data are used by policymakers in the U.S. Congress and the administration, by medical researchers, and by others in the health community.

http://obssr.od.nih.gov/scientific_areas/translation/dissemination_and_implementation/index.aspx. This site provides information on NIH opportunities to support implementation and dissemination research, including research to advance measures of key constructs.

http://conferences.thehillgroup.com/obssr/DI2011/index.html. This site provides information on a series of annual conferences on the science of dissemination and implementation in health. Abstracts are periodically available, including several that address measurement issues.

http://www.delicious.com/implementation.science/implementation-research. Implementation Science is an open-access, peer-reviewed, online journal that aims to publish research relevant to the scientific study of methods to promote the uptake of research findings into routine health care in both clinical and policy contexts. The Web site provides links to articles, many of which address measurement issues in implementation research, as well as links to questionnaires for measuring key constructs in implementation research.

http://www.queri.research.va.gov/ciprs.cfm. Center for Implementation Practice and Research Support, The VA Center for Implementation Practice and Research Support (CIPRS) is a new QUERI resource center that aims to facilitate accelerated improvement in the quality and performance of the VA health care delivery system through enhanced VA implementation practice and research. CIPRS programs include education, technical assistance, and consultation to VA implementation practitioners and researchers, and development of implementation theory and methods. CIPRS also facilitates better linkages and partnerships between VA implementation researchers and VA clinical practice and policy leaders. CIPRS collaborates with CIDER, HERC, and VIReC in assessing and meeting the needs of the VA implementation community

■ ACKNOWLEDGMENTS

Preparation of this chapter was supported by P30 MH068579 and UL1 RR024992. The authors acknowledge the following individuals, who contributed ideas or insights about measurement of dissemination and implementation outcomes: Graham Colditz, Lauren Gulbas, Curtis McMillen, Susan Pfefferle, and Martha Shumway.

■ REFERENCES

1. Kerner J, Rimer B, Emmons K. Dissemination research and research dissemination: How can we close the gap? *Health Psychol*. 2005;24(5):443–446.
2. Meissner HI. Proceedings from the 3rd annual NIH Conference on the Science of D & I: *Methods and Measurements*. Bethesda, MD. 2010. Office of Behavioral and Social Science Research.
3. Rabin BA, Glasgow RE, Kerner JF, Klump MP, Brownson RC. Dissemination and implementation research on community based cancer prevention: A systematic review. *Am J Prev Med*. 2010;38(4):443–456.
4. Institute of Medicine Committee on Quality of Health Care in America. *Crossing the quality chasm: A new health system for the 21st century*. Washington, DC: Institute of Medicine, National Academy Press. 2001.

5. Institute of Medicine Committee on Crossing the Quality Chasm. *Adaptation to mental health and addictive disorder: Improving the quality of health care for mental and substance-use conditions.* Washington, DC: Institute of Medicine, National Academies Press. 2006.

6. Brownson RC, Chriqui JF, Stamatakis KA. Understanding evidence-based public health policy. *Am J Public Health.* Sep 2009;99(9):1576–1583.

7. Proctor EK, Landsverk J, Aarons G, Chambers D, Glisson C, & Mittman B. Implementation research in mental health services: An emerging science with conceptual, methodological, and training challenges. *Adm Policy Ment Health.* 2009;36(1): 24–34.

8. Proctor EK, Silmere H, Raghavan R, et al. Outcomes for implementation research: Conceptual distinctions, measurement challenges, and research questions. *Adm Policy Ment Health.* 2011;38:65–76.

9. Grimshaw J, Eccles M, Thomas R, et al. Toward evidence-based quality improvement: Evidence (and its limitations) of the effectiveness of guideline D & I strategies 1966–1998. *J Gen Intern Med,* 2006;21S:S14–S20.

10. Rychetnik L, Hawe P, Waters E, Barratt A, Frommer M. A glossary for evidence based public health. *J Epidemiol Community Health.* Jul 2004;58(7):538–545

11. Brownson RC, Fielding JE, Maylahn CM. Evidence-based public health: A fundamental concept for public health practice. *Annu Rev Public Health.* Apr 21 2009;30: 175–201.

12. Glasgow RE, Green LW, Klesges LM, et al. External validity: We need to do more. *Ann Behav Med.* Apr 2006;31(2):105–108.

13. Green LW, Glasgow RE. Evaluating the relevance, generalization, and applicability of research: Issues in external validation and translation methodology. *Eval Health Prof.* Mar 2006;29(1):126–153.

14. Bickman L. A measurement feedback system (MFS) is necessary to improve mental health outcomes. *J Amer Acad Child Adolesc Psychiatry.* 2008;47(10):1114–1119.

15. Department of Health and Human Services. Dissemination and Implementation Research in Health (R01). Grants Website. http://grants.nih.gov/grants/guide/pa-files/PAR-10-038.html. Updated December 1, 2009. Accessed November 21, 2011.

16. Mittman BS, Tonesk X, Jacobson PD. Implementing clinical practice guidelines: Social influence strategies and practitioner behavior change. *Qual Rev Bull.* 1992; 18(12):413–422.

17. Dingfelder HE, Mandell DS. Bridging the research-to-practice gap in autism intervention: An application of diffusion of innovation theory. *J Autism Dev Disord.* 2010; 40(5):597–609

18. Rabin BA, Brownson RC, Kerner JF, Glasgow RE. Methodologic challenges in disseminating evidence-based intervention to promote physical activity. *Am J Prev Med.* 2006; 31(4S):S24–S34.

19. Dowda M, Sallis JF, McKenzie TL, Rosengard P, Kohl III HW. Evaluating the sustainability of SPARK physical education: A case study of translating research into practice. *Res Q Exerc Sport* 2005;76(1):11–19.

20. Shojania KG, Ranji SR, Shaw LK, Charo LN, Lai JC, Rushakoff RJ, McDonald KM, Owens DK. Diabetes Mellitus Care. Vol. 2 of : Shojania KG, McDonald KM, Wachter RM, Owens DK. Closing The Quality Gap: A Critical Analysis of Quality Improvement Strategies. Technical Review 9 (Contract No. 290–02-0017 to the Stanford University–UCSF Evidence-based Practice Center). AHRQ Publication

No. 04-0051-2. Rockville, MD: Agency for Healthcare Research and Quality. September 2004.

21. Magnabosco JL. Innovations in mental health services implementation: A report on state-level data from the U.S. evidence-based practices project. *Implement Sci.* 2006;1(13).

22. Michie S, Johnson M, Abraham C, Lawton R, Parker D, Walker A. Making psychological theory useful for implementing evidence based practice: A consensus approach. *Qual Saf Health Care.* 2005;14(1):26-33.

23. Michie S, Fixsen D, Grimshaw J, Eccles M. Specifying and reporting complex behavior change interventions: The need for a scientific method. *Implement Sci.* 2009;4(1):40.

24. Kottke TE, Isham GJ. Measuring health care access and quality to improve health in populations. *Preven Chron Dis.* 2010;7(4):1-8.

25. Rabin BA, Brownson RC, Haire-Joshu D, Kreuter MW, Weaver NL. A glossary for dissemination and implementation research in health. *J Public Health Manag Pract.* 2008;14(2):117-123.

26. Rye CB, Kimberly JR. The adoption of innovations by provider organizations in health care. *Med Care Res Rev.* 2007;64(3):235-278.

27. Klein KJ, Sorra JS. The challenge of innovation implementation. (Special topic forum on the management of innovation). *Acad Manage Rev.* 1996;21(4):1055-1081.

28. Karsh BT. Beyond usability: Designing effective technology implementation systems to promote patient safety. *Qual Saf Health Care.* 2004;13:388-394.

29. Dusenbury L, Brannigan R, Falco M, Hansen WB. A review of research on fidelity of implementation: Implications for drug abuse prevention in school settings. *Health Educ Res.* 2003;18(2):237-256.

30. Mihalic S. The importance of implementation fidelity. *J Emot Behav Disord.* 2004;4: 83-86.

31. Dane AV, Schneider BH. Program integrity in primary and early secondary prevention: Are implementation effects out of control? *Clin Psychol Rev.* 1998;18:23-45.

32. Stiles PG, Boothroyd RA, Snyder K, Zong X. Service penetration by persons with severe mental illness: How should it be measured? *J Behav Health Serv Res* 2002; 29(2):198.

33. Glasgow RE. *The RE-AIM model for planning, evaluation and reporting on implementation and dissemination research.* Paper presented at the NIH Conference on Building the Science of D & I in the Service of Public Health: Bethesda, MD. September 2007.

34. Johnson K, Hays C, Center H, Daley C. Building capacity and sustainable prevention innovations: A sustainability planning model. *Eval Program Plann.* 2004;27: 135-149.

35. Turner KMT, Sanders MR. Dissemination of evidence-based parenting and family support strategies: Learning from the triple p-positive parenting program system approach. *Aggress Violent Behav.* 2006;11(2):176-193.

36. Glasgow RE, Vogt TM, Boles SM. Evaluating the public health impact of health promotion interventions: The RE-AIM framework. *Am J Public Health.* 1999;89:1322-1327.

37. Goodman RM, McLeroy KR, Steckler AB, Hoyle RH. Development of level of institutionalization scales for health promotion programs. *Health Educ Q.* 1993;20(2):161-179.

38. Raghavan R, Bright C, Shadoin A. Toward a policy ecology of implementation of evidence-based practices in public mental health settings. *Implement Sci.* 2008;3:26.

39. Frost M, Reeve B, Liepa A, Stauffer J, Hays R. Mayo/FDA Patient-Reported Outcomes Consensus Meeting Group. What is sufficient evidence for the reliability and validity of patient-reported outcome measures? *Value Health.* 2007;10(S2):S94–S105.

40. Luke DA. *Multilevel modeling.* Sage University Papers Series on Quantitative Applications in the Social Sciences. Thousand Oaks, CA: Sage. 2004.

41. Bates DM, Sarkar D. *lme4: Linear mixed-effects models using S4 classes,* R package version 0.99875–6. 2007.

42. Shumway M, Saunders T, Shern D, et al. Preferences for schizophrenia treatment outcomes among public policy makers, consumers, families, and providers. *Psychiatr Serv.* 2003;54:1124–1128.

43. Chamberlain P, Brown, CH, Saldana L, et al. Engaging and recruiting counties in an experiment on implementing evidence-based practice in California. *Adm Pol Ment Health.* 2008;35:250–260.

44. Waldorff F, Steenstrup A, Nielsen B, Rubak J, Bro F. Diffusion of an e-learning programme among Danish general practitioners: A nation-wide prospective survey. *BMC Fam Pract.* 2008;9(1):24.

45. Adily A, Westbrook J, Coiera E, Ward J. Use of on-line evidence databases by Australian public health practitioners. *Med Inform Internet Med.* 2004;29(2):127–136.

46. Fischer MA, Vogeli C, Stedman MR, Ferris TG, Weissman JS. (2008). Uptake of electronic prescribing in community-based practices. *J Gen Intern Med.* 2008;23(4): 358–363.

47. Cooke M, Mattick R P, Walsh RA. Implementation of the "fresh start" smoking cessation programme to 23 antenatal clinics: A randomized controlled trial investigating two methods of dissemination. *Drug Alcohol Rev.* 2001;20:19–28.

48. Woolf, S.H. (2008). The meaning of translational research and why it matters. *J Am Med Assoc.* 299(2):211–213.

49. Repenning NP. A simulation-based approach to understanding the dynamics of innovation implementation. *Organ Sci.* 2002;13(2):109–127.

50. Hovmand PS, Gillespie DF. Implementation of evidence based practice and organizational performance. *J Behav Health Serv Res.*2008; 37(7): 79–97

51. Klein KJ, Knight AP. Innovation implementation: Overcoming the challenge. *Curr Dir Psychol Sci.* 2005;14(5):243–246.

52. Rogers EM. *Diffusion of innovations* (4th ed.). New York: The Free Press; 1995.

53. Aarons GA, Covert J, Skriner LC, et al. The eye of the beholder: Youths and parents differ on what matters in mental health services. *Adm Policy Ment Health.* 2010; 37(6): 459–467.

54. Chambers D. Advancing the science of implementation: A workshop summary. *Adm Policy Ment Health.* 2008 35(1–2):3–10.

55. Kimberly J, Cook JM. Organizational measurement and the implementation of innovations in mental health services. *Adm Policy Ment Health.* 2008;35(1–2): 11–20.

56. National Advisory Mental Health Council. *The road ahead: Research partnerships to transform services.* A report by the National Advisory Mental Health Council's Workshop on Services and Clinical Epidemiology Research. Washington, DC: National Institutes of Health, National Institute of Mental Health. 2006.

57. Shumway M. Comparison of direct and indirect methods for measuring preferences for schizophrenia outcomes: Comprehension and decision strategies in three assessment methods. *Men Health Serv Res.* 2001;5(3):121–135.

58. Shumway M, Sentell T, Chouljian T, Tellier J, Rozewicz F, Okun M. Assessing preferences for schizophrenia outcomes: Comprehension and decision strategies in three assessment methods. *Men Health Serv Res.* 2003;5(3):121–135.

59. Swartz MS, Swanson, JW, van Dorn, RA, Elbogen EB, Shumway M. Patient preferences for psychiatric advance directives. *Int J Forensic Ment Health.* 2006;5:67–81.

60. Palinkas LA. Nutritional interventions for treatment of seasonal affective disorder. *Neurosci Ther.* 2010;16(1):3–5.

14 Fidelity and Its Relationship to Implementation Effectiveness, Adaptation, and Dissemination

■ JENNIFER D. ALLEN,
LAURA A. LINNAN,
AND KAREN M. EMMONS

■ INTRODUCTION

Effective dissemination and implementation (D&I) of evidence-based interventions (EBIs) assume that program strategies and methods will be conducted with "fidelity." Fidelity has been defined as the "extent to which the intervention was delivered as planned. It represents the quality and integrity of the intervention as conceived by the developers."[1] Careful measurement of fidelity allows researchers and program implementers to fully appreciate whether outcomes of an intervention are related to the quality or extent of implementation, or whether some other factors—unrelated to the intervention—may account for observed outcomes. In the case of interventions that do not achieve expected outcomes, fidelity is critical to understanding whether the failure of an intervention is attributable to poor or inadequate implementation (termed "Type III error")[2] or to intervention program theory failure, or some combination thereof. There is growing evidence that the fidelity with which an intervention is implemented is highly associated with success in achieving change in targeted outcomes.[3–6] Poor or inadequate implementation is likely a cause of inadequate translation of EBIs into practice.[7] Therefore, maximizing fidelity is crucial for successful D&I of interventions that will have long-term public health impact.

Foundational work on the topic of fidelity has largely emerged from the field of community psychology and education.[8–13] More recently, fidelity has received increased attention in trials of behavioral interventions.[14–16] The purpose of this chapter is to discuss the importance of fidelity for D&I research, to propose a framework for considering factors that influence fidelity, and to describe strategies for producing high fidelity in interventions. We also share an example of a community-based intervention and various attempts to assess fidelity, highlighting several key factors, processes, and challenges. We conclude by summarizing implications of fidelity and adaptation issues on intervention dissemination for practitioners, researchers, and policymakers. Our goal is to add conceptual clarity regarding fidelity across the study design spectrum.

Defining Fidelity

A variety of terms have been used interchangeably with fidelity in the literature, including "implementation fidelity,"[3,17-20] "treatment fidelity,"[5,21-23] and "treatment integrity."[24,25] The looseness with which the term "fidelity" is used can lead to lack of clarity in terms of both conceptual and design parameters. Fidelity is often viewed as a unitary/singular construct, considered most commonly in efficacy trials. In actuality, it applies to all types of studies, from tightly controlled efficacy studies to D&I studies, although the nature and focus on fidelity may vary across each type of study.

In this chapter, we focus on fidelity as it relates to the effective implementation of core intervention elements in the context of D&I research. "Core" intervention elements are those components of an intervention that were tested through rigorous research designs and linked with desired outcomes. These are considered fundamental to programmatic impact—directly responsible for intervention effects. They are the "essential ingredients" that represent the internal logic of the intervention.[11] As such, fidelity requires that core elements be implemented in the manner intended by program developers. In contrast to core elements, "adaptive" elements do not change the internal logic or core aspects of the intervention, such that their modification is not believed to alter the impact of the intervention.[11] In fact, such adaptations typically reflect cultural or contextual "translations" that are critical to successful D&I efforts in nonresearch settings.

In our conceptualization of fidelity, we build on prior work,[1,3,11,12] which has described five elements: adherence, dose, quality of delivery, participant responsiveness, and program differentiation. *Adherence* involves consideration of the intervention *dose* or *exposure*—the amount, frequency, and/or duration of intervention delivered. *Quality of delivery* reflects how well an intervention is implemented, both in terms of content and process. Quality is often assessed by comparing actual delivery with a standard, benchmark, or theoretical ideal.[3] *Participant responsiveness* is the extent to which the target audience engages with and accepts or is satisfied with the intervention. This is a concept analogous to the dose of "intervention received."[1] *Program differentiation* reflects the underlying mechanisms by which the intervention exerts its influence. It is the unique features and/or core elements of the intervention and the extent to which they are elucidated and described.[3] Some investigators urge that all five elements of fidelity be measured,[12] while others suggest that each of these elements may provide alternative means for assessment of fidelity.[3,18] In reality, it is often necessary to prioritize which elements will be measured. Decisions about the most relevant measures require consideration of the nature of the intervention and its objectives, as well as the personnel and resources available.

■ FIDELITY AS A RESEARCH DESIGN ELEMENT

Fidelity is an important consideration of research design planning for a number of reasons. Perhaps most obvious is fidelity's effects on validity.[14] *Internal validity* is adversely affected if an intervention is not administered as intended, as it becomes impossible to know if observed effects are due to the intervention or to external factors. In essence, if fidelity is not maintained, then internal validity is compromised and a true test of the intervention cannot be conducted. Described in detail in Chapter 15, *external validity* is also impacted by fidelity, in that standardized implementation procedures are needed to ensure that an intervention can be replicated in other settings. If the intervention is effective but the procedures for implementing and/or adapting the intervention occur without attention to fidelity, there may be limits on its generalizability to other settings, populations, and/or health issues.

Efforts to enhance one type of validity may result in a diminution of the other. As more emphasis is placed on tightly controlling core intervention elements that may enhance internal validity, the intervention is likely to be more difficult to translate or adapt to diverse settings and populations. As the field of community-based health promotion was developing and trying to establish its legitimacy alongside a rich tradition of clinical trials research, an emphasis on internal validity was essential. However, now that health promotion has a rich body of research in its own right, we argue for a shift in emphasis to external validity. Only then can EBIs move into routine use to fully inform practice and be disseminated and implemented on a wide-scale basis.

Indeed, as the field of D&I research grows, there is increasing recognition of this struggle between internal and external validity in study design.[26,27] For example, if in the design of an efficacy study for weight loss the focus is primarily on internal validity (e.g., use of highly intensive, tightly controlled interventions within clinical settings, run-in phases that emphasize enrollment of highly motivated health clinics that are willing to manage research and intervention requirements, exclusion of individuals with any comorbid conditions, enrollment of only highly motivated participants who demonstrate their ability to participate in the intervention requirements through a detailed run-in prior to enrollment), then built in to this study design are features that threaten the ability to maintain intervention fidelity in a broader dissemination effort, where real-world clinic settings and populations may not be this ideal.

The intervention elements in efficacy studies are typically designed to maximize change and thus may require considerable effort from individual participants, organizations, and study personnel. When dissemination is the goal, maintaining fidelity to such intensive, complex interventions can be extremely challenging. In a community-based setting such as a low-income/subsidized housing community, implementing a very complex intervention with high fidelity for one health issue may result in decreased attention to other health issues that are equally or more important for the health of the population. Further, demanding fidelity to a protocol that may ultimately be offensive or impractical for a new group of participants or population subgroup may yield frustration/resentment and ultimately will lead to implementation or dissemination failure. Identifying the core elements of an intervention that must be included to maintain high fidelity and thus increase the likelihood of successful implementation, adaptation, and/or dissemination will ultimately make it possible to create initial and ongoing fidelity as efficacy/effectiveness is established and we move to dissemination. Thus, it is critically important to consider these core factors from the earliest phases of research and intervention design.[28]

Involving those who are likely to be the intended beneficiaries of the intervention to assist with implementation, adaptation, and dissemination will help maximize effectiveness at each stage and can help to preserve high levels of fidelity.[29,30] For example, if health care providers from community health settings are included as partners in the design of interventions that will ultimately be used in that setting, it is much more likely that high intervention fidelity will be achieved and maintained through the dissemination process, since practical considerations of the context and issues important to the EBI implementers have been considered.

Fidelity is also important by virtue of its impact on *effect size* and *statistical power.* The power to detect a difference between intervention and control/comparison groups in most study designs is a function of minimizing random variability and increasing intended variability between study groups.[14] If an intervention is not delivered as intended, particularly if there is more variability, less *dose* delivered, or intended recipients do not engage with the intervention (low *participant responsiveness*), all of these factors are likely to reduce the potential effect size and diminish statistical power to detect differences between the groups.

A key consideration for implementation efforts is to identify the minimal "dose" of intervention or the "active ingredients" that are required to produce desired change.[31] Thus, the ability to evaluate *dose effects* is also important, so that the minimal amount of dose needed for a specific amount of change can be estimated. Monitoring fidelity enables estimation of the impact of specific intervention doses.[16] For example, it may be useful to determine whether outcomes were comparable when three of five core elements were delivered versus when five core elements were delivered. The recent focus on comparative effectiveness research may allow investigators to design studies that will help to evaluate these types of empirical questions.[32] Also needed are studies that address the process and minimal dose required for effective D&I of policy interventions.[33]

When fidelity is actively and accurately monitored, it is also possible to detect problems with intervention quality or deviations from the intervention protocol, to make midcourse corrections, and to provide encouragement, reward, or recognition for efforts produced. This type of feedback, when incorporated in the study design as a routine part of intervention delivery, has been found to be a key part of maximizing provider engagement in real-world settings and contributing to effective dissemination efforts. For example, intermediate feedback on the quality and adherence to protocol of a worksite-based intervention was provided to managers as way of encouraging peer competition that enhanced participation and increased ownership of the intervention effort in the Working Well Trial. This resulted in increased fidelity.[34]

Beyond establishing a feedback loop between intervention practitioners and researchers during initial efficacy testing, improved communication between these parties within the context of D&I efforts could have a substantial impact on successful translation of research to practice. As discussed later, implementers should be involved in "*designing for fidelity,*" as they have experience and expertise about the types of interventions that may be acceptable, feasible, and effective for the populations with whom they work. Effective efforts to design for fidelity are consistent with the idea of developing an opportunity for practitioners to be integrally involved with building "practice-based evidence."[35]

Finally, *assessment of fidelity* plays a key role in interpretation of study results. If significant intervention results are not found, knowing whether the intervention was delivered as intended makes it possible to eliminate variation in intervention delivery as a contributor to the findings. Particularly in the context of dissemination efforts, null outcomes from an EBI that was delivered with high fidelity would suggest that the intervention itself may not be addressing the key behavioral mediators or most salient contextual factors facing the treatment settings and/or intervention participants. Such findings may suggest the need for a fundamental reevaluation of the intervention theory or implementation effort.

■ FACTORS THAT INFLUENCE FIDELITY

Understanding factors that influence the fidelity with which interventions are implemented is vital to efforts to measure and maximize its occurrence. A growing body of literature documents factors that influence implementation processes.[36] We propose a schematic, as shown in Figure 14–1, which categorizes potential sources of influence. Our goal is to provide researchers and practitioners with a framework to consider when planning, implementing, and/or evaluating dissemination efforts. Consideration of these factors will enable practitioners and researchers to identify designs and methods/measures that will address and document these issues, and to anticipate potential unintended consequences of the intervention by considering the broad range of influences early in the process. Moreover, it gives both researchers and practitioners an opportunity to discuss these influences upfront, before use of resources, time, or expertise is expended in ways that are not efficient or practical.

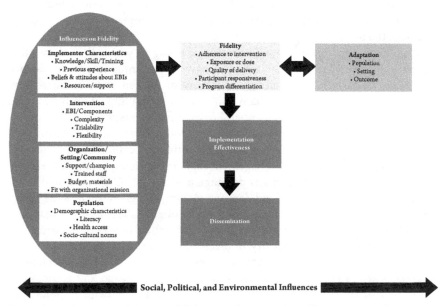

Figure 14–1 Factors influencing fidelity, implementation effectiveness and dissemination.

The schema depicts four categories of influence and their interrelationships. First, *implementer characteristics* can impact ability to implement EBIs with fidelity. For example, a novice practitioner or researcher may have limited awareness about existing EBIs and may be less able to anticipate and problem-solve implementation challenges. Thus, fidelity may be compromised when an implementer has less skill, experience, training, or confidence, resulting in diminished amount, type, or quality of intervention delivered. Alternatively, highly experienced implementers may be more confident in their abilities to modify intervention elements and, therefore, less likely to implement them in a manner consistent with original ideals. Implementation research of health education efforts in schools reveals great variability in implementation of "required" intervention curriculum based on school, teacher, and student characteristics that would not be apparent unless carefully documented.[37-39]

Second, *characteristics of the intervention* will influence fidelity. As discussed in Chapter 3, factors such as intervention complexity, trialability, and the extent to which one intervention provides a relative advantage over the current program/status quo are all important influences on fidelity. These and other features were first described by Rogers in his seminal work on Diffusion of Innovations.[40] For example, highly complex interventions that have a large number of core elements are more difficult to implement than those with fewer, less complex elements. Furthermore, interventions that allow greater flexibility and are amenable to adaptation may be easier for practitioners to implement without omitting or changing core elements. Interventions that are adequately described for the purposes of replication are also more likely to be implemented (*program differentiation*). Similarly, those that are easily accessible to implementers, such as interventions posted on RTIPs (Research Tested Intervention Programs, a website with evidence-based cancer prevention and control interventions)[41] may be more likely to be implemented with fidelity because of the detail and materials provided.

Third, characteristics of the *organization or setting* in which the intervention is to be implemented or disseminated can have a substantial impact on fidelity. Organizational resources, including availability of trained staff, financial capital, and existence of a program "champion" exert a strong impact on the manner in which programs can be implemented. For example, worksites that have at least one staff person who has designated time and responsibility for implementing wellness programs are 10 times more likely to report offering a comprehensive worksite wellness program.[42] Moreover, management support has an important influence on implementation effectiveness in a wide range of settings.[43] Organizational structure, communication channels, and decision-making processes, such as the ability to make strategic decisions "on the frontlines" can also affect implementation.[36] Weiner has recently noted that the "readiness" of a particular organization to adopt a new initiative can influence fidelity, implementation, and dissemination.[44]

Fourth, the *population* for whom the intervention is intended will impact fidelity. Differences across populations influence the relevance, impact, and appropriateness of core or adaptive intervention elements. For example, demographics (age, gender, socioeconomic status, education levels), sociocultural norms, and literacy levels can all influence *participant responsiveness* to the intervention and are all key population factors that are linked to the appropriateness and feasibility of implementing core elements. Such factors will require serious attention when adaptation and dissemination are considered. Kumanyika and Yancey[45] eloquently discuss the tensions between fidelity and the necessary adaptations required so that cultural and ethical/moral issues that influence health equity and justice are considered. Adaptations for setting-specific issues and cultural considerations are considered in detail elsewhere in this book.

Maximizing Fidelity

Given that it can have a significant moderating effect on intervention impact, concerted efforts to maximize fidelity should be undertaken. We advocate efforts to maximize fidelity by attending to the four categories of influence described in Figure 14–1 (*implementer characteristics, characteristics of the intervention, organizational setting, and population*), which can all exert both independent and combined effects on fidelity and the need for adaptation. Fidelity should be a consideration at the time of intervention design, during intervention delivery, and at the time of analysis, as well as at all stages along the research continuum (i.e., efficacy, effectiveness, implementation).

While methods to measure and maximize fidelity to core intervention elements have been discussed in the literature for more than a decade,[46] they are often inconsistently applied. In this section, we begin by discussing strategies to maximize fidelity. Next, we identify strategies for measuring and monitoring fidelity, so that it can be taken into consideration in analysis and interpretation of intervention effects, prior to widespread dissemination efforts.

As noted, efforts toward maintaining fidelity should begin with the initial process of intervention development. Despite tension created by the need to deliver the maximum dose of a highly intensive intervention so as to achieve significant change in primary outcomes, it is also necessary to consider whether such an approach could be scalable for widespread dissemination. *Designing for fidelity* refers to the consideration of the extent to which tested intervention approaches could be applied in "real-world settings," as well as providing adequate documentation of the theoretical basis, mediating and moderating factors, and description of activities so that they can be replicated. Not surprisingly, interventions described with a high degree of specificity are more easily and effectively implemented with fidelity than complex interventions that are insufficiently described.[3,11]

Implementing with fidelity entails putting mechanisms in place to assure that implementers have the knowledge, skills, and resources required to deliver the intervention as planned (*quality of intervention delivery*). This can be accomplished in a number of ways, including providing standardized training for implementers, ensuring that implementers have the requisite knowledge and skills following training (e.g., pencil-and-paper test, return demonstration), and development of detailed implementation protocols or program manuals that clearly specify core intervention components and strategies.[3,14] Moreover, providing implementers with intervention scripts (e.g., for one-to-one or group interactions), standardized materials that help to ensure consistency of message delivery (e.g., flip charts, tip sheets, Q and A's), or checklists can also be useful. It is also important to anticipate the potential for "intervention drift," a phenomenon where either implementer skills or adherence to protocol diminishes over time.[14] Intervention drift can be counteracted by planning periodic booster training sessions, instituting quality control protocols that provide regular feedback to implementers, and providing problem-solving support targeted at potential reasons for drift.

A variety of generic strategies for measuring fidelity exist,[15] categorized as direct or indirect (see Table 14–1). *Direct methods* are generally implemented by trained observers or auditors. This method has traditionally been the gold standard for measuring fidelity because independent observers are less prone to biased reporting.[11,15] Examples of direct assessment include in-person observation (e.g., completed with a checklist outlining key components), "shadowing" implementers (e.g., as in the case of one-to-one interventions), and audio or videotaping intervention events for coding completion of key components at a later time. Advantages of direct observation include the fact that they can yield highly accurate and valid data. Main disadvantages include cost and feasibility. Direct observation may be less feasible in large-scale dissemination initiatives. However, with carefully constructed sampling procedures, it may be feasible to do this on a limited basis.[15]

Indirect measures may include self-reports by implementers, who may complete intervention logs, diaries, or checklists designed to document delivery of core elements, or may involve self-report by program participants. For example, participants may be asked about receipt of core intervention components and/or their level of satisfaction with the intervention (which may reflect *quality of delivery, participant responsiveness*). In-person data collection (e.g., interviews, focus groups) may be utilized, or participants may be asked to complete self-administered data collection forms (e.g., pencil-and-paper rating forms).[15] New technologies and social networking programs offer interesting options for quick feedback from participants via web-based, Facebook, texting, or Twitter.[47]

The main advantages of indirect methods are that they are generally less costly, time consuming, and labor intensive. Moreover, the collection of data from implementers or participants can provide helpful insights about the intervention (i.e., factors that influence fidelity, participant responsiveness) that would not otherwise be available. Disadvantages relate to the accuracy of data (i.e., potential for overreporting, social desirability bias) and the possibility of missing data (e.g., either reports not completed or failure to document information about contextual or situational factors that may impact fidelity).

Considerations when selecting a data collection method should include cost, feasibility, efficiency, validity/reliability of data, reactivity, and ability to collect sufficient "samples" (i.e., intervention delivery) to accurately assess fidelity over time.[15] Additional considerations may include type of intervention delivery (e.g., in-person, telephone), characteristics and skill levels of implementers, as well as population characteristics (e.g., willingness to be observed).

Accurate measurement requires predefined, highly specific core intervention elements against which fidelity can be judged. Unfortunately, the level of description of specificity with which core intervention elements are described in the literature is rarely sufficient for this purpose.[7] Recently, a number of authors have published

TABLE 14-1   *Direct and Indirect Strategies for Measuring Fidelity*

Direct	Advantages	Disadvantages
Trained observers or independent auditors using checklists, rating scales	– Generally considered most accurate	– Observer variability possible; intensive training may be required – More costly and labor intensive than indirect methods – In vivo observation may alter implementer behaviors. – Observer may "miss" seeing subtle events. – Difficult to capture rare events – Not feasible for large-scale dissemination – May not be appropriate for some forms of intervention (e.g., counseling)
Audio or videotape	– May be as accurate as in vivo observation – Possible to establish interrater reliability; raters view same video or listen to same audio – Possible to review intervention delivery more than once – Can be used as tool for providing implementers with feedback about their performance – Less likely to impact implementer behaviors than direct observation	– Less costly than having an auditor present at intervention delivery – Potential to miss important nonverbal or contextual cues – Observer variability possible; intensive training may be required – Video recording equipment is costly; audio equipment is less costly. – May be logistically difficult to bring equipment to setting of intervention delivery – Equipment malfunction may occur.
Indirect		
Data from implementers (e.g., intervention logs, diaries)	– Relatively inexpensive Less time consuming – Can include implementer insights about factors that influenced fidelity, participant responsiveness	– Prone to bias, overreporting – Completion rates may be low. – Recall may be inaccurate, particularly if documentation doesn't occur immediately after intervention delivery.
Data collected from intervention participants (e.g., exit interviews, paper-and-pencil surveys, e-based communication such as Twitter, Facebook)	– Enables assessment of participant responsiveness, perceived quality of delivery – Less costly and time consuming than direct methods	– Participants may want to reflect well on implementer; social desirability. – Participants may not be able to recognize or distinguish between intervention components. – Potential for low completion rates, depending on participant motivation

Adapted in part from Breitenstein et al. 2010[15].

measurement instruments for assessing intervention-specific aspects of fidelity.[19,20] However, a recent review of instruments designed to measure fidelity for behavioral interventions for addiction found that the majority did not establish psychometric properties.[48] While the availability of intervention-specific rating instruments is a step in the right direction, Breitenstein et al.[15] note that such measures do not allow for standardization or cross-comparison of findings across studies. They argue that intervention-specific instruments hinder the ability to compare similar interventions sharing theoretical underpinnings and core components. They suggest that more general assessments of fidelity that can be utilized across interventions and settings may be more valuable in terms of advancing implementation and dissemination science.[15] Setting-specific fidelity measures and sample data collection instruments for interventions that take place in schools, worksites, and a variety of community-based settings have been summarized from several intervention studies by Linnan and Steckler.[1]

Monitoring fidelity during initial implementation, after adaptation, and prior to dissemination is essential. Monitoring should involve ongoing review of fidelity data from direct or indirect measurement and with a feedback loop ensuring that feedback is provided to those responsible for intervention delivery. If not undertaken, deviations or drift from protocol may go unnoticed until it is too late to make revisions or corrections.

A final matter is that of *analyzing fidelity.* Data collected in the process of intervention implementation provides essential information about the extent to which the intervention was implemented as planned, which can be valuable in the analysis of program effects. One manner in which this can be done is to calculate a proportion of core elements that are completed as dictated in protocol and compute a "fidelity score." For example, Lobb et al.[49] measured the proportion of participants who received each set of key intervention components as planned, and then created a multi-item index of protocol completion.[49] Such an index can be included in analyses as an independent variable to help explain unexpected findings or variability of intervention effects.[15]

■ ADAPTATION—EFFORTS TO PRESERVE FIDELITY AND ENHANCE DISSEMINATION

While maximizing fidelity to core intervention elements is a goal of EBI dissemination, there are many instances when adaptation of the original intervention may be warranted or desired. EBIs may need to be adapted for a new setting, population, and/or health outcome. There are important contextual factors (e.g., sociocultural, political, economic, and/or environmental) that will influence fidelity in the "real world." As discussed, characteristics of the population or audience, those responsible for its delivery (implementers), intervention, and issues inherent to the organization/setting, must also be take into account, as they can directly influence initial fidelity.[21]

Balancing the need for fidelity, while maintaining sufficient flexibility to accommodate differences across implementation settings, populations, and situational contexts, is a major challenge. It is not feasible or desirable to "reinvent" interventions for specific settings and populations. There is a tension between the need for standardized implementation, and the flexibility or adaptability that is needed in the provision of community-based, culturally appropriate approaches.[21] Likely, the ability to achieve this balance has major implications for whether or not an EBI will be implemented, disseminated, and/or sustained over time.[50]

In the process of initial identification of EBIs for implementation, practitioners need to be cognizant of the factors that influence fidelity, as well as those that may impact the need for adaptation (see Figure 14–1). Consideration of the population for whom the intervention was originally developed, the original setting in which it was implemented, the characteristics of the intervention and resources required for its implementation, and implementer skills and experiences required are all essential. Finding the right "fit" between community needs and existing EBIs can be a challenge. Even when an EBI for a similar population or setting is available, community members and practitioners may feel a need to customize interventions for their particular setting or audience—as a way to take ownership of the program or better align with "real-world" contexts.[50,51] For example, many school-based EBI interventions have a required curriculum as part of the core elements. However, teachers in any given school, especially experienced teachers, will often decide to adapt the curriculum in ways that are consistent with his/her teaching approach and lesson plans. This "ownership" may make it more likely for schools to agree to implement the intervention, but will often make it less likely that it is done with high fidelity, which may alter the outcomes associated with that intervention.

Two prevailing views about the extent to which EBIs can be adapted for D&I studies have been described.[13,21] One view is that complete fidelity, with strict adherence to intervention protocol, is required under all circumstances.[21,23,52] Indeed, in this view, successful replication is defined by not allowing modification of standardized content.[50] As noted earlier, this approach maximizes the potential for internal validity yet may reduce external validity.

An alternate view is that "adaptation happens." EBIs are rarely implemented in the exact manner of the original trial[10,27] in large part because adaptations are often needed to ensure that the intervention is feasible (administratively, logistically, and financially). Adaptation can help improve the sociocultural "fit" between the intervention, population, and setting. This approach is weighted to favor external validity over internal validity. Still, proponents of this view recognize that adaptations must not compromise the essence of the intervention, and major changes in "core elements" are discouraged.

An excellent example of a program that has grappled with this issue is Peers for Progress, a global initiative focused on accelerating best practices in peer support for diabetes. A key focus of the initiative has been to operationalize the core functions of peer support: (1) assistance in applying disease management of prevention plans in daily life (e.g., goal setting, skill building, practice/rehearsal of behaviors, and problem solving), (2) emotional and social support (e.g., encouragement in use of skills, dealing with stress, talk about emotions), (3) linkage to clinical care (liaison to clinical care, patient activation, etc.), and (4) ongoing support (e.g., proactive, flexible, as-needed, on-demand, and extended over time).[53] Being implemented across several settings and in multiple countries, this project has "designed for fidelity" from its inception, allowing local adaptation in how the core elements are implemented. Careful documentation of the core functions associated with peer support and how peer supporters, participants with diabetes, and health care providers engage with the program around these core functions will allow comparisons of intervention implementation (and outcomes) across the studies.

To promote effective D&I research, it is essential to provide practitioners with evidence-based strategies for guiding adaptation, so as maintain high fidelity and avoid decrements in intervention impact. Until recently, there has been relatively little guidance in this area. Presently, a number of models have emerged to help guide the adaptation process. For example, the Centers for Disease Control and Prevention

(CDC) have developed the "Replicating Effective Programs" as a roadmap for effectively implementing EBIs through a combination of intervention "packaging" (i.e., translation of protocols into user-friendly manuals), technical assistance, and training, as well as other strategies to improve the likelihood of effective implementation and sustainability.[54] Lee et al.[50] proposed "Planned Adaptation" as an approach to help practitioners consider factors that may necessitate modification of existing EBIs, while retaining change-producing mediating mechanisms (core elements). "Cultural adaptation" refers to modifications to EBIs that are responsive to culturally derived beliefs, norms, and customs.[55] The goal of this process is to create "culturally equivalent" interventions based on EBIs that are sensitive and responsive to the unique needs, priorities, and concerns of a cultural group.[55]

A very thoughtful description of this process has been undertaken by the CDC in their efforts to adapt EBIs for HIV prevention to different settings and populations. The result of this work is "ADAPT-ITT," which is an adaptation process that has evolved over several rounds of work with practitioners, policymakers, and academics. What began as a five-step process (assess, select, prepare, pilot, and implement)[56] has evolved into an eight-step adaptation process with multiple feedback loops and decision steps[57,58] that has proved extremely helpful for doing cost-effective adaptation of HIV EBIs. These approaches generally share the following processes: (1) identification of existing EBIs with high potential for "fit" with the population, setting, and available resources; (2) determination of core intervention elements; (3) anticipation of barriers to effective implementation and generation of potential solutions; (4) establishment of mechanisms for measuring and monitoring fidelity on an ongoing basis. Some[54] also incorporate a step for feedback and refinement of the EBI so as to further the potential for wide-scale dissemination.

We believe that fidelity should be monitored so that when adaptation occurs, every step is taken to document these changes and the effects they have on fidelity over time. If adaptations occur and no effort to assess fidelity of the adapted intervention is made, then it is entirely possible that initial intervention effectiveness may be compromised, and dissemination efforts may not lead to the intended outcomes. While it would be ideal to measure all five elements of fidelity, consideration of available resources, the nature of intervention, and issues of feasibility require consideration, as noted above. At a minimum, adaptations should be observed, documented, and understood in order to enhance translation of EBIs into practice.[21,59] We encourage researchers and practitioners to take the time needed to reestablish fidelity after adaptation and provide continuous monitoring to ensure effective intervention implementation and dissemination.

■ CASE EXAMPLE

Adaptation of Cosmetologist (Stylist) Training Workshops for Barbers Enrolled in the Trimming Risk in Men (TRIM) Research Study

Here, we will introduce a real-world community-based intervention example from our own work, which may illustrate directly some of the challenges associated with measuring fidelity as part of implementation effectiveness, adaptation, and dissemination.

Background

Cancer-related disparities exist, and African Americans suffer a disproportionately high incident and mortality burden for nearly all types of cancer nationally, and in North Carolina (NC). Interventions in beauty salons and barbershops take advantage of a setting where customers spend between 30 minutes and several hours each visit, return often, focus on personal health and appearance, and develop a unique and trusted bond with the barber/stylist. The barbershop and beauty salons are a unique and historically cherished place that African Americans consider "safe havens" as well as places of trust and social exchange.[60,61] Dr. Linnan and colleagues have worked in collaboration with licensed African American stylists and barbers in NC to offer a wide range of research studies with barbers or stylists as "natural helpers" to deliver health information and services to promote physical activity, healthy eating, weight control, and a variety of cancer screenings.[62]

Context

This case example focuses attention on a training workshop for licensed cosmetologists that had been found to increase stylist knowledge, self-efficacy, and intention to deliver key health messages to customers (eat at least five fruits/vegetables and get regular physical activity). The BEAUTY (Bringing Education and Understanding to You) intervention prompted changes in self-reported customer behavior immediately postintervention and at a 12-month follow-up assessment.[63] Moving from this initial efficacy trial, we describe factors that influenced fidelity when we took that evidence-based intervention approach (training workshop) and adapted it for use in Trimming Risk in Men (TRIM) with a new population (barbers), in a new setting (barbershops), and with a new health topic (informed decision-making about prostate/colorectal cancer screening).

Given the need for extensive adaptation, we used a systematic approach starting with the messages/materials and training curriculum we had tested successfully with licensed stylists. We worked closely with members of the BEAUTY and Barbershop Advisory Board to develop the overall adaptation approach, followed the NCI's Stage of Health Communications process[64] (and Figure 14–2), and a series of formative research steps to adapt the barber-training workshop for barbers. Specifically, we first conducted four focus groups with AA (African-American) men to assess the perceptions about health, cancer, and potential interest in getting health information in the barbershop. Next we interviewed 21 barbershop owners and barbers to ascertain their interest in sharing health information generally and, specifically, information about how to make informed decisions about prostate and colorectal cancer screening. Finally, we conducted observations using established protocols[65] in 11 barbershops to better understand who initiates conversations between barbers/customers, and common topics of conversation in the shop, including health-related topics. Building on these data and the findings

Sample Training Workshop (4 hrs)

- Welcome/Introductions/Objectives
  Test Your Knowledge About Cancer Screening (Game/Quiz)

- Why Are We Here? – Understanding Cancer Disparities among Black Men

- Why Barbershops for Promoting Health/Reducing Cancer Disparities

- Cancer – The Facts... plus ... "Ask the Doc" to Address Myths/Misconceptions

- Lunch with a Special Guest – A Cancer Survivor Tells His Story

- Introductions to the TRIM Campaign Messages/Materials

- Demonstration – How to Weave the Key Messages into a Typical Shop Visit

- Role Play Activity – Barbers Try It Out at the Tarheel Shop

- General Discussion – How to Make This Work/The Challenges/Wrap-Up/Personal Promises

- Follow-up Cancer Screening Knowledge Quiz & Final Evaluation

Figure 14–2 Sample TRIM barber training workshop agenda.

of BEAUTY, we looked for intervention leverage points for the best way to introduce the messages during a typical barbershop visit. Once we gathered information from these sources, we developed a series of messages to start a conversation that could be delivered by barbers during a typical customer appointment in the barbershop. Two separate campaign messages and materials, as well as two separate barber-training workshops, were developed, implemented, and evaluated as part of the TRIM Study—one for colorectal cancer, and one for prostate cancer. A sample agenda for the final prostate cancer training workshop is found in Figure 14–2.

To test the effects of the adapted barber training workshop, we conducted a pilot workshop with eight barbers for each cancer target and measured changes in knowledge, self-efficacy, and intention to deliver key messages to customers using pre/post-test training workshop evaluation forms. We also gathered information about barber satisfaction with the training workshops and interest in attending future workshops, which were key fidelity indicators compared with the initial beauty salon training workshops. A similar set of tests was conducted separately with the colorectal cancer training workshop and materials. Each of these assessments was completed prior to a larger effectiveness trial.

Findings and Lessons Learned

During the process of collecting information to adapt the stylist training workshops for the barbershop environment, we identified key elements of the training intervention: (1) describing the role of the stylist/barber as a "natural helper" and wise adviser capable of promoting health among customers; (2) dispelling myths and misconceptions; (3) learning the facts about cancer and the good news about cancer prevention; (4) reviewing key health messages/materials provided by the research team; (5) demonstrating how to introduce messages/materials by the research team; (6) role play activity with hypothetical customers, including feedback; and, (7) pre/post-test knowledge quiz. Compared with pretest, posttest results indicated that participating barbers improved in all areas, including knowledge about CRC/prostate cancer, increased self-reported knowledge, comfort in providing information, self-confidence to give customers key messages, and confidence of making an informed decision about getting the CRC/prostate cancer screening tests. In addition, 91% of participating barbers reported that they were extremely or very interested in attending future trainings. We also assessed each training component on dimensions of barber-perceived helpfulness and satisfaction. All scores at posttest were 3.55 or greater on a 5-point Likert scale (1 = not at all, 5 = extremely). Thus, the transition from stylist to barber training met an initial set of fidelity expectations by demonstrating increased knowledge, self-efficacy, and improved self-reported informed decision making about CRC and PC screening tests—the key desired outcomes. In addition, barbers reported high levels of satisfaction and helpfulness, as well as interest in attending future workshops.

Several challenges emerged as part of this adaptation effort. First, there was no previous research or published literature to guide the barber-training effort, so we drew on adult learning principles and social cognitive theory, which were used to guide the initial stylist-training effort. Second, barbers are extremely busy, so we were mindful of that fact and made our training time (4 hrs) concise and incentivized them by offering a healthy dinner and a $50 stipend plus travel costs to attend the training. We also recognized that barbers spend far less time with their customers than the typical stylist does with her customers, so that key health messages had to be brief and suited to the type of interactions that take place in barbershops. We linked our messages to other common topics discussed in the barbershop—women, cars, sports, and politics. Finally, because print materials were less common in barbershops than beauty salons, we placed the key health messages on the back of a business card for the barber, which had the added benefit of promoting the barber and his shop.

A number of important lessons were learned about adapting the stylist workshops for the barbers/barbershops that have the potential for impacting fidelity, implementation effectiveness, and potential for dissemination. Regarding *population issues*, we learned that barbers (men) are different from stylists (women) in a number of important ways that influence intervention efforts. First, barbers are less likely to talk about personal issues with their customers, spend less time with a customer in the chair, and are simply less likely to talk with a customer at all, compared with stylists. As a result, delivering health messages may be less likely during the interaction in the chair. Barbers were more willing to refer a customer to a poster or other materials that might be strategically placed in the barbershop than to deliver the health message directly. Thus, our training and materials were modified to accommodate this difference in population attributed to gender differences. Lessons learned during adaptation addressed *setting* issues by recognizing that barbershops are very open, social places and offer less privacy between customer and barber than is typically found in beauty salons.[65] As a result, we created other ways for barbers to encourage customers to get desired messages, including a display turnstile, business cards, and wrist bands for the barbers to prompt brief message exchanges. And, a lesson learned about adapting to new *health* issues was that providing colorectal and prostate cancer information was far more sensitive than encouraging healthy eating or physical activity (our health focus in the stylist trainings). To address this issue, we included a physician in the barber training workshops to answer all types of questions the barber might have. This proved to be an excellent new addition to the training that barbers appreciated and found helpful.

■ CONCLUSIONS AND RECOMMENDATIONS

Increased D&I of EBIs could result in significant public health gains. While the availability of EBIs is increasing, study of implementation, adaptation, and dissemination is in its infancy. To date, insufficient attention has been given to the issue of fidelity. Consideration of fidelity is necessary to balance need for internal and external validity across the research continuum. There is need for a more robust literature to increase knowledge about factors that influence fidelity, strategies for maximizing fidelity, and methods for measuring and analyzing fidelity.

We echo the recommendations of others[14,21] who advocate for designing interventions with dissemination in mind and having a comprehensive plan for maximizing fidelity throughout intervention delivery, as well as a system for documenting what, how, and why adaptations are made. As discussed above, there are a growing number of models designed to facilitate adaptation of EBIs while maintaining fidelity. It will be important to study the utility and feasibility of these models across different settings, populations, and health issues.

Ultimately, efforts to advance the science of D&I research with a particular focus on fidelity will require the involvement of researchers, practitioners, funders, and policymakers (Table 14-2). Researchers must lead the charge by: designing interventions that can be implemented with fidelity in practice settings, developing standardized methods and measures for assessing fidelity, evaluating strategies for maximizing fidelity, analyzing the impact of fidelity on program outcomes, making explicit the core elements in interventions, ensuring availability of appropriately "packaged" intervention materials, examining the efficacy of strategies for maximizing fidelity, and analyzing emerging models for EBI adaptation.

Practitioners must be responsible for identifying available EBIs that are suitable for their populations and settings. They can make significant contributions to D&I research by communicating the challenges they encounter when delivering EBIs, the reasons for adaptation when this occurs, and for utilizing newly emerging models for adaptation that retain a focus on fidelity to core intervention elements. Such communication will help to build "practice-based evidence" that can advance both science and practice.

Policymakers can play a role in helping to create the infrastructure required for increased communication and exchange between researchers, practitioners, and intervention developers. Web-based technologies—LISTSERVS and databases supported by the NIH and/or CDC—could be a logical infrastructure home for this dialogue. Funders can require attention to fidelity in research applications

TABLE 14-2 *Roles for Practitioners, Researchers, Policymakers, and Funders*

Practitioners	Researchers	Policymakers/Funders/Journal Editors and Reviewers
• Be proactive in learning about available EBIs; know where to search for information about EBIs (e.g., NCI[41]; HHS[66]; The Cochrane Collaboration[67]; Cancer Control PLANET[68]; NREPP[69]). • Choose EBIs that are appropriate to specific audience, setting, implementer skills/ knowledge, health issues, available resources. • Contact researchers to gain access to information about core elements and what might be required for effective implementa- tion, adaptation, and/or dissemination. • If adaptations are made, avoid modifying core elements. Consider one of the adaptation models and/ or do what is necessary to understand your audience and setting so that adap- tation is appropriate and done with fidelity prior to dissemination. • Partner with research- ers and/or evaluators to provide input into how EBIs can be implemented in practice, and how barriers to implementation may be overcome.	• Design interventions with dis- semination in mind—increased attention to external validity to enhance the ability of practitio- ners to implement interventions in "real-world" settings. • Depict interventions with explicit logic models to enhance understanding of the intended process and outcomes. Be sure to clarify core versus adaptive ele- ments. Be explicit about theory that guides the intervention and show key constructs/elements on the logic model. • Carefully measure and analyze fidelity. Consider undertaking component analysis or other post hoc analyses to examine impact of specific intervention elements. • Consider a conceptual frame- work for examination of factors that influence fidelity (see Figure 14–1) and integrate specific initiatives to maximize fidelity • Collect and summarize information and "lessons learned" from "first generation" implementers; provide to "second generation" imple- menters and integrate their feedback on what is feasible and acceptable for implementation in the settings and for the popu- lations with whom they work. • Package EBIs for implementa- tion and dissemination. Provide access to intervention protocols to implementers; include sufficient detail so that activities can be replicated with fidelity. Develop and make available intervention protocols that max- imize and measure fidelity. • Build a more robust literature on fidelity. Specifically address in key publications: Which factors in our conceptual model are most important in terms of ensuring and maintaining fidelity? What are the best methods for maximizing fidelity?	• Funders: Require assessment of and provide adequate funding for evaluation of fidelity in all phases of the research continuum. • Policymakers: Advocate for implementation of EBIs with emphasis on initial fidelity as well as allow for measuring/monitoring fidelity when EBIs are adapted for new health outcomes, settings, or populations. • Journal editors: Assess and report fidelity in guidelines for reporting of interventions (e.g., CONSORT).

across the research continuum and provide targeted funds for examination of the research questions that are needed to build a more robust literature in this field. Journal editors could require increased reporting of issues related to fidelity in publications (along the lines of CONSORT guidelines),[70] and reviewers could be asked to pay increased attention to fidelity in the manuscript review process.

SUGGESTED READINGS

Bellg AJ, Borrelli B, Resnick B, et al.. Enhancing treatment fidelity in health behavior change studies: best practices and recommendations from the NIH Behavior Change Consortium. Health Psychol. 2004;23(5):443–451.

> *This article describes a multisite initiative by the Treatment Fidelity Workgroup of the National Institutes of Health Behavior Change Consortium to conceptualize and address fidelity and its measurement. They offer recommendations for improving treatment fidelity, including strategies for monitoring and improving provider training, delivery and receipt of treatment, and enactment of treatment skills. Authors emphasize the need for funding agencies, reviewers, and journal editors to make treatment fidelity a standard component in reporting of health intervention research.*

Breitenstein SM, Gross D, Garvey CA, Hill C, Fogg L, Resnick B. Implementation fidelity in community-based interventions. Res Nurs Health. 2010;33(2):164–173.

> *This article defines implementation fidelity, offers rationale for its importance in implementation science, describes data collection strategies and tools, and provides recommendations for advancing the study of implementation fidelity. Authors provide a comprehensive description of methods for measuring fidelity, including the advantages and limitations of each.*

Carroll C, Patterson M, Wood S, Booth A, Rick J, Balain S. A conceptual framework for implementation fidelity. Implement Sci. 2007;2:40–49.

> *This article critically reviews literature on implementation fidelity (2002–2007) and presents a new framework for conceptualizing and evaluating fidelity. The authors define five elements of fidelity (adherence to intervention, exposure or dose, quality of delivery, participant responsiveness, and program differentiation) and suggest that two additional elements be included in the conceptualization of fidelity: intervention complexity and facilitation strategies.*

Durlak JA, DuPre EP. Implementation matters: a review of research on the influence of implementation on program outcomes and the factors affecting implementation. Am J Community Psychol. 2008;41(3–4):327–350.

> *This review examines studies that assess the impact of implementation fidelity on program outcomes, and identifies factors that affect the implementation process. Authors describe the Interactive Systems Framework and argue that elements of this framework, including organizational capacity, training, and technical assistance are central to effective implementation.*

Dusenbury L, Brannigan R, Falco M, Hansen WB. A review of research on fidelity of implementation: implications for drug abuse prevention in school settings. Health Educ Res. 2003;18(2):237–256.

> *This review examines literature on drug abuse prevention programs in school settings over a 25-year period, focusing on ways that fidelity has been defined and measured during this time. They conclude that the field is hindered by a lack of consistency in definitions and measures and offer recommendations for development of standardized methods for assessment*

and analysis. Authors conclude by discussing the tension between fidelity and reinvention/ adaptation and offer suggestions for achieving balance.

Hawe P, Shiell A, Riley T, Gold L. Methods for exploring implementation variation and local context within a cluster randomized community intervention trial. *J Epidemiol Community Health.* 2004;58:788–793.

Noting that variability in implementation of interventions is inevitable, this paper stresses the importance of assessing contextual factors that affect implementation fidelity. Authors present a combination of quantitative and qualitative methods for assessing contextual factors in a large-scale trial of an intervention to promote material health following childbirth, based in primary care and community settings in Australia.

Klimes-Dougan B, August GJ, Lee CYS, et al. Practitioner and site characteristics that relate to fidelity of implementation: the early risers prevention program in a going-to-scale intervention trial. *Prof Psychol Res Pr.* 2009;40(5):467–475.

This article discusses the translation of research to real-world practice settings, including how individual practitioner or organization characteristics can aid or impede effective implementation. The authors stress that a lack of fidelity to the original intervention can change the ultimate outcomes of prevention programs.

Linnan L, Steckler A. Process evaluation and public health interventions: An overview. In: Steckler A, and Linnan L, eds. *Process Evaluation in Public Health Interventions and Research.* San Francisco: Jossey-Bass; 2002.

This book provides a rationale and detailed description of how to plan and implement a comprehensive process evaluation effort for a public health intervention that takes place in a wide range of settings. A detailed overview chapter defines key terms of a process evaluation, and a process for undertaking the development of process evaluation. Chapters follow that provide detailed examples of process evaluation for worksite, school, and other community settings where sample data collection tools, key results, and lessons learned are offered. Additional chapters on process tracking data management systems and process evaluation for media campaigns are included, which should benefit practitioners and researchers alike.

SELECTED WEBSITES AND TOOLS

Using What Works: Adapting Evidence-Based Programs to Fit Your Needs. http:// cancercontrol.cancer.gov/use_what_works/start.htm

This website provides a train-the-trainer course designed for health promoters and educators on the national, regional, State, and local levels. The goal is to instruct users on how to plan a health program using evidence-based programs (aka "research-tested programs") for cancer prevention and control.

U.S. Department of Health & Human Services: Agency for Healthcare Research and Quality Evidence-Based Practice. http://www.ahrq.gov/.

AHRQ aims to improve the delivery of clinical preventive health care by developing tools, resources, and materials to support health care organizations and engage the entire health care delivery system. The Research in Action syntheses section of the webiste provides an interpretation of findings from AHRQ-sponsored studies and demonstrates how results can be used in practice.

Research Tested Intervention Programs (RTIPs). http://rtips.cancer.gov/rtips/ index.do

RTIPs is a searchable database of cancer control interventions and program materials and is designed to provide program planners and public health practitioners easy and immediate access to research-tested materials.

Substance Abuse and Mental Health Services Association's National Registry of Evidence-based Programs and Practices. http://nrepp.samhsa.gov/.

NREPP is an online registry of interventions and programs supporting mental health and substance abuse prevention and treatment. The site facilitates connections between intervention developers and members of the public so they can learn how to implement these intervention and program approaches in their communities.

The Cochrane Collaboration. Cochrane Reviews. http://www2.cochrane.org/reviews/.

This site houses systematic reviews of research in human health care and health policy conducted by the Cochrane Collaboration, an international network established to assist healthcare providers, policymakers, patients and their advocates make well-informed decisions about human health care by preparing, updating and promoting the accessibility of evidence.

■ ACKNOWLEDGMENTS

This work was supported in part by cooperative agreements among the Centers for Disease Control and Prevention (CDC) and the National Cancer Institute (NCI) (Allen, U48-DP000064; Linnan U48DP000311); by the NCI (Linnan, R21-CA126373; Emmons, KO5-CA124415, RO1-CA126596, RO1-CA123228), and by the American Cancer Society (Linnan, TURSG-02-190-01-PBP).

■ REFERENCES

1. Linnan L, Steckler A. Process evaluation and public health interventions: An overview. In: Steckler A, Linnan L, eds. *Process Evaluation in Public Health Interventions and Research*. San Francisco: Jossey-Bass; 2002:1–23.
2. Dobson K, Singer AR. Definitional and practical issues in the assessment of treatment integrity. *Clin Psychol*. 2005;12:384–387.
3. Carroll C, Patterson M, Wood S, et al. A conceptual framework for implementation fidelity. *Implement Sci*. 2007;2:40.
4. Durlak JA, DuPre EP. Implementation matters: a review of research on the influence of implementation on program outcomes and the factors affecting implementation. *Am J Community Psychol*. 2008;41(3–4):327–350.
5. Eames C, Daley D, Hutchings J, et al. The Leader Observation Tool: a process skills treatment fidelity measure for the Incredible Years parenting programme. *Child Care Health Dev*. 2008;34(3):391–400.
6. Johnson-Kozlow M, Hovell MF, Rovniak LS, et al. Fidelity issues in secondhand smoking interventions for children. *Nicotine Tob Res*. 2008;10(12):1677–1690.
7. Fixsen D, Naoon SF, Blasé KA, et al. *Implementation Research: A Synthesis of the Literature*. Tampa, Fl: Louis de la Parte Florida Mental Health Institute; 2005.
8. Moncher F, Prinz FJ. Treatment fidelity in outcome studies. *Clin Psychol Rev*. 1991;11: 247–266.

9. Lichstein K, Reidel BWA, Grieve R. Fair tests of clinical trials: A treatment implementation model. *Adv Behav Res Thery*. 1994;16:1–29.

10. Blakely C, Mayer JP, Gottschalk RG, et al. The fidelity-adaptation debate: implications for the implementation of public sector social programs. *Am J Community Psychol*. 1987;15:253–268.

11. Dusenbury L, Brannigan R, Falco M, Hansen WB. A review of research on fidelity of implementation: implications for drug abuse prevention in school settings. *Health Educ Res*. 2003;18(2):237–256.

12. Dane AV, Schneider BH. Program integrity in primary and early secondary prevention: are implementation effects out of control? *Clin Psychol Rev*. 1998;18(1): 23–45.

13. Bauman LJ, Stein RE, Ireys HT. Reinventing fidelity: the transfer of social technology among settings. *Am J Community Psychol*. 1991;19(4):619–639.

14. Bellg AJ, Borrelli B, Resnick B, et al. Enhancing treatment fidelity in health behavior change studies: best practices and recommendations from the NIH Behavior Change Consortium. *Health Psychol*. 2004;23(5):443–451.

15. Breitenstein SM, Gross D, Garvey CA, et al. Implementation fidelity in community-based interventions. *Res Nurs Health*. 2010;33(2):164–173.

16. Resnick B, Bellg AJ, Borrelli B, et al. Examples of implementation and evaluation of treatment fidelity in the BCC studies: where we are and where we need to go. *Ann Behav Med*. 2005;29(Suppl):46–54.

17. Byrnes HF, Miller BA, Aalborg AE, Plasencia AV, Keagy CD. Implementation fidelity in adolescent family-based prevention programs: relationship to family engagement. *Health Educ Res*. 2010;25(4):531–541.

18. Mihalic S. The importance of implementation fidelity. *Emotional and Behavioral Disorders in Youth*. 2004;4(4):83–105.

19. Gingiss PM, Roberts-Gray C, Boerm M. Bridge-it: a system for predicting implementation fidelity for school-based tobacco prevention programs. *Prev Sci*. 2006;7(2): 197–207.

20. Rohrbach LA, Gunning M, Sun P, Sussman S. The Project Towards No Drug Abuse (TND) dissemination trial: implementation fidelity and immediate outcomes. *Prev Sci*. 2010;11(1):77–88.

21. Cohen DJ, Crabtree BF, Etz RS, et al. Fidelity versus flexibility: translating evidence-based research into practice. *Am J Prev Med*. 2008;35(5 Suppl):S381–S389.

22. Hogue A, Henderson CE, Dauber S, et al. Treatment adherence, competence, and outcome in individual and family therapy for adolescent behavior problems. *J Consult Clin Psychol*. 2008;76(4):544–555.

23. Spillane V, Byrne MC, Byrne M, et al. Monitoring treatment fidelity in a randomized controlled trial of a complex intervention. *J Adv Nurs*. 2007;60(3):343–352.

24. DiGennaro F, Martens BK, McIntyre LL. Increasing treatment integrity through negative reinforcement: effects on teacher and student behavior. *School Psych Rev*. 2005;34:220–231.

25. Noell G. Research examining the relationships among consultation process, treatment integrity and outcomes. In: Erchul WP, Sheridan SM eds. *Handbook of Research in School Consultation: Empirical Foundations for the Field*. Mahwah, NJ: Lawrence Erlbaum; 2008:323–342.

26. Glasgow RE. What types of evidence are most needed to advance behavioral medicine? *Ann Behav Med*. 2008;35(1):19–25.

27. Glasgow RE, Klesges LM, Dzewaltowski DA, Bull SS, Estabrooks P. The future of health behavior change research: what is needed to improve translation of research into health promotion practice? *Ann Behav Med.* 2004;27(1):3–12.

28. Kerner J, Rimer B, Emmons K. Introduction to the special section on dissemination: dissemination research and research dissemination: how can we close the gap? *Health Psychol.* 2005;24(5):443–446.

29. Israel BA, Parker EA, Rowe Z, et al. Community-based participatory research: lessons learned from the Centers for Children's Environmental Health and Disease Prevention Research. *Environ Health Perspect.* 2005;113(10):1463–1471.

30. Minkler N, Wallerstein N. *Community-Based Participatory Research for Health.* San Franscisco: Jossey-Bass; 2003.

31. Brownson RC, Fielding JE, Maylahn CM. Evidence-based public health: a fundamental concept for public health practice. *Annu Rev Public Health.* 2009;30:175–201.

32. Horn SD, Gassaway J. Practice-based evidence study design for comparative effectiveness research. *Med Care.* 2007;45(10 Suppl 2):S50–S57.

33. Brownson RC, Chriqui JF, Burgeson CR, Fisher MC, Ness RB. Translating epidemiology into policy to prevent childhood obesity: the case for promoting physical activity in school settings. *Ann Epidemiol.* 2010;20(6):436–444.

34. Linnan L, Thompson B, Kobetz E. The working Well Trial: Selected process evaluation results. In: Steckler A, Linnan L, eds. *Process Evaluation for Public Health Interventions and Research.* San Francisco: Jossey Bass Inc; 2002:155–183.

35. Green LW. From research to "best practices" in other settings and populations. *Am J Health Behav.* 2001;25(3):165–178.

36. Greenhalgh T, Robert G, Macfarlane F, Bate P, Kyriakidou O. Diffusion of innovations in service organizations: systematic review and recommendations. *Milbank Q.* 2004;82(4):581–629.

37. Davis M, Baranowski T, Hughes M, et al. Using children as change agents to increase fruit and vegetable consumption among lower income African American parents: Process evaluation results of the Bringing It Home Program. In: Steckler A, Linnan L, eds. *Process Evaluation for Public Health Interventions and Research.* San Francisco: Jossey Bass Inc; 2002:249–267.

38. Steckler A, Ethelba B, Jane Martin C, et al. Lessons learned from the Pathways Process Evaluation. In: Steckler A, Linnan L, eds. *Process Evaluation for Public Health Interventions and Research..* San Francisco: Jossey-Bass; 2002:268–288.

39. Markham C, Basen-Engquist-K, Coyle K, Addy RC, Parcel GS. Safer Choices, a school-based HIV, STD, and pregnancy prevention program for adolescents: Process evaluation issues related to curriculum implementation. In: Steckler A, Linnan L, eds. *Process Evaluation For Public Health Interventions and Research.* San Francisco: Jossey-Bass; 2002:209–248.

40. Rogers E. *Diffusion of Innovations.* 5th ed. New York: Free Press; 2003.

41. National Cancer Institute. Research-Tested Intervention Programs (RTIPs). http://rtips.cancer.gov/rtips/index.do. Accessed August 10, 2010.

42. Linnan L, Bowling M, Childress J, et al. Results of the 2004 National Worksite Health Promotion Survey. *Am J Public Health.* 2008;98(8):1503–1509.

43. Helfrich CD, Weiner BJ, McKinney MM, Minasian L. Determinants of implementation effectiveness: adapting a framework for complex innovations. *Med Care Res Rev.* 2007;64(3):279–303.

44. Weiner BJ. A theory of organizational readiness for change. *Implement Sci.* 2009;4:67.

45. Kumanyika SK, Yancey AK. Physical activity and health equity: evolving the science. *Am J Health Promot.* 2009;23(6):S4–S7.
46. Backer T. *Finding the Balance—Program Fidelity and Adaptation in Substance Abuse Prevention: A State-of-the-Art Review.* Rockville, MD: Center for Substance Abuse Prevention; 2001.
47. Lee CY, August GJ, Realmuto GM, et al. Fidelity at a distance: assessing implementation fidelity of the Early Risers prevention program in a going-to-scale intervention trial. *Prev Sci.* 2008;9(3):215–229.
48. Baer JS, Ball SA, Campbell BK, et al. Training and fidelity monitoring of behavioral interventions in multi-site addictions research. *Drug Alcohol Depend.* 2007;87(2–3): 107–118.
49. Lobb R, Gonzalez Suarez E, Fay ME, et al. Implementation of a cancer prevention program for working class, multiethnic populations. *Prev Med.* 2004;38(6): 766–776.
50. Lee SJ, Altschul I, Mowbray CT. Using planned adaptation to implement evidence-based programs with new populations. *Am J Community Psychol.* 2008;41(3–4): 290–303.
51. Castro FG, Barrera M, Jr., Martinez CR, Jr. The cultural adaptation of prevention interventions: resolving tensions between fidelity and fit. *Prev Sci.* 2004;5(1):41–45.
52. Dumas JE, Lynch AM, Laughlin JE, Phillips Smith E, Prinz RJ. Promoting intervention fidelity. Conceptual issues, methods, and preliminary results from the EARLY ALLIANCE prevention trial. *Am J Prev Med.* 2001;20(1 Suppl):38–47.
53. Boothroyd RI, Fisher EB. Peers for progress: promoting peer support for health around the world. *Fam Pract.* 2010;27(Suppl 1):i62–i68.
54. Kilbourne AM, Neumann MS, Pincus HA, Bauer MS, Stall R. Implementing evidence-based interventions in health care: application of the replicating effective programs framework. *Implement Sci.* 2007;2:42.
55. Kumpfer KL, Alvarado R, Smith P, Bellamy N. Cultural sensitivity and adaptation in family-based prevention interventions. *Prev Sci.* 2002;3(3):241–246.
56. McKleroy VS, Galbraith JS, Cummings B, et al. Adapting evidence-based behavioral interventions for new settings and target populations. *AIDS Educ Prev.* 2006; 18(4 Suppl A):59–73.
57. Wingood GM, DiClemente RJ. The ADAPT-ITT model: a novel method of adapting evidence-based HIV Interventions. *J Acquir Immune Defic Syndr.* 2008;47(Suppl 1): S40–S46.
58. Latham TP, Sales JM, Boyce LS, et al. Application of ADAPT-ITT: adapting an evidence-based HIV prevention intervention for incarcerated African American adolescent females. *Health Promot Pract.* 2010;11(3 Suppl):53S–60S.
59. Glasgow RE. RE-AIMing research for application: ways to improve evidence for family medicine. *J Am Board Fam Med.* 2006;19(1):11–19.
60. Linnan LA, Ferguson YO. Beauty salons: a promising health promotion setting for reaching and promoting health among African American women. *Health Educ Behav.* 2007;34(3):517–530.
61. Linnan LA, Reiter PL, Duffy C, Hales D, Ward D, Viera A. Assessing and promoting physical activity in African American barbershops: results of the FITStop pilot study. *Am J Mens Health.* 2010;5(1):38–46.
62. Linnan L, Rose J, Carlisle V, et al. The North Carolina BEAUTY and Health Project: overview and baseline results. *The Community Psychologist.* 2007;40(2):61–66.

63. Linnan LA, Ferguson YO, Wasilewski Y, et al. Using community-based participatory research methods to reach women with health messages: results from the
North Carolina BEAUTY and Health Pilot Project. *Health Promot Pract.* 2005;6(2):
164–173.
64. National Cancer Institute. Pink Book—Making Health Communication Programs
Work. http://www.cancer.gov/cancertopics/cancerlibrary/pinkbook. Accessed August
10, 2010.
65. Solomon FM, Linnan LA, Wasilewski Y, et al. Observational study in ten beauty
salons: results informing development of the North Carolina BEAUTY and Health
Project. *Health Educ Behav.* 2004;31(6):790–807.
66. U.S. Department of Health & Human Services: Agency for Healthcare Research
and Quality. Evidence-Based Practice. http://www.ahrq.gov/. Accessed August 10,
2010.
67. The Cochrane Collaboration. Cochrane Reviews. http://www2.cochrane.org/
reviews/. Accessed August 10, 2010.
68. Cancer Control PLANET. http://cancercontrolplanet.cancer.gov/. Accessed August
10, 2010.
69. NREPP: SAMHSA'S National Registry of Evidence-based Programs and Practices.
http://nrepp.samhsa.gov/. Accessed August 10, 2010.
70. Zwarenstein M, Treweek S, Gagnier JJ, et al. Improving the reporting of pragmatic
trials: an extension of the CONSORT statement. *BMJ.* 2008;337:a2390.

15 Furthering Dissemination and Implementation Research: The Need for More Attention to External Validity

■ LAWRENCE W. GREEN
AND MONA NASSER

■ INTRODUCTION

The channels and tools of dissemination have become ever more efficient (though not necessarily effective), accessible, and omnipresent in their indexing, distributing, and searching capacity. Practitioners have seldom complained that they can find nothing to read on their issue at hand, unless it is a truly emergent disease, condition, population, or setting. They complain, if at all, that the literature is overwhelmingly voluminous, unsorted, and often dubiously related to their own setting, problem, or population. They seem to be saying that they are drowning in information but starved for relevance. Increasingly, systematic reviews of public health interventions (e.g., the Guide to Community Preventive Services) provide an array of viable intervention options and synthesize the essence of numerous original studies. The problem may be less with disseminating systematic reviews than with relevance of the original research for health practice or policy. We heartily endorse the suggestion in another chapter in this book (Chapter 11) that this problem could be addressed in part with the development of a system of channels linking the generation of original research (not just its synthesis) with the end-user practitioners,[1] and emphasizing "best processes" as much as "best practices."[2,3]

A related perspective that this chapter takes questions the assumption that greater rigor or scientific control increases the certainty that the studies available demonstrate that intervention X will cause the change in outcome Y when applied in other settings, populations, or circumstances. Overriding the set of considerations of experimental design and statistical certainty, or "internal validity," when it comes to adopting and applying an intervention with "proven" efficacy is whether it was proved under circumstances and in populations similar to those in which one would consider applying the intervention. Indeed, we may have fallen into a trap in our excessive use of the words *proof, proved,* or *proven* to apply to what are essentially probabilistic and conditional relationships between X and Y, limited in their generalizability to a narrow range of populations, settings, treatment conditions, and outcomes originally sampled and observed.

With these considerations, D&I research will do well to consider supplementing and complementing these now established sources of evidence-based practices with more practice-based evidence. Until practitioners and policymakers see more evidence that is generated in circumstances like their own, they will remain skeptical of the applicability, relevance, and fit of the evidence. Even greater perceived relevance would be gained if the practice-based research were generated through more participatory research processes, with more engagement of representative end users in specification of the research questions and variables, and interpretation of the research findings.

With this as a backdrop, this chapter has as its main objective to examine ways to tilt the balance of emphasis for D&I research in health from the preoccupation seen in most journals and systematic reviews with a pipeline from studies with exquisite internal validity to a greater emphasis on external validity. We offer, as the essential core of the D&I research strategy to do this, an approach that (1) engages practitioners or policymakers more actively in the research process, and (2) asks not how can we get practitioners to adopt and implement evidence (with "fidelity" to the form of intervention in the original studies), but how can we study the adaptations and innovations that emerge from their attempts to do so, and what the trade-offs are between the original efficacy-tested forms of interventions and the adapted forms.

What Is External Validity?

Rothwell captured the problem most tersely and compellingly with his finding that "Lack of consideration of external validity is the most frequent criticism by clinicians of RCTs (randomized controlled trials), systematic reviews, and guidelines."[4] Most of those clinicians might not have used the term "external validity" in expressing their criticism of the scientific literature on interventions, but for Rothwell it came down to that technical term in summarizing what the practitioners found lacking or problematic in the literature they were given to apply to their practices. One hears this complaint at least as much, if not more, among public health professionals and policymakers, whose applications must be to yet more diverse settings, populations, outcomes, and treatments. Their treatments are usually more complex programs rather the discrete interventions tested in most randomized trials; their populations more diverse insofar as they constitute a wider range of well and ill people, not just patients; and their settings likely to have fewer resources and time to devote to the interventions and less training and supervision of intervention staff than in the experimental trials.

When we combine that perspective with the first perspective that dissemination is not the barrier to implementation, we are forced to consider whether more efficient dissemination of what practitioners find unusable is self-defeating.[5] We have a case for looking not so much down the science-to-practice pipeline at the failure of practitioners to take the final step to adoption and implementation, but rather up the pipeline at the production end of the science and the processes by which we vet the science through the pipeline. This chapter will acquaint the reader with the ways in which research is strengthened to meet the needs of scientists for internal validity and their peer review and systematic review processes, and the ways in which some of these processes undermine the external validity or relevance of scientific results for the settings, populations, and circumstances in which they would be used.

Campbell and Stanley, in their classic work on *Experimental and Quasi-Experimental Designs for Research*[6] distinguished internal validity from external validity, putting primary emphasis on internal validity as "the basic minimum without which any experiment is uninterpretable: Did in fact the experimental treatments make a difference in this specific experimental instance?" (p. 5). Campbell and Stanley go on to distinguish external validity as that which asks "To what populations, settings, treatment variables, and measurement variables can this effect be generalized?" (p. 5). They also acknowledge that "Both types of criteria are obviously important, even though…features increasing one may jeopardize the other" (p.5). To be sure, one cannot expect much external validity without internal validity, and our plea in this chapter for more attention to external validity is not an appeal to sacrifice much internal validity to achieve it. But for applied health research, one must ask the "so what?" question if a study is air tight with its internal validity but has nowhere to go with its lack of external validity. The argument here is not to abandon the efficacy studies that establish internal validity, but to supplement them with on-site studies of the adaptation or substitution and implementation of components of the efficacy-tested interventions to make them fit local circumstances and to enhance their implementability.

External validity is one of two sources of generalizability of research. The other is *construct validity*. This is of more theoretical concern and refers to the degree to which the specific intervention, or the specific population sampled to study it, or the specific setting in which it was conducted, or the specific outcome measures can be generalized to a more generic construction of any one of these concepts about the intervention, population, setting, or outcome. It is a question of generalizing to the widest possible range of one or more of these elements of a study: types of people, types of settings, types of related outcomes measured, and types of intervention. For example, Egbert and colleagues (Egbert et al., 1964)[7] conducted an RCT in which the intervention arm of patients was visited before their surgery by an anesthesiologist to explain what they should expect and what they could do postsurgically to minimize their symptoms and to hasten their discharge. The reduction in hospital days before discharge was attributed to the rapport developed by the visit between a doctor and a patient. But the inference of that outcome might be generalized to any presurgical patient education delivered by any hospital staff member, or to any anesthesiologist visit to patients before surgery with a general anxiety-reducing or self-efficacy-increasing message, or to the specific information imparted to the patient, which might have been by pamphlet or audio recording. Depending on the theory used to develop the intervention, or the theory invoked to explain the effect, this study would have had more or less construct validity.

Constructs are the stuff of theorizing in that they describe an inference about cause and effect in a more general class of the objects or processes. The theory is confirmed or disconfirmed by the study (not "proved"), and the theory is usually a highly generalized statement about the causal relationship between the treatment and the outcome with applicability across most if not all settings and populations, as well as variable forms of the treatment and various measures of the outcome.

Insofar as theory development or testing is not the main purpose of this book, we will focus here on the other problem of generalizing from experimental studies—external validity.

External validity is concerned not with experiments as a test of whether a theoretical construct generalizes to most, if not all, units of people, treatments, observations, or settings. These are the four elements identified by Cronbach and colleagues[8] and by Cronbach[9] with the acronym "UTOS" of generalization: Units, Treatments, Outcomes, and Settings. External validity is more concerned with whether a causal relationship can be expected to apply *across various (typical or representative) persons, settings, treatments, and outcomes*. It is the range of these things that becomes the concern of external validity, and more so as the persons, settings, treatments, and outcomes of experiments become less representative of the "real-world" of the practitioners or policymakers who would apply the findings. As Shadish et al. (p. 18)[10] have said, "Most experiments are highly localized and particularistic...but have general aspirations." If it were not the investigators of each experiment who aspired to generalization, then the growing army of systematic review teams, meta-analytic reviewers, and "best practice" guideline producers would seek to make the findings of multiple studies more generalizable by combining numerous cases of similar studies on the same class of treatment and outcome, but with variations in the units/populations, treatments, settings, and sometimes with different measures of the outcome.

Specific Threats to External Validity

We made mention of the classic distinction offered by Campbell and Stanley[6] among sources of invalidity in experiments. They identified eight threats to internal validity that can arise in the various generic evaluation designs, including three "preexperimental" designs, three "true experimental" designs (p. 8), and eight "quasi-experimental" designs (pp. 40 & 56). For each of these 16 designs, they also identify four threats to external validity that are either presented by the specific design or avoided by it. In a later edition, Shadish et al. (2002, pp. 86–93)[10] further divided the four threats into five. Here, paraphrased and highly condensed from Campbell and Stanley (pp. 16–22) and from Shadish et al. (pp. 86–93) are the threats to external validity, where X refers to the experimental intervention and its causal relationship to outcomes:

1. *Interaction of testing and X.* This refers to the ways in which a baseline or ongoing measure ("testing" before or during the experimental intervention) can cause the subjects of the experiment to be more prepared for, or more sensitive to, or more reactive to the intervention, and thus the results cannot be generalized to situations in which the intervention would not be accompanied by a pretest or other testing during the intervention. Physical exams, blood tests, written tests, interviews, questionnaires, audio- or videotaping administered before or during an experimental intervention is usually sensitizing in ways that make generalization about the intervention invalid. This threat to validity could be especially biasing of

results in dissemination or implementation studies insofar as the experimental subjects would be made more aware of the innovation to be adopted or implemented. With their focus on educational and social intervention evaluations, Campbell and his colleagues[6] would not have anticipated the extensive use made of pretests of many kinds in behavioral medicine, most of them sufficiently obtrusive, even invasive, as to surely compromise the generalizability of results. Indeed, the demand by peer reviewers for baseline data to assure equivalence of experimental and control groups seems to have forgotten that equivalence of these groups was the main point of random assignment.

2. *Interaction of selection and X (interaction of units with the causal relationship).* This threat to external validity refers to ways in which the sampling is not representative, screening might produce a further degradation of representativeness, and differential attrition or retention (especially between experimental and control groups) of subjects for the experiment or evaluation create a readiness or resistance to the intervention that biases the result toward or against the intervention. This has become a major concern with the increasingly controlled screening and selectivity of subjects for clinical studies seeking to minimize threats to internal validity by eliminating confounding factors associated with patients or subjects who have any complications (medical or social) that might interact with the relationship between X and the outcomes. This pursuit of homogeneity and simplicity of the profile of subjects makes for less complicated designs and statistical adjustments but also makes the study results less generalizable. For an experiment requiring inconvenience for subjects or institutions in which they are to be found, the refusal of some to participate produces a biased sample of the universe of people or institutions to which one would want to generalize the results.

3. *Reactive arrangements (interaction of settings with the causal relationship).* Besides testing, many of the other circumstances of experimentally controlled study settings and arrangements create a reactivity of subjects (and staff who would implement the intervention) that would not occur in normal circumstances to which the results are to be generalized. Informed consent requirements are just the beginning of a series of arrangements that produce either a "Hawthorne effect" or an "I'm a guinea pig" response among subjects, a vigilance or a receptivity, a predisposition to behave as one assumes the researchers want one to behave. These reactive arrangements, combined with the preceding "interaction of selection with X" has led us to recommend that more of the scientific evaluation of innovations for D&I should be conducted within the routine and circumstances of normal, representative practice settings with representative practitioners as the deliverers of the X. More generally, an effect that is found in one setting might not generalize to other settings.

4. *Multiple-X interference (interaction of treatment variations with the causal relationship).* This threat arises when the treatment cannot be replicated, cannot be adequately described, takes various forms with different personnel implementing them, or produces variations of effect with various combinations, dosages, or sequencing of the interventions. These situations arise with complex

interventions, typical of public health or community interventions that pride themselves as having ecological robustness and systems thinking inherent in their construction. The ecological aspect means they recognize the necessity of intervening simultaneously at several levels of individual behavior, family or social norms and groups, organizations, and sometimes whole-community policy or environmental change. The systems aspect similarly recognizes that every system, for example, a family or an organization, is a subsystem of another system, and that change in one will produce a feedback loop with adjustments and change in the other. Such interventions become more difficult to generalize in part because each of the components is interdependent with the others, and because they go quickly beyond the experimental control of the investigators who study them.

5. *Context-dependent mediation.* This added dimension of threats to external validity in Shadish et al.[10] acknowledges that studies of intervention effects seldom assume a direct relationship between interventions and outcomes, but rather mediated relationships. The mediating variables are transferring the effect of the intervention to the outcome, such as an educational intervention intended to effect behavior change through mediators of increased awareness of the action that is needed, knowledge of actions and how to take them, beliefs that the actions are important and effective, and possession of the ability and resources to take them. Each of these mediators may take on more or less strength, depending on the context in which another set of variables, moderating variables, may influence the relationship between the intervention and the mediating variables and/or the relationship between the mediators and the outcomes, as shown in Figure 15–1. Moderators might be context-dependent variables such as the demographic and socioeconomic characteristics of the community or population in which the intervention is applied; the level of threat presented by the outcome in the community or population, and the availability of media to transmit the educational messages. If they are context dependent, the context in which the study of the intervention was conducted will be more or less generalizable to other contexts.

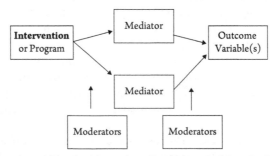

Figure 15–1. The place of mediating and moderating variables, the latter generally controlled rather than assessed in RCTs.
Source: Green LW, Kreuter MW, *Health Program Planning: An Educational and Ecological Approach.* 4th ed. New York: McGraw-Hill, 2005, p. 204

Alternative Ways to Generalize

Two ways in which studies can be made more generalizable are to assess them on two dimensions of external validity: (a) generalizability of alternative measures of the program or the outcomes; (b) generalizability to or across people, settings, and time.[11,12]

A much neglected and fruitful level of analysis to gain insight on external validity is on alternative or intermediate measures of the outcome, as in construct validity. This asks of a study whether the obtained results would occur if the program or the outcomes were measured in a different way, or the sampling design of the study had given it sufficient statistical power to detect significant differences between experimental and control groups on alternative outcomes. Studies that take multiple measures of the outcomes tend to do it on the basis of a logic model for the program, with interventions shown to influence intermediate or mediating variables (such as behavioral or environmental changes), and from there to ultimate outcomes (such as health outcomes) as shown generically in Figure 15–1. They tend to use the ultimate outcome, if possible, as the basis for setting a sample size sufficient to detect statistical differences between experimental and control groups. This sample size is often sufficient to assess the significance of differences on mediating variables as well because the ultimate outcome has a lower probability of occurring than its determinants among the mediating variables within the time frame of most studies. But after publishing the main effects on the ultimate outcome, too many studies never get to the analysis or at least to the reporting of secondary analyses of effects on mediating variables. This is often because of space limitations and the preferences of journal editors.

With D&I studies, the mediating and moderating variables have been extensively reviewed and catalogued by the late Everett Rogers over five editions of his book on *Diffusion of Innovations*.[13] The historical evolution of Rogers's theory is covered in Chapter 3. The mediating and moderating variables can be summarized in the following adaptation showing the mediating variables in the arrows and the moderating variables in "prior conditions," the characteristics of the "decision-unit," and the characteristics of the "innovation" (Figure 15–2).

More attention in the studies of D&I to measuring each of these stages and their associated moderating variables would allow for greater interpretation of the generalizability of the study results, in addition to the ultimate outcome or end point of interest.

The second form of external validity concerns generalizability across populations. This could be strengthened with systematic analyses of subgroups within a study or group of studies. This use of subgroup analysis within studies fell into disrepute especially after the Multiple Risk Factor Intervention Trial (MRFIT or Mister Fit) of the 1970s obtained disappointing aggregate results, and the investigators set about to examine subgroups within the study to see which groups benefitted or not, even though the average benefits were not statistically significant. An outcry arose from statisticians who objected to the subgroup analysis on the grounds that the subgroups were not randomly assigned to the interventions. The technical truth in this obscures the waste of information when clear differences in outcomes

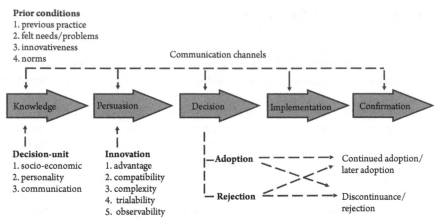

Figure 15–2. Stages and influences in the Innovation-Decision-Adoption-Implementation-Maintenance process.
Source: Rogers E. *Diffusion of Innovations.* 5th Ed. New York: Free Press, 2003, p.170.

between subgroups could lead to hypotheses, at least, and guides to practitioners at best on whether the results might apply to their populations. It also denies the utility of the wide range of nonrandomized evaluations of programs and policies in real time and with situations that do not lend themselves to ethical or feasible random assignment. In short, applying this criterion to the legitimacy of subgroup analysis would eliminate from credibility all of the literature based on quasi-experimental designs.[14–16] It would also preclude the closer inspection of results for subgroups of studies that were published with positive main effects comparing experimental and control groups. Examples are studies in which the significant main effects were examined further for comparison of the relative outcomes between low- and high-risk groups[17] and relative effects for different age groups.[18]

Another way in which past studies could serve more fruitfully to answer the applicability questions of practitioners and policymakers that otherwise fail to get addressed in primary research is to ask what became of the people over a longer period of time than the primary studies were funded originally to run. Often, such follow-up studies can be performed with death records, hospitalization records, school records, employee benefits or insurance claim records, primary care records in medical group plans such as Kaiser-Permanente, or linked medical records in the case of some jurisdictions in Canada, the UK, and other national health care systems. These systems preclude the necessity of pursuing the original study's subjects themselves, which is often too expensive or otherwise not feasible if many have died, or by informed consent limitations or other ethics rules. Examples of this are two other cases from the hypertension literature. One is the follow-up study by Morisky et al.[19] and Levine et al.[20] of the mortality in subjects of a randomized factorial design study on three hypertension control interventions.[21] The original study showed reductions in blood pressure, but the five-year follow-up study was also able to show reductions in morbidity and mortality in the original study subjects who had been exposed to various combinations of the three interventions.

A similar, but more dramatic, example of follow-up opportunities to answer practitioners' and policymakers' questions brings us back to the issue of subgroup analyses of the erstwhile MRFIT data, and follow-up opportunities that lie in such data sets when combined with other sources. Practitioners and policymakers are often challenged to defend their programs or proposed programs on the basis of benefits beyond the specific disease they are intended to control. Hypertension is known to cause strokes and contributes to other cardiovascular diseases and deaths. Terry et al.[22] assessed the association of blood pressure with specific types of "accidental" death. They examined data from baseline interviews and 25 years of mortality follow-up (1973–1999) for 347,978 men screened for MRFIT, comparing associations of blood pressure with all external causes of death and individual causes. Men with Stage 2 hypertension had nearly twice as many deaths from falls and nearly 1.5 times as many deaths from motor vehicle injuries.

The point of these examples is to illustrate ways to compensate for the absence of external validity in some studies, or to squeeze some relevance and generalizability from them, where scientific concerns for internal validity have squeezed much of the relevance to practice out of them. Until the priorities of research funding and publishing practices, and the demands of systematic reviews, all of which generally place a premium on internal validity at the expense of external validity, give greater attention to relevance of the research for practice and policy, these are ways to extract some relevance from them.

Related Sources of the External Validity Problem for D&I Research

Besides external validity in the strict sense defined above, many if not most of the research studies conducted with RCT designs that qualify them for systematic reviews and guidelines for evidence-based practice are conducted under such controlled (and often enriched) circumstances that they cannot be replicated or afforded in other settings or taken to scale in multiple, varied settings.

Two of the most prominent problems produced by excessive levels of control in RCTs relate to the inclusion and exclusion of units or subjects in the original studies. The studies are typically conducted in one setting, rather than in a random sample of settings. It is usually a setting over which the academic investigators have some control, such as clinics in the university's teaching hospital, or community settings in which the research grant provided funding for the interventions or evaluation such that the academic investigators could negotiate a greater degree of control over the training and supervision of those who would be the interventionists. The very act of agreeing to open the staff, patients, students, employees, or clients of an organization to the rigors of a controlled trial, especially a randomized controlled trial, makes that clinic, school, worksite, or other service-providing organization a special—possibly ungeneralizable—case. A remedy called "practical trials" has been proposed and now increasingly implemented to overcome this problem.[23] Practice-Based Research Networks (PBRNs) have also developed standing arrangements for the experimental testing of new or routine practices in more natural medical, nursing, and dental settings.[24] A growing emphasis on practice-based and participatory research among the Prevention Research Centers funded by CDC has suggested ways to build greater reality testing and representativeness into multisite studies of D&I.[25]

The screening of subjects to minimize confounding factors makes the samples of patients or subjects in most published studies further unrepresentative of the populations in which the interventions would be applied. They often eliminate patients, for example, who have multiple diagnoses or multiple risk factors. This exclusion is to minimize the confounding of the study results. Such homogenization of the study sample makes it unlike most of the patients or other populations to which one might wish to apply the treatment and to generalize the results. The problem of representativeness of the population sampled is compounded by the differential attrition or drop-out from experimental and control groups, especially when the experimental treatment requires effort or inconvenience from the subjects to the point that those who remain in the study to be measured at the end are not representative of the population enrolled, much less of other populations who might be enrolled. Furthermore, they are no longer as equivalent as a group to the control group as they were when randomized to the experimental treatment.

The homogeneity of the samples after screening and attrition adds another threat to external validity: most interventions in the "real world" will not be so restrictive in their responsiveness to the wider range of people eligible for, needing, or interested in the intervention, and the greater heterogeneity produced in the real-life samples changes the nature of the required intervention processes, forms, duration, or intensity. If a study of interventions to increase hypertension self-management eliminates from the study all the hypertension patients who also have diabetes, for example, the results will not apply to the many hypertension patients in most clinical settings who have those two comorbidities.

The term "randomized controlled trials" refers neither to the random *sampling* of the population of units or people, nor to the random *sampling* of settings, but to the use of random *assignment* of units or subjects within the cooperating units or settings to experimental and control groups. This distinction between random sampling and random assignment is not lost on practitioners who often look first to the setting and population of the study to decide whether it is relevant to their own practice. When they look for more detail on the setting and population, or if satisfied with those as relevant, more detail on the description of the intervention, they are often disappointed to find too little detail to make an informed decision on whether the intervention and its results apply to their setting, population, and resources. Health science journals and their editors have tended, when print space limits are exceeded, to require cuts in the description of the intervention.

Many of the problems described above are compounded when the interventions are complex, multilevel, and comprehensive and have other features known to be important to effective community or population-level programs. We can summarize these and other departures of the RCT circumstances in producing evidence for *population health interventions*, from the types of evidence needed in practice, in Table 15–1. The left column lists the widely acknowledged conditions that produce effective interventions (more likely programs and policies combined to produce a comprehensive set of synergistic interventions), and a matched list in the right

TABLE 15-1. *The Major Features of Successful Community Interventions, and the Constraining Features of Randomized Controlled Trials for Each*

The Imperatives of Population Health versus RCT Rules of Evidence	
What We Know Is Needed	What RCTs Often Seek and Test
• Comprehensive	• Isolation of independent variable
• Ecological	• Randomizable experimental units
• Upstream determinants	• Focus on proximal determinants
• Multisectoral intervention	• Intervention controlled
• Participatory	• Blinded, double-blinded...
• Adapted to cultures, contexts	• Tests based on averages; results standardized for everyone
• Tailored to individuals	• "Fidelity" to the tested form
• Professional discretion	• Protocol controlled
• Social justice	• Informed consent

column of what randomized controlled trials demand and produce. The conditions that produced the great public health successes with tobacco control in the last third of the 20th century, for example, were demonstrated with systematic evaluations of the statewide, comprehensive programs of California and Massachusetts, in particular. These states were not randomized, but their experience confirmed much of what was becoming the cumulative, practice-based wisdom of public health programs addressing the complex issues of lifestyle and social factors influencing population health.[26] The nine characteristics of "Best Practices for Comprehensive Tobacco Control Programs" were compiled by CDC from these states and others to produce a document by this name.[27]

But even at the clinical and other organizational levels of intervention, more comprehensive, ecological, upstream, multisectoral, participatory, culturally adapted, individually tailored, professionally guided, and socially just programs and interventions are generally found to be more effective, but difficult to evaluate using the strict criteria of RCTs.

How the Neglect of External Validity Relates to D&I Practice

The places and populations seen in diffusion theory and in D&I practice as hardest to reach, late adopters, and the underserved are the ones often underrepresented in much of the intervention research providing "evidence-based practices." The local decision makers, program planners, and practitioners who would be expected as first-line adopters of the evidence find the undigested original research publications to have too little detail on the interventions (because of journal publication practices) to apply them systematically, much less to replicate them with "fidelity."[28] As Rothwell pointed out, "...researchers, funding agencies, ethics committees, the pharmaceutical industry, medical journals, and governmental regulators alike all neglect external validity, leaving clinicians to make judgments...[R]eporting of the determinants of external validity in trial publications and systematic reviews is usually inadequate".[4(p.82)]

When described with greater detail on the intervention, the local would-be adopters find the studies often lacking in relevance or applicability to their population, patients, or practitioners, or to their local circumstances, resources, capabilities, or culture. They also find too little information on the numbers or proportion of eligible people who were or could be reached—not just how effective the intervention was with those who *were* reached and who agreed to participate in the study. They also find too little information on how acceptable the intervention is or was to the organization that must adopt it, and to the practitioners in that organization who must implement it, and how well it was maintained after adoption.

In an attempt to address these problems of reporting of original experimental studies in professional and scientific journals, a set of criteria based on the RE-AIM model (see Chapter 16) were proposed,[29] and a group of editors and associate editors of 13 leading professional journals were convened to review the criteria and to consider the merits and possible ways to incorporate them into their guidelines to authors or peer review processes for their journals.[30] Among the journals represented, two ran editorials acknowledging the importance of the issue,[31,32] two others commented on the issue in more general editorials, and two invited editorials from the conference organizers and others.[33,34] One, *Annals of Behavioral Medicine*, has added referral to the methodology article[29] in its manuscript preparation guidelines for authors. Several have indicated plans to increase their website pages to accommodate richer description of interventions. There is hope, then, that the publishing end of the pipeline is beginning to give greater attention to the need for authors of published articles to give greater description to the interventions and the methods for readers to judge the relevance and applicability of the findings of research for their actual practice population, setting, and interventions (Table 15-2).

Before publication, however, are the funding and conduct of the research. The journal editors noted that unless the funding priorities and peer review of research grant applications provide for more attention to external validity in funded research, there would be little point in expecting the journals or their authors to report more on it. Priorities for federal funding have turned notably in the direction of greater attention to participatory research,[35] which should be expected to increase the relevance of the research to the needs of communities, practitioners, and policymakers (see Chapter 10). The Robert Wood Johnson Foundation has made community-based participatory research a requirement of its Clinical Scholars Program.[36] The Centers for Disease Control have made community-based participatory research a central expectation of funding for its Prevention Research Centers, which also puts an emphasis on making the research more practice based.[37]

Finally, there is the point downstream from publication in the research-to-practice pipeline where evidence from multiple individual studies are indexed, compiled, and systematically reviewed, and recommendations derived for "evidence-based practice" guidelines for practitioners, program planners, and policymakers. These guidelines become the justification or requirement for funding of programs, thereby limiting funding to those interventions that can be shown to have this source justification. The systematic reviews have a history of development and institutionalization in the tradition of evidence-based medicine, which places its emphasis on internal validity, based on the *strength* of evidence. It less often reports data to judge the *weight* of evidence across settings, populations, and times that would bear on the applicability of the results of the systematic reviews.[38]

TABLE 15-2. *Guidelines for Conduct and Reporting of Trials to Assure Greater Attention to External Validity*

1. Settings and populations

    A. Participation: Are there analyses of the participation rate among potential (a) settings, (b) delivery staff, and (c) patients (consumers)?

    B. Target audience: Is the intended target audience stated for adoption (at the intended settings such as worksites, medical offices, etc.) and application (at the individual level)?

    C. Representativeness—Settings: Are comparisons made of the similarity of settings in the study to the intended target audience of program settings—or to those settings that decline to participate?

    D. Representativeness—Individuals: Are analyses conducted of the similarity and differences between patients, consumers, or other subjects who participate versus either those who decline, or the intended target audience?

2. Program or policy implementation and adaptation

    A. Consistent implementation: Are data presented on the level and quality of implementation of different program components?

    B. Staff expertise: Are data presented on the level of training or experience required to deliver the program or quality of implementation by different types of staff?

    C. Program adaptation: Is information reported on the extent to which different settings modified or adapted the program to fit their setting?

    D. Mechanisms: Are data reported on the process(es) or mediating variables through which the program or policy achieved its effects?

3. Outcomes for decision making

    A. Significance: Are outcomes reported in a way that can be compared to either clinical guidelines or public health goals?

    B. Adverse consequences: Do the outcomes reported include quality of life or potential negatives ?

    C. Moderators: Are there any analyses of moderator effects—including of different subgroups of participants and types of intervention staff—to assess robustness versus specificity of effects?

    D. Sensitivity: Are there any sensitivity analyses to assess dose–response effects, threshold level, or point of diminishing returns on the resources expended?

    E. Costs: Are data on the costs presented? If so, are standard economic or accounting methods used to fully account for costs?

4. Time: Maintenance and institutionalization

    A. Long-term effects: Are data reported on longer-term effects, at least 12 months following treatment?

    B. Institutionalization: Are data reported on the sustainability (or reinvention or evolution) of program implementation at least 12 months after the formal evaluation?

    C. Attrition: Are data on attrition by condition reported, and are analyses conducted of the epresentativeness of those who drop out?

Source: Green LW, Glasgow RE. Evaluating the relevance, generalization, and applicability of research: issues in external validation and translation methodology. *Eval Health Prof.* Mar 2006;29(1):126–153.

Regression, Construct Validity, and External Validity in Systematic Reviews

Systematic reviews of health interventions use systematic methods to minimize bias in identifying, evaluating, and synthesizing primary research. A systematic approach toward considering construct validity and external validity can enhance the applicability of the systematic reviews in the later steps of the research-to-practice pipeline. One such approach is to use more regression analysis with meta-analytic techniques in systematic reviews to understand and explain the heterogeneity in effects across subsets of the data. These could be especially informative in knowing where and with whom the effects are more or less effective, rather than the usual point estimates that imply fixed effects of the interventions. This could address some of the external validity concerns and needs of practitioners and policymakers by adding a multistudy dimension to the subgroup analyses of individual studies, discussed elsewhere in this chapter, but often the multiple studies required for a meta-regression analysis are not available. Even when they are, Hauck et al. "recommend that the primary analyses adjust for important prognostic covariates in order to come as close as possible to the clinically most relevant subject-specific measure of treatment effect. Additional benefits would be…improved external validity. The latter is particularly relevant to meta-analyses."[39]

Construct validity

The existing theoretical frameworks on the inference between cause and effect can help systematic reviewers in defining the purpose and the eligibility criteria of studies for the review. Besides quantitative studies, qualitative studies can help in defining how and why participants' characteristics or contextual factors can influence effectiveness and how broad or narrow the question should be.[40] For example, the Agency for Healthcare Research and Quality (AHRQ) uses an "analytical framework" in its comparative effectiveness research program to provide an overview of the clinical concepts underlying the health topic.[41] Similarly, the Task Force on Community Preventive Services develops a detailed logic model or "logic framework" to guide each systematic review and updates of previous reviews. These logic models identify the presumed sequence of determinants, interventions, and mediating and moderating variables, while distinguishing the connecting arrows between each pair of these according to whether that causal link was included in the review or not.[42] An example of such a logic model used to develop the review and published with the Task Force recommendations is shown in Figure 15–3.[43]

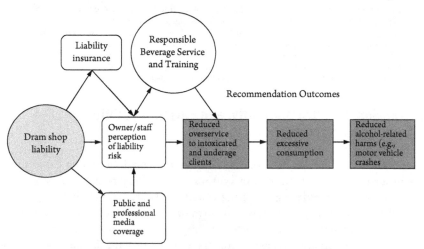

Figure 15–3 A logic model showing the variables included in a systematic review. *Source*: Task Force on Community Preventive Services. Recommendations for reducing excessive alcohol-related harms by limiting alcohol outlet density. *Am J Prev Med*. Dec 2009;37(6):570–571.

External validity

As with primary research studies, systematic reviewers evaluate whether the causal relation from intervention to outcome is generalizable to different units, treatments, outcomes, and settings (UTOS). Currently no universal approach exists to deal with it, but reviewers can make adjustments in their review to achieve this:

1. *Using external validity tools to evaluate the conduct and reporting of the included research studies in a systematic review:* External validity tools can help reviewers assess the extent to which these UTOS dimensions are considered in the included primary trials and how it might affect the recommendation based on the synthesis of the trials. Tools vary from single question as part of a quality assessment tool or reporting checklist[44] to a validated and comprehensive checklist for evaluating external validity of trials.[29] For example, Klesges et al. applied the Green & Glasgow tool for external validity in a review of studies of childhood obesity prevention, examining dimensions of reach and representativeness, implementation and adaptation, outcomes of decision making, and maintenance and institutionalization.[45] Depending on the question of the review, reviewers might also decide to develop a specific external validity tool for the research question of the review.[46]

2. *Differentiating pragmatic and explanatory trials:* Randomized trials can be differentiated as efficacy versus effectiveness trials or explanatory versus pragmatic trials. These refer to conducting trials under ideal testing environments and circumstances (efficacy or explanatory trials) versus conducting trials under usual situations. Although studies are not purely one or another, reviewers could determine the position of the trial in the pragmatic-explanatory continuum in comparison to each other.[47]

3. *Exploring heterogeneity across population, setting, treatment variations, and outcomes:* Systematic reviews provide an opportunity to investigate the effectiveness of the intervention across different populations, different contexts, treatment variations, and outcomes. Subgroup analyses[48] and meta-regression are two quantitative methods to explore the heterogeneity across different groups; however, they have pitfalls and need to be carefully interpreted, as noted in the previous section of this chapter.

Individual patient data meta-analysis can be an asset in exploring the interaction between interventions and patient-level characteristics. A Cochrane systematic review evaluating home safety education and provision of safety equipment for injury prevention was able to access individual patient data for certain research studies and therefore could estimate not only a total summarized effect but also variations in the intervention effect across social variables, child age, gender, ethnic groups, single-parent family, and measures of deprivation.[49,50]

Reviewers could also investigate the effect of intervention across different levels of disadvantage in groups and can inform programs aiming to reduce health inequalities. Disadvantaged groups can be identified, depending on the question of the review, by place of residence, race or ethnicity, occupation, gender, religion, education, socioeconomic position (SES) and social capital, sexual orientation, disability, and age.[51–53]

4. *Mediating factors in the interaction between intervention and outcome (context-dependent mediation and moderators).* Reviewers could identify and report potential modifying contextual moderators and mediating factors on the causal relationship of intervention to outcomes, provide a framework on how they can change the intervention, and finally provide research evidence about such context and modifying factors.[54] For example, a Cochrane systematic review on the effect of pharmaceutical pricing and purchasing policies on drug use, health care utilization, health outcomes, and costs also listed a summary of factors that could affect reference pricing like equivalence of the drug, incentives, and drug availability, and provided available evidence or a rational for them.[55-57]

■ SUMMARY

This chapter has raised questions about the reliability of much "evidence-based practice" disseminated from the original studies and systematic reviews of those studies, insofar as they were often conducted and reviewed with inadequate attention to external validity. Many important issues are raised for D&I researchers. Indeed, the pressure on investigators to provide for increasingly rigorous controls on threats to internal validity, and to exclude studies that fall below standards for internal validity, has made many such sources of evidence more suspect in their external validity and less credible to the practitioners or policymakers who would adopt them. Dissemination of such evidence as best practices for application "with fidelity" in wide-ranging settings, populations, and circumstances may imply that local discretion and professional judgment in adapting such interventions should be suppressed. Greater attention is needed to ways to incorporate considerations of external validity into studies and in systematic reviews of studies to produce more generalizable evidence, on one hand, and greater attention to practice-based evidence that can complement the more formal evidence-based practices in the process of implementing and evaluating the dissemination and implementation process, on the other hand.

SUGGESTED READINGS

Armstrong R, Waters E, Doyle J (editors). Chapter 21: Reviews in health promotion and public health. In Higgins JPT, Green S (editors). *Cochrane Handbook for Systematic Reviews of Interventions* Version 5.0.1 (updated September 2008). The Cochrane Collaboration, 2008. Available from www.cochrane-handbook.org.

The methods guide of the Cochrane public health review group to conduct systematic reviews of public health includes how to consider ethics, inequalities, context, sustainability, applicability, and transferability.

Deeks JJ, Higgins JPT, Altman DG (editors). Chapter 9: Analysing data and undertaking meta-analyses. In: Higgins JPT, Green S (editors). *Cochrane Handbook for Systematic Reviews of Interventions* Version 5.0.1 (updated September 2008). The Cochrane Collaboration, 2008. Available from www.cochrane-handbook.org.

The methods guide of the Cochrane Collaboration on how to synthesize data from primary trials in systematic reviews includes methods to deal with heterogeneity.

Lavis JN, Oxman AD, Souza NM, Lewin S, Gruen RL, Fretheim A. SUPPORT Tools for evidence-informed health policymaking (STP) 9: Assessing the applicability of the findings of a systematic review. *Health Res Policy Syst.* 2009 Dec 16;7(Suppl 1):S9.

Part of a series of articles to help people responsible for making decisions about health policies and to provide a guide on assessing the applicability of the findings of a systematic review to a specific setting.

Schünemann HJ, Fretheim A, Oxman AD. Improving the use of research evidence in guideline development: 13. Applicability, transferability and adaptation. *Health Res Policy Syst.* 2006 Dec 8;4:25.

A background paper on applicability, transferability, and adaptation of guidelines for the World Health Organization (WHO) advisory committee on Health research.

Schünemann HJ, Oxman AD, Vist GE, et al. Chapter 12: Interpreting results and drawing conclusions. In: Higgins JPT, Green S (editors), *Cochrane Handbook for Systematic Reviews of Interventions* Version 5.0.1 (updated September 2008). The Cochrane Collaboration, 2008. Available from www.cochrane-handbook.org.

The methods guide of the Cochrane Collaboration to interpret the result of synthesizing data in systematic reviews includes the methods to judge the applicability of the results.

Thorpe KE, Zwarenstein M, Oxman AD, et al. A pragmatic-explanatory continuum indicator summary (PRECIS): A tool to help trial designers. *CMAJ.* 2009 May 12;180(10):E47–E57.

A tool to determine the extent to which a clinical trial is pragmatic or explanatory.

Tugwell P, Petticrew M, Kristjansson E, et al. Assessing equity in systematic reviews: Realising the recommendations of the Commission on Social Determinants of Health. *BMJ.* 2010 Sep 13;341:c4739. DOI: 10.1136/bmj.c4739.

Guidance on assessing equity for users and authors of systematic reviews of interventions.

Welch V, Tugwell P, Petticrew M, et al. How effects on health equity are assessed in systematic reviews of interventions. *Cochrane Database Syst Rev.* 2010 Dec 8;12:MR000028.

A systematic review of methods to assess effects of health equity in systematic reviews of effectiveness of health care interventions.

West SL, Gartlehner G, Mansfield AJ, et al. Comparative effectiveness review methods: Clinical heterogeneity. In: Agency for Healthcare Research and Quality. Comparative Effectiveness Review Methods: Clinical Heterogeneity. Posted 09/28/2010. Available at http://effectivehealthcare.ahrq.gov/.

Summary and review of the current methods for addressing clinical heterogeneity in systematic reviews and comparative effectiveness research.

SELECTED WEBSITES AND TOOLS

Cancer Control P.L.A.N.E.T. <http://cancercontrolplanet.cancer.gov/index.html>. Cancer Control P.L.A.N.E.T. acts as a portal to provide access to data and resources for designing, implementing, and evaluating evidence-based cancer control programs. The site provides five steps (with links) for developing a comprehensive cancer control plan or program.

Task Force on Community Preventive Services <http://www.thecommunityguide.org>. The Community Guide provides a repository of the 200+ systematic reviews conducted by the Task Force, an independent, interdisciplinary group with staff support by the Centers for Disease Control and Prevention. Each review gives attention to the "applicability" of the conclusions beyond the study populations and settings in which the original studies were conducted.

Cochrane Collaboration. <http://www.cochrane.org/>. The Cochrane Collaboration prepares Cochrane Reviews and aims to update them regularly with the latest scientific evidence. Members of the organization (mostly volunteers) work together to assess evidence to help people make decisions about health care practices and policies. Some people read the health care literature to find reports of randomized controlled trials; others find such reports by searching electronic databases; others prepare and update Cochrane Reviews based on the evidence found in these trials; others work to improve the methods used in Cochrane Reviews; others provide a vitally important consumer perspective.

RE-AIM. <http://www.RE-AIM.org>. The acronym refers to Reach, Effectiveness, Adoption, Implementation, and Maintenance, all important dimensions in the consideration of D&I research and in the external validity or applicability of research results in original studies for the alternative settings and circumstances in which they might be applied. These were applied in the development of a set of guidelines for assessing and reporting external validity in reference 29 below.

The Center of Excellence for Training and Research Translation. <http://www.center-trt.org/>. The Center of Excellence for Training and Research Translation seeks to increase the public health impact of programs and policies to prevent obesity, heart disease, stroke, and other chronic diseases. The Center addresses these issues via training and intervention translation initiatives that extend their reach, improve their effectiveness, strengthen their adoption in real-world settings, improve the quality of their operations, and sustain their efforts over time.

Making research more relevant, useful and actionable in policy, program planning and practice. <http://rwjcsp.unc.edu/resources/articles/S187-S191.pdf>. This review and commentary on participatory and other strategies to increase external validity introduced a series of papers in a special issue of the *American Journal of Preventive Medicine*, December 2009, with a series of reports from community-based participatory research projects conducted under the Robert Wood Johnson Foundation's Clinical Scholars Program.

REFERENCES

1. Kreuter MW, Bernhardt JM. Reframing the dissemination challenge: A marketing and distribution perspective. *Am J Public Health*. 2009;Dec;99(12):2123–2127.
2. Mercer SL, MacDonald G, Green LW. Participatory research and evaluation: From best practices for all states to achievable practices within each state in the context of the Master Settlement Agreement. *Health Promot Pract*. 2004;July;5(3):167S–178S.
3. Green LW. From research to "best practices" in other settings and populations. *Am J Health Behav*. 2001;25:165–178.
4. Rothwell PM. External validity of randomised controlled trials: "To whom do the results of this trial apply?" *Lancet* 2005;365:82–93, quote from p. 82.
5. Green LW, Ottoson JM, Garcia C, Hiatt R. Diffusion theory and knowledge dissemination, utilization and integration. *Ann Rev Public Health*. 2009;30:151–174.
6. Campbell DT, Stanley JC. *Experimental and Quasi-Experimental Designs for Research*. Chicago: Rand McNally, 1963.

7. Egbert LD, Battit GE, Welch CE, Bartlett MK. Reduction of postoperative pain by encouragement and instruction of patients. A study of doctor-patient rapport. *N Engl J Med.* 1964;270:825–827.

8. Cronbach LJ, Ambron SR, Dornbusch SM, et al.. *Toward Reform of Program Evaluation.* San Francisco: Jossey-Bass, 1980.

9. Cronbach LJ. *Designing Evaluations of Educational and Social Programs.* San Francisco: Jossey-Bass, 1982.

10. Shadish WR, Cook TD, Campbell DT. *Experimental and Quasi-Experimental Designs for Generalized Causal Inference.* Boston, New York: Houghton Mifflin Co., 2002.

11. Cook TJ, Campbell DT, Eds. *Quasi-Experimentation, Design and Analysis Issues for Field Settings.* Chicago: Rand McNally, 1979.

12. Green LW, Lewis FM. *Measurement and Evaluation in Health Education and Health Promotion.* Palo Alto, CA: Mayfield Publishing Co., 1984.

13. Rogers EM. *Diffusion of Innovations.* New York, London, Toronto, Sydney: Free Press, 2003.

14. Mercer SM, DeVinney BJ, Fine LJ, Green LW, Dougherty D. Study designs for effectiveness and translation research: Identifying trade-offs. *Am J Prev Med.* 2007;33(2):139–154.

15. Sanson-Fisher RW, Bonevski B, Green LW, D'Este C. Limitations of the randomized controlled trial in evaluating population-based health interventions. *Am J Prev Med.* 2007;33(2):155–161.

16. Hawkins NG, Sanson-Fisher RW Shakeshaft A, D'Este C, Green, LW. The multiple-baseline design for evaluating population-based research. *Am J Prev Med.* 2007; 33(2):162–168.

17. Morisky DE, Levine DM, Green LW, Russell RP, Smith C. The relative impact of health education for low- and high-risk patients with hypertension. *Prev Med.* 1980;9:550–558.

18. Morisky DE, Levine DM, Green LW, Smith C. Health education program effects on the management of hypertension in the elderly. *Arch Intern Med.* 1982;142:1835–1838.

19 .Morisky DE, Levine DM, Green LW, Shapiro S, Russell RP, Smith CR. Five-year blood pressure control and mortality following health education for hypertensive patients. *Am J Public Health* 1983;73:153–162.

20. Levine DM, Green LW, Morisky D. Effect of a structured health education program on reducing morbidity and mortality from high blood pressure. *Bibl Cardiol.* 1987;48:8–16.

21. Levine DM, Green LW, Deeds SG, Chwalow AJ, Russell RP, and Finlay J. Health education for hypertension patients. *J Am Med Assoc.* 1979;241:1700–1703.

22. Terry PD, Abramson JL, Neaton JD; MRFIT Research Group. Blood pressure and risk of death from external causes among men screened for the Multiple Risk Factor Intervention Trial. *Am J Epidemiol.* 2007;165(3):294–301.

23. Tunis SR, Stryer DB, Clancey CM. Practical clinical trials: Increasing the value of clinical research for decision making in clinical and health policy. *JAMA* 2003;290:1624–1632.

24. Green LA, Hickner J. A short history of primary care practice-based research networks: From concept to essential research laboratories. *J Am Board Fam Med.* 2006;19:1–10.

25. Katz D, Murimi M, Gonzalez A, Nijike V, Green LW. From clinical trial to community adoption: The Multi-site Translational Community Trial (mTCT). *Am J*

*Public Health.*Published online ahead of print June 16, 2011:e1–e11. DOI:10.2105/AJPH.2010.300104.

26. Green LW, Kreuter MW. *Health Program Planning: An Educational and Ecological Approach.* New York: McGraw-Hill, 2005.

27. Centers for Disease Control and Prevention. *Best Practices for Comprehensive Tobacco Control Programs—August 1999.* Atlanta, GA: U.S. Department of Health and Human Services, Centers for Disease Control and Prevention, National Center for Chronic Disease Prevention and Health Promotion, Office on Smoking and Health, 1999.

28. Cohen DJ, Crabtree BF, Etz RS, et al.. Fidelity versus flexibility: Translating evidence-based research into practice. *Am J Prev Med.* 2008;35(5 Suppl):S381–S389.

29. Green LW, Glasgow RE. Evaluating the relevance, generalization, and applicability of research: Issues in external validation and translation methodology. *Eval Health Prof* 2006;29(1):126–153.

30. Green LW, Glasgow RE, Atkins D, Stange K. Making evidence from research more relevant, useful, and actionable in policy, program planning, and practice: Slips "twixt cup and lip." *Am J Prev Med.* 2009 Dec;37(6S1)S187– S191. Available at: http://rwjcsp.unc.edu/resources/articles/S187-S191.pdf.

31. Patrick K, Scutchfield FD, Woolf SH. External validity reporting in prevention research. *Am J Prev Med.* 2008;34(3):260–262.

32. Steckler A, McLeroy KR. The importance of external validity. *Am J Public Health.* 2008 Jan;98(1):9–10.

33. Glasgow RE, Green LW, Klesges LM, et al. External validity: We need to do more. *Ann Behav Med.* 2006 Apr;31(2):105–108.

34. Glasgow RE, Green LW, Ammerman A. A focus on external validity. *Eval Health Prof.* 2007;30(2):115–117.

35. Mercer, SL Green, LW. Federal funding and support for participatory research in public health and health care. In Minkler M, Wallerstein N (Eds.). *Community-Based Participatory Research in Health.* 2nd ed. San Francisco: Jossey-Bass, 2008, pp. 399–406.

36. Armstrong K, Green LW, Hayward RA, Rosenthal MS, Wells KB (Eds.). *Bridging Clinical Scholarship and Community Scholarship: New Directions for the Robert Wood Johnson Foundation's Clinical Scholars Program.* Special Issue of *Am J Prev Med.* 2009;37(6S1):S187–S191.

37. Green LW. The Prevention Research Centers as models of practice-based evidence: Two decades on. *Am J Prev Med* 2007;33(1S):S6–S8.

38. Ahmad N, Boutron I, Dechartres A, Durieux P, Ravaud P. Applicability and generalisability of the results of systematic reviews to public health practice and policy: A systematic review. *Trials.* 2010 Feb 26;11:20.

39. Hauck WW, Anderson S, Marcus SM. Should we adjust for covariates in nonlinear regression analyses of randomized trials? *Control Clin Trials.* 1998;19(3):249–256.

40. Harris J. Using qualitative research to develop robust effectiveness questions and protocols for Cochrane systematic reviews. In: Noyes J, Booth A, Hannes K, Harden A, Harris J, Lewin S, Lockwood C, eds. *Supplementary guidance for inclusion of qualitative research in Cochrane Systematic Reviews of interventions.* Version 1 (updated August 2011). Cochrane Collaboration Qualitative Methods Group, 2011. Available at: http://cqrmg.cochrane.org/supplemental-handbook-guidance.

41. Helfand M, Balshem H. AHRQ series paper 2: Principles for developing guidance: AHRQ and the effective health-care program. *J Clin Epidemiol.* 2010 May;63(5): 484–490. Epub 2009 Aug 27.

42. Zaza S, Briss PA, Harris KW. (Eds. for the Task Force on Community Preventive Services). *The Guide to Community Preventive Services: What Works to Promote Health?* New York: Oxford University Press, 2005.

43. The Task Force on Community Preventive Services. Recommendations for reducing excessive alcohol-related harms by limiting alcohol outlet density. *Am J Prev Med.* 2009;37(6):570–571.

44. Schulz KF, Altman DG, Moher D, CONSORT Group. CONSORT 2010 statement: Updated guidelines for reporting parallel group randomised trials. *PLoS Med* 2010;7(3):e1000251. DOI:10.1371/journal.pmed.1000251.

45. Klesges LM, Dzewaltowski DA, Glasgow RE. Review of external validity reporting in childhood obesity prevention research. *Am J Prev Med.* 2008;34(3):216–223.

46. Haraldsson B, Gross A, Myers CD, et al. Massage for mechanical neck disorders. *Cochrane Database of Systematic Reviews* 2006;Issue 3. Art. No.: CD004871. DOI: 10.1002/14651858.CD004871.pub3.

47. Thorpe KE, Zwarenstein M, Oxman AD, et al. A pragmatic-explanatory continuum indicator summary (PRECIS): A tool to help trial designers. *CMAJ.* 2009 May 12;180(10):E47–E57.

48. Sun X, Briel M, Busse JW, et al. Subgroup Analysis of Trials Is Rarely Easy (SATIRE): A study protocol for a systematic review to characterize the analysis, reporting, and claim of subgroup effects in randomized trials. *Trials.* 2009 Nov 9;10:101.

49. Stewart LA, Tierney JF, Clarke M. Chapter 19: Reviews of individual patient data. In: Higgins JPT, Green S (Eds.), *Cochrane Handbook for Systematic Reviews of Interventions* Version 5.0.1 (updated September 2008). The Cochrane Collaboration, 2008. Available from: www.cochrane-handbook.org.

50. Kendrick D, Coupland C, Mulvaney C, Simpson J, Smith SJ, Sutton A, Watson M, Woods A. Home safety education and provision of safety equipment for injury prevention. *Cochrane Database Systematic Reviews.* 2007 January 24;(1):CD005014. Review.

51. Armstrong R, Waters E, Doyle J (Eds.). Chapter 21: Reviews in health promotion and public health. In Higgins JPT, Green S (Eds.). *Cochrane Handbook for Systematic Reviews of Interventions.* Version 5.0.1 (updated September 2008). The Cochrane Collaboration, 2008. Available from: http://www.cochrane.org/resources/handbook.

52. Kavanagh J, Oliver S, Lorenc T (2008). Reflections on developing and using PROGRESS-Plus. Equity Update 2: 1–3 [online]. Available from: http://equity.cochrane.org/Files/Equity_Update_Vol2_Issue1.pdf [accessed 13 February 2009].

53. Berkey CS, Hoaglin DC, Mosteller F, Colditz GA. A random-effects regression model for meta-analysis. *Stat Med.* Feb 28 1995;14(4):395–411.

54. Fisher EB. The importance of context in understanding behavior and promoting health. *Ann Behav Med.* 2008;35:3–18.

55. Aaserud M, Austvoll-Dahlgren A, Kösters JP, Oxman AD, Ramsay C, Sturm H. Pharmaceutical policies: Effects of reference pricing, other pricing, and purchasing policies. *Cochrane Database of Systematic Reviews* 2006;Issue 2. Art. No.: CD005979. DOI: 10.1002/14651858.CD005979.

56. Lavis JN, Oxman AD, Souza NM, Lewin S, Gruen RL, Fretheim A. SUPPORT Tools for evidence-informed health Policymaking (STP) 9: Assessing the applicability of the findings of a systematic review. *Health Res Policy Syst.* 2009 Dec 16; 7(Suppl 1):S9.
57. Schünemann HJ, Oxman AD, Vist GE, et al. Chapter 12: Interpreting results and drawing conclusions. In: Higgins JPT, Green S (Eds.). *Cochrane Handbook for Systematic Reviews of Interventions* Version 5.0.1 (updated September 2008). The Cochrane Collaboration, 2008. Available from: www.cochrane-handbook.org.

16 Evaluation Approaches for Dissemination and Implementation Research

■ BRIDGET GAGLIO
AND RUSSELL E. GLASGOW

■ INTRODUCTION

This chapter focuses on evaluation issues and approaches to assessing dissemination and implementation (D&I) research. An important take-home point is that evaluation should be considered an ongoing process, rather than a one-time, post hoc activity. Like planning for dissemination, best results are obtained by an integrated series of evaluation activities stretching from initial needs assessment to formative evaluation, ongoing process evaluation, and finally summative evaluation, all of which are interactive and provide feedback to key stakeholders and decision makers. There is moderate overlap between this chapter and others on related topics, including those that focus on external validity, measurement issues, fidelity and adaptation, and designing for dissemination.

After a brief overview of the scope of evaluation activities relevant to D&I, several key evaluation approaches are reviewed, including their unique foci and contributions. The chapter focuses most heavily on the RE-AIM model,[1,2] including discussion of its evolution and status, followed by an exemplary case study applying RE-AIM to a translational project. Finally, we summarize the status of current research/practice and future directions in D&I-related evaluation. There is also an appendix that lists evaluation resources, including planning tools, websites, and an annotated bibliography.

■ ROLE OF EVALUATION IN TRANSLATIONAL RESEARCH

Preparation for dissemination should begin at the planning phase of a project or program and continue throughout and after implementation. For effective translation, it is necessary to bridge and integrate traditionally different evaluation approaches for evaluability and formative, process, and outcome/summative evaluations.[3] Evaluability assessments early on can also be useful in that they allow for preliminary evaluation of program design so that modifications can be made if necessary prior to full-scale implementation and subsequent evaluation.[3,4] In the future, we can look for increasing use of modeling, including simulations of the potential outcomes of proposed interventions under different assumptions, before large-scale trials are conducted.

Likewise, team science collaborations, which include cross-discipline and mixed-methods approaches to analyzing and evaluating research questions, should be considered.[5] Team science collaborations can take on many forms ranging from multidisciplinary versus interdisciplinary versus transdisciplinary.[5] Multidisciplinary refers to a process where researchers in different fields work independently, from their individual field's perspective, eventually coming together with others to blend their efforts to address the same research question.[5] Interdisciplinary differs in that researchers work together, drawing from their respective disciplines to address the same research question.[5] Transdisciplinary refers to researchers working together to create a shared theoretical frameworks and models that are a blend of all disciplines involved to address a research question.[5] Deciding which approach to use depends on the extent to which the research question of interest is suited for a collaborative approach. Having a transdisciplinary approach increases the potential to speed the rate at which a research program or project is translated into practice.[6] With a greater emphasis on the need for realistic evaluation of interventions[7] to address the multifactoral causes of health disparities, it makes sense that a transdisciplinary approach would also be needed in evaluation and translation of research.[8]

Evaluation should include a realist approach, an approach that is comprehensive in identifying how, and for whom, a program might work, as well as understanding the implementation of the program as proposed by Pawson and Tilley.[7] A broad array of techniques (both quantitative and qualitative) should also be included to best assess the quality and effectiveness of a particular program or policy. The goal of evaluation should be to understand the nature of the program, the context in which it was delivered, and the extent of limits on external validity.[7,9] Pawson and Tilley[7] propose that to fully understand the relationship between the intervention and outcome questions of the following form need to be asked, "What intervention is most effective, for whom (representativeness of participants/clients), under what circumstances (setting characteristics and staff delivering the program)?"[10,11] While identifying and describing the contextual environment is often key to understanding why an intervention did not work, evaluators are challenged with the task of studying complex interventions, settings, and participants, yet must be able to summarize the results in simple, understandable language for decision makers and the lay public. The frameworks and models reviewed throughout this chapter discuss the need to identify, describe, and understand the context in which a program or policy is implemented in order to understand outcomes.

■ EVALUATION APPROACHES

Many interventions found to be effective in health services research studies fail to translate into meaningful patient care outcomes, or across different contexts.[12] Barriers to implementation arise at multiple levels of health care delivery: the patient, the provider team or group, the organizational, and the policy levels.[13] Formative, process, and mixed-methods evaluations are useful to assess the extent to which implementation is effective in a specific context to optimize intervention benefits, prolong sustainability of the intervention in that context, and inform dissemination into other contexts.[14] While this chapter does not provide an exhaustive list, the following is a summary of several key evaluation frameworks that have been proven to be practical in translation of research findings. Some of the frameworks are intended to help guide both the development and evaluation of an intervention, while others are designed solely for evaluation.

Performance of Routine Information System Management (PRISM)

The PRISM framework is a comprehensive evaluation of routine health information systems. PRISM consists of a logic-model-like conceptual framework and data collection tools to assess, design, and evaluate routine health information. The framework proposes that inputs (technical and behavioral determinants of process and performance) influence processes (data collection, data transmission, data analyses, and quality), which in turn effect outputs (information use), outcomes (improved health system performance), and impact (improved health status).[15] The framework's underlying assumption is that routine information system management is a system with a defined performance and that performance is determined by the information management process. This process is influenced by three contextual factors: technical (i.e., complexity of reporting), organizational (i.e., governance, training, supervision), and behavioral (i.e., competence in tasks, motivation, data demand). The framework assesses whether these three factors act directly to influence the routine information system management process and performance, or if technical and organizational factors act indirectly through behavioral factors.[15] In addition to describing the relationship of these three key factors to the performance of routine information system management, the framework measures their importance as well as evaluates the impact on health system performance and health status. We note that this framework is different from the PRISM framework of Feldstein and Glasgow,[16] who have added explicit organizational roles to the RE-AIM model discussed below to develop their PRISM model.

Cost per Quality Adjusted Life Year (QALY)

Is it cost-effective? This question is increasingly asked about health interventions as we attempt to achieve the greatest benefit from limited health care resources[17] and has typically been least often reported in evaluation efforts.[18,19] Increasingly, cost-effectiveness analysis (CEA), which attempts to identify how much good is achieved for each dollar spent, is playing a greater role in the evaluation of health interventions. One form of cost-effectiveness analysis is the quality-adjusted life year (QALY). QALY is an economic evaluation used in CEA to compare relevant health outcomes from different health interventions.[17,20] The measure combines both quantity and quality into a single measure, such as cost per pound lost or cost per smoker who quits. Although not really a model of D&I, QALY-related concepts have been influential in driving the D&I field and are included in most evaluation models, either implicitly or explicitly. We note that QALY approaches have recently become quite controversial and are actually proscribed from being used in at least some federally funded comparative effectiveness research for political reasons.[21]

Evaluability Assessment

Evaluability assessment was developed in the late 1970s in response to the challenge of dealing with programs that were unsuitable for evaluation.[4] This assessment method consists of six steps to be conducted prior to investing in a large-scale project: (1) involving the intended users of evaluation information, (2) clarifying the intended program, (3) exploring program reality, (4) reaching agreement on needed changes in activities or goals, (5) exploring alternative evaluation designs, and (6) agreeing on evaluation priorities and intended uses of information. This model is participatory in that it involves stakeholders using an iterative process to create a logic model that represents the expectations, goals, and rationale for the project.[4] Once the logic model is completed, a plausibility assessment is conducted. This involves assessment on whether outcomes are achievable given the context of the project, time frame, resources available and allocation, and implementation efforts of the project. Plausibility analysis lays the ground work for the formal evaluation. While evaluability assessment has its roots in the core functions of public health, it is now being used in translating research into practice. As evidence-based programs are being implemented, evaluability assessment can test assumptions about the program being tested in a new context and setting. This method can guide adaptations to real-world conditions or raise a warning early on that constraints are too great for implementation.[4]

Realist Evaluation

A realist approach to evaluation, while not specific to D&I, stresses a number of contextual factors and philosophy-of-science approaches congruent with it. The realist approach to evaluation and reviews of the literature[7,22] emphasizes contextual factors, considering data from a variety of types of designs. It places value on qualitative as well as quantitative data, on factors influencing implementation, and in particular, on not assuming that intervention results generalize across settings, staff, implementers, or different patient subgroups. Their approach is summarized as attempting to answer the questions in the form: "Which intervention conducted by what staff, conducted under what conditions, is most effective, in producing what outcomes?"[7]

Promoting Action on Research Implementation in Health Services (PARiHS)

The Promoting Action on Research Implementation in Health Services framework is a framework for guiding the implementation of evidence-based practice and was originally proposed by Kitson et al.[23] as an alternative to existing linear and unidimensional models of research to practice. The framework consisted of three elements: (1) evidence, (2) context, and (3) facilitation. Instead of a hierarchy or linearity cause-and-effect model, all of the dimensions are considered simultaneously.[23]

Each element in the framework (evidence, context, and facilitation) includes a number of subelements that were revisited in 2002.[24,25] The revision included content analysis by critically reviewing the literature to further develop the subelements included within the framework. Evidence consists of research, clinical experience, and patient experience; context consists of leadership, culture, and evaluation; and high facilitation includes a match between the purpose and role of facilitation with the skills and attributes of the facilitator. Each of the elements is ranked on a scale from low to high. Several empirical studies have provided support for the PARiHS framework by demonstrating that successful implementation is a function of evidence, context, and facilitation.[26–28] However, it is still unclear if the elements or subelements have equal weighting in getting evidence into practice.[29]

Pragmatic-Explanatory Continuum Indicator Summary (PRECIS)

The Pragmatic-Explanatory Continuum Indicator Summary (PRECIS) tool is used to assist researchers in designing trials by identifying and quantifying research study characteristics that differentiate pragmatic and explanatory trials.[30] A pragmatic trial attempts to answer the question "Does this intervention work under usual conditions?" whereas an explanatory trial addresses the question "Does this intervention work under ideal conditions?" The PRECIS tool consists of 10 domains identified as being critical to distinguishing pragmatic trials from explanatory trials. The domains are: (1) participant eligibility criteria, (2) flexibility of experimental intervention, (3) experimental intervention—practitioner expertise, (4) flexibility of the comparison intervention, (5) comparison intervention—practitioner expertise, (6) follow-up intensity, (7) primary trial outcome, (8) participant compliance with "prescribed" intervention, (9) practitioner adherence to study protocol, and (10) analysis of the primary outcome. The tool consists of a "spoke-and-wheel plot" where the explanatory end of the continuum is the hub, and the pragmatic end is the outside edge. Each spoke is labeled with a domain. Each domain is then marked along the range of the spoke to indicate how pragmatic versus explanatory (using a 0 to 4 rating scale) the trial is on that dimension. The dots are then connected to create a visual representation of where a trial falls along the continuum (Figure 16–1).[30,31] We view PRECIS as an important advance to help us get beyond arguments of efficacy versus effectiveness or demonstration trials, and of randomized controlled trials versus alternative designs. It also helps to facilitate transparency in reporting, and to emphasize that no trial is completely explanatory or completely pragmatic. We hope that, since it is promoted by the CONSORT Work Group on Pragmatic Trials, the PRECIS scale and associated diagrams will be widely adopted for planning and reporting studies.

■ CASE STUDY

Quality Enhancement Research Initiative (QUERI)—U.S. Department of Veterans Affairs (VA)

QUERI was launched in 1998 as a key component of the Veterans Health Administration's efforts to systematically examine and improve its quality of care.[32]

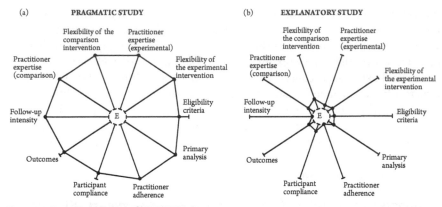

Figure 16–1. Examples of PRECIS diagrams.

QUERI is a combination of clinical care delivery, health services research, and policy actions intended to identify and implement best practices in all VA health care settings. The QUERI process consists of six steps:

1. identify high-risk, high-volume diseases or problems,
2. identify best practices,
3. define existing practice patterns and outcomes across the VA and current variation from best practices,
4. identify and implement interventions to promote best practices,
5. document that best practices improve outcomes, and
6. document that outcomes are associated with improved health-related quality of life.[32,33]

Within Step 4, implementation efforts follow a series of four phases to ensure the spread of effective and sustainable implementation programs across the VA system. These include: (a) single-site pilot, (b) small-scale, multisite implementation trial, (c) large-scale, multiregion implementation trial, and (d) system-wide rollout.[33]

The VA currently uses nine, condition-specific QUERI centers across the United States to identify gaps in quality of care and performance and has recently funded a new cross-condition eHealth QUERI focused on the Veteran's Administration health portal, My Healthy Vet.

QUERI Centers:

* Chronic Heart Failure
* Diabetes Mellitus
* HIV/Hepatitis
* Ischemic Heart Disease
* Mental Health
* Polytrauma and Blast-Related Injuries
* Spinal Cord Injury
* Stroke
* Substance Use Disorders

The QUERI process is iterative and was designed to improve and accelerate the systematic translation of evidence-based practices throughout the VA system and to improve patient outcomes. Much has been written on the VA's experiences and lessons learned on their system-wide implementation and translation efforts. The focus of the current literature has been on Steps 1–5 of the QUERI process and Phases 1 and 2.[34] It is clear that through the QUERI process, the VA has systematically and dramatically improved both the quality and the outcomes of care for many illnesses.[35–39] These improvements are one of the great success stories of the D&I field.

PRECEDE-PROCEED Model

PRECEDE-PROCEED is a planning and evaluation model that combines educational approaches with ecological approaches to the assessment and strategy planning for public health interventions and population-based health programs.[40] The original PRECEDE model was developed in the 1970s and has probably been more widely used than any other model to plan and evaluate public health interventions (http://www.lgreen.net/precede.htm). The acronym PRECEDE means—Predisposing, Reinforcing, and Enabling Constructs in Educational/ Environmental Diagnosis and Evaluation. This part of the model recognizes the need for assessment prior to intervention planning. In the early 1990s, PROCEED was added to the model.[40] The acronym PROCEED stands for—Policy, Regulatory, and Organizational Constructs in Educational and Environmental Development. These factors were added to the model to recognize the importance of environmental and contextual factors as determinants of health, and they seem particularly applicable today with the recent focus on social and built environment determinants of health behavior. The model was revised in 2005 and now consists of six phases: (1) social assessment and situational analysis, (2) epidemiological assessment, (3) educational and ecological assessment, (4) administrative and policy assessment and intervention alignment, (5) implementation, and (6) process evaluation (short-term and long-term outcomes). Due to the flexibility and scalability of this model, it has been widely used to guide the design and evaluation of many public health programs. PRECEDE-PROCEEED provides a structured framework to apply health behavior theories at all levels.[41] Moreover, the model stresses a multidisciplinary approach and evaluation of the multitude of factors that impact health and well-being.

Getting to Outcomes (GTO)

The Getting to Outcomes (GTO) framework of Chinman and colleagues helps users plan and implement programs that are more likely to produce their intended outcomes in real-world settings[42,43] GTO was developed to address the gap between prevention research and practice by building capacity at both the individual and program levels for planning, implementing, evaluating, and sustaining evidence-based practices. The GTO framework has users respond to a series of 10 accountability questions. Each question is associated with a specific step in the GTO process. Six questions are associated with planning, two with process and outcome evaluation, and two on the use of data to improve and sustain programs.[43] The 10 questions are:

1. What are the underlying needs and conditions in the community?
2. What are the goals, target populations, and objectives?
3. Which evidence-based models and best practice programs can be useful in reaching the goals?
4. What actions need to be taken so the selected program "fits" the community context?
5. What organizational capacities are needed to implement the plan?
6. What is the plan for this program?
7. How will the quality of the program and/or initiative implementation be assessed?
8. How well did the program work?
9. How will continuous quality improvement strategies be incorporated?
10. If the program is successful, how will it be sustained?

The unique value of the GTO framework is that it keeps the focus on outcomes and on the impact of processes on outcomes—rather than being concerned primarily with fidelity to a fixed protocol.

Consolidated Framework for Implementation Research (CFIR)

Finally, as summarized in Table 16–1, the CFIR is a meta-theoretical framework that consists of five domains that can be used to guide how implementation is planned, organized, and conducted.[12] It has been developed relatively recently and is intended to synthesize key aspects of earlier models of implementation and evaluation. The five domains of the CFIR are: the intervention, inner setting (internal context), outer setting (external context), the individuals involved, and the process by which implementation is accomplished[12] Within each of the five domains, constructs from implementation are classified. The framework provides a synthesis of published models, theories, and frameworks from within the health care field. In addition, it offers a consistent terminology and set of definitions for the field of implementation.[12] The intervention refers to the characteristics of the intervention (core components and adaptable periphery) being implemented into a particular site or organization. The outer setting includes the social, economic, and political context within which a site exists, and the inner setting includes characteristics of cultural, structural, and political contexts through which the implementation process will occur. The individuals involved with the intervention and/or implementation process impact the intervention, consciously and unconsciously. Finally, understanding the process by which implementation occurs helps to explain and inform outcomes. This framework can be used to: (1) identify potential influences of implementation and to make comparisons across studies through the different stages of assessment prior to implementation, (2) adaptation of the intervention to sites, (3) real-time observation of implementation fidelity and progress toward outcome goals, and (4) evaluation of sustainability and prospects for wider dissemination after the study is completed.[12]

TABLE 16–1. *Summary of Selected Evaluation Approaches for Dissemination and Implementation Research*

Evaluation Method	Acronym	Summary
Performance of Routine Information System Management Framework	PRISM[15]	* The framework consists of inputs (determinants of process and performance), processes (data collection, data transmission, data analyses, and quality), outputs (information use), outcomes (improved health system performance), and impact (improved health status) * Promotes objective measurement of data quality and the degree to which the information is used in evidence-based decisions * Application in diverse countries
Cost Per Quality Adjusted Life Year	QALY[20]	* QALY is an economic evaluation used in cost-effectiveness analysis to compare across health outcomes from different health interventions * The measure combines both cost and primary outcomes into a single measure
Evaluability Assessment	N/A[4]	* Was developed in the late 1970s in response to the challenge of dealing with programs that were unsuitable for evaluation * Consists of six steps: (1) involving the intended users of evaluation information, (2) clarifying the intended program, (3) exploring program reality, (4) reaching agreement on needed changes in activities or goals, (5) exploring alternative evaluation designs, and (6) agreeing on evaluation priorities and intended uses of information * This model is participatory in that it involves stakeholders using an iterative process to create a logic model that represents the expectations, goals, and rationale for the project
Realist Evaluation	N/A[7]	* Emphasizes importance of context and does not assume broad generalization * Answers question of what intervention for what type of patient in what setting delivered under what conditions is most effective on what outcome?
Promoting Action on Research Implementation in Health Services	PARiHS[29]	* Successful implementation is defined as a function of evidence, context, and facilitation. * Evidence consists of research, clinical experience, and patient experience. * Context consists of leadership, culture, and evaluation. * Facilitation includes a match between the purpose and role of facilitation with the skills and attributes of the facilitator.

(continued)

TABLE 16-1. *Continued*

Evaluation Method	Acronym	Summary
Pragmatic-Explanatory Continuum Indicator Summary	PRECIS[30]	* A tool to assess and identify the position of any given trial along the pragmatic-explanatory continuum * Identifies 10 domains for study design decisions to determine the degree to which a trial is pragmatic or explanatory * Intended to inform trial design and systematic reviews
U.S. Department of Veterans Affairs - Quality Enhancement Research Initiative	QUERI[14,32,33]	* Large-scale, multidisciplinary quality improvement initiative designed to ensure excellence in all areas where the VA provides health care services * A six-step process is utilized where researchers collaborate with VA policy and practice leaders, clinicians, and operations staff to implement evidence-based practices into routine care.
PRECEDE-PROCEED Planning Model	PRECEDE-PROCEED[40]	* Model that links intervention planning and evaluation into one integrated framework * Comprehensive model emphasizing a multidisciplinary approach assessing the multiple factors that impact and influence health * Six phase model: (1) social assessment and situational analysis, (2) epidemiological assessment, (3) educational and ecological assessment, (4) administrative and policy assessment and intervention alignment, (5) implementation, and (6) process evaluation (short-term and long-term outcomes)
Getting to Outcomes	GTO[42,43]	* Was developed to address the gap between prevention research and practice by building capacity at both the individual and program levels * Ten accountability questions * Emphasis is on planning, implementation, evaluation, and sustainment.
Consolidated Framework for Implementation Research	CFIR[12]	* Emphasis is on identifying and understanding potential influences on implementation. * Comprises common constructs from published implementation theories—"meta-theoretical" * Consists of five major domains: the intervention, inner and outer settings, the individuals involved, and the process by which implementation is accomplished
Reach, Effectiveness, Adoption, Implementation, and Maintenance	RE-AIM[1]	* Emphasizes five dimensions that together determine public health impact * Places equal emphasis on external and internal validity * Evaluates results at both the setting/contextual and individual levels

In summary, while each framework and model has its unique strengths and limitations, all of the conceptual models for D&I tend to emphasize several common themes. First, implementation is heavily dependent on context, and one needs to conduct a needs assessment and be sensitive to local conditions, history, and resources. Second, as discussed in more detail in Chapter 14 on fidelity adaptation, quality of implementation is a frequent challenge, and programs are almost never implemented exactly as they were designed or tested in efficacy studies. Third, both implementation and dissemination are complex multilevel undertakings, not easily explained by simplistic models or appropriately evaluated by reductionistic designs. Finally, traditional evaluation and research methods tend to ignore or undervalue the importance of several D&I factors such as reach and engagement of the target audience in partnership research;[44] the need to consider setting, delivery staff, organizational and individual factors and their interactions;[45] and the issue of cost and cost effectiveness. The important point from our perspective is not to argue about the minor differences among approaches or to say which one is "best," but rather to have program developers and evaluators select a framework, or combination of frameworks, that fits their question and needs and to use the framework(s) consistently to evaluate results—including collecting data on factors hypothesized by the model to produce outcomes. Next, following a discussion of the importance and need for greater incorporation of qualitative methods, we consider in detail the history, development, and application of the RE-AIM model, the conceptual approach with which we have worked most intensively.

Qualitative Methods in Evaluation

Qualitative evaluation methods are an essential part of the range of tools that evaluators can draw upon. Certain questions, problems, and purposes are more fitting with qualitative methods than with others, and these approaches can almost always be used to help understand and explain quantitative findings. Qualitative methods can be used in evaluation work to provide detail and context to the interpretation of statistical data.[46] Qualitative approaches to evaluation are themselves diverse. They can range from formative studies, to outcome evaluation, to process studies, to implementation evaluation, to program comparisons, to documenting development over time, to investigating system change, and to conducting "postmortem" exams to explore unanticipated results.[46] Qualitative evaluations often rely on a handful of data collection methods. Methods include focus groups, case studies, in-depth interviews, and observational field notes. Integrating qualitative methods with more traditional quantitative evaluation methods lends depth and clarity to understanding outcomes.

■ RE-AIM PLANNING AND EVALUATION FRAMEWORK

Initial Years: 1999–2003

The RE-AIM framework, which is an acronym for Reach, Effectiveness, Adoption, Implementation, and Maintenance, is just over 10 years old. The first RE-AIM publication was in late 1999.[1] The model grew out of frustration with the lack of reporting on key issues related to implementation, replication, and generalizablity of much of the health care research literature.[2] RE-AIM was developed partially as a response to trends toward research conducted under optimal efficacy conditions (e.g., studying highly motivated patients with only one medical condition admitted to the study; intensive and costly interventions implemented by content experts in world-class medical or academic settings). The problem was not so much that this type of research was being conducted, but that it was increasingly being considered the only type of valid research and was always the "gold standard" for decision making and guidelines. In addition, the results of one "stage" of research, such as efficacy, were also assumed to necessarily also be the best candidate for later stages in the then popular Greenwald-Cullen[47] or Flay[48] stages of research model.[9] Although intended to be used at all stages of research from planning through evaluation, RE-AIM elements do follow a logical sequence beginning with adoption and reach, followed by implementation and efficacy/effectiveness, and finishing with maintenance, as shown in Figure 16–2.

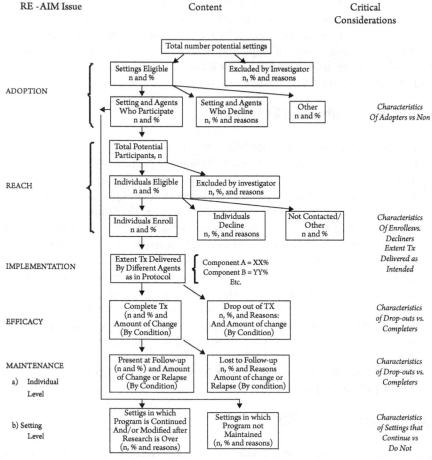

Figure 16–2. Extended CONSORT diagram.

The goal of RE-AIM is to address several key issues in program or policy delivery and results that, together, dramatically increase the probability that it can be successfully implemented and sustained in a large number of settings. An important point is that RE-AIM includes elements related to both internal and external validity. It was intended to help program developers, researchers, and decision makers needing to evaluate a program focus on five key issues necessary for success. The definitions of each of these five elements are given in Table 16–2 and explained in more detail elsewhere.[2,49] Several issues that are commonly misinterpreted about RE-AIM are emphasized here:

1. RE-AIM addresses issues at both the individual level (Reach, Effectiveness) and the setting/staff level (Adoption and Implementation). The maintenance dimension has components on both levels.
2. Consistency (or lack of consistency) of results is important at each level. Thus, RE-AIM is concerned not only with overall mean results, but also with impacts on subgroups related to health disparities, by different implementation staff, in different settings, and so on. RE-AIM requires that robustness or generalizability across these and other key dimensions be demonstrated and reported—not just assumed.
3. Cost is important in the RE-AIM model.[2,50,51] It is considered under the implementation factor as cost is one of the key questions decision makers have when considering practical issues such as who can implement a program, what resources it requires, and so on.
4. RE-AIM is congruent with, and not opposed to, efficacy research. It simply asks that researchers report transparently (for example, using TREND—Transparent Reporting of Evaluations with Nonrandomized Designs or

TABLE 16–2. *RE-AIM Guidelines for Developing, Selecting, and Evaluating Programs and Policies Intended to Have a Public Health Impact*

RE-AIM Element	Guidelines and Questions to Ask
REACH Percent and representativeness of participants	Can the program attract a large and representative percent of the target population? Can the program reach those most in need and most often left out (i.e., the poor, low-literacy- and numeracy, complex patients)?
EFFECTIVENESS Impact on key outcomes, quality of life, unanticipated outcomes and subgroups	Does the program produce robust effects across subpopulations? Does the program produce minimal negative side effects and increase quality of life or broader outcomes (i.e., social capital)?
ADOPTION Percent and representativeness of settings and staff that participate	Is the program feasible for the majority of real-world settings (costs, expertise, time, resources, etc.)? Can it be adopted by low-resource settings and typical staff serving high-risk populations?
IMPLEMENTATION Consistency and cost of delivering program and adaptations made	Can the program be consistently implemented across program elements, different staff, time, etc.? Are the costs—personnel, up-front, marginal, scale-up, equipment costs—reasonable to match effectiveness?
MAINTENANCE Long-term effects at individual and setting levels, modifications made	Does the program include principles to enhance long-term improvements (i.e., follow-up contact, community resources, peer support, ongoing feedback)? Can the settings sustain the program over time without added resources and leadership?

See www.re-aim.org or http://www.center-trt.org/index.cfm?fa=webtraining.reaim for more information.

PRECIS—Pragmatic-Explanatory Continuum Indicator Summary) on the procedures used and detail both inclusions and exclusions made at the contextual levels of settings and staff, as well as at the patient level. As seen in Figure 16–2, this extends the usual CONSORT reporting and figure to include actions taken and results both before the typical CONSORT requirements[52] in terms of selection of settings and staff, and also at the end of program to report on longer-term sustainability at both setting and individual levels.

Another focus of RE-AIM has been on the multiple levels of participants (patients or end users; citizens), providers or staff; and settings (workplaces, schools, communities). The issues of selections, exclusions, participation rates, and representativeness at the setting and staff levels are just as important as at the individual participant level but receive much less research attention.

RE-AIM was developed by thinking through the issues related to program impact at each phase of conducting a program or policy, beginning with a logic model of hypothesized effects[2] and then sequentially working through the process of recruitment (at the sequential setting, staff, and patient levels), implementation, and short-term and longer-term outcomes. As can be seen in Figure 16–2, this logical process resulted in a slightly different acronym of "ARIEM" (sequentially the "steps" of Adoption, Reach, Implementation, Effectiveness, and Maintenance). However, the initial RE-AIM developers of Glasgow et al.[1] decided that such a tongue-twisting acronym that did not have any intuitive connotation would not be likely to be recalled, so opted for the RE-AIM acronym.

In the early years, RE-AIM focused primarily on summative and quantitative evaluations and emphasized the need to include information on reach in reporting intervention outcomes.[1,53,54] Although RE-AIM was always intended to apply to evaluation of all types of interventions, including programs, policies, and environmental interventions, it was primarily operationalized in evaluating face-to-face behavioral interventions in its initial applications. These first applications were predominantly focused on research reports by the original RE-AIM team and their colleagues and dealt with health behavior change in areas such as smoking cessation, dietary and physical activity change, and diabetes self-management.

Phase 2 of RE-AIM: Expansion, Reviews, and Website

The first explicit funding received to support and develop the RE-AIM model was from the Robert Wood Johnson Foundation (RWJF), and coordinated with our foundation partner Dr. Robin Mockenhaupt, as part of the National Institutes of Health (NIH)–sponsored Behavior Change Consortium (BCC).[55] The RWJF grant funded a BCC cross-grant RE-AIM translation workgroup and added colleagues including Drs. Sheana Bull, David Dzewaltowski, Paul Estabrooks, Lisa Klesges, Marcia Ory, Lisa Strycker, and Deborah Toobert. Members of this group, along with Dr. Glasgow, conducted several reviews of the health behavior change literature in different settings including worksites, health care settings, schools, and communities. The key findings and lessons learned from these reviews were summarized in Glasgow et al.[18] and included findings that: an increasing number of studies reported on participant recruitment rates; no standard definitions of reach were used, and there were few reports of the representativeness of participants; many studies reported on maintenance at the individual level, but almost none at the setting level; and there were very few reports of adoption at the setting or staff level. As part of this review, we called for more transparent reporting of results throughout all phases of a study, and for more reports to including quality-of-life outcomes, unanticipated results, and program delivery costs.[18]

This BCC workgroup, along with other researchers, also expanded the range of content areas to which RE-AIM was applied to include healthy aging, policy change interventions,[56] medication safety, cancer screening, depression, and quality improvement. One of the key products of the BCC translation work group was the creation of the RE-AIM website, www.re-aim.org, originally hosted at Kansas State University, and currently hosted at the National Cancer Institute, Rockville, Maryland. The website is intended to provide resources, tools, and guidance for applying the RE-AIM model for program planning and evaluation, as well as in reporting of results and conducting literature reviews using the model. This version of the website included separate sections for researchers and practitioners, a list of RE-AIM-related publications, and presentations. This phase also included the first use of interactive tools, specifically the "RE-AIM Self-Rating Quiz" (http:// tools.re-aim.org/quiz/intro.html) to help individuals to conduct "virtual reviews" of their intended interventions before, during, and after their implementation to identify areas of potential limitation and provide suggestions for remediation.[57]

Although always intended to be used for both program and policy planning as well as post hoc evaluation, until 2004, the vast majority of RE-AIM applications were retrospective uses of the model for analyzing outcomes. The first proactive use of the model to help implementers evaluate programs while they were ongoing and adaptations were possible was as part of the Active for Life Program, funded by the RWJF and directed by Dr. Marcia Ory.[58] Members of the BCC Translation Workgroup met individually with the funded sites and assisted grantees with RE-AIM computer applications, including the self-rating quiz and other newly developed interactive applications such as the reach (http://www.re-aim.org/tools/ calculations/use-the-reach-calculator.aspx) and adoption (http://www.re-aim. org/tools/calculations/use-the-adoption-calculator.aspx) calculators.

This middle period also saw the first application of RE-AIM in requests for grant applications. The model was used as part of several CDC calls for proposals, and the most comprehensive and prescribed use was as part of the RWJF Prescription for Health Program[59] (http://www.prescriptionforhealth.org/). Applicants were required to include RE-AIM in their evaluation plans, which focused on practical applications to address multiple health behaviors (e.g., smoking, eating patterns, regular physical activity, risky drinking) in primary care–based research networks.[60,61]

Finally, as the RE-AIM model achieved greater exposure, new questions were raised about its application to community and nonindividual-focused applications. Many of these issues were addressed in the manuscript on policy by Jilcott et al.[56] Several of the RE-AIM definitions and measures transferred directly, but adaptations were made concerning adoption and implementation dimensions. The RE-AIM framework clarifies why policies are often more impactful than programs at community or target population levels, because of their greater reach and ease of implementation, but also points out dangers of "unfunded mandates," when sufficient resources are not provided or regulatory policies are allowed to "sunset."

The other issue that emerged around this time was that of "summary metrics" to characterize the overall public health impact of a program. At presentations and in website queries, colleagues would ask, "Which of the RE-AIM dimensions is the most important?" or "Some programs are better on some dimensions, while others are better on others; so which has the most public health impact?" This later question was, in fact, illustrated by the results of the few studies on which there were enough data across RE-AIM dimensions to compare different programs.[50]

From the original conceptualization of RE-AIM, we had intended that all dimensions receive equal weight, or were treated as equally important. In fact, our original paper contained a proposal to provide a summary score by multiplying RE-AIM scores across the five dimensions, but this was rejected by reviewers as too speculative. In 2006, a group of RE-AIM investigators[51] proposed several "RE-AIM metrics" or summary scores, depending upon the purpose, audience, and use to be made of the summary score. We cannot review all the background, rationale, or formulas proposed in that article (which contained both more detailed calculations for each of the five dimensions, as well as ways to combine the dimensions) but mention four summary metrics here:

1. *The Individual Impact Summary Score*: This metric is calculated by multiplying the "Composite Reach" indicator (0–1 score of participation ratio adjusted to account for representativeness and health disparities) by the "Composite Effectiveness" score (0–1) indicator on the primary outcome minus any negative impacts on quality of life or other measures and adjusted for variation in impact across participant subgroups.
2. *The Efficiency Score*, which is the cost of the intervention divided by the Individual Impact score.
3. *The Setting Level Impact Score*, which multiplies the composite Adoption score (0–1 adjusted for representativeness of settings and staff that participate) by the Implementation composite score (0–1 adjusted for inconsistencies across settings, staff, time, and program elements), and finally
4. Graphical or bar chart comparisons of the 0–1 RE-AIM scores on the different dimensions.

It was felt that each of these summary indices had advantages and limitations. The first two scores were recommended for cases in which stakeholders were more comfortable with calculations and composite scores and demanded a quantitative outcome. The more "transparent" and straightforward visual displays were recommended for settings such as community groups and especially for planning purposes when no actual data were available, but estimates and decisions needed to be made.

This issue of overall or summary scores is in need of further research, as none of the solutions above are completely satisfactory. The current formulas in Glasgow et al.[50,51] are not particularly user friendly, they have no absolute anchor or norms for interpretation, and are not possible to calculate if there are missing values.

Phase 3 of RE-AIM: 2008–Present: Website Revision and Broader Application

Recently, the RE-AIM model has been applied more widely, both to more diverse content areas and by research teams in over 30 countries including Australia, Canada, the United Kingdom, The Netherlands, and Taiwan. The RE-AIM model is now 10 years old from the date of the first publication in late 1999, and in early 2010, we located what was to our knowledge the 100th publication on RE-AIM that used the model to frame the article or analyze results (many others and numerous grants mention RE-AIM in the introduction or discussion but have not yet operationalized or presented data or addressed methods issues using the model).

Figure 16–3 summarizes the growth in RE-AIM publications over the past decade. As can be seen, there has been a gradually increasing trend in the number of publications using the model. As of this writing, we are aware of a total of 137 publications that have substantively used the model, and we have identified RE-AIM publications by 69 different primary authors. Citations for these articles, and related abstracts when available, are listed by year in the new version of the RE-AIM website (www.re-aim.org), which was revised in early 2010.

The revised website also contains an updated list of recent talks and presentations, and notices of upcoming and recent conferences related to RE-AIM issues. As shown in Figure 16–4, this revision makes more information available in one or two clicks. It is now easier to find interactive tools; the "Self-Rating Quiz" is more prominently displayed; RE-AIM related figures, graphs, and images as well as quotes on the site are rotated upon each new visit. We now include a list of the pages and content most frequently accessed over the past week, and it is easier to directly access information on the five key RE-AIM dimensions. Use of

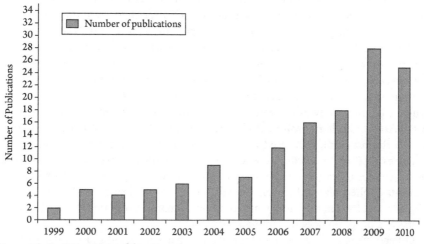

Figure 16–3. RE-AIM publications by year.

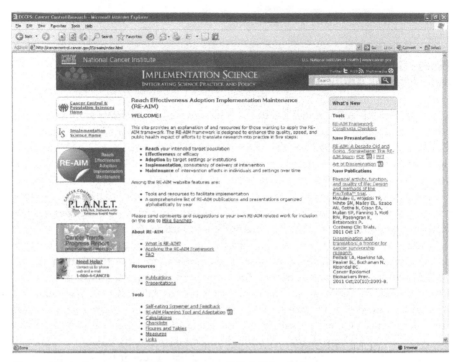

Figure 16-4. Screen shot of home page—RE-AIM website.

the website has gradually increased, and spikes in use are typically seen when new RE-AIM talks or publications appear, or the model is referred to in an RFA or Call for Papers. Over the last several months, approximately 3,500 different users visited the site per week.

In recent years the RE-AIM model has been used by more applied and community organizations. Of particular note are the CDC Healthy Aging Program, which developed a monograph based on RE-AIM for their state programs[62] and developed and cosponsored RE-AIM resources at a national meeting on aging at the Rosalynn Carter Institute; and the Kaiser Permanente Colorado Community Benefit Program, which provides grants to communities to enhance healthy eating and active living[63] and uses RE-AIM to work with grantees to collaboratively develop and evaluate their programs. Work on the Kaiser Community Benefit Program led indirectly to a recently published manuscript detailing the application of RE-AIM to built environment change programs.[64] Dr. Diane King, lead evaluator on the program, partnered with other RE-AIM researchers and community benefit evaluators to discuss how RE-AIM can be operationalized to fit environmental change programs and be accessible to community groups[40,44] Most RE-AIM elements applied reasonably well, but adaptations needed to be made as targets for adoption and implementation of environmental change programs changed over the course of a program or policy implementation.[64]

Other more recent trends include greater emphasis on mixed and qualitative methods to supplement quantitative measures. In particular, qualitative analysis of the context in which interventions are attempted have been emphasized in recent writings. There also is increasing congruence between RE-AIM and other approaches such as the PRECIS criteria from the CONSORT pragmatic trials work group and publications on practical and pragmatic trials[30,31] and complex interventions,[65] all of which place enhanced emphasis on external validity, feasibility, application to real-world settings, and transparency in reporting.

The cost of delivering programs and polices has been discussed as part of implementation in RE-AIM for several years but is now receiving substantially greater attention. Dr. Ritzwoller, in particular, has focused on replication cost issues, and on including costs of recruitment, as well as training, implementation, and maintenance in programs intended for wider application.[66,67] One of the most recent developments is that colleagues at the University of North Carolina–Chapel Hill have developed an online training for RE-AIM that consists of four different "lessons." The training is available without charge, but registration is required at http://courses.sph.unc.edu/tms/centertrt.

In summary, RE-AIM began a little over 10 years ago and was used initially by a small group of investigators primarily to do quantitative, post hoc evaluations of individually focused, health behavior change.[68] Today, it is used for planning, simulating,[69] and conducting ongoing "checks" to inform progress;[70] analyzing complex outcomes; reporting results;[51] and conducting reviews of complex issues.[71] As of this writing, at least 129 peer-reviewed publications have used RE-AIM across a wide variety of content areas, including policy, environmental change, and multilevel community interventions, with contributions from an increasingly diverse set of investigators, including anthropological, contextual, and qualitative scientists; pharmacists; and community coalitions in many different countries. We have recently attempted to provide a central registry and resources related to the RE-AIM model on the revised website at www.re-aim.org.

■ CASE STUDY

Applying RE-AIM to Plan, Implement, Evaluate, and Report Outcomes: The Smoking Less, Living More Study

Overview

The *Smoking Less, Living More* study was conducted in the Kaiser Permanente Colorado health care system with individuals 18 years of age and older. It was a year-long intervention in which individuals were randomized into one of two conditions. The intervention was a six-month program consisting of four telephone counseling calls and five tailored print materials all focused on smoking reduction. The control condition was usual care from the health care system and included access to a number of online and in-person cessation resources, as well as the state telephone Quitline. Assessments were conducted at baseline, three, and twelve months. The RE-AIM framework was used throughout all phases of the study as summarized in Table 16–3. The intervention was a tailored phone- and print-based intervention integrated around the "teachable situation" created when a person experienced outpatient surgery or a diagnostic procedure.[72,73]

RE-AIM was used in planning the intervention to enhance public health impact by recruiting a population-based sample of smokers scheduled for colonoscopy, sigmoidoscopy, mammography, or other outpatient procedure using the health plan's electronic medical record and designing the intervention to be conducted entirely by phone and mail. In addition, we partnered with the health plan's prevention department to create a smoking reduction program that would fit with what was offered smokers in terms of smoking cessation. Finally, lay individuals were used to deliver the counseling calls to reduce costs and increase potential dissemination by not requiring trained counselors to conduct the intervention.

Application of Framework

Reach was assessed by the number and characteristics of smokers who were identified as being eligible, the number who chose to participate versus not, and those who chose cessation versus reduction. We also calculated the percentage of individuals who received at least one intervention call as well as the attrition rate for the study at each intervention and assessment time point. *Effectiveness* was measured using three-month and 12-month self-reported quitting, reduction, biochemical measures of smoking, and quality of life. *Implementation* was measured using the number of intervention sessions delivered to study participants and the costs of the program. *Adoption* was measured by whether or not the health plan incorporated a reduction option into its current menu of cessation offerings following the completion of the trial. *Maintenance* was measured by 12-month reduction rates.

Results

Reach

We enrolled 30% of eligible known smokers, which is high for population-based recruitment studies. There were few differences among members of four self-selected groups (smoking reduction participants, those who initially agreed but did not complete baseline assessment, those who declined to participate, those who chose to quit). The majority of participants were over 50 years of age, female, smoked approximately a pack a day, and had smoked for over 30 years. The only significant difference was that Latinos were more likely to choose cessation over reduction or other options ($P < 0.05$). We had challenges maintaining participation throughout the study. More intervention than control participants dropped out (37% vs. 18%) by the 12-month assessment, and this was addressed using imputation analyses.

Effectiveness

Short-term behavioral and biochemical effects were promising. A chi-square analysis revealed that significantly more intervention than control participants achieved

TABLE 16–3.   Case Study Summary—Application of RE-AIM Framework to the Smoking Less, Living More Study

	Planning	Implementation	Evaluation	Outcomes
Reach	Use of EMR to identify and invite largest number of potentially eligible individuals to participate.	Enrolled 30% of known eligible smokers. Generally representative sample of 320 smokers scheduled for a outpatient procedure. No significant difference between conditions. Average age was 55. Participants generally were female, white, smoked approximately a pack a day, and had smoked on average almost 40 years.	More intervention than control withdrew from the study by the three-month assessment period (35% vs. 12%).	More intervention than control withdrew from the study by the 12-month assessment period (37% vs. 18%).
Effectiveness	Decision to use number of cigarettes per day and quit rates as practical outcomes. Used biochemical measures (expired CO and saliva cotinine) for assessment of unanticipated outcomes.	Counseling calls were scheduled at the convenience of the participant. Newsletters were tailored to individual participant's success and/or failure at reduction.	Three-month outcomes: Differences in achieving a 50% reduction in smoking was significant between conditions (15.9% vs. 7.7%). No difference in quit rates between both conditions.	12-month outcomes: Differences in achieving a 50% reduction in smoking was no longer significant between conditions (6.7% vs. 4.4%). Moderator analyses revealed that outcomes were generally consistent across a wide range of potential factors including dependence, smoking rate, health literacy, and depression screener scores.
Adoption	Study was designed to fit with current menu of offerings at health plan and involved Director of Prevention Services. Trained lay people to conduct counseling calls to test feasibility and make for easier adoption and dissemination.	Worked with several different clinical settings—i.e., outpatient surgery and radiology. Adapted to change in health plan's EMR during course of study.	Talks began at three-month assessment about incorporating reduction option into health plan offerings to smokers.	Not adopted by health plan.
Implementation		79% of all intervention participants received three or more of the four counseling calls (96% of those who did not withdraw from the study). 73% received four or more newsletters (89% of those who did not withdraw).	Competing contextual factors during course of study: (1) Colorado increased tobacco tax, (2) Colorado implemented a state-wide indoor smoking ban, and (3) State Quitline started offering two months free nicotine replacement therapy.	Cost of delivering intervention: $652 marginal cost per intervention participant relative to usual care. This translated to approximately $7132 per participant that cut smoking by 50%. Major costs were recruitment and overhead.
Maintenance				Smoking reduction rates seen at three months were not maintained by either condition at 12 months but were still better than baseline rates.

a 50% reduction in number of cigarettes per day ($P = 0.008$). Imputation analyses using missing-at-random assumptions were also significant (22.3% vs. 9.9%, $P < 0.05$). Analyses of the percent of participants who achieved at least a 50% reduction in CO levels were significant for the complete cases (chi-square, $P < 0.05$), but not for intent-to-treat or imputation analyses (although relative risks did favor intervention participants [RR = 1.9 and 2.4, respectively, NS]). Finally, there were no differences between conditions on quitting-related variables. Twenty-three percent of participants in each condition reported having attempted to quit by the three-month follow-up, but few of those were successful. As would be expected, significantly more intervention (96%) than control participants (81%) reported attempting smoking reduction ($P = 0.0005$). Interaction analyses (moderator variable × treatment condition) were significant for those having a chronic illness and had greater reductions in both number of cigarettes smoked ($P = 0.004$) and CO level ($P = 0.009$) than those without a chronic illness, and those who reported purchasing cigarettes by the carton at baseline (vs. by the pack) made greater reductions in both cigarettes smoked ($P = 0.019$) and CO levels ($P = 0.022$). Intervention effects appeared robust across a variety of other potential moderators including income, ethnicity, health literacy, education, gender, age, the depression screener, and type of medical procedure. Long-term behavioral and biomedical effects were disappointing. None of the significant differences observed between conditions at the three-month assessment period held at the 12-month assessment.

Adoption

The program was ultimately not used by the health care plan, which preferred to retain the more conventional cessation oriented options.

Implementation

The program was well implemented, with all of the intervention participants receiving at least three of the four phone calls (96% of those who did not withdraw from the program), and 73% receiving four or more newsletters (89% of those who did not withdraw).

Maintenance

At the individual level, effects seen at three months were not sustained at the 12-month time period. Again, there were no differences in cessation rates, and more intervention participants reduced their smoking by at least 50% (22.3% vs. 9.9%, $P < 0.05$) but this difference was no longer significant.

Summary

The *Smoking Less, Living More* study used RE-AIM throughout all phases of the study to plan the intervention, assess intervention consistency, and assess outcomes on each of the five dimensions. Using the RE-AIM framework when planning, designing, and evaluating intervention programs may lead to the development of studies and programs that have greater public health impact and are more likely to enhance translation of evidence-based interventions into real-world settings. At minimum, as illustrated in this case study, RE-AIM should enhance transparency of reporting and identify both strengths and limitations of programs on key issues such as recruitment, implementation, costs, and outcomes important to decision and policymakers.

■ CONCLUSIONS AND FUTURE ISSUES

It is never too early to start planning for dissemination (see Chapter 6). Whether using RE-AIM or one of the other models in Table 16–1, the D&I framework should be used in an ongoing manner before, during, and after implementation.[74]

Before large expenditures of time and effort are made, it is increasingly possible to conduct simulations, ranging from complex statistical or system dynamic modeling of probable outcomes and including sensitivity analyses[75,76] to simple "thought exercises" such as the interactive RE-AIM self-rating quiz tool to estimate potential outcomes to see if such an investment is likely to pay off. Such simulations could save a great deal of research dollars and also identify unanticipated outcomes that would not otherwise be considered.

Use of D&I models during implementation implies the need for adaptive research designs in which intervention is modified as needed based on initial results.[77] Such "adaptive designs" are now being considered by the FDA[78] and signal a movement to bring research and practice closer together. In our experience, adjustments both minor and sometimes major are frequently made to recruitment procedures, interventionist training or supervision, intervention details, collection of measures, or other aspects of a study but are seldom reported. In our view, such adjustments should be expected and are appropriate—as long as they are reported. We should learn from rather than hide such changes. The complex issue of what types of adaptations and customizations are appropriate and what kind are likely to be detrimental is complex and discussed in Chapters 11 and 14.

One of the most important issues for future D&I research involves developments such as the CONSORT group PRECIS criteria[30] and the RE-AIM "extended CONSORT reporting criteria" (www.re-aim.org), which should enhance the transparency of reporting and will substantially increase the percent of studies that report information such as reach, adoption, consistency of implementation, and generalization of outcomes across different settings and key subgroups related to health disparities.[79]

Several of the D&I evaluation models in Table 16–1 can help address the complex and challenging health and health care issues facing us today. D&I evaluation approaches that sensitize evaluators, policymakers, and consumers to the importance of contextual factors can greatly help close the research–practice and quality chasms.[80] A "realist" emphasis on issues such as who participates, engages, and benefits and under what conditions[7] can help identify and reduce health inequities. These approaches should also be very useful in the new comparative effectiveness research programs, as long as they are used to compare two real-world alternative interventions, as recommended in practical trials.[10,11,19]

In conclusion, both the challenges of and the opportunities for D&I research are great. The realist D&I questions of the future will take the form of "which complex intervention for what type of complex patients (which will include genomics) delivered by what type of staff or interactive modalities will be most cost effective, under what conditions (and in what environments) for what outcomes, and how does it come about?"

SUGGESTED READINGS

Damschroder LJ, Aron DC, Keith RE, Kirsh SR, Alexander JA, Lowery JC. (2009). Fostering implementation of health services research findings into practice: a consolidated framework for advancing implementation science. *Implement Sci.* 2009;4:50.

> *This article describes the Consolidated Framework for Implementation Research (CFIR), promoting implementation by finding what methods will apply across multiple contexts. The authors suggest using the CFIR model to guide formative evaluations and enhance implementation knowledge.*

Glasgow RE, Vogt TM, Boles SM. Evaluating the public health impact of health promotion interventions: the RE-AIM framework. *Am J Public Health.* 1999;89(9): 1322–1327.

> *In this seminal article, Glasgow et al. evaluate public health interventions using the RE-AIM framework. The model's five dimensions (reach, efficacy, adoption, implementation, and maintenance) act together to determine a particular program's public health impact. The article also summarizes the model's strengths and limitations, and suggests that failure to evaluate on all five dimensions can result in wasted resources.*

Glasgow RE, Nelson CC, Stryker LA, King D. Using RE-AIM metrics to evaluate diabetes self-management support interventions. *Am J Prev Med.* 2006;30:67–73.

> *This article demonstrates the use of proposed RE-AIM summary scores to estimate public health impact. Using the summary scores could assist practitioners in identifying the programs that are most likely to have a significant public health impact.*

Green LW, Ottoson JM, Garcia C, Hiatt RA. Diffusion theory and knowledge dissemination, utilization, and integration in public health. *Annu Rev Public Health.* 2009;30:151–174.

> *Green et al. provide a rigorous review of the public health implications of diffusion, dissemination, and implementation to improve public health practice and guide the design of future research. The article suggests a decentralized approach to dissemination and implementation, as well as ways diffusion may be combined with other theories.*

Jilcott S, Ammerman A, Sommers J, Glasgow RE. Applying the RE-AIM framework to assess the public health impact of policy change. *Ann Behav Med.* 2007;34:105–114.

> *This article evaluates health policies using the RE-AIM framework. The authors suggest using the framework to compare different policies, plan more successful policies, and assess policy impact on public health.*

Klesges LM, Estabrooks PA, Dzewaltowski, DA, Bull SS, Glasgow RE. Beginning with the application in mind: designing and planning health behavior change interventions to enhance dissemination. *Ann Behav Med.* 2005;29:66S–75S.

> *This article describes the use of RE-AIM for planning and design studies. The authors conclude that use of the RE-AIM framework does not guarantee an intervention's success, but it can inform future efforts at program dissemination.*

Leviton LC, Khan LK, Rog D, Dawkins N, Cotton D. Evaluability assessment to improve public health polices, programs, and practices. *Annu Rev Public Health.* 2010;31:213–233.

> *This article describes the rationale, history, and evolution of evaluability assessment. It serves a number of important purposes in public health, including giving constructive staff feedback, developing realistic program goals, and translating research into practice and practice into research.*

Pawson R, Greenhalgh T, Harvey G, Walshe K. Realist review: a new method of systematic review designed for complex policy interventions. *J Health Serv Res Policy.* 2005;10:S21–S39.

> *Pawson et al. suggest an alternative approach to systematic reviews and evidence that emphasizes context and external validity. This approach to evidence review seeks to answer questions such as which intervention, for which problem, for which set of patients is the intervention most effective, and for producing what outcome?*

SELECTED WEBSITES AND TOOLS

Cancer Control P.L.A.N.E.T. <http://cancercontrolplanet.cancer.gov/index.html> Cancer Control P.L.A.N.E.T. provides access to data and resources for designing, implementing, and evaluating evidence-based cancer control programs. The site proves five steps (with links) for developing a comprehensive cancer control program.

Measure Evaluation. <http://www.cpc.unc.edu/measure/tools/monitoring-evaluation-systems/prism>. The Measure Evaluation website provides additional information on PRISM: Performance of Routine Information System Management. Additional resources such as toolkits, checklists, and case studies are available.

The PRECEDE-PROCEED Model of Health Program Planning and Evaluation. <http://www.lgreen.net/precede.htm>. The PRECED-PROCEED Model of Health Promotion and Planning Evaluation website provides an overview of the PRECED-PROCEED model and provides additional references and resources.

RE-AIM website. < http://cancercontrol.cancer.gov/IS/reaim/>. The RE-AIM website provides an explanation of and resources for those wanting to apply the RE-AIM framework. It contains: self-rating quiz on RE-AIM dimensions:<http://tools.re-aim.org/quiz/intro.html> walks individuals through a thought process related to program aspects that are often ignored, or considered after a program concludes.

Reach calculator:

<http://tools.re-aim.org/reach.aspx> assists the user with calculations related to determining the participation rate of a project or program.

Adoption calculator:

<http://tools.re-aim.org/adoption.aspx> assists the user with calculations related to determining the adoption rate among program or project settings.

RE-AIM on-line training:

<http://www.center-trt.org/index.cfm?fa=webtraining.reaim> is a web-based training module available through the Center of Excellence for Training and Research Translation (Center-TRT). The module includes four lessons that provide instruction on

the five dimensions of the RE-AIM framework and that use case examples to illustrate the application of RE-AIM to behavior change and policy/environmental change interventions. This training is appropriate for anyone interested in considering the overall public health impact of health promotion interventions including researchers, program planners, evaluators, funders, and policymakers.

■ REFERENCES

1. Glasgow RE, Vogt TM, Boles SM. Evaluating the public health impact of health promotion interventions: The RE-AIM framework. *Am J Public Health* 1999;89: 1322–1327; PMID 10474547.
2. Glasgow RE, Linnan LA. Evaluation of theory-based interventions. In: Glanz K, Rimer BK, Viswanath K, eds. *Health behavior and health education: Theory, research, and practice.* 4th ed. San Francisco, CA: Jossey-Bass; 2008;487–508.
3. Wholey JS. Evaluability assessment. In: Wholey JS, Hatry HP, Newcomer KE, eds. *Handbook of practical program evaluation.* 2nd ed. San Francisco, CA: John Wiley and Sons; 2004;33–62.
4. Leviton LC, Khan LK, Rog D, Dawkins N, Cotton D. Evaluability assessment to improve public health policies, programs, and practices. *Annu Rev Public Health* 2010;31:213–233.
5. Stokols D, Hall KL, Taylor BK, Moser RP. The science of team science: Overview of the field and introduction to the supplement. *Am J Prev Med* 2008;35:S77–S89.
6. Emmons KM, Viswanath K, Colditz GA. The role of transdisciplinary collaboration in translating and disseminating health research: Lessons learned and exemplars of success. *Am J Prev Med* 2008;35:S204–S210.
7. Pawson R, Tilley N. *Realistic evaluation.* Thousand Oaks, CA: Sage Publications; 1997.
8. Abrams DB. Applying transdisciplinary research strategies to understanding and eliminating health disparities. *Health Educ Behav* 2006;33:515–531.
9. Green LW. Making research relevant: If it is an evidence-based practice, where's the practice-based evidence? *Fam Pract* 2008;25 Suppl 1:i20–i24.
10. Glasgow RE, Magid DJ, Beck A, Ritzwoller D, Estabrooks PA. Practical clinical trials for translating research to practice: Design and measurement recommendations. *Med Care* 2005;43:551–557; PMID 15908849.
11. Tunis SR, Stryer DB, Clancey CM. Practical clinical trials: Increasing the value of clinical research for decision making in clinical and health policy. *JAMA* 2003;290:1624–1632; PMID 14506122.
12. Damschroder LJ, Aron DC, Keith RE, Kirsh SR, Alexander JA, Lowery JC. Fostering implementation of health services research findings into practice: A consolidated framework for advancing implementation science. *Implement Sci* 2009;4:50.
13. Ferlie EB, Shortell SM. Improving the quality of health care in the United Kingdom and the United States: A framework for change. *Milbank Q* 2001;79:281–315.
14. Stetler CB, Legro MW, Wallace CM et al. The role of formative evaluation in implementation research and the QUERI experience. *J Gen Intern Med* 2006;21 Suppl 2: S1–S8.
15. Aqil A, Lippeveld T, Hozumi D. PRISM framework: A paradigm shift for designing, strengthening and evaluating routine health information systems. *Health Policy Plan* 2009;24:217–228.

16. Feldstein AC, Glasgow RE. A practical, robust implementation and sustainability model (PRISM) for integrating research findings into practice. *Jt Comm J Qual Patient Saf* 2008;34:228–243.

17. Gold MR, Patrick DL, Torrance GW et al. Identifying and valuing outcomes. In: Gold MR, Siegel JE, Russell LB, Weinstein MC, eds. *Cost-effectiveness in health and medicine*. New York: Oxford University Press; 1996;82–123.

18. Glasgow RE, Klesges LM, Dzewaltowski DA, Bull SS, Estabrooks P. The future of health behavior change research: What is needed to improve translation of research into health promotion practice? *Ann Behav Med* 2004;27:3–12; PMID 14979358.

19. Glasgow RE, Emmons KM. How can we increase translation of research into practice? Types of evidence needed. *Ann Rev Public Health* 2007;28:413–433.

20. Boome J. QALYS. *J Public Econ* 1993;50:149–167.

21. Congress of the United States, Congressional Budget Office. *Research on the comparative effectiveness of medical treatments: Issues and options for an expanded federal role.* Washington, DC: Congressional Budget Office; 2007.

22. Pawson R, Greenhalgh T, Harvey G, Walshe K. Realist review: A new method of systematic review designed for complex policy interventions. *J Health Serv Res Policy* 2005;10:S21–S39.

23. Kitson A, Harvey G, McCormack B. Enabling the implementation of evidence based practice: A conceptual framework. *Qual Health Care* 1998;7:149–158.

24. Harvey G, Loftus-Hills A, Rycroft-Malone J et al. Getting evidence into practice: The role and function of facilitation. *J Adv Nurs* 2002;37:577–588.

25. McCormack B, Kitson A, Harvey G, Rycroft-Malone J, Titchen A, Seers K. Getting evidence into practice: The meaning of "context." *J Adv Nurs* 2002;38:94–104.

26. Cummings GG, Hutchinson AM, Scott SD, Norton PG, Estabrooks CA. The relationship between characteristics of context and research utilization in a pediatric setting. *BMC Health Serv Res* 2010;10:168.

27. Ellis I, Howard P, Larson A, Robertson J. From workshop to work practice: An exploration of context and facilitation in the development of evidence-based practice. *Worldviews Evid Based Nurs* 2005;2:84–93.

28. Brown D, McCormack B. Developing postoperative pain management: Utilising the promoting action on research implementation in health services (PARIHS) framework. *Worldviews Evid Based Nurs* 2005;2:131–141.

29. Kitson AL, Rycroft-Malone J, Harvey G, McCormack B, Seers K, Titchen A. Evaluating the successful implementation of evidence into practice using the PARiHS framework: Theoretical and practical challenges. *Implement Sci* 2008;3:1.

30. Thorpe KE, Zwarenstein M, Oxman AD et al. A pragmatic-explanatory continuum indicator summary (PRECIS): A tool to help trial designers. *CMAJ* 2009;180: E47–E57.

31. Treeweek S, Zwarenstein M. Making trials matter: Pragmatic and explanatory trials and the problem of applicability. *Trials* 2009;10:37.

32. McQueen L, Mittman BS, Demakis JG. Overview of the Veterans Health Administration (VHA) Quality Enhancement Research Initiative (QUERI). *J Am Med Inform Assoc* 2004;11:339–343.

33. Yano EM. The role of organizational research in implementing evidence-based practice: QUERI Series. *Implement Sci* 2008;3:29.

34. Graham ID, Tetroe J. Learning from the U.S. Department of Veterans Affairs Quality Enhancement Research Initiative: QUERI Series. *Implement Sci* 2009;4:13.

35. Jha AK, Perlin JB, Kizer KW, Dudley RA. Effect of the transformation of the Veterans Affairs Health Care System on the quality of care. *N Engl J Med* 2003;348: 2218–2227.
36. Asch SM, McGlynn EA, Hogan MM et al. Comparison of quality of care for patients in the Veterans Health Administration and patients in a national sample. *Ann Intern Med* 2004;141:938–945.
37. Goetz MB, Bowman C, Hoang T et al. Implementing and evaluating a regional strategy to improve testing rates in VA patients at risk for HIV, utilizing the QUERI process as a guiding framework: QUERI Series. *Implement Sci* 2008;3:16.
38. Krein SL, Bernstein SJ, Fletcher CE et al. Improving eye care for veterans with diabetes: An example of using the QUERI steps to move from evidence to implementation: QUERI Series. *Implement Sci* 2008;3:18.
39. Smith JL, Williams JW, Jr., Owen RR, Rubenstein LV, Chaney E. Developing a national dissemination plan for collaborative care for depression: QUERI Series. *Implement Sci* 2008;3:59.
40. Green LW, Kreuter MW. *Health program planning: An educational and ecological approach*. 4th ed.New York: McGraw-Hill; 2005.
41. Gielden AC, McDonald EM, Gary TL, Bone RL. Using the Precede-Proceed Model to apply health behavior theories. In: Glanz K, Rimer BK, Viswanath K, eds. *Health behavior and health education: Theory, research, and practice*. 4th ed. San Francisco, CA: Jossey-Bass; 2008;407–433.
42. Chinman M, Hunter SB, Ebener P et al. The getting to outcomes demonstration and evaluation: An illustration of the prevention support system. *Am J Community Psychol* 2008;41:206–224.
43. Chinman M, Imm P, Wadersman A. *Getting to outcomes 2004: Promoting accountability through methods and tools for planning, implementation, and evaluation. Technical Report*. Santa Monica, CA: Rand Corporation; 2004.
44. Minkler M, Wallerstein N, Wilson N. Improving health through community organization and community building. In: Glanz K, Rimer BK, Viswanath K, eds. *Health behavior and health education*. 4th ed. San Francisco, CA: John Wiley; 2008;287–312.
45. Schensul JJ. Community, culture and sustainability in multilevel dynamic systems intervention science. *Am J Community Psychol* 2009;43:241–256.
46. Patton MQ. *Qualitative research and evaluation methods*. 3rd ed. Thousand Oaks, CA: Sage Publications; 2002.
47. Greenwald P, Cullen JW. The new emphasis in cancer control. *J Natl Cancer Inst* 1985;74:543–551.
48. Flay BR. Efficacy and effectiveness trials (and other phases of research) in the development of health promotion programs. *Prev Med* 1986;15:451–474.
49. Glasgow RE. RE-AIMing research for application: Ways to improve evidence for family practice. *J Am Board Fam Pract* 2006;19:11–19; PMID 16492000.
50. Glasgow RE, Nelson CC, Strycker LA, King DK. Using RE-AIM metrics to evaluate diabetes self-management support interventions. *Am J Prev Med* 2006;30:67–73; PMID 16414426.
51. Glasgow RE, Klesges LM, Dzewaltowski DA, Estabrooks PA, Vogt TM. Evaluating the overall impact of health promotion programs: Using the RE-AIM framework to form summary measures for decision making involving complex issues. *Health Educ Res* 2006;21:688–694; PMID 16945984.

52. Moher D, Schulz KF, Altman DG, for the CONSORT Group. The CONSORT statement: Revised recommendations for improving the quality of reports. *JAMA* 2001;285:1987–1991.

53. Glasgow RE, McKay HG, Piette JD, Reynolds KD. The RE-AIM framework for evaluating interventions: What can it tell us about approaches to chronic illness management? *Patient Educ Couns* 2001;44:119–127; PMID 11479052.

54. Glasgow RE. Outcomes of and for diabetes education research. *Diabetes Educ* 1999;25:74–88.

55. Ory MG, Jordan PJ, Bazzare T. The Behavior Change Consortium: Setting the stage for a new century of health behavior change research. *Health Educ Res* 2002;17: 500–511.

56. Jilcott S, Ammerman C, Sommers J, Glasgow RE. Applying the RE-AIM framework to assess the public health impact of policy change. *Ann Behav Med* 2007;34:105–114.

57. Klesges LM, Estabrooks PA, Glasgow RE, Dzewaltowski D. Beginning with the application in mind: Designing and planning health behavior change interventions to enhance dissemination. *Ann Behav Med* 2005;29:66S–75S; PMID 15921491.

58. Ory MG, Mier N, Sharkey JR, Anderson LA. Translating science into public health practice: Lessons from physical activity interventions. *Alzheimers and Dement* 2007;Apr;3:S52–S57.

59. Green LA, Cifuentes M, Glasgow RE, Stange KC. Redesigning primary care practice to incorporate health behavior change: Prescription for Health Round 2 results. *Am J Prev Med* 2008;35:S347–S349.

60. Nutting PA, Beasley JW, Werner JJ. Practice-based research networks answer primary care questions. *JAMA* 1999;281:686–689.

61. Agency for Health Care Research and Quality. Practice-Based Research Networks. *http://pbrn.ahrq.gov/portal/server.pt*; accessed 5/25/10.

62. Centers for Disease Control and Prevention. *Assuring healthy caregivers, a public health approach to translating research into practice: The RE-AIM framework*. Neenah, WI: Kimberly-Clark Corporation; 2008.

63. Kaiser Permanente. Community Health Initiatives. *http://info.kp.org/community benefit/html/our_work/global/our_work_3_ahtml*; accessed 5/15/2010.

64. King DK, Glasgow RE, Toobert DJ et al. Self-efficacy, problem solving, and social-environmental support are associated with diabetes self-management behaviors. *Diabetes Care* 2010;33:751–753.

65. Campbell M, Fitzpatrick R, Haines A et al. Framework for design and evaluation of complex interventions to improve health. *Br Med J* 2000;321:694–696.

66. Ritzwoller DP, Sukhanova A, Gaglio B, Glasgow RE. Costing behavioral interventions: A practical guide to enhance translation. *Ann Behav Med* 2009;Apr 37:218–227.

67. Ritzwoller DP, Toobert D, Sukhanova A, Glasgow RE. Economic analysis of the Mediterranean Lifestyle Program for Postmenopausal women with diabetes. *Diabetes Educ* 2006;32:761–769; PMID 16971709.

68. Glasgow RE, Whitlock EP, Eakin EG, Lichtenstein E. A brief smoking cessation intervention for women in low-income Planned Parenthood Clinics. *Am J Public Health* 2000;90:786–789.

69. Dzewaltowski D, Glasgow RE, Klesges LM, Estabrooks PA, Brock E. RE-AIM: Evidence based standards and a web resource to improve translation research into practice. *Ann Behav Med* 2003;Oct;28:75–80.

70. King DK, Glasgow RE, Leeman-Castillo B. RE-AIMing RE-AIM: Using the model tp plan, implement, evaluate, and report the impact of environmental change approaches to enhance population health. *Am J Public Health*. 2010;100(11):2076–2084.

71. Klesges LM, Dzewaltowski DA, Glasgow RE. Review of external validity reporting in childhood obesity prevention research. *Am J Prev Med* 2008;34:216–223.

72. Glasgow RE, Gaglio B, Estabrooks PA et al. Long-term results of smoking reduction program. *Med Care* 2008;47:115–120; PMID 19106739.

73. Glasgow RE, Estabrooks PA, Marcus AC et al. Evaluating initial reach and robustness of a practical randomized trial of smoking reduction. *Health Psychol* 2008;27: 780–788.

74. Ottoson JM, Hawe P (Editors). *Knowledge utilization, diffusion, implementation, transfer, and translation: Implications for evaluation: new directions for evaluation.* Hoboken, NJ: Wiley; 2009.

75. National Cancer Institute. Cancer Intervention and Surveillance Modeling Network (CISNET). *http://cisnet.cancer.gov; accessed 5/11/10.*

76. Stern M, Williams K, Eddy D, Kahn R. Validation of prediction of diabetes by the Archimedes model and comparison with other predicting models. *Diabetes Care* 2008;31:1670–1671.

77. Lei X, Yuan Y, Yin G. Bayesian phase II adaptive randomization by jointly modeling time-to-event efficacy and binary toxicity. *Lifetime Data Anal*. 2011;17(1):156–174.

78. U.S.Department of Health and Human Services, Food and Drug Administration, Center for Drug Evaluation and Research (CDER), Center for Biologics Evaluation and Research (CBER). *Guidance for industry: Adaptive design clinical trials for drugs and biologics.* February—Clinical/Medical ed. Washington DC: US Dept of Health and Human Services; 2010.

79. Woolf SH, Johnson RE, Fryer GE, Jr., Rust G, Satcher D. The health impact of resolving racial disparities: An analysis of US mortality data. *Am J Public Health* 2008;98:S26–S28.

80. Institute of Medicine, Committee on Quality of Health Care in America. *Crossing the quality chasm: A new health system for the 21st Century.* Washington, DC: National Academy Press; 2001.

Setting- and population-specific dissemination and implementation

17 Dissemination and Implementation Research in Community and Public Health Settings

■ KATHERINE A. STAMATAKIS,
CYNTHIA A. VINSON, AND
JON F. KERNER

■ INTRODUCTION

Dissemination and implementation (D&I) research in community and public health (C&PH) settings holds great promise for widespread improvements in population health by closing the gap between scientific evidence and public health action. The goal of public health is centered on implementing preventive measures intended to decrease morbidity and mortality from a broad array of infections, chronic diseases, mental illness, abusive substances, and injuries. Public health action may take the form of programs and policies that intervene broadly at national levels or that specifically address regional or local issues.

Settings for public health are as diverse as the contexts in which public health-related action occurs. The Institute of Medicine report *The Future of Public Health* defined the concept of a public health system as "what we as a society do collectively to assure the conditions in which people can be healthy."[1] This definition expands the notion of public health outside of government agencies, to encompass other sectors and settings including the community at large, mass media, and worksites, as well as more traditional public health agencies.[2,3] In addition, the transfer and integration of evidence-based interventions to communities occurs both through institutions and organizations and directly to community members, defining the two main groups of audiences. Given that both types of audiences may be found in community and public health settings, D&I strategies may range from those that target "implementers" (e.g., public health practitioners and policymakers) to interventions aimed at improving dissemination directly to "end users" (e.g., members of the community). This heterogeneous mix of settings and levels can be viewed as comprising a linked system, albeit with varying degrees of integration across components, which offers opportunities not only to strengthen the translation of scientific discoveries into practice settings, but equally important, for research to be informed by the needs and priorities of practitioners and policymakers.

For the purpose of this chapter, we focus on government public health systems in the United States and Canada, highlighting characteristics relevant for D&I research. Other settings relevant for public health described in detail in other chapters of this book include social services (Chapter 18), health care delivery systems (Chapter 19), schools (Chapter 20), and policy-making settings (Chapter 21).

In the United States, governmental public health agencies are considered the backbone of the public health system,[4] structured by laws, regulations, and organizational components, and driven by human, informational, and fiscal resources.[5] At the national level, public health agencies play an important role in setting the nation's agenda for public health (e.g., Healthy People objectives), securing funding, dispersing resources at state and local levels, and policy making, although primary authority for public health in the United States resides at the state level.[5]

Dispersal of community health resources occurs through local agencies, including local public health departments and health care centers. The Community Health Centers (CHC) program (supported by the Health Resources and Services Administration [HRSA]) funds Federally Qualified Health Centers (FQHC), FQHC "Look-Alikes" (FQHCLA), and outpatient health programs/facilities operated by tribal organizations focused on medically underserved populations and areas. In 2009, over 1,100 CHCs operated more than 7,900 clinics (half in rural areas) and served almost 19 million patients.[6] Local health departments (LHDs) implement community and public health programs and provide services directly or in partnership with other agencies and organizations, often serving as a bridge linking state and federal infrastructure and resources with local communities. In addition, LHDs are organizations where population-based interventions often mix with health care provision in the same setting (i.e., as FQHCLA), with many agencies directly providing or contracting preventive health care services. There are almost 2,800 LHDs in the United States.[7]

As in the United States, the public health "system" in Canada might be best described as a grouping of multiple systems with varying roles, strengths, and linkages. Each province has its own public health legislation, although the age and content of these vary considerably. In most provinces and territories, public health is delivered through regional and/or municipal health authorities or the provincial/territorial government.[8] At the federal level, Health Canada and the Public Health Agency of Canada are the two leading federal funders of public health services. They are also the primary supporters of public health services in Canada's three territories and funders of services for the indigenous populations of Canada (i.e., First Nations, Inuit, and Métis).

While there are a number of systematic reviews and compilations of evidence-based practices for community health promotion and disease prevention, such as the Guide to Community Preventive Services,[9] the demand for and readiness to implement and maintain evidence-based practice varies across settings. Furthermore, the potential efficacy of evidence-based practice designed and tested under ideal research conditions is likely to differ from the effectiveness when applied in real-world practice. Dissemination and implementation research grounded in strong research–practice–policy linkages offers many opportunities to address these challenges.

In this chapter, we will discuss the evidence base, theories, and other important themes guiding current D&I research in C&PH settings, and provide some case examples that highlight gaps and opportunities for future work in this area.

■ EVIDENCE-BASED PRACTICES FOR COMMUNITY AND PUBLIC HEALTH SETTINGS

A growing number of resources and tools have been developed in the past 10 years to enhance the ease with which public health and clinical practitioners can find and use evidence-based programs and practices. These range from systematic reviews of public health intervention and policy approaches to IT tools to help practitioners find evidence-based resources for planning and implementation. Key research questions in D&I research revolve around examining how and to what extent practitioners are using these tools, identifying barriers, and testing the relative effectiveness of strategies for disseminating and integrating research into practice (e.g., Brownson et al.[10]).

Some of the tools designed for use by practitioners and policymakers are described below.

Guide to Community Preventive Services

In 1996, the U.S. Department of Health and Human Services established the Task Force for Community Preventive Services to develop guidelines for evidence-based practice based on the systematic review of community-based health promotion and disease prevention interventions.[11] The Guide to Community Preventive Services[9] is an online resource for identifying interventions that have been evaluated, the intervention effect, the intervention aspects that users can identify as most appropriate for their respective communities, and the intervention cost and return on investment. Interventions are rated as "recommended," "recommended against," or "insufficient evidence," with those that are recommended also rated according to the strength of the evidence, as "strong" or "sufficient." The rigorous systematic review methods employed by the Task Force[12,13] are described straightforwardly on the website. Practitioners can browse the website by following links to various health topics, which are broken down further according to results of systematic reviews in specific areas of each topic. Users are also given guidance as to various ways the information on the website can be applied, for developing policies, programs, funding proposals, research, education, and other general uses.

National Registry of Evidence-Based Programs and Practices

In 1997, the Substance Abuse and Mental Health Services Administration (SAMHSA) launched the National Registry of Effective Prevention Programs (NREPP)[14] as a resource to help practitioners identify and implement substance abuse prevention programs. Under the initial NREPP program 1,100 programs were externally peer reviewed and were identified as "model," "effective," or "promising" programs and made available online. Programs that were deemed as "model" programs were provided additional resources from SAMSHA to facilitate dissemination of the program by enhancing program materials and expanding program training.

The NREPP site expanded to include mental health and substance abuse prevention and treatment interventions in 2004 and also modified the rating and review criteria they had been using.

The NREPP was updated in 2007 with the new name of National Registry of Evidence-Based Programs and Practices (NREPP). This version no longer labels programs as "model" or "effective." Practitioners can search online by topic area for more than a 150 programs and can evaluate the evidence base of the programs by examining the programs' individual outcome ratings (reliability, validity, fidelity, missing data/attrition, confounding variables, and data analysis). The new NREPP also provides ratings on readiness for dissemination, which include scores on implementation materials, training and support, quality assurance, and an overall rating on dissemination readiness.[14]

Cancer Control P.L.A.N.E.T. (Plan, Link, Act, Network with Evidence-Based Tools)

Launched in 2003, the Cancer Control P.L.A.N.E.T.[15] is a web portal designed to provide cancer control practitioners with stepwise access to data and evidence-based resources to assist in planning and implementation of evidence-based programs. The site is co-sponsored by the National Cancer Institute (NCI), Centers for Disease Control and Prevention (CDC), Agency for Healthcare Research and Quality (AHRQ), SAMHSA, American Cancer Society (ACS), and the Commission on Cancer (CoC). The Canadian Partnership Against Cancer partnered with the NCI and adapted Cancer Control P.L.A.N.E.T. into a Canadian version of the site and launched it in English in 2008 and in French in 2009.[16] Cancer Control P.L.A.N.E.T. Canada is also supported by associates from the Canadian Association of Provincial Cancer Agencies, Canadian Cancer Research Alliance, Canadian Cancer Society, North American Association of Central Cancer Registries, the Public Health Agency of Canada (PHAC), and Statistics Canada. Practitioners in both countries can access state- and county- or provincial-level cancer incidence, access mortality and prevalence data from the State or Provincial Cancer Profiles websites (Step 1), and create easy-to-understand jurisdiction-specific maps, graphs, and tables in seconds. Potential research partners working in different aspects of cancer control can be found on Step 2 of both sites. Step 3 of the sites provides access to research reviews currently available from the Guide to Community Preventive Services, the U.S. Preventive Health Services, and in the United States, the Evaluation of Genomic Applications in Practice and Prevention (EGAPP), and, in Canada, the Cochrane Library of systematic evidence reviews and the Canadian Taskforce on Preventive Healthcare. Step 4 provides access to the Research-Tested Intervention Programs website and, in Canada, the Canadian Best Practices Portal, both described below. The fifth step provides access to U.S. state, tribal, territorial, and Pacific Island Jurisdiction cancer control plans, and in Canada, national and provincial cancer control plans as well as a searchable database of federal, provincial, and territorial cancer and chronic disease prevention policies.

Research-Tested Interventions Programs (RTIPs) Website

In 2002, the NCI began developing the Research-Tested Interventions Programs website[17] to provide cancer control practitioners access to programs that had been conducted in peer-reviewed, grant-funded studies, had positive outcomes published in peer-reviewed journals, and had materials that could be disseminated (by NCI or the developer) and adapted for use in community or clinical settings. NCI chose not to label programs as "model" or "effective" but, rather, provided sufficient information so that practitioners could make an informed decision about a program fit based on the level of evidence, and the appropriateness for the specific community level of resources required for implementation. The NCI partnered with SAMHSA, modified the criteria from the NREPP program, and began posting programs on the RTIPs website in April 2003. Similar to the NREPP program, the RTIPs website evolved over time. The site currently contains over 100 programs in breast, cervical, and colorectal cancer screening, informed decision making for cancer screening, diet/nutrition, physical activity, public health genomics, sun safety, survivorship, and tobacco control, with a majority of the programs focused on community or public health settings. The eligibility criteria for posting programs on the site were modified in 2009 to allow programs that were not evaluated in a peer-reviewed, grant-funded, research project. However, all programs included must have had outcomes published in peer-reviewed journals and must have utilized an experimental or quasi-experimental evaluation design.[17]

Canadian Best Practices Portal

After five years of development work, including reviews of other best practice tools and resources internationally, and surveys of public health researchers and practitioners in Canada, the PHAC officially launched the Canadian Best Practices Portal for Health Promotion and Chronic Disease Prevention in 2006. The content of the Portal reflected a population health approach and, for a resource (e.g., best practice intervention, a systematic review site) to be included, it had to address one of the eight elements of the Population Health Template (see Figure 17–1) and involve an evidence-informed decision-making process.[18] Plans were put in place to expand the evidence available on the Portal including current (e.g., physical activity) and new topics (e.g., obesity prevention), and a broader range of practices, programs, and policies (Phase II), and later (Phase III) to monitor the uptake of Portal content and its influence on health promotion practice. This latest focus on monitoring the uptake and impact of evidence-based interventions is one of the most complex evaluation challenges facing the field of knowledge translation.

Diffusion of Effective Behavioral Interventions (DEBI) Website

HIV prevention researchers and practitioners have been pioneers in dissemination and implementation of evidence-based interventions. Beginning in 1999, the CDC conducted a systematic review of evidence-based HIV prevention interventions and published a compendium of tested interventions that currently includes over

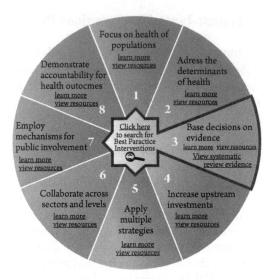

Figure 17–1. Canada's Population Health Template for the Best Practices Portal.

60 programs that have been proven effective in research studies, utilized experimental or quasi-experimental study design, and have materials packaged and ready for dissemination.[19] To enhance the dissemination process, the DEBI project staff provides training and technical assistance for the programs posted in the compendium, which is seen as essential for building the capacity of individuals, organizations, and communities.[20]

Center of Excellence for Training and Research Translation (UNC)

A hybrid of research-tested and practice-tested interventions can be found at the Center of Excellence for Training and Research Translation site sponsored by the University of North Carolina–Chapel Hill in collaboration with the CDC's Well-Integrated Screening and Evaluation for Woman Across the Nation (WISEWOMAN) program and the Nutrition and Physical Activity Program to Prevent Obesity and Other Chronic Diseases.[21] Criteria for inclusion of an intervention on this site are similar to RTIPs and DEBI for research-tested interventions. Practice-tested interventions are included as a separate category, recognizing that varying levels of evidence exist and providing access to interventions that have been evaluated in practice but not tested in formal research studies. Both the research-tested and practice-tested interventions and programs are reviewed based on the criteria from the RE-AIM framework (reach, effectiveness, adoption, implementation, and maintenance).

■ D&I CHALLENGES IN COMMUNITY AND PUBLIC HEALTH SETTINGS

Infrastructure and Workforce Issues

Community and public health settings have the potential to play an important role in the widespread application of evidence-based programs and policies, although they vary greatly in size and resources, and in many areas, lack the capacity to implement a full array of public health services.[22] In the United States, state and local health departments are positioned to serve as a link between producers of research evidence (i.e., federal agencies and academia) and sources of tacit knowledge (e.g., local practitioners, community members),[23,24] by cultivating community advocacy and partnerships[25] and adapting and developing programs and policies to the unique context of the organizations and communities that may influence their effective application over time.[26,27]

A number of studies have discussed a set of barriers that practitioners have identified as impeding the use of evidence-based practice in public health settings. These include both personal and institutional barriers, such as lack of time, inadequate funding, absence of cultural and managerial support (especially the absence of incentives),[28–32] and the perception of institutional priority for evidence-based practices and actual use of research to inform program adoption and implementation.[29,33] While some barriers, particularly personal barriers, may be overcome by improving training opportunities,[31] progress in dissemination research will be made by involving practitioners in all steps of the research process, from identifying barriers and setting priorities to designing strategies for improved D&I.[34,35]

There is little systematic information available on the functioning of public health systems. A working group of the Advisory Committee on Population Health assessed the capacity of the Canadian public health system in 2001 through a series of key informant interviews and literature reviews.[8] The consistent finding was that public health had experienced a loss of resources, and there was concern for the resiliency of the system infrastructure to respond consistently and proactively to the demands placed upon it. Significant disparities were observed between "have" and "have not" provinces and regions in their capacity to address public health problems. This is particularly important since these jurisdictions often have the highest rates of unhealthy behaviors and chronic diseases.

The pervasive concern regarding Canada's public health system prompted a review of alternative international models for organizing and funding essential public health programs and services that Canada might want to consider in restructuring its national, provincial/territorial, regional, and locally based public health programs and services. Background documents and key informant interviews were conducted for the following countries: England, Australia, New Zealand, and the United States. The development of the provincial public health system in Quebec was also reviewed.[8]

Based on these reviews and the collective experience of Committee members, the following key infrastructure elements of a national public health system need to be achieved:

- Clearly defined essential functions of public health;
- Defined roles and responsibilities at each level of the system (national, provincial/territorial, regional/local);
- Consistent, modern legislation within each jurisdiction across the country to support those functions, roles, and responsibilities;
- Appropriate delivery structures to accomplish functions, roles, and responsibilities within each jurisdiction;

- Appropriate funding levels and mechanisms that ensure equitable availability of public health services to all Canadians;
- Appropriate numbers of well-trained staff;
- Appropriate information systems to support assessment and surveillance;
- Access to expertise and support to develop a prospective vision, carry out these responsibilities expertly and efficiently, and promote innovation and evaluation; and
- Accountability mechanisms at each level of the system.

These recommendations provided by the Canadian committee parallel those identified in the United States by the Institute of Medicine (IOM) committee in 1988[1] and were reiterated in the 2003 follow-up report,[4] which also emphasized the importance of other sectors outside of government in promoting the public's health. For example, whether tobacco, nutrition, or physical activity, the private sector plays a key role in facilitating or helping to inhibit unhealthy behaviors. Similarly, NGOs play a key role in promoting the utilization of public health services (e.g., screening), as well as advocating for public health policy change (e.g., increased tobacco excise taxes). The complex interrelationship between government, the private sector, and nongovernmental organizations (NGOs), and the different resources each sector can bring to bear to effect change, makes for a highly variable set of conditions within public health both over time and across jurisdictions. Given this diversity and complexity, we have provided two case studies described below that highlight partnerships between government and academia, and across government, NGOs, and the private sector.

Practice Implications / Fundamental Issues for Practitioners

Most government research–funding agencies are mandated to share the information generated from the research they fund, and similarly NGOs who fund research also select research findings to communicate to the public and their donor populations. Historically, government research funding agencies have used three broad approaches to move science into practice: (1) communication and diffusion of research findings (e.g., conferences, publications, press releases), (2) dissemination campaigns to alter knowledge and behavior, and (3) large-scale demonstration projects.[36] All three approaches share some characteristics in that funding for these efforts is usually time limited (constraining sustainability) and proportionately small compared with the major investments in the primary mission of these agencies (research), and the level of agency support varies depending on the agency's annual budget. Application, practice, and service support agencies (e.g., Health Resources and Service Administration, Public Health Agency of Canada) often use similar diffusion and dissemination approaches. Given that the bulk of their funding supports service delivery, the proportion of the budget available to link science with service is also relatively small.[37]

Research results are most commonly communicated through the peer-reviewed publication of research findings. With respect to the communication of research results to the public, the news media are regularly contacted by research funding agencies to alert the public of new findings. As such, both the news media and the research community may be more focused on novelty rather than the public health or clinical significance of new scientific knowledge.

The high level of public and private investment in health research, in combination with the current funding emphasis on basic discovery research, creates an interesting information dissemination paradox. On the one hand, enormous amounts of information are being generated through research, published in thousands of discipline-specific journals and presented in hundreds of discipline-specific professional meeting venues. On the other hand, so much information is being pushed out through this passive process of information diffusion that a "signal-to-noise" ratio problem exists with respect to translating research into practice and policy.[37]

The massive and largely passive diffusion approach used in science may also raise unrealistic expectations in the practice community. Many individual research reports, while suggesting exciting new innovations that may lie ahead, have little or no immediate application in practice. Thus, it may be difficult for the practice community to distinguish the signal about what is currently important to practice from the noise of what may or may not become important in the future.[38]

In the past several years, a number of NGOs have begun including a focus on utilizing evidence-based interventions as a condition of receiving funding. This is a shift from a focus on funding innovative interventions that may not yet be based on research evidence of efficacy or effectiveness. For example, the Susan G. Komen foundation partnered with the NCI's Cancer Information Service (CIS) between 2007 and 2009 on a pilot project to increase the knowledge and skills of potential community grantees around identifying, adapting, and implementing evidence-based interventions. Several of the Komen regions participated in the pilot by modifying their funding announcements to focus on incorporating evidence-based interventions and collaborating on in-person training for potential grantees.

While it is often assumed that the demand for evidence-based health promotion and disease prevention interventions is high, many in the public health, clinical practice, and public policy communities do not hold with this assumption, albeit privately, and there are equal and often opposing forces to the dissemination and implementation of new knowledge gained from research.[35] These include the mass of tacit knowledge gained from practice and policy experience,[39,40] as well as the complex service delivery and political policy-making contextual factors that constrain the acceptance, adaptation, and implementation of innovations based on research.[41] Thus, it has been posited that to close the gap between scientific discovery and service delivery, if we want more evidence-based practice, we need more practice-based evidence.[42]

Dissemination of research evidence about new approaches to promote health and prevent disease to public health practitioners should take into account: (1) the level of training of most public health practitioners (e.g., master's or bachelor's) for translating information into practical knowledge that can be applied in public health practice contexts, (2) the variation in resources in international, national, state/provincial, and local public health practice contexts that influence the implementation of public health interventions based on new health promotion information, and (3) the extent to which public health practitioners working in resource-limited practice contexts may or may not be amenable to change.

Ferlie and Dopson[43] argue that a shift to evidence-based practice in health, as an example of organizational change, is highly context dependent and not at all generic in nature. However, they also contend that there are core context factors that produce low-level patterning, if not predictive laws. So, for example, health care (and presumably health promotion) delivery contexts vary across time and place, so that D&I strategies that work in a country or at a time when there is universal access to health care (e.g., Canada) may not apply where universal access is not available (e.g., United States). They also note that there are significant differences in roles, provider relationships, and practices from one service sector to another, as well as different histories, cultures, and capabilities for learning and change across service sectors, all of which may be key modifiers of the impact of translating and implementing evidence-based interventions in practice. A key challenge for the emerging field of D&I research will be to develop reliable measures of these contextual factors and use them across service contexts to sort out the extent to which there are general principles for how contextual factors influence dissemination and implementation.[18]

■ OVERVIEW OF RESEARCH IN C&PH SETTINGS

Summary of Existing Research

While a large number of intervention studies exist that contribute to the evidence base for interventions applied in D&I research, there are few studies in community and public health settings that are explicitly D&I research studies. Much of the research in community settings has been conducted in schools (subject of Chapter 20), with other notable examples in government public health agencies, worksites, churches, and private sector settings.

Two studies have employed quasi-experimental or experimental designs to examine the impact of D&I strategies in government public health agencies. Brownson et al.[10] studied the effect of providing workshops on guidelines (Community Guide) for evidence-based practice in physical activity promotion in state and local health departments in the United States, resulting in improvements in end points including awareness and adoption, though important differences at state and local levels were found. More recently, Dobbins et al.[44] employed a randomized-controlled trial to examine the relative impacts of various knowledge translation and exchange strategies to increase the use of evidence-informed healthy–body weight programs and policies in a national sample of health departments in Canada. A treatment effect on the number of programs and policies was observed only for tailored, targeted messages (the other two strategies were providing a knowledge broker and online access to informational resources), with notable moderation by organizational culture.

Some D&I research has also been conducted in churches, worksites, and other private sector settings. An evaluation of a national dissemination campaign of the church-based Body & Soul intervention is currently underway (funded by NCI as part of their strategic dissemination initiative of research-tested intervention programs), with preliminary results indicating that repeated contact with knowledgeable staff has been key to early dissemination efforts.[45] Results from the Working Well Trial found that the maintenance of tobacco control activities in study worksites over time was related to the degree of institutionalization, which included the existence of assigned committees and budget allotments.[46] Research on dissemination and implementation of skin cancer interventions has been conducted in a number of private sector settings, including swimming pools and zoos.[47–49] With respect to relative impact of various strategies, more intensive did not always result in better outcomes; in some cases, more intensive, "enhanced" treatment groups exhibited better outcomes,[49] while in others, the less intensive (generic materials) treatments showed relatively better results.[44,48]

Research-tested interventions that are posted on several of the previously noted resources are not designed to be disseminated and require significant modifications to be ready for widespread use. Programs posted on the RTIPs website are not currently required to include information on core program components primarily due to the fact that researchers do not test or report on this in outcome publications. However, implementation guides have been developed for programs posted on the site to assist users with maintaining fidelity to the original studied intervention. An evaluation of the Cancer Control P.L.A.N.E.T. site in 2007 found that more than 50% of users incorporated components of programs posted on the site into existing or developing programs.[50] A similar finding was found from a pilot project called Team-Up: Cancer Screening Saves Lives that was designed to encourage the use of research-tested interventions by creating partnerships in counties experiencing high cervical cancer mortality rates. The pilot was sponsored by NCI, the American Cancer Society, and the CDC, and an evaluation was conducted in 2008. The evaluation found that there were challenges among practitioners concerning what constituted an evidence-based program. Questions arose over whether a program had to be implemented with fidelity to be considered evidence based and to what extent teams could modify tested interventions by using only certain components based on demographic and geographic characteristics of the women they were trying to reach. For complex, multicomponent interventions, partnerships often selected the components that they felt would be most appropriate for their audience and were affordable to implement.[51]

Generating Evidence of What Works from D&I Research

In 2005, the National Institutes of Health initiated a trans-NIH funding opportunity focused on dissemination and implementation research, which was open to international investigators. By 2010, 18 dissemination and implementation projects in community and public health settings had been funded, all of which are in the United States, comprising 45% of the total number of D&I funded projects under this initiative (Figure 17–2). Topics being addressed in these grants include tobacco control, alcohol and substance abuse, nutrition and physical activity, cancer screening, HIV/STIs, mental health, flu vaccinations, palliative care, bone health, and chronic back pain.

The Centers for Disease Control and Prevention (CDC) subsequently initiated three different funding opportunities since 2007 focused on what they labeled as

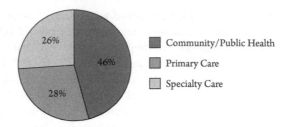

Figure 17–2. Funded
NIH Dissemination and
Implementation Research in
Health Grants (2005–2009).

translational research. A total of 35 of these translational research projects focused on community and public health settings, comprising approximately 65% of the total number of funded projects between 2007 and 2009 (Figure 17–3). Topics addressed in the CDC grants include asthma, diabetes, HIV, mental health, obesity, nutrition, cardiovascular disease, physical activity, substance abuse, tobacco control, emergency preparedness, motor vehicle safety, vaccinations, and cancer prevention.[52]

In Canada, the Canadian Institutes for Health Research's (CIHR) knowledge translation (KT) activities focus on areas where they can make a unique contribution on the basis of their recognized core competencies: researcher training and research funding; their close relationship with the health research community; their ability to develop integrated, strategic national research agendas; and their credibility as a forum for consideration of complex health research issues. CIHR builds on past and ongoing KT planning, programs, and activities, incorporating what has been learned to promote KT through activities designed to: (1) support research on KT concepts and processes; (2) contribute to building KT networks of researchers and research users; (3) strengthen and expand KT at CIHR by improving the capability to support KT research and, with partners, KT itself; and (4) support and recognize KT excellence by building and celebrating a culture of KT.

Theories and Conceptual Frameworks in D&I Research

Previous chapters have described the different theories and approaches used in D&I research. It has been noted that there is no single underlying theory base or conceptual framework driving the field. Rather, D&I research draws on a range of theories and practices depending on the project underway.

For example, researchers applying for D&I research grant funding frequently combine multiple theories and models or create a hybrid theory/model to meet specific project needs (Table 17–1). The NIH's D&I Research in Health grants have

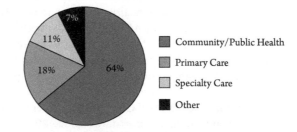

Figure 17–3. Funded CDC
Translational Research
Grants (2007–2009).

TABLE 17-1.   *Theories/Models Cited in NIH Dissemination and Implementation Research in Health Grants (2005–2009)*

	Diffusion of Innovations	RE-AIM	Systems/ Network Theory	Community-based Participatory Research	Quality Improvement	Organizational Theory	Other Theory/ Model	Combined Theories/ Models
Community/ Public Health (18)	28%	17%	17%	17%	0%	0%	28%	50%
Primary Care (11)	18%	36%	9%	0%	36%	0%	36%	36%
Specialty Care (10)	10%	0%	0%	0%	20%	30%	50%	20%

encouraged grantees to focus on conceptual frameworks when designing their research studies, and it is interesting to examine the theories that have been used in the various research programs and how D&I research in public or community health research differs from those in primary care or specialty care. In an analysis of these awards, community and public health researchers utilized Rogers's Diffusion of Innovations theory[53] most frequently while researchers focused on specialty care cited it the least.

The RE-AIM model was the most frequently cited model for researchers focused on primary care, which may be related to the RE-AIM site having formerly been hosted solely by Kaiser Permanente (it is currently also hosted on the NCI Implementation Science website).[54,55] RE-AIM, systems, and network theory were present in both community/public health and primary care D&I research but were not cited at all in specialty care D&I research. Community-based participatory research was a model frequently used by community and public health D&I research while quality improvement models were more frequently utilized by clinical D&I research. Other theories and models that were cited in grants included health marketing, decision-making theory, knowledge integration theory, and Practical Robust Implementation and Sustainability Model (PRISM).[56] Organizational theories were most frequently cited in specialty care D&I research but were not utilized at all community and public health D&I research. A majority of community and public health D&I research projects combined multiple theories and models.

As noted previously, the CDC has also been funding grants to improve the translation of research into practice. Between 2007 and 2009, they had three different initiatives focused on what they labeled translational research: (1) Improving Public Health Practice through Translation Research, (2) Elimination of Health Disparities through Translation Research, and (3) Translating Research to Protect Health through Health Promotion, Prevention, and Preparedness. In an analysis limited to information in publicly available abstracts from 54 funded grants, the majority of abstracts did not identify the theoretical construct in the research. Ten of those that mentioned theories or models in their abstracts incorporated the RE-AIM model in their research design and a couple cited *Diffusion of Innovations*.

D&I research being conducted in community and public health settings by and large do not appear to be initiated by community partners. Organizations that received funding for the 18 NIH D&I Research in Health grants focused on community and public health were all academic and/or research organizations. While they all had partners in the community, the funding was awarded through well-established research entities with histories of successfully applying for federal research grants. In the limited abstract analysis of the CDC-funded translation grants, 3 of the 54 awarded grants went to local government agencies (city or county), and 1 went to a community organization, while the rest were awarded to academic and/or research organizations. With the majority of D&I research largely based in academia, this raises the question of how likely it is that the findings from this research will be incorporated into community and public health practice settings if they are rarely the lead on the project.

■ GOVERNMENT/ACADAMIC CASE STUDY: PREVENTION RESEARCH CENTERS

Background

In 1984 the U.S. Congress enacted Public Law 98–551, which established a program for Centers for Research and Demonstration of Health Promotion and Disease Prevention, currently known as the Prevention Research Center (PRC) program of the CDC. The program has evolved since its inception, expanding into 37 academic centers, which maintain research–practice linkages with community members, practice, and policy settings in their respective communities.[42,57] In 1997 the IOM commissioned a report that reviewed the program's progress and discussed a vision for the future that explicitly placed dissemination research as one of its goals.[58] Dissemination research activities were included in the CDC's evaluation of the PRC program,[59] though as noted in the evaluation report, tracking indicators in dissemination and implementation has been difficult and highlights one area where further investment in D&I research activities can help sustain the program.

Context

The Cancer Prevention and Control Research Network (CPCRN) is one of five thematic research networks in the PRCs and is supported collaboratively by the Division of Cancer Prevention and Control at the CDC and the Division of Cancer Control and Population Science at the NCI. The CPCRN began in 2002 with a goal of accelerating the adoption of evidence-based cancer prevention and control in communities. The network provides the infrastructure to allow the 10 funded research institutions and one coordinating center to collaborate on community-based, participatory D&I cancer research that spans academic and geographic boundaries (Figure 17–4).

Lessons Learned

The CPCRN has collaborated on research grant applications and has been able to partner on many D&I research projects. During the first funding cycle (2004–2009), the network produced 28 collaborative publications, partnered on

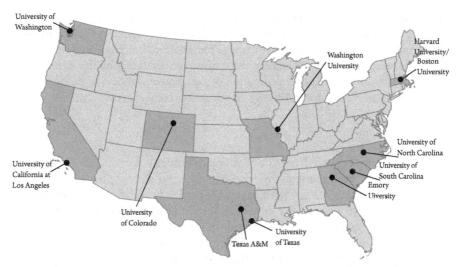

Figure 17–4. Cancer Prevention and Control Research Network (CPCRN) Map.

47 grant applications that received grant funding in excess of $26 million, and had 125 collaborative research activities.[60] One example of a successful research project is the partnership with national 2–1-1 hotlines. 2–1-1 is a nationally designated three-digit telephone number (like 9–1-1 for emergencies) that provides callers with access to information on social and health services in their community. A pilot project was initially developed in 2007 by the Washington University Network Center with the Missouri 2–1-1 hotline. The results of this pilot found that callers to the hotline were receptive to receiving health information and had greater cancer risk factors than the average person (higher smoking rates, lower screening rates, and lower rates health insurance coverage).[61,62]

In 2008, after a successful initial pilot in Missouri, additional CPCRN centers from Harvard, University of North Carolina, University of Texas, and University of Washington began working with 2–1-1 Centers in their states. The expanded pilot included giving callers a cancer control needs assessment and providing referrals for free or low-cost services as appropriate. In 2009, the University of Texas Network Center received funding to examine the use of phone navigators to provide counseling and navigation services to increase cancer screening and human papilloma virus (HPV) vaccination rates by 25%. Results of the studies have not yet been published.

▪ NGO CASE STUDY: CANADIAN PARTNERSHIP AGAINST CANCER

Background

The Canadian Partnership Against Cancer (the Partnership) is a nongovernmental organization, albeit fully funded by the federal government (Health Canada) to accelerate action on cancer control for all Canadians. The organization is made up of a partnership of cancer experts from academia; charitable organizations; federal, provincial, and territorial governments; patients and survivors; and the private sector determined to bring change to the cancer control domain. The Partnership works together to stimulate the generation of new knowledge and to accelerate the implementation of existing knowledge about cancer control across Canada.

Context

The Partnership evolved from the Canadian Strategy for Cancer Control—a volunteer-driven coalition working to counteract the growing burden of cancer on Canadian society. The coalition drafted Canada's first national cancer control plan and advocated successfully for its funding in 2007.[63] From its inception, the Partnership recognized that vital information for cancer control is being generated every day both in research and real-world settings throughout Canada.

Knowledge management efforts of the Partnership, including knowledge translation and knowledge exchange, aim to maximize the value of this constantly evolving information, through the establishment of collaborative networks, with the ultimate goal of using these resources to solve common challenges in cancer control. While technology plays a crucial role in this work to foster the creation, exchange, and application of accurate, timely information, the Partnership has also made substantial investments in what might be labeled "high-touch" (in addition to "hi-tech") approaches to knowledge management. One such effort in the public health arena of the prevention and early detection of cancer and other chronic diseases is Coalitions Linking Action & Science for Prevention (CLASP).

Lessons Learned

CLASP is an initiative of the Partnership that aims to improve the health of communities and of all Canadians. CLASP does this by bringing together government and NGO and private sector organizations across two or more provinces and territories, forming research, practice, and policy coalitions to integrate cancer prevention with strategies to prevent other chronic diseases. CLASP recognizes that many aspects of healthy living and a healthy environment (e.g., behavioral and policy approaches) can reduce the risk not only of many cancers but also of chronic diseases such as diabetes and lung and heart disease.

As Figure 17–5 indicates, CLASP was viewed as a systems change initiative in that it builds bridges for networking, communication, coordination, and eventually collaboration[64] across jurisdictions, chronic diseases, and research, practice, and policy sectors, in order to broaden the reach and deepen the impact of existing cancer and chronic disease prevention initiatives in Canada.

Together with its funding partners, the Public Health Agency of Canada and the Heart and Stroke Foundation, the Partnership is providing a total of $15.5 million to seven CLASP projects over a period of two and a half years. Beyond funding specific coalitions to address multiple cancer and chronic disease risk factors, the Partnership is providing ongoing collaboration opportunities to further support

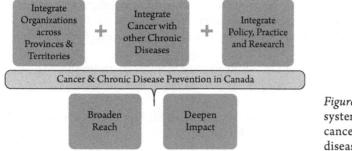

Figure 17–5. A systems approach to cancer and chronic disease prevention.

the prevention community in sharing knowledge across practices and in cultivating additional research, practice, and policy partnerships. Key to this funding initiative has been the commitment to knowledge exchange among jurisdictions, chronic diseases, and research, practice, and policy specialists across government, NGO, academic, and private sectors in the implementation phases of CLASP.

There were three phases to implementing the CLASP initiative: (1) knowledge exchange (KE) consultations across Canada to help develop the RFP, (2) program review of letters of intent from, and evaluation support for, potential applicants, as well as significant support for KE among the research, practice, and policy peer reviewers about the RFP review criteria *before* they received their applications to review, and (3) semiannual knowledge exchange meetings among the seven funded CLASP coalitions, quarterly conference calls by cross-CLASP working groups on KE, sustainability, and evaluation, and a cross-CLASP web-based collaborative workspace to increase opportunities for knowledge exchange. This unprecedented level of commitment to collaboration and knowledge exchange both before and after the CLASP funding is being evaluated at each phase of the CLASP implementation process to determine the value added by this substantial commitment to KE.[65,66]

■ DIRECTIONS FOR FUTURE RESEARCH

The variability in structure, resources, and function of public health systems creates challenges as well as opportunities for D&I research. For example, while uniformity can facilitate the transfer of research-tested interventions across settings, variability creates "laboratories" for testing interventions under different conditions. A recent review of community-based D&I research in cancer prevention,[67] which extended the work of a previous review by the AHRQ,[68] provides these recommendations for future research and practice that apply broadly to D&I research in community and public health settings:

- Standardize the terminology for D&I research;
- Evaluate the D&I of effective interventions targeting diverse populations and various community settings;
- Develop and use reliable and valid measures of D&I constructs;
- Use a combination of quantitative and qualitative data from multiple sources;

- Measure the real-world impact of D&I studies using standardized measures of stages of the D&I process, moderators, mediators, and outcomes;
- Apply appropriate study designs; RCT is not always the most appropriate or feasible; and
- Active and multimodal D&I strategies are more likely to be effective than passive, single-modal strategies.

Other fields of research also hold promise in the future development of D&I research in community and public health settings. Community-Based Participatory Research (CBPR) has been defined as "a collaborative approach to research that equitably involves all partners in the research process and recognizes the unique strength that each brings."[69] The strong focus on social and economic justice places it as a key concept in the development, implementation, and evaluation of interventions that address social determinants of health inequities.[70] Placed in the more general context of participatory research, core elements have been described as building mutual trust and respect, building capacity, empowerment and ownership, and accountability and sustainability.[71] Given the heterogeneous settings for community health, applying CBPR methods by involving the community in early stages of study design should enhance success of the later stages of D&I.

The nascent but growing field of public health services and systems research (PHSSR) attempts to capitalize on the variability inherent in public health systems by investigating factors such as organization, workforce, financial resources, and other characteristics of components of the public health system in relation to performance and outcomes.[72,73] A central focus of enhancing growth in the field has been the development of data resources,[74,75] including the PHSSR subset of the National Library of Medicine's health services research (HSR) database.[76]

Both the review in this chapter of what we know and the case examples of what is being done to close the gap between research discovery and program and policy delivery suggest that a very small portion of the overall investment in research, practice, and policy work is being used to link the lessons learned from science with the lessons learned from policy and practice. From the research-funding agency perspective, the NIH, CDC, and the Canadian Institutes for Health Research (CIHR) have supported dissemination and implementation research (United States) and knowledge translation research (Canada) for the past several years. From the practice/policy funding perspective, the CDC and the Public Health Agency of Canada have also provided support for such linkages as well as providing forums and IT tools to disseminate evidence-based intervention approaches and best practices across their respective countries and internationally. However, as has been noted elsewhere,[35] these relatively small steps at their current level of support, and in and of themselves, are unlikely to accelerate closing the discovery–delivery gap.

To make significant change, each and every sector involved in public health will need to examine its funding priorities and decide what proportion of the investments will be focused on what it can do on its own versus what it should do in partnership with other sectors. For example, even as academic organizations recognize the potential for peer-reviewed funding and publications in this nascent field in public health, will they be willing to also provide academic credit and career advancement for faculty who choose to invest their time and energy in building coalitions and collaborating with public health practice and policy partners outside academia?

Similarly, government research and practice–funding agencies face a similar choice: continue to expend most of their resources on their own initiatives, within their mission frameworks and comfort zones, versus making a significant investment in collaborative funding initiatives and sharing the credit and the responsibility for working together across departments, ministries, and jurisdictions. While it is much easier to network and coordinate than to cooperate and collaborate,[64] absent a significant effort at redesigning and increasing investments in D&I research and knowledge translation on the part of science and service–funding agencies, and a similar change in the academic rewards for research, practice, and policy partnerships, integrating the lessons learned from research with those learned from practice and policy, the ideal of research influencing practice and policy and vice versa, will remain a side show to our seemingly unquenchable thirst for discovery.

"You must be the change you wish to see in the world."—Mahatma Gandhi

SUGGESTED READINGS

Brownson RC, Fielding JE, Maylahn CM. Evidence-based public health: a fundamental concept for public health practice. *Annu Rev Public Health.* 2009;30:175–201.

Reviews the evolution of the concept of evidence based public health and provides a typology of scientific evidence for public health practice. Also discusses organizational, political, and structural barriers to implementing evidence-based practice in public health settings, and strategies for enhancing workforce competencies.

Dobbins M, Hanna SE, Ciliska D, et al. A randomized controlled trial evaluating the impact of knowledge translation and exchange strategies. *Implement Sci.* 2009;4:61.

A randomized trial to evaluate the effectiveness of three different implementation strategies for improving knowledge translation and exchange in health departments.

Rabin BA, Glasgow RE, Kerner JF, Klump MP, Brownson RC. Dissemination and implementation research on community-based cancer prevention: a systematic review. *Am J Prev Med.* 2010;38(4):443–456.

A systematic review of recent dissemination and implementation research of evidence-based interventions in smoking, health diet, physical activity, and sun protection.

Contandriopoulos D, Lemire M, Denis JL, Tremblay E. Knowledge exchange processes in organizations and policy arenas: a narrative systematic review of the literature. *Milbank Q.* 2010;88(4):444–483.

A narrative literature review that provides a framework for analyzing context with respect to developing knowledge exchange strategies in organizations and policy arenas. Emphasizes the importance of contextual factors in three domains and the limitations of context-independent evidence resulting from randomized trials, providing direction to address some of the limitations discussed in Dobbins et al. 2009.[44]

SELECTED WEBSITES AND TOOLS

Title	Description	Website
Guide to Community Preventive Services	Federally sponsored website that provides guidance on selecting community-based programs and policies to improve health and prevent disease that are based on systematic reviews of the evidence	http://www.thecommunityguide.org/index.html
National Registry of Evidence-Based Programs and Practices	Online registry of tested interventions that support mental health promotion, substance abuse prevention, and mental health and substance abuse treatment	http://www.nrepp.samhsa.gov/
Cancer Control P.L.A.N.E.T. (Plan, Link, Act, Network with Evidence-Based Tools)	Web portal designed to provide cancer control practitioners with stepwise access to data and evidence-based resources to assist in planning and implementing evidence-based plans and programs (available in the United States and Canada)	http://cancercontrolplanet.cancer.gov/ and http://cancercontrolplanet.ca/
Research-Tested Interventions Programs (RTIPs) website	Searchable database of cancer control interventions and program materials, designed to provide program planners and public health practitioners easy and immediate access to research-tested materials	http://rtips.cancer.gov/rtips/index.do
Canadian Best Practices Portal	A virtual front door to community and population health interventions related to chronic disease prevention and health promotion	http://cbpp-pcpe.phac-aspc.gc.ca/
Diffusion of Effective Behavioral Interventions (DEBI) website	Website designed to bring science-based, community-, group-, and individual-level HIV prevention interventions to community-based service providers and state and local health departments	http://www.effectiveinterventions.org/en/home.aspx
Center of Excellence for Training and Research Translation (UNC)	Website focused on enhancing the impact of the WISEWOMAN program and the Nutrition and Physical Activity Program to Prevent Obesity and Other Chronic Diseases	http://www.center-trt.org/

REFERENCES

1. Institute of Medicine. *The Future of Public Health.* Washington, DC: National Academies Press; 1988.
2. Aday LA. *Reinventing Public Health.* San Francisco: Jossey-Bass; 2005.
3. Scriven A. *Public Health: A Social Context and Action.* Berkshire, UK: One University Press; 2007.
4. Institute of Medicine. *The Future of the Public's Health in the 21st Century.* Washington, DC: The National Academies Press; 2003.
5. Turnock BJ. *Public Health: What It Is and How It Works.* 4 ed. Sudbury, MA: Jones and Bartlett Publishers LLC; 2009.
6. U.S. Department of Health and Human Services. HRSA Health Center National Data. October 11, 2010. http://www.hrsa.gov/data-statistics/health-center-data/index.html.
7. National Association of County and City Health Officials. *2008 National Profile of Local Health Departments.* Washington, DC: National Association of County and City Health Officials; 2009.
8. Frank J, DiRuggerio E, Muloughney B. The Future of Public Health in Canada: Developing a Public Health System for the 21st Century. http://www.cihr.ca/e/19573.html. Published Last December 1, 2003. Accessed July 21, 2011.
9. The Community Guide Branch, Epidemiology Analysis Program Office (EAPO), Office of Surveillance, Epidemiology, and Laboratory Services (OSELS), Centers for Disease Control and Prevention. Guide to Community Preventive Services. http://www.thecommunityguide.org/index.html. Accessed July 28, 2010.
10. Brownson RC, Ballew P, Brown KL, et al. The effect of disseminating evidence-based interventions that promote physical activity to health departments. *Am J Public Health.* Oct 2007;97(10):1900–1907.
11. Truman BI, Smith-Akin CK, Hinman AR, et al. Developing the Guide to Community Preventive Services—overview and rationale. The Task Force on Community Preventive Services. *Am J Prev Med.* Jan 2000;18(1 Suppl):18–26.
12. Mullen PD, Ramirez G. The promise and pitfalls of systematic reviews. *Annu Rev Public Health.* 2006;27:81–102.
13. Zaza S, Briss PA, Harris KW, eds. *The Guide to Community Preventive Services: What Works to Promote Health?* New York: Oxford University Press; 2005.
14. National Registry of Evidence-Based Programs and Practices. June 7, 2010. http://www.nrepp.samhsa.gov. Accessed June 19, 2010.
15. Cancer Control P.L.A.N.E.T. http://cancercontrolplanet.cancer.gov/index.html. Accessed July 28, 2010.
16. Cancer Control P.L.A.N.E.T. Canada. http://www.cancercontrolplanet.ca. Accessed July 22, 2010.
17. Research-Tested Interventions Programs. April 16, 2010. http://rtips.cancer.gov/rtips/index.do. Accessed June 19, 2010.
18. Jetha N, Robinson K, Wilkerson T, Dubois N, Turgeon V, DesMeules M. Supporting knowledge into action: The Canadian Best Practices Initiative for Health Promotion and Chronic Disease Prevention. *Can J Public Health.* Sep–Oct 2008;99(5):11–18.
19. Division of HIV/AIDS Prevention, National Center for HIV/AIDS, Viral Hepatitis, STD, and TB Prevention, Centers for Disease Control and Prevention. 2009

Compendium of Evidence-Based HIV Prevention Interventions. December 18, 2009. http://www.cdc.gov/hiv/topics/research/prs/evidence-based-interventions. htm. Accessed July 28, 2010.

20. Danya International, Inc. Diffusion of Effective Behavioral Interventions. http://www.effectiveinterventions.org/en/AboutDebi.aspx. Accessed June 15, 2010.

21. Center of Excellence for Training and Research Translation. http://www.center-trt. org/. Accessed July 28, 2010.

22. National Association of County and City Health Officials. *2005 National Profile of Local Health Departments.* Washington, DC: National Association of County and City Health Officials; 2006.

23. Brownson RC, Fielding JE, Maylahn CM. Evidence-based public health: a fundamental concept for public health practice. *Annu Rev Public Health.* Apr 29 2009;30:175–201.

24. Colditz GA, Emmons KM, Vishwanath K, Kerner JF. Translating science to practice: community and academic perspectives. *J Public Health Manag Pract.* Mar–Apr 2008;14(2):144–149.

25. Yancey AK, Fielding JE, Flores GR, Sallis JF, McCarthy WJ, Breslow L. Creating a robust public health infrastructure for physical activity promotion. *Am J Prev Med.* Jan 2007;32(1):68–78.

26. Dearing JW. Evolution of diffusion and dissemination theory. *J Public Health Manag Pract.* Mar–Apr 2008;14(2):99–108.

27. Green LW, Ottoson JM, Garcia C, Hiatt RA. Diffusion theory, and knowledge dissemination, utilization, and integration in public health. *Annu Rev Public Health.* 2009; 30:151–174.

28. Baker EA, Brownson RC, Dreisinger M, McIntosh LD, Karamehic-Muratovic A. Examining the role of training in evidence-based public health: a qualitative study. *Health Promot Pract.* Jul 2009;10(3):342–348.

29. Dobbins M, Cockerill R, Barnsley J, Ciliska D. Factors of the innovation, organization, environment, and individual that predict the influence five systematic reviews had on public health decisions. *Int J Technol Assess Health Care.* 2001;17(4): 467–478.

30. Dreisinger M, Leet TL, Baker EA, Gillespie KN, Haas B, Brownson RC. Improving the public health workforce: evaluation of a training course to enhance evidence-based decision making. *J Public Health Manag Pract.* Mar–Apr 2008;14(2):138–143.

31. Jacobs JA, Dodson EA, Baker EA, Deshpande AD, Brownson RC. Barriers to evidence-based decision making in public health: a national survey of chronic disease practitioners. *Public Health Rep.* Sep–Oct;125(5):736–742.

32. Maylahn C, Bohn C, Hammer M, Waltz EC. Strengthening epidemiologic competencies among local health professionals in New York: teaching evidence-based public health. *Public Health Rep.* 2008;123 (Suppl 1):35–43.

33. Brownson RC, Ballew P, Dieffenderfer B, et al. Evidence-based interventions to promote physical activity: what contributes to dissemination by state health departments. *Am J Prev Med.* Jul 2007;33(1 Suppl):S66–S73; quiz S74–S68.

34. Glasgow RE, Marcus AC, Bull SS, Wilson KM. Disseminating effective cancer screening interventions. *Cancer.* Sep 1 2004;101(5 Suppl):1239–1250.

35. Kerner JF. Integrating science with service in cancer control: closing the gap between discovery and delivery. In: Elwood M, Sutcliffe S, eds. *Cancer Control.* Oxford: Oxford University Press; 2010:81–99.

36. National Cancer Institute. Community-Based Interventions for Smokers: The COMMIT Field Experience; 1995.
37. Kerner JF, Hall KL. Research dissemination and diffusion: translation within science and society. *Res Soc Work Pract.* 2009;19(5):519–530.
38. Kerner JF, Rimer BK, Emmons KM. Dissemination research and research dissemination: how can we close the gap? *Health Psychology.* 2005;24(5):443–446.
39. Kerner JF. Knowledge translation versus knowledge integration: a "funder's" perspective. *J Contin Educ Health Prof.* Winter 2006;26(1):72–80.
40. Kerner JF. Integrating research, practice, and policy: what we see depends on where we stand. *J Public Health Manag Pract.* Mar–Apr 2008;14(2):193–198.
41. Dopson S, Fitzgerald L. The active role of context. In: Dopson S, Fitzgerald L, eds. *Knowledge to Action? Evidence-Based Health Care in Context.* Oxford: Oxford University Press; 2005:79–103.
42. Green LW. The prevention research centers as models of practice-based evidence two decades on. *Am J Prev Med.* Jul 2007;33(1 Suppl):S6–S8.
43. Ferlie E, Dopson S. Study complex organizations in health care. In: Dopson S, Fitzgerald L, eds. *Knowledge to Action? Evidence-Based Health Care in Context.* Oxford: Oxford University Press; 2005:8–26.
44. Dobbins M, Hanna SE, Ciliska D, et al. A randomized controlled trial evaluating the impact of knowledge translation and exchange strategies. *Implement Sci.* 2009;4:61.
45. Campbell MK, Hudson MA, Resnicow K, Blakeney N, Paxton A, Baskin M. Church-based health promotion interventions: evidence and lessons learned. *Annu Rev Public Health.* 2007;28:213–234.
46. Sorensen G, Thompson B, Basen-Engquist K, et al. Durability, dissemination, and institutionalization of worksite tobacco control programs: results from the Working Well trial. *Int J Behav Med.* 1998;5(4):335–351.
47. Glanz K, Steffen A, Elliott T, O'Riordan D. Diffusion of an effective skin cancer prevention program: design, theoretical foundations, and first-year implementation. *Health Psychol.* Sep 2005;24(5):477–487.
48. Lewis E, Mayer JA, Slymen D, et al. Disseminating a sun safety program to zoological parks: the effects of tailoring. *Health Psychol.* Sep 2005;24(5):456–462.
49. Rabin BA, Nehl E, Elliott T, Deshpande AD, Brownson RC, Glanz K. Individual and setting level predictors of the implementation of a skin cancer prevention program: a multilevel analysis. *Implement Sci.* 2010;5:40.
50. Sood R, Ho PS, Tornow C, Frey W. *Cancer Control P.L.A.N.E.T. Evaluation Final Report.* Division of Cancer Control and Population Sciences, National Cancer Institute; 2007.
51. Breslau ES, Rochester PW, Saslow D, Crocoll CE, Johnson LE, Vinson CA. Developing partnerships to reduce disparities in cancer screening. *Preventing Chronic Disease: Public Health Research, Practice and Policy.* May 2010 2010;7(3):A62.
52. Centers for Disease Control and Prevention. Advancing Excellence and Integrity of CDC Science. April 28, 2010. http://www.cdc.gov/od/science/index.htm. Accessed June 1, 2010.
53. Rogers EM. *Diffusion of Innovations.* New York: Free Press; 2003.
54. RE-AIM. http://cancercontrol.cancer.gov/IS/reaim/index.html. Accessed July 21, 2011.
55. Dzewaltowski DA, Glasgow RE, Klesges LM, Estabrooks PA, Brock E. RE-AIM: evidence-based standards and a web resource to improve translation of research into practice. *Ann Behav Med.* 2004;28(2):75.

56. Feldstein AC, Glasgow RE. A practical, robust implementation and sustainability model (PRISM). *Jt Comm J Qual Patient Saf.* April 2008;34(4):228–243.
57. National Center for Chronic Disease Prevention and Health Promotion. *Prevention Research Centers: Building the Scientific Research Base with Community Partners.* Atlanta, GA: Centers for Disease Control and Prevention; 2010.
58. Stoto M, Green L, Bailey L. *Linking Research and Public Health Practice: A Review of CDC's Program of Centers for Research and Demonstration of Health Promotion and Disease Prevention.* Washington, DC: Institute of Medicine; 1997.
59. Centers for Disease Control and Prevention. *Prevention Research Centers Program. Evaluation Results: Program Indicators.* Atlanta: U.S. Department of Health and Human Services; 2010.
60. Williams R. *Cancer Prevention and Control Research Network Summary Progress Report: 9-30-04 to 9-29-09.*
61. Cancer Prevention and Control Research Network. www.cpcrn.org. Accessed July 15, 2010.
62. Ribisi K. CPCRN: Your partner in cancer control. Paper presented at: Presentation to CDC, May 24, 2010; Atlanta, GA.
63. Canadian Partnership Against Cancer. http://www.partnershipagainstcancer.ca. Accessed June 29, 2010.
64. Himmelman AT. On coalitions and the transformation of power relations: collaborative betterment and collaborative empowerment. *Am J Community Psychol.* Apr 2001;29(2):277–284.
65. Lobb R, Petermann L, Manafo E, Keen D, Kerner J. Multi-disciplinary collaborations to reduce incidence of cancer and chronic disease: case study of a Canadian initiative. (*Manuscript in preparation.*)
66. Manafo E, Petermann L, Lobb R, Keen D, Kerner J. Research, practice and policy partnerships in Pan-Canadian Coalitions for cancer and chronic disease prevention. (*Manuscript in preparation.*)
67. Rabin BA, Glasgow RE, Kerner JF, Klump MP, Brownson RC. Dissemination and implementation research on community-based cancer prevention: a systematic review. *Am J Prev Med.* Apr 2010;38(4):443–456.
68. Agency for Healthcare Research and Quality. *Diffusion and dissemination of evidence-based cancer control interventions.* Rockville, MD: AHRQ; 2003.
69. Minkler M, Wallerstein N. *Community Based Participatory Research for Health.* San Francisco: Jossey-Bass; 2003.
70. Brennan Ramirez L, Baker E, Metzler M. *Promoting Health Equity: A Resource to Help Communities Address Social Determinants of Health.* Atlanta: U.S. Department of Health and Human Services, Centers for Disease Control and Prevention; 2008.
71. Cargo M, Mercer SL. The value and challenges of participatory research: strengthening its practice. *Annu Rev Public Health.* 2008;29:325–350.
72. Mays GP, Halverson PK, Scutchfield FD. Behind the curve? What we know and need to learn from public health systems research. *J Public Health Manag Pract.* May–Jun 2003;9(3):179–182.
73. Mays GP, Smith SA, Ingram RC, Racster LJ, Lamberth CD, Lovely ES. Public health delivery systems: evidence, uncertainty, and emerging research needs. *Am J Prev Med.* Mar 2009;36(3):256–265.
74. Scutchfield FD, Bhandari MW, Lawhorn NA, Lamberth CD, Ingram RC. Public health performance. *Am J Prev Med.* Mar 2009;36(3):266–272.

75. Scutchfield FD, Lawhorn N, Ingram R, Perez DJ, Brewer R, Bhandari M. Public health systems and services research: dataset development, dissemination, and use. *Public Health Rep.* May–Jun 2009;124(3):372–377.

76. National Information Center on Health Services Research and Health Care Technology (NICHSR). http://wwwcf.nlm.nih.gov/hsrr_search/index.cfm. Accessed July 28, 2010.

18 Dissemination and Implementation in Social Service Settings

■ CURTIS MCMILLEN

Social service sectors of care are uniquely positioned to influence the dissemination and implementation (D&I) of health prevention and intervention protocols to reach vulnerable populations. Current D&I efforts in the social services are often geared to implement complex protocols in complicated systems of care and possess interesting implications for D&I work and research in other sectors of care. Before addressing these larger points, some boundaries around the social services, and thus this chapter, are proposed.

The collective use of the term "social services" confuses many, even those who work within them. This is because the term is commonly used to represent a number of different sectors of care, a class of nonmedical services designed to increase social well-being. Generally, the social services are thought to encompass:

- child maltreatment investigations and remediation efforts, including foster care and adoption;
- juvenile justice services (delinquency prevention, services to offending children, juvenile detention, residential services);
- some adult justice services, such as probation, parole, and job assistance;
- income transfer programs for the poor, such as (in the United States), Temporary Aid for Needy Families and the Supplemental Nutritional Assistance Program (formerly food stamps);
- some housing programs for people who are poor or homeless;
- community long-term care services for older adults, generally designed to keep older adults living in the community and out of long-term care facilities;
- and services for victims of interpersonal violence.

■ THE POTENTIAL OF DISSEMINATION AND IMPLEMENTATION EFFORTS IN THE SOCIAL SERVICES

Developing structures and strategies to disseminate and implement health-focused prevention and intervention protocols in the social services is justified for three main reasons. First, there is often a primacy of relationships between social service workers and their clients. Second, social service clients often possess high need for improved health. Third, it is often of self-interest to social service systems of care to improve the health of their clients.

Another Primary Care

For many children, youth, and families deeply involved in social service sectors of care, the professional most primary to them—chief in importance, most frequently seen, and first seen in a sequence of help seeking behaviors—is a social service provider. In some sectors of care, the social services case manager explicitly serves as the gatekeeper of other services, including medical care.[1] In these sectors, the social services case manager can be thought of as the primary care provider, a term usually reserved for a patient's first-line physician.

In other sectors of care, the combination of a frequency of contact between the social services professional and a social services client and the degree of impairment of the service client places the social services case manager in an important role of influence. These workers know what is going on with their clients, and the clients may not be capable of accessing care without the social service worker's assistance.

High Need

The second reason to consider a role for the social services in the D&I of health prevention and treatments is the level of need among social service clients. While we are all at risk of some diseases no matter our neighborhood, social class, or ethnic group, two common denominators of health problems are emerging from a vast and complex literature—low income and early life adversity. People who grew up in families with little income and high levels of adversity like maltreatment, parental substance abuse, and incarceration are at high risk of both social service involvement and health problems. This convergence points to the social services as a natural entry point for health interventions.

In many countries, including the United States, income and health are negatively and consistently related.[2,3] Also, studies like the Adverse Childhood Experiences Study are providing convincing evidence that early adversity is predictive of a wide range of later health problems.[4,5] Increasingly, a life course perspective is taken to understand inequalities in health,[6,7] showing how low income and early adversity unfold over the life course to leave adults vulnerable to poor health. Some social services, like income transfer programs, are designed to lessen the impact of hardship. Others, like foster care and juvenile justice systems, strive to provide turning points that alter life courses in positive ways. In this sense, theoretically, the social services are situated to see large numbers of people with health problems in a helping context.

The literature on the health needs of social service clients is underdeveloped, segmented by service sector, and largely hidden from traditional literature searches in government reports. But my field of practice, foster care services for older youth, can be exemplary. Estimates are that 35% of these young people are obese,[8] cigarette smoking is twice as common as among other teens,[9,10] and rates of past year major depression for foster youth[11] are three times as high as that of other youth.[12]

Self-Interest

Health is not the raison d'être of these social service sectors and thus rarely the primary focus of social service systems. Still, the D&I of evidence-supported health interventions might assist social service agencies in fulfilling their main functions. Income assistance programs are motivated to help their clients budget their meager means to last through the month. Therefore, they may want to help their clients stop smoking, in order for the financial assistance they provide to go further. They also want to help move their clients from the welfare rolls to employment. Therefore, they may want to help some clients lose weight, as high body weight may be a barrier in gaining employment.[13] The intersection between health concerns and service system mission will be different for each sector of care. An agency that provides in-home services to older adults may not be interested in smoking cessation, for example, but may be interested in depression-focused interventions, as preventing or treating depression may help keep older adults in their homes.

■ WHAT COULD AND SHOULD BE DISSEMINATED AND IMPLEMENTED IN THE SOCIAL SERVICES?

The justification for D&I work in the social services provided above suggests that there should be broad interest within social service sectors for health prevention and intervention protocols with the highest potential for affecting multiple disease processes. These protocols would target increased physical activity levels, healthy eating, and the cessation or prevention of tobacco use. In some of these sectors of care (e.g., juvenile justice, child welfare, probation and parole), HIV prevention could also be prioritized.

There are programs for each of these targets developed for other sectors of care that could be adapted for social service settings. Yet, in most social service sectors of care, there has been little activity surrounding these health targets. For example, on its website, the U.S. Office of Juvenile Justice and Delinquency Prevention lists 175 model programs in 26 categories that it promotes for dissemination in juvenile justice settings (http://www.ojjdp.gov/mpg/). Only one, *Not on Tobacco,* is focused on physical activity, healthy eating, or tobacco control.

To date, the D&I action in the social services has been mostly focused on implementing complex protocols for multifaceted, difficult-to-treat conditions. Substance abuse, conduct disorder, depression, and posttraumatic stress disorder are the most common targets. The juvenile justice sector exemplifies this theme. In this sector, the most promoted programs are designed to decrease and prevent youth conduct problems. Many of these programs are proprietary, and the most promoted are complex clinical programs that possess substantial evidence of their efficacy generated through multiple, randomized clinical trials, including *Multisystemic Therapy (MST), Multidimensional Treatment Foster Care, Functional Family Therapy,* and *Promoting Alternative Thinking Strategies.* The exception to this trend is in the sector of community services for older adults, where programs promoted for dissemination include those for physical activity and health eating.

■ WHAT GROUPS HAVE COMPILED, DISSEMINATED, AND ENDORSED PROGRAMS FOR DISSEMINATION IN THE SOCIAL SERVICES?

Some of the social service sectors have established websites and organizations designed to increase awareness of information about known, evidence-supported interventions that are available for implementation within the sector. One model organization is the California Evidence-Based Clearinghouse for Child Welfare (CEBC). It is unique in several ways. First, it is state funded, through the California Department of Social Services. Second, it uses scientific experts to rate the quality and type of published, peer-reviewed research associated with a program. Third, it rates the relevance of the program for child welfare populations. Fourth, it also conducts reviews of programs in areas that are important to child welfare practice, but for which there are not yet evidence-supported interventions. It does this to inform administrators and consumers about programs that may market themselves as evidence based, when they are not. As of August 2010, the Clearinghouse had reviewed 156 intervention programs in 25 topic areas. Sixteen of the rated programs received their best scientific rating of "well-supported by research." Activity levels, healthy eating, and smoking cessation are not among the topic areas covered to date.

Numerous organizations have compiled and disseminated evidence-supported programs in the juvenile justice sector. The *Blueprints for Violence Prevention* program, affiliated with the University of Colorado at Boulder, aims to identify and promote a small number of programs with a very high scientific standard of effectiveness aimed at reducing substance use and violent behavior. According to its website (as of October 26, 2010), it had assessed over 800 programs and certified 11 as model programs and 19 as promising programs. It uses staff reviews followed by scientific reviews from an advisory board (http://www.colorado.edu/cspv/blueprints/). The U.S. Office of Juvenile Justice and Delinquency Prevention, on the other hand, lists 175 model programs in 26 categories that it promotes for dissemination in juvenile justice settings. It rates 39 of these programs as "exemplary," its highest rating. Despite the number of available programs for dissemination, estimates are that only about 5% of juvenile offenders have the opportunity to benefit from programs with demonstrated efficacy or effectiveness.[14]

In the sector of community long-term care services for older adults, the private nonprofit National Council on Aging maintains a list of a small number of evidence-based programs on its website. It promotes four programs: *Healthy Moves for Aging Well*, a program to promote physical activity, *Health Changes*, a diabetes self-management program, *Healthy Eating for Successful Living*, and *Healthy Ideas*, a depression care management program.

In mental health, the Substance Abuse and Mental Health Services Administration (SAMHSA) maintains a National Registry of Evidence-Based Programs and Practices for the prevention and treatment of mental health and substance abuse problems. As of October 26, 2010, its registry included 160 programs. Program developers can self-nominate their programs for inclusion. The Registry does not rate for effectiveness; instead, it rates programs on the quality of the research conducted on the program and its readiness for dissemination.

To date, efforts to disseminate health prevention and intervention protocols through the social services have been focused on the juvenile justice, child welfare, mental health, and community long-term care services for older adults sectors of care. Professionals working in other social service sectors of care may need to rely on compilations of evidence-supported protocols that are health topic specific. There are a number of these. Some are reviewed in several other chapters in this book.

■ DISSEMINATION AND IMPLEMENTATION MODELS IN THE SOCIAL SERVICES

No one model of D&I has taken hold in the social services. Most efforts described in the literature are what can be referred to as blended models; they use multiple implementation strategies, often targeting multiple levels of an organization or system. Few of these models have been named or branded. This review starts with three that are.

ARC

Charles Glisson's ARC model (Availability, Responsiveness, Continuity; Glisson and Schoenwald, 2005)[15] is a complex implementation model that blends interventions at three levels—community, administration, and clinical teams—and guides organizations through 12 components in three stages of work lasting 1 to 3 years. ARC components are (1) building organizational leadership, (2) building personal relationships, (3) accessing and facilitating organizational networks, (4) building teamwork in frontline clinical teams, (5) providing information and training related to a clinical innovation, (6) team decision making and technical support, (7) establishing a data feedback mechanism, (8) implementing participatory decision making in frontline teams, (9) resolving staff conflicts, (10) goal setting and continuous quality improvement, (11) redesigning jobs, and (12) ensuring self-regulation and stabilization. Theoretically, ARC is designed to affect implementation through improved agency culture and climate, partnered with the introduction of new systems to monitor progress and confront problems as they are experienced. In a Tennessee-based randomized clinical trial, ARC was tested in conjunction with implementation of MST in a large public agency, with counties randomized to ARC or implementation as usual. Youth who received MST in ARC counties experienced significantly greater decreases in problem behavior than youth in implementation-as-usual counties.[16]

The California Institute of Mental Health Community Development Team Model

The manual for the Community Development Model[17] describes a process that involves (a) outreach to agency directors to drum up interest in evidence-supported interventions, (b) partnerships with treatment developers to deliver clinical training, (c) agency-developed implementation plans, (d) individualized, technical assistance from centralized staff to agencies on issues of implementation, and (e) the development of peer-to-peer networks of agency staff who are implementing evidence-supported interventions to jointly problem-solve implementation barriers and to share successful strategies. This model is being used in a large clinical trial, of *Multidimensional Treatment Foster Care* in California and Ohio counties, with the counties randomized to receive implementation as usual or implementation using the Community Development Team Model (Chamberlain et al., 2008).[18]

The KIT (Knowledge Informing Transformation) Program of the Substance Abuse and Mental Health Services Administration

The KIT program is based on the notion of a toolkit. SAMSHA, working with treatment developers, has developed toolkits for several different, complex, evidence-supported intervention programs. The toolkits include introductions to the importance of evidence-supported interventions, implementation tips for agency administrators, training modules for practitioners, outcomes and fidelity measures to be used by program staff in monitoring quality and outcomes, and multimedia products (DVDs and slide presentation tools) to introduce the intervention to stakeholders, including staff, consumers, and family members. These tools are available free of charge on the SAMSHA website (http://mentalhealth.samhsa.gov/cmhs/ CommunitySupport/toolkits). SAMSHA also supports implementation through large, competitive grants to states, designed to transform service systems by integrating the recommended interventions.

The other models discussed here have been named for the purpose of this article.

Awareness-Based Web Dissemination

Perhaps the most common dissemination tool is the web-based compilation of best practices. Several were described earlier in this chapter. Most of these efforts are simply trying to get the word out that there are programs available for D&I.

The Purveyor Organization

Several intervention developers working in social service sectors use separate training and technical assistance organizations to aid with dissemination and implementation. An existing organization may agree to take on this task, or a new, separate organization may be developed. Care for Elders, a Houston-based TA agency for *Healthy Ideas*, is an example of the former. Examples of purveyor organizations created explicitly for D&I work include Behavioral Tech, LLC, to disseminate *Dialectical Behavior Therapy*, TFC, Inc., to disseminate *Multidimensional Treatment Foster Care*, and MST Services to disseminate *Multisystemic Therapy* (see Case Study). Some of these are nonprofit and others are incorporated for-profit organizations.

The interventions these organizations disseminate tend to be complex enough to require substantial start-up assistance. In all known cases, the demand for training far outweighed the ability of the clinical innovator to provide it. These separate organizations are in charge of the dissemination and implementation activities associated with the clinical innovation and thus allow the original treatment developers to create new innovations and run clinical trials. For this chapter, two different models are described that operate within these purveyor organizations, though there are undoubtedly other variations in operation.

Training + Implementation Technical Assistance

Some purveyor organizations provide substantially more implementation guidance than can be found in a typical SAMSHA toolkit. These developers have created implementation standards and guidance that they distribute to organizations that are adopting their intervention. Care for Elders, the disseminator of *Healthy Ideas*, offers a free initial consultation and readiness assessment tools for organizations interested in adopting their intervention. Once an adoption decision has been made, Care for Elders, for a one-time fee, will visit the organization; provide monthly telephone consultation on implementation designed to ensure that ongoing training, quality assurance, and fidelity measurement have been instituted; and provide program and implementation manuals, training videos, a variety of other tools and unlimited e-mail technical assistance.

Training + Consultation + Certification

Some of the purveyor organizations have more of a focus on consultation for clinical services. As an example, TFC, Inc., trains clinical teams in their treatment foster care model during a week-long training program in Oregon, provides consultation on start-up and recruiting foster parents, then provides weekly supervision to the team by phone from their offices in Oregon for the first year of clinical services. During this year, clinical team and foster parent team meetings are audiorecorded and reviewed by the TFC, Inc., consultant, who provides guidance on adhering to the model. Some of the dissemination and implementation organizations offer a certification or accreditation process that designates an organization as officially capable of delivering the intervention. After a year of ongoing consultation with TFC, Inc., and a site visit by the TFC, Inc., consultant, a *Multidimensional Treatment Foster Care* team can be certified to provide these services for a specified period of time without TFC, Inc., consultation or additional site visits. Such designations may prove useful in efforts to get funders to pay for the clinical service. For example, a state Medicaid office may agree to pay a lump sum for providing *Multidimensional Treatment Foster Care* services but will only offer reimbursement to provider organizations certified by TFC, Inc. This keeps other organizations, theoretically those providing lesser services at lower costs, from being able to bill as providing the evidence-supported program.

■ DESIGNING D&I INTERVENTIONS FOR THE SOCIAL SERVICES

The consolidated framework for implementation science proposed by Damschroder and colleagues[19] offers a useful tool for discussing the special considerations needed to disseminate and implement health interventions in social service settings. They propose five domains of influences on D&I: intervention characteristics, the outer setting, the inner setting, characteristics of individuals, and process. We will discuss the first four of these domains.

Intervention Characteristics

Rogers's Diffusion of Innovation Theory[20] proposed that innovations that have greater *relative advantage, compatibility, trialability,* and *observability,* along with less *complexity,* generally will be adopted over innovations that do not. There is no doubt that the complexity of the evidence-supported interventions now being implemented in the social services may challenge the most robust implementation strategies. *Multidimensional Treatment Foster Care,* for example, is a 24-hour-per-day, 7-day-per-week, 365-day-per-year intervention delivered in teams of six program staff (a supervisor, therapist, family therapist, skills coach, foster parent recruiter, daily caller), plus foster parents, serving 10 clients at a time. Many of these interventions require intense training and substantial consultation through the learning phase. The *trialability* of this kind of intervention is exceptionally low.

The expense of these interventions is compounded by the complexity of the implementation strategies needed to make them work in the long term. Retraining, booster training, and ongoing monitoring of intervention processes for quality assurance are typical implementation requirements for complex interventions. For organizations that successfully implement these interventions, mounting less complex protocols, like smoking cessation programs, might be easier than for other organizations. On the other hand, organizations that attempt to launch these complex programs and fail might be hesitant to try to implement a less complex protocol.

Complex, expensive interventions with low trialability require high competitive advantage and high observability in order for adoption to take place. At this juncture, with low dissemination of evidence-supported programs, agencies may receive substantial competitive advantage just by advertising their adoption of an evidence-based program. Over time, however, documented improved outcomes will likely be required to sustain these programs.

Outer Setting Considerations—Social Service Consumers

Think about two kinds of social service consumers—chronic and temporary. Many people use a social service for a short time. Rank and Hirschl,[21] for example, found that half of Americans use food stamps at some point in their lifetime. Far fewer need food stamps for years at a stretch. Temporary users of social services can be thought of as resourceful, capable, often resilient adults who experience a tough patch along the life course and turn to the social services for help. The social services may not be the most likely access point for delivering evidence-supported health interventions for the temporary social service client. They can be reached through other means.

It is the longer-term users of a social service who will consider the social service case manager their "primary carer," and for whom the influence of this case manager to move clients toward evidence-supported health interventions is greatest.

However, chronic users of social services need these services for reasons. They have fewer resources. They come from more difficult circumstances. They have more comorbid problems. These complicating factors make implementing programs of any type more difficult. Will a weight loss program work for a client on psychotropic medications known to lead to weight gain? Will a smoking cessation program work for a person with poor emotional regulation? Will a chronic disease management program work for a client who lives on the streets for weeks at a time?

Some social service consumers may also have less competence in daily living and organizational skills than health service providers are accustomed to or that some health protocols require. Social service consumers also enter health intervention activities with long service histories. While some are sensitized to respond to professional intervention through prior service successes, others may have a history of service failures that may need to be addressed in any new intervention effort.

These complexities introduced by the nature of social service consumers may require substantial program adaptation. These adaptations might include adding assessments for readiness, adding motivational interviewing to intervention protocols, using materials that require less literacy, parsing the intervention into less complicated processes, and scheduling changes. Some of these adaptation strategies may be uncovered by active attempts to gather consumer and service provider inputs into implementation planning.

Other Outer Setting Considerations

Moving evidence-supported health protocols into the social services faces one challenge that overshadows all others. Who will pay for it? Other pressures can be leveraged to advocate for increased access to evidence-supported health interventions—from advocacy groups, consumer groups, and the press—but without means to pay for these interventions, they will likely not be adopted and sustained by social service agencies. Health interventions moved into social service settings will either need to pay for themselves—with a business case laid out before adoption—or they need to have payment worked out in advance.

Complex interventions, like those often implemented in social service sectors, bring complex payment options. Medicaid is the most common payer for many of the health interventions discussed in this chapter. Complex protocols can sometimes be broken down into billable parts using existing billing codes. *Multidimensional Treatment Foster Care*, for example, can bill some of its services as psychotherapy. On other occasions, agencies can arrange for reimbursement for the entire package of a multicomponent intervention, through paying per case or per day;[22] often, this occurs when the Medicaid agency is eager to support evidence-based approaches and the agency provider possesses good advocacy skills. Even more rare are instances where Medicaid provides a reimbursement sufficient to cover both the intervention and the necessary implementation strategies needed to adopt and sustain it.

Inner Setting Considerations

Local context is a valid consideration in every implementation effort. Social service agencies vary, however, on every possible dimension. Some dimensions that may have the most relevance for D&I work include size, financial resources, accessibility to information, presence of a professionalized quality assurance and improvement workforce, history of successful implementation efforts, electronic case records, and leadership commitment. Public agencies often have difficulty freeing money from compartmentalized funding streams to innovate. Private agencies often operate with small margins on their service contracts and operate with limited reserves that can be tapped to move new initiatives forward.

Provider Considerations

The level of staff motivation needs to be assessed as part of any implementation effort in the social services. Social service employees are often stereotyped as underpaid and overworked. Social service caseworkers who are overworked are not good candidates for new innovations. They will only participate if the new intervention reduces their workload.

Skill and educational levels vary in the social services. Juvenile justice and child welfare services are often delivered by frontline staff with bachelor's degrees. Intervention activities have to be commensurate with staff skill and allow sufficient time in training.

For all of these considerations, the D&I of evidence-supported health and health prevention into the social services will require careful collaboration. Community-Based Participatory Research (CBPR) models of research have poignant relevance in the social services.[23,24] Social services consumers and providers will be skeptical that researchers without practical experiences in their worlds will understand the social realities embedded in these sectors of care and will welcome efforts to establish partnerships of equals that promote colearning, address health from both positive and ecological perspectives, and disseminate findings and knowledge to all partners.

■ CASE STUDY: MULTISYSTEMIC THERAPY (MST)

Like other interventions being implemented in the social services, MST is a complicated clinical intervention being implemented in a sector of care not necessarily known for high-quality service—juvenile justice. Also typical of work in the social services, MST is disseminated through a purveyor organization. MST is atypical in at least three ways. Its intervention model is more intense than most. MST has been the focus of substantial implementation science. And, its dissemination story is described in the literature.[21]

What is Being Disseminated

MST is a manualized, complex, clinical intervention designed for youth with conduct problems and a history of juvenile offenses.[25] It is short term (3–5 months), intense, and includes 24/7 therapist availability. There is daily contact between MST therapists and families, and an MST therapist sees only three to six families at a time. MST is focused on changing sequences of behavior between and among systems that maintain problem behaviors. It is strength based and action focused, and it targets well-specified problems. It uses behavioral, cognitive, and systems concepts in its intervention protocol.

The Vehicles of Dissemination

MST has two primary vehicles for dissemination, MST Services and MST Network Partners. Like many other efforts, the dissemination of MST began ad hoc, with its treatment developers providing training on a moonlighting basis, supplementing their regular academic jobs at the Medical University of South Carolina. This led to a training agreement with the state of South Carolina (using the state's federal family preservation block grant dollars) to disseminate MST across the state. Out-of-state training continued ad hoc, until the demand became too great and the treatment developers sought a new solution. The result was a university-licensed, for-profit organization, MST Services, launched in 1996 in the name of technology transfer. Through MST Services, agencies purchase training, consultation, and quality assurance services from MST Services, and MST Services licenses agencies to use their program.

By 2000, some agencies expressed a desire to train their own MST teams using a train-the-trainer model and expand their own programs. A new dissemination system, MST Network Partners, was developed to allow established MST organizations to carry out the entire MST dissemination and implementation process.[21] In some cases, MST Services helps states and organizations start an MST program and then transfers oversight to a nearby MST network partner.

Dissemination and Penetration Process

MST Services works with agencies and state governments to develop the appropriate framework and context for MST service delivery. This includes assessment of agency finances, beliefs, other services and community support for MST. The assessment procedures are used to build support for MST implementation and to identify unique barriers to be overcome and strengths to use in the implementation effort.[26] Novel foci include developing agency human resources policies that support a 24/7 service delivery model and developing a financial plan that puts into place reimbursement mechanisms that will allow MST to function.[21] This up-front work on financial arrangements is one thing that sets MST's dissemination efforts apart from others and likely contributes to longer-term sustainment.

The MST implementation model likely fits in the training + consultation + certification category described earlier, but with some additional components. Training in MST includes an initial 5-day on-site training, quarterly booster trainings, and weekly on-site supervision by a member of MST Services as well as weekly phone consultations with an MST expert. What may truly set MST's implementation model apart from others, however, is its heavy accent on monitoring and quality assurance. Therapist adherence to MST has consistently predicted consumer outcomes (e.g., Henggeler et al.[27]; Schoenwald et al.[28]). Their data also show that the fidelity of the MST consultant to the model contributes to consumer outcomes.[29] Therefore, MST Services and their network partners accent adherence to MST protocols more than almost any other known implementation effort. Clinicians are monitored with consumer measures of adherence, supervisors are monitored with clinician measures of adherence, and consultants are monitored with measures completed by clinicians and supervisors.

Reach and Penetration

One hundred MST teams were established in the first 5 years, with approximately a 25% increase in the subsequent 7 years, with 425 teams trained by 2008.[21] Schoenwald,[21] however, suggests that even with these teams, a very small percentage of juvenile offenders receive MST.

■ DIRECTIONS FOR FUTURE RESEARCH

Everything that can be written about the need for further D&I research in other settings can be written about D&I research in the social services. There is a need for better specification of implementation outcome measurement, a need for studying implementation over time, a need for comparative effectiveness studies of implementation strategies, a need for testing theoretical models of implementation, and so on. Also, almost every research question important to the field of D&I in health could be addressed in research that is conducted in social service settings. Other questions can be generated from this brief review of D&I work in the social services. I'll mention four.

Are social service sectors of care interested in health intervention and prevention protocols? Given the competing demands inherent in doing health work in the social services, what is the acceptability of this work in social service settings to the different social service stakeholders? How are health concerns prioritized among other demands in these sectors? Given similar efforts to disseminate, are adoption and uptake rates of these interventions similar to those found in other sectors of care?

Are intervention and prevention protocols designed for other sectors of care effective when implemented through social service sectors of care? What are the common adaptations needed to bring health prevention and intervention protocols into social service settings? Can successful implementation of health intervention and prevention protocols in the social services change the outcomes of most interest to social service administrators?

Are implementation protocols developed for complex social service systems of care effective in implementing intervention and prevention protocols in other sectors of care? Can the lessons learned, say, about fidelity in juvenile justice settings by the MST research teams, be transported to medical settings of care?

What are the active ingredients of complex, blended implementation efforts? Given some of the difficulties of bringing complex intervention protocols into less than ideal settings, the implementation strategies in use in the social service sectors have tended to be multifaceted, multiphased efforts. It is important to know what components of these interventions are the most important to successful implementation.

■ CONCLUSION

Social service settings offer numerous complexities in their staffing, consumers, and payer mix that require careful consideration in designing dissemination and implementation efforts. But the social services access to vulnerable populations with health problems may prove vital in efforts to improve the health status of many of our citizens. While a number of well-developed, blended dissemination and implementation models are being used in social service settings, they all require additional documentation, research, and field experience. Nonetheless, the lessons learned in the social services may help organizations in other sectors better implement health interventions with complex consumers in complex settings.

SUGGESTED READINGS

Cargo M, Mercer SL. The value and challenges of participatory research: strengthening its practice. *Annu Rev Public Health.* 2008; 29:325–350.

> *This thorough and sophisticated article on CBPR in the health field provides a critical review of the literature, followed by an "integrative practice framework" highlighting key domains including values and drivers (such as knowledge transfer and self-determination), partnership processes, and the interpretation and application of research outcomes.*

Damschroder LJ, Aron DC, Keith RE, Kirsh SR, Alesander JA, Lowery JC. Fostering implementation of health services research findings into practice: a consolidated framework for advancing implementation science. *Implement Sci.* 2009; 4:50–65.

> *This influential integrative article provides practitioners and researchers a useful framework to think through some of the issues that they might confront when taking on a D&I project in the social services.*

Israel BA, Schulz AJ, Parker EA, Becker AB. Review of community-based research: assessing partnership approaches to improve public health. *Annu Rev Public Health.* 1998; 19:173–202.

> *This paper introduces CBPR and its core principles, as well as some of the challenges entailed in their implementation. In addition to providing a review of the literature, this work uses early lessons of the Detroit Community-Academic Research Center to explicate CBPR principles and their implementation.*

Weisz JR, Kazdin AE. *Evidence-based psychotherapies for children and adolescents.* 2nd ed. New York: Guilford; 2009.

> *The second edition of this book not only provides an introduction to interventions for children and adolescents that have substantial research support but also offers eight chapters on D&I work related to several of these interventions.*

SELECTED WEBSITES AND TOOLS

The website for *Blueprints for Violence Prevention* (http://www.colorado.edu/cspv/blueprints), a project of the Center for the Study and Prevention of Violence at the University of Colorado, serves as a resource for governments, foundations, businesses, and other organizations trying to make informed judgments about their investments in violence and drug prevention programs. The project has reviewed the research for violence and drug prevention programs and promotes the use of specific model programs with detailed program descriptions, introductory videos, and contact information.

The *California Evidence-Based Clearinghouse for Child Welfare* (http://www.cebc4cw.org) provides professionals access to information about the research evidence for programs being used or marketed. It rates programs on the strength of their evidence and their relevancy to child welfare populations and categorizes programs by content area. It has become a force in the dissemination world such that a new positive rating or an improved rating based on updated research drives requests for training from purveyor organizations.

The Community Tool Box (http://ctb.ku.edu). Created by the Work Group for Community Health and Development at the University of Kansas, and over 6,000 pages in length, this well-organized website offers numerous tools for participatory community assessment and evaluation, as well as other aspects of CBPR and related approaches.

Community-Campus Partnerships for Health (www.ccph.info). This site is a portal to a wide array of resources for partnerships undertaking CBPR, including sample memoranda of understanding, tools for collaborative asset and risk mapping, research dissemination, and articles and workbooks on the translation of findings into policy and practice change.

The *National Implementation Research Network* website (http://www.fpg.unc.edu/~nirn) is designed to provide information for service providers in the human services about implementation science. It provides links to evidence-supported interventions, bibliographies on select topics on implementation, and links to reports on implementation science of relevance to the social services.

■ REFERENCES

1. Stiffman AR, Psecosolido B, Cabassa L. Building a model to understand youth service access: The Gateway Provider Model. *Mental Health Services Research*. 2004; 6 (4):189–198.
2. Wilkinson RG. Putting the picture together: Prosperity, redistribution, health and welfare. In Marmot M, Wilkinson RG, eds. *The social determinants of health*, 2nd ed. Oxford, UK: Oxford University Press. 2006:256–273.
3. Williams RB. Lower socioeconomic status and increased mortality: Early childhood roots and the potential for successful interventions. *JAMA*. 1998; 279: 1745–1746.
4. Anda RF, Felitti VJ, Bremner JD et al. The enduring effects of abuse and related adverse experiences in childhood: A convergence of evidence from neurobiology and epidemiology. *European Archives of Psychiatry and Clinical Neuroscience*. 2006; 256: 174–186.
5. Dube SR, Felitti VJ, Dong M, Giles WH, Anda RF. The impact of adverse childhood experiences on health problems: Evidence from four birth cohorts dating back to 1900. *Preventive Medicine*. 2003;37:268–277.
6. Blane D. The life course, the social gradient, and health. In: Marmot M, Wilkinson RG, eds. *The social determinants of health*, 2nd ed. Oxford, UK: Oxford University Press. 2006:54–77.
7. Kuh D, Ben-Shlomo Y. *A life course approach to chronic disease epidemiology: Tracing the origins of ill health from early to adult life*, 2nd edition. Oxford, UK: Oxford University Press; 2004.
8. Steele JS, Buchi KF. Medical and mental health of children entering the Utah foster care system. *Pediatrics*. 2008;1122:e703–e709.

9. Monitoring the Future. http://monitoringthefuture.org/data/09data.html#2009 data-cigs (accessed August 16, 2010).

10. Vaughn M, Ollie M, McMillen JC, Scott LD, Munson, MR. Substance use and abuse among older youth in foster care. *Addictive Behaviors.* 2007;32:1929–1935.

11. McMillen JC, Zima BT, Scott LD et al. The prevalence of psychiatric disorders among older youths in the foster care system. *Journal of the American Academy of Child and Adolescent Psychiatry.* 2005;44:88–95.

12. Reinherz HZ, Giacona RM, Lefkowitz ES, Pakiz B, Frost AK Prevalence of psychiatric disorders in a community sample of older adolescents. *Journal of the American Academy of Child and Adolescent Psychiatry.* 1993;32:369–377.

13. Cawley J, Danziger S. *Obesity as a barrier to the transition from welfare to work.* Cambridge, MA: National Bureau of Economic Research Working paper # W10508; 2004.

14. Greenwood P. Prevention and intervention programs for juvenile offenders: The benefits of evidence-based practice. *The Future of Children.* 2008;18:11–36.

15. Glisson C, Schoenwald SK. The ARC organizational and community intervention strategy for implementing evidence-based children's mental health treatments. *Mental Health Services Research.* 2005;7(4):243–259.

16. Glisson C, Schoenwald SK, Hemmelgarn A et al. Randomized trial of MST and ARC in a two-level evidence-based treatment implementation strategy. *Journal of Consulting and Clinical Psychology.* 2010;78:537–550.

17. Sosna T, Marsenich L. *Community Development Team Model: Supporting the model adherent implementation of programs and practices.* Sacramento, CA: California Institute for Mental Health; 2006.

18. Chamberlain P, Brown CH, Saldana L et al. Engaging and recruiting counties in an experiment on implementing evidence-based practice in California. *Administration and Policy in Mental Health and Mental Health Services Research.* 2008;35:250–260.

19. Damschroder LJ, Aron DC, Keith RE, Kirsh SR, Alesander JA, Lowery JC. Fostering implementation of health services research findings into practice: A consolidated framework for advancing implementation science. *Implementation Science.* 2009:4, 50–65.

20. Rogers E. *Diffusion of innovation,* 4th edition. New York: Free Press; 1995.

21. Rank MR, Hirschl T. Likilihood of using food stamps during the adulthood years. *Journal of Nutrition Education and Behavior.* 2005;37:137–146.

22. Schoenwald SK. From policy pinball to purposeful partnership: The policy contexts of Multisystemic Therapy transport. In Weisz JR, Kazdin AE, eds. *Evidence-based psychotherapies for children and adolescents,* 2nd edition. New York: Guilford Press; 2010:538–553.

23. Cargo M, Mercer SL. The value and challenges of participatory research: Strengthening its practice. *Annual Review of Public Health.* 2008;29:325–350.

24. Israel BA, Schulz AJ, Parker EA, Becker AB. Review of community-based research: Assessing partnership approaches to improve public health. *Annual Review of Public Health.* 1998;19:173–202.

25. Henggeler SW, Schoenwald SK, Borduin CM, Rowland MD, Cunningham PB. *Multisystemic treatment of antisocial behavior in children and adolescents.* New York: Guilford Press; 1998.

26. Edwards DL, Schoenwald SK, Henggeler SW, Strother KB. (2001). A multi-level perspective on the implementation of multisystemic therapy (MST): Attempting

dissemination with fidelity. In Bernfield GA, Farrington DP, Leschied AW, eds. *Offender rehabilitation in practice: Implementing and evaluating effective programs.* London: Wiley; 2001:97–120.

27. Henggeler SW, Pickrel SG, Brondino MJ. Multisystemic treatment of substance abusing and dependent delinquents: Outcomes, treatment fidelity, and transportability. *Mental Health Services Research.* 1999;1:171–184.

28. Schoenwald SK, Carter RE, Chapman JE, Sheidow AJ. Therapist adherence and organizational effects on change in youth behavior problems one year after multisystemic therapy. *Administration and Policy in Mental Health and Mental Health Services Research.* 2008;35:84–97.

29. Schoenwald, SK, Sheidow AJ, Letourneau, EJ. Toward effective quality assurance in evidence-based practice: Links between expert consultation, therapist fidelity, and child outcomes. *Journal of Clinical Child & Adolescent Psychology.* 2004;33:94–104.

19 Implementation Science in Health Care

■ BRIAN S. MITTMAN

■ INTRODUCTION

Among the many domains and sectors studied by implementation researchers during the past 30–40 years, the variety of settings and volume of implementation science activity in the domain of health care are arguably among the richest and most diverse. Health care implementation science has contributed valuable theory and empirical evidence and has advanced efforts to identify and address important conceptual and methodological challenges in implementation research. Implementation research in health care has also helped stimulate increased policy and practice interest and has facilitated the field's continuing transformation into a coherent, integrated body of research encompassing multiple disciplines and domains. Yet implementation science in health care continues to confront the full range of challenges facing the field more broadly, including lack of consensus and underdevelopment of concepts and terminology; shortcomings in the availability and application of relevant theory; debates over appropriate research approaches, designs, and methods; and gaps in research attention to key phenomena. This chapter briefly reviews key stages in the evolution and development of implementation science in health care, describes the range of settings and effective practices of interest to implementation researchers—and the implementation strategies and programs developed to facilitate improvements in health care processes and outcomes—and examines key challenges and future directions in the field. A case study of an integrated program of implementation research in schizophrenia illustrates many of the ideas discussed in the chapter.

■ EVIDENCE BASE AND THEORY

The field of implementation science in health care comprises a broad range of studies and literature, much of which developed through separate streams of activity and has only recently begun to coalesce into a more unified whole. Early implementation research within the field of health services research during the 1970s, 1980s, and continuing into the 1990s studied strategies for "changing physician behavior"[1,2] and was conducted primarily by physician researchers and a smaller group of social and behavioral scientists. Driven largely by concerns over excessive resource utilization and costs (e.g., duplicative or nonindicated diagnostic testing), this research assumed that individual physician decisions were the primary driver of most clinical practices and health care resource utilization, and that effective strategies for changing physician behavior were key to improving adherence to recommended practices and thus to improving quality and efficiency.

Much of the early research in this period examined the effectiveness of information dissemination and conventional educational strategies such as continuing medical education,[3] based on the implicit assumption that physicians' clinical practices are driven primarily by information, knowledge, and education.[4] Other strategies studied during this period included financial incentives[1] and manual (chart-based) and reminder systems[5,6] intended to incentivize and prompt physicians to follow recommended practices and apply the knowledge they obtained via education and information dissemination strategies. Accumulating evidence showing the lack of effectiveness of these methods helped stimulate a series of articles (beginning in the late 1980s and 1990s) discussing the limitations of passive information dissemination and education and examining the role of professional norms and related factors in influencing physician practices,[7,8] particularly in light of the high levels of uncertainty inherent in clinical decision making.[9] These insights led to the development and testing of strategies such as opinion leader methods,[10] academic detailing,[11] and others based on principles of social influence rather than models of rational, analytical decision making.[12] Positive results from many of these studies, in contrast to the largely negative findings of studies evaluating educational strategies, prompted increased interest and continued research on social influence approaches.[13,14]

In addition to concerns over cost and resource utilization (e.g., excessive test ordering), studies evaluating strategies for changing physician practices were also driven by research documenting significant geographic variations in health care practices and outcomes and a related body of research conceptualizing and measuring the quality of health care. Early research documenting variations in care across health care delivery settings and geographic regions[15] led to further studies producing evidence that many variations reflected inappropriate use of specific medical procedures and services.[16] Research to define and measure "quality of care" began in the 1960s and accelerated in the 1970s and 1980s,[17,18] producing specific measures of quality, such as hospital mortality rates,[19] and the accumulation of additional evidence demonstrating gaps and deficiencies in health care quality and outcomes, including widely cited reports from the Institute of Medicine and other groups in the United States and abroad.[20,21,22,23]

Interest in the development of strategies for addressing quality problems was also strengthened by the introduction of appropriateness criteria,[24] clinical practice guidelines[25,26] and "practice parameters,"[27] and other tools and approaches associated with the emerging field of evidence-based medicine.[28] These tools summarized applicable clinical evidence supplemented by expert consensus to specify the desired clinical practices that proponents of improved clinical practice strove to achieve. They offered detailed clinical recommendations and decision aids that could serve as the focus of behavior change and quality improvement strategies, and provided specific benchmarks for measuring health care quality and progress in its improvement. A significant share of implementation research in health care continues to focus on guideline implementation[29,30,31] targeting guidelines compiled in repositories such as the National Guidelines Clearinghouse and the International Guidelines Database maintained by the Guidelines International Network, as well as implementation of specific evidence-based programs and practices and evidence syntheses produced by entities such as Cochrane Collaboration review groups, AHRQ Evidence-based Practice Centers, and the UK University of York Center for Reviews and Dissemination. Recent interest in comparative effectiveness research (CER) and the establishment of the Patient-Centered Outcomes Research Institute (PCORI) in the United States will generate additional clinical evidence and evidence-based guidance for health care practice, prompting additional implementation research to guide CER implementation efforts.[32,33] Priorities for CER and support by PCORI are also expected to stimulate expanded research activity in implementation science: the 100 priorities for CER developed by a U.S. Institute of Medicine committee convened to offer guidance for U.S. CER efforts lists numerous implementation-related priorities and highlights the importance of implementation and the need for better guidance and evidence regarding implementation strategies and processes.[34]

Concurrent with the growth of interest in health care quality and evidence-based medicine, the prevailing emphasis on individual clinician practices during the early decades of implementation science in health care was replaced by a focus on the role of organizational structures and policies ("systems") in the 1980s and 1990s, with an accompanying transition away from efforts to change individual physician behavior and toward strategies such as "continuous quality improvement" and "total quality management" employed in the manufacturing and service sectors in the United States and abroad.[35,36] This trend led to replacement of the label "changing physician practices" with the term "quality improvement research" to describe activity now labeled "implementation research." This period also witnessed a significant increase in the volume of policy, practice, and research activity in health care quality improvement and significant growth in quality improvement research funding (e.g., following establishment of the Agency for Health Care Policy and Research in 1989, later renamed the Agency for Healthcare Research and Quality). Several new journals were established in this period as well, including the *American Journal of Medical Quality*, 1986; *International Journal for Quality in Health Care*, 1989; and *Quality in Health Care*, 2000, subsequently retitled *Quality and Safety in Health Care* and later *BMJ Quality and Safety*.

The development and application of theories and conceptual frameworks guiding implementation strategies, and the use of specific techniques for changing behavior, evolved together with changes in emphasis from individual clinicians to organizations. Theories of individual decision making and behavior change were augmented by theories drawn from management research and by conceptual frameworks linked to the dominant quality improvement techniques such as continuous quality improvement and total quality management. Although key theories from the fields of management research and organizational behavior have been harnessed to design and study implementation strategies and processes,[37-42] the volume of activity to catalogue and explore the role and application of organizational theories in implementation lags that devoted to psychological theories,[43-45] which continue to dominate published implementation science literature in health care. Rogers's Diffusion of Innovations theory[46] and extended versions[47] have featured prominently in implementation studies throughout the history of the field, but additional theoretical frameworks have become increasingly prevalent, including the PARiHS framework[48], as well as broader planning and conceptual frameworks such as PRECEDE-PROCEED[49] and RE-AIM.[50]

The streams of research activity discussed above represent only a portion of the overall body of activity comprising implementation science in health care. Developing largely in parallel with the quality improvement–oriented work in the domain of health care implementation research, additional bodies of implementation research activity in health were underway within related fields such as nursing research, health psychology, and health promotion research, as well as research on substance use disorders, patient safety, health equity and disparities, and others. This research continues to proceed under labels such as "research utilization" (most commonly within nursing research[51,52]), "technology transfer" (substance use disorders research[53]), "operations research"[54] (research in global health and improvement of health systems), and others.[55] Overlapping bodies of research captured by the labels "dissemination and implementation research in health" in the United States, "knowledge translation" (largely in Canada), and related labels in Europe and elsewhere embody theories, research approaches, and empirical studies closely related to work labeled "quality improvement research in health." In the United States, the label "quality improvement research" tends to be more common in studies funded by the Agency for Healthcare Research and Quality and by key foundations supporting quality improvement and patient safety work (e.g., Robert Wood Johnson Foundation, Commonwealth Fund), whereas "dissemination and implementation research" is more commonly seen in studies supported by the National Institutes of Health. The latter body of studies often differs in some respects from quality improvement studies, in their focus on implementation of research evidence and evidence-based practices to overcome the "translational roadblocks" identified by the Institute of Medicine Clinical Research Roundtable[56,57] and serving as a key motivation for the development of the NIH Roadmap Initiative,[58,59] the NIH Clinical and Translational Science Award program, and related initiatives. Despite minor differences in stated policy and practice foundations and goals (e.g., an emphasis on improving quality and reducing quality gaps vs. an emphasis on increasing adoption of research- and evidence-based practices and innovations), each of these subfields of implementation science in health encompasses common theories, research approaches, and methods and pursues common research aims, questions, and hypotheses.

■ DESIGNING DISSEMINATION AND IMPLEMENTATION PROGRAMS AND STRATEGIES

Guidance in selecting and designing implementation strategies in health care is available from a variety of sources. Early work in the field employed an approach representing a form of "empirical treatment" in which single-component, narrowly focused physician behavior change or quality improvement strategies found to be effective in changing clinical practices in earlier studies were selected for use in subsequent studies despite differences between the clinical and quality problems, settings, and other features of the earlier versus subsequent studies. This approach was based on an implicit assumption that specific behavior change strategies were inherently and broadly effective or ineffective, independent of the implementation problem to be addressed or the features of the setting or other factors. This "magic bullet" approach was eventually replaced by recognition that implementation strategies must be selected on the basis of (1) identified causes of quality and implementation gaps and (2) an assessment of barriers and facilitators to practice change, as well as (3) guided by appropriate behavior change theory and conceptual models and (4) sensitive to features of the context and settings in which the implementation effort will occur. Furthermore, because most implementation or quality gaps have multiple causes and involve multiple barriers to change, implementation programs must generally include multiple components, each designed to address one or more identified causes of poor quality or barriers to adoption of recommended practices, and each guided by relevant theory from the social and behavioral sciences. Recognition and responses to these challenges were gradual, however, with an early transition away from single-component to multicomponent implementation approaches, but only a more gradual recognition of the need for the multicomponent approaches to be guided by theory, careful diagnosis, and identification of the underlying causes of quality and implementation gaps and selected to match specific features of the target settings.

The field's evolution from single-component studies to multicomponent approaches to theory-based and problem-based approaches was relatively slow in part because early studies found multicomponent approaches to be superior to single-component strategies even in the absence of careful selection and matching of components to barriers. In many cases this might have been caused by the simple fact that a multicomponent approach is more likely to successfully address one or more key barriers merely because including more components increases the odds of a fortuitous match to key barriers. Subsequent findings suggesting that multicomponent approaches were not always superior to single-component approaches helped trigger recognition that individual components must be carefully selected. Although only limited evidence is available regarding the benefits of tailoring[60] and directly comparing a randomly selected package of implementation strategies to a package consisting of components explicitly selected to match identified barriers to change, the argument that intentional design of an implementation program based on a thorough diagnosis of observed quality or implementation gaps has considerable face validity and is a feature of key frameworks and published guidance for implementation in health care.[61,62] Increased use of behavioral and social science theory[63-65] and formative and process evaluation in evaluations of implementation programs[66] supports improved selection, application, and tailoring of implementation strategies to underlying implementation gaps and settings.

Researchers and practice leaders interested in selecting and combining individual implementation methods have only limited guidance. The Cochrane Collaboration Effective Practice and Organization of Care (EPOC) review group[67] has published approximately 70 systematic reviews (as of November 2010) of implementation strategies in health care, including strategies incorporating financial incentives, educational programs, organizational policy and structure changes, and others. The EPOC collection includes systematic reviews focused on specific single-component implementation strategies and reviews examining strategies studied in reference to a specific type of implementation program or care setting. In the United States, the federal Agency for Healthcare Research and Quality (AHRQ) Evidence-based Practice Center program[68] has published several systematic reviews of implementation strategies under the topic "Quality Improvement and Patient Safety," including a multivolume series entitled "Closing the Quality Gap: A Critical Analysis of Quality Improvement Strategies." The range of potential strategies and multicomponent (multistrategy) implementation programs (packages of strategies) is limitless, however, and continues to grow as research continues. A useful tool for selecting individual strategies and planning a multicomponent implementation program is the Cochrane EPOC review group's typology of practice change interventions,[69] adapted from a typology employed in a published systematic review.[70]

■ BARRIERS TO DISSEMINATION AND IMPLEMENTATION

Recognition of the importance of identifying and overcoming barriers to implementation in health care is well established: many of the key frameworks for planning and conducting implementation research in health care include specific research phases and activities in which barriers are explicitly assessed and analyzed,[61] and several empirical studies have documented and classified barriers to implementation (e.g., Cabana et al. 1999).[71] Although specific barriers vary across the range of health care delivery settings (e.g., small physician practices, hospitals), most result from a common set of fundamental characteristics of health care, including (1) high levels of uncertainty in diagnostic and treatment decision making and in identifying causal links between treatment activities and outcomes, (2) the resulting dominance of professionals and professional norms and culture in health care delivery, and (3) the diverse range of constraints and influences on health care practices.

Professionals and Professional Norms

The central role of professionals in health care delivery and the implications of professionalism for practice change were recognized at an early point in the development of the field. For implementation efforts targeting individual, autonomous clinicians (e.g., physicians in solo and small practices and working in community hospitals under traditional fee-for-service reimbursement), effective implementation requires changes in professional norms in addition to changes in individual clinicians' knowledge and beliefs, economic incentives, and other factors. Professional norms are typically highly stable and not easily influenced by outsiders. Physician resistance to improvement efforts led by insurers and other outside stakeholders is high: clinical practice guidelines developed by physicians' peers and professional communities (e.g., medical societies) are seen as more credible than those developed by government bodies or insurance companies.[72,73] Traditional norms of professionalism favor individual professional judgment and patient-by-patient decisions over standardized, codified policies and procedures, leading physicians to rely more heavily on their own individual judgment rather than clinical practice guidelines, evidence-based practices documented in systematic reviews, and other summaries of research and guidance. This led to early organized resistance to clinical practice guidelines by the American Medical Association, which employed the label "practice parameters" rather than "clinical practice guidelines" to convey the belief that guidelines should offer a voluntary, advisory set of parameters for use in clinical decisions rather than a more explicit form of guidance. Although more accepted now than during the 1990s, guidelines and other tools of evidence-based medicine continue to face strong resistance among many physicians and other health care professionals.

Professionalism and professional autonomy represent significant barriers to implementation in large, organized delivery systems as well as individual settings. Conventional approaches to management employed in traditional complex organizations, in which authority increases in relation to higher positions in a traditional, pyramid-shaped organization, are not applicable in health care delivery organizations (and other "professional bureaucracies"[74]) in which frontline workers at the bottom of traditional organizational pyramids are highly educated, professional clinicians whose decisions and practices are more heavily influenced by outside professional communities and peers rather than organizational rules and policies. Although quality improvement strategies such as continuous quality improvement have been adapted successfully to accommodate the unique hierarchical features of health care organizations, the dominance of external professional norms over internal organizational policies remains a significant barrier to implementation efforts within organizations.

Uncertainty

The importance of professional autonomy and individual judgment in professionals' clinical decision making and practices is reinforced by high levels of uncertainty in health care delivery and in cause–effect relationships.[6] High levels of variability in treatment outcomes, combined with the effects of psychological processes such as belief perseverance,[75] contribute to clinical inertia[76] and to considerable stability and resistance to change in clinicians' beliefs regarding clinical practices. Conservatism and resistance to change are reinforced by the prevalence of contradictory findings from clinical research:[77,78] clinicians trained prior to the era of meta-analyses and systematic reviews appropriately downgrade the weight of individual studies, and thus published guidance, and approach clinical practice guidelines and other forms of published guidance with the same inherent skepticism.

Multilevel Influences

Another significant source of challenges to implementation in health care is the multilevel nature of influences and constraints on health care practices. Several authors[79–81] have noted that health care practices are influenced by a broad range of factors operating at the level of the individual patient and patient–clinician dyad; at the level of clinical microsystems, clinics and larger organizations; within professional communities and regions; and at the national policy level. Individual implementation efforts typically involve behavior change strategies aimed at one or two levels (e.g., patients and clinicians); implementation researchers, clinical leaders, and others attempting to change clinical practices lack sufficient leverage and authority to influence the full range of factors constraining and influencing the target practices. Although the need for multilevel, coordinated approaches to implementation is increasingly recognized and has led to innovative programs such as the Robert Wood Johnson Foundation "Aligning Forces for Quality" initiative,[82] it remains a fundamental challenge and barrier to success.

■ QUALITY IMPROVEMENT CASE STUDY

Frameworks guiding the design and conduct of implementation studies and portfolios of implementation research[61] and texts offering broad overviews of implementation science in health[83,84] describe a series of desirable research activities and study features important for achieving success in identifying, diagnosing, and closing quality and implementation gaps. Table 19–1 summarizes much of this guidance by listing important research activities and selected features of these activities.

Many of the key features of implementation research in health care are illustrated by a rich program of implementation studies targeting quality improvement for schizophrenia. Conducted by Alexander Young and colleagues based at the VA Greater Los Angeles Healthcare System and UCLA, this research encompasses a series of studies documenting and diagnosing gaps in quality and outcomes, and evaluating specific strategies for closing these gaps through implementation of evidence-based practices and other innovations in care delivery.

The origins of this research program include studies documenting significant gaps in the quality of health care received by patients with schizophrenia.[85–87] This evidence, including more recent updated data on quality, implementation, and equity gaps,[88,89] has stimulated and guided a program of research to develop and evaluate quality improvement strategies to improve care, guided by a careful assessment of the key research needs and challenges and a roadmap specifying the research activities to be conducted.[90]

Consistent with frameworks for preimplementation and implementation studies, Young et al. supplemented initial research to identify and quantify quality gaps with studies examining the determinants, and thus potential causes, of these gaps[87] and research to assess key stakeholders' views and recommendations regarding potential approaches for closing these gaps.[91,92] Additional preimplementation and methods development research included studies developing and assessing the validity of key measures of implementation program impacts such as quality of care,[93] clinician competencies,[94] and additional tools, methods, and measures required for implementation studies.[95]

A series of interventional implementation studies launched by Young and colleagues illustrates many of the desirable features of such studies, including extensive formative and process evaluation to examine implementation barriers, facilitators, and processes and thus to supplement and explain analyses of implementation program effectiveness. The research portfolio has included studies examining individual elements of a multicomponent approach to implementation, such as a computerized decision support system,[96] a consumer-led strategy targeting clinicians,[97] and a family targeted intervention.[98] Additional studies (EQUIP-1, EQUIP-2) are evaluating

TABLE 19–1. *Key Features of a Comprehensive Implementation Research Portfolio and Features of Individual Studies*

Research Activity	Desirable Features and Comments
Preimplementation Studies	
Clinical effectiveness research to develop evidence-based, innovative practices	Research design, methods, sampling, and other features should maximize external validity and policy/practice relevance to increase acceptability to target clinicians and leaders.
Development of evidence-based clinical practice guidelines	Guideline development processes should follow published recommendations for appropriate use of evidence, involvement of key stakeholder groups, sponsorship, etc.[72,73]
Development of other innovations	Innovation characteristics should facilitate adoption, incorporating features identified by research on the diffusion of innovations.[47]
Development of methods and measures for implementation studies	Important research tools include validated, casemix-adjusted measures of implementation outcomes (adherence, adoption) and appropriate data sources; study designs for quantitative impact evaluation with adequate external validity; and research approaches and methods for process evaluation.
Documentation of current practices and their determinants	Observational studies to understand current clinical practices and their influences incorporating quantitative and qualitative methods
Measurement and diagnosis of quality or implementation gaps	Observational studies to compare current practices to desired practices and to identify determinants or "root causes" of quality and implementation gaps
Observational Implementation Studies	
Studies of naturally occurring (policy- and practice-led) implementation processes	Observational studies maximize external validity, avoid artificial elements of researcher-led implementation trials, and offer opportunities to develop insights into barriers, facilitators, and key influences on routine implementation processes and success. Strong research designs are needed to achieve adequate internal validity.
Interventional Implementation Studies	
Phase 1 pilot studies of implementation programs	Pilot studies offer opportunities to develop initial evidence regarding the feasibility, acceptability, and potential effectiveness of implementation strategies and to begin to identify key contextual influences and other factors influencing effectiveness. Emphasis on formative evaluation to modify the implementation program based on frequent measurement of impact and operation.
Phase 2 efficacy-oriented, small-scale trials of implementation programs	Trials of implementation programs under idealized (efficacy-oriented) conditions, such as active research team facilitation and support for participating sites and grant funding for added costs, are designed to assess implementation program effectiveness under best-case conditions. Phase 2 studies feature initial formative evaluation to refine implementation programs followed by emphasis on fidelity (with site-level adaptation guided by a predeveloped adaptation protocol).
Phase 3 effectiveness-oriented, large trials of implementation programs	Larger trials of implementation programs under routine conditions (e.g., limited or no research team technical assistance or grant support to participating sites) are designed to assess implementation program effectiveness when deployed under real-world conditions. Phase 3 studies feature site-level adaptation guided by a predeveloped adaptation protocol, and measurement of sustainability, scale-up/spread potential, costs and cost effectiveness, and a broad range of outcomes (implementation outcomes and, where feasible, system-level as well as clinical and patient outcomes, e.g., clinical, functional, quality of life, etc.).
Phase 4 "postmarketing" study of implementation programs	Research-led monitoring and evaluation of policy/practice-led scale-up and spread of an effective implementation program. Phase 4 studies generate feedback to policy/practice leaders to guide their management of an implementation and spread effort.

multicomponent, multilevel implementation programs building on the prior studies of individual components.[99,100] This sequence illustrates the progression from small-scale to larger implementation trials, as well as the value and use of extensive formative and process evaluation and other key features of implementation research portfolios and studies.

■ RESEARCH GAPS AND DIRECTIONS FOR FUTURE RESEARCH

Recent growth in funding, interest, and activity in health care implementation research offers considerable promise for progress in addressing the field's key challenges. Increased attention from researchers trained in a broader range of disciplines and employing a broader range of research approaches and methods will help enrich the methodological toolkit, the range of theoretical perspectives, and the breadth of research epistemologies applied to the field's key questions, while simultaneously helping to increase the volume of empirical evidence and insights and the range of implementation problems and settings studied.

Future activity in the field is likely to help address several identified gaps and advance a number of key debates regarding the future of the field and the need for new ideas and approaches.[101] Important gaps include (1) the limited amount of research attention to barriers and strategies for achieving sustainability and routine scale-up and spread of effective practices following their initial adoption; (2) the need for increased research examining naturally occurring implementation processes (vs. investigator-led implementation); and (3) greater attention to implementation processes and mechanisms via process evaluation and theory-based evaluation, to complement and help understand and interpret the results of impact-oriented research. Key challenges to progress in addressing these research gaps include ongoing debates regarding the role of theory in implementation science and the need for research to inventory, classify, and guide the selection and effective use of theory; debates regarding research approaches and the nature of evidence required to better understand implementation processes and the effectiveness of alternative implementation strategies and programs; and the need for improved methods for observational research on implementation.

Sustainability, Scale-up, and Spread

Interest in barriers and facilitators to sustainability and scale-up and spread has increased recently, based on recognition that successful implementation of effective practices through short-term, research-led efforts targeting a limited number of research sites does not naturally lead to sustained adoption in the participating sites nor broader adoption in additional sites. Interventional implementation studies comparing an intensive, investigator-led multifaceted implementation strategy deployed in a sample of health care organizations against a low-intensity "usual-care" implementation approach in a matched sample of settings can produce significant increases in rates of adoption of the target health care practice. Yet much of this increase might be due to temporary factors such as high levels of researcher attention, technical assistance and support for participating sites, grant funding for additional staff and resources (e.g., IT support for implementation), and others. Studies measuring long-term sustainability of resulting practice changes after withdrawal of these resources are rare, despite considerable evidence from management theory and related fields suggesting that professional and organizational changes may be temporary. Theory and research on phenomena such as organizational learning[102,103] and institutionalization offer considerable value in explaining and predicting long-term patterns of behavior change, and should be explored as part of a broader program of theory development and empirical research to better understand sustainability phenomena and to guide efforts to design improved implementation strategies to increase the likelihood that short-term successes in changing health care practices will be sustained.

A similar need exists for increased attention to scale-up and spread barriers, processes, and strategies. A range of factors limit the external validity and transferability of the findings from interventional implementation studies assessing effectiveness of an investigator-led implementation program in a small number of sites. Factors limiting sustainability, such as temporary researcher attention and technical assistance and grant-provided funds for staff and IT, serve to limit the spread of effective practices beyond sites participating in time-limited implementation research projects as well: responsibility for deploying effective implementation strategies on a large-scale, including provision of technical assistance and other forms of facilitation and support provided by research teams in grant-funded implementation studies, is often unclear. Other factors contribute to limited spread, including nonrepresentativeness of sites participating in research studies: these sites are often high-resource organizations whose ability to successfully adopt effective practices is likely to be high even in the absence of research support and the use of carefully designed practice change strategies. Research to understand barriers and facilitators to scale-up and spread and to develop effective scale-up strategies will help identify and characterize these and other limitations of current approaches to implementation research and will help develop new guidance for successful scale-up and spread.

Observational Studies

Increased research attention to sustainability and scale-up and spread processes will help stimulate growth in observational research examining naturally occurring spread, as well as phased implementation research programs[61,104] involving progression from small-scale efficacy-oriented implementation trials (involving high levels of researcher technical assistance and support for participating sites) to larger-scale effectiveness-oriented trials and observational studies in which researchers have little or no role in facilitating implementation but serve mainly to evaluate the implementation process. Researcher-led implementation efforts are often highly artificial, addressing quality and implementation gaps viewed as important by researchers but not necessarily by participating sites, and involving a range of practice change strategies led by an external research team rather than internal staff. Insights into barriers and facilitators to practice change from research-led implementation efforts have limited external validity. Better insights are needed from appropriately designed[105,106] observational studies of large-scale implementation efforts conducted by policy and practice entities, such as CDC and HRSA and Medicare Quality Improvement Organizations in the United States, as well as practice-driven implementation efforts conducted by integrated health care delivery systems such as the VA, Kaiser Permanente, and national health systems outside the United States.

Impact versus Process and Mechanism Focus

Much of the research examining implementation in health care has pursued questions of implementation strategy effectiveness and has employed well-established experimental and quasi-experimental research approaches for assessing the effectiveness of various implementation strategies. Researchers are increasingly recognizing that effectiveness of implementation strategies is often highly dependent on contextual factors and features of the manner in which the implementation strategies are delivered and managed.[107] As a result the main effect of an implementation strategy is often weak and dominated by a large number contextual and delivery factors, limiting the ability of standard evaluation approaches to estimate effectiveness of the core implementation program. Recent interest and efforts to define, conceptualize, and measure contextual factors[108,109] and to develop better analytical methods for examining their effects[110] are addressing the challenge of weak main effects, but the sample size requirements and other barriers to estimating implementation strategy effectiveness when main effects are small and the number of significant contextual factors is large will continue to challenge the field. In extreme (although arguably common) situations in which outcomes of implementation efforts are driven almost entirely by contextual factors and the manner in which implementation strategies are delivered, with essentially no detectable main effect of the implementation strategy, implementation research efforts must focus on developing insights into the processes and mechanisms of action, pursuing questions such as how, when, where, and why an implementation strategy is effective, rather than whether it is effective.[111–113] Research efforts to develop appropriate methods and approaches for these questions, including theory-based evaluation and realistic evaluation, and debates over the role and value of these approaches in quality improvement and implementation research, will help broaden the portfolio of such research and increase the likelihood that valid, useful insights and guidance will emerge and better contribute to ongoing efforts to reduce quality and implementation gaps and enhance the performance and beneficial impacts of health care delivery and health services.

SUGGESTED READINGS

Eccles MP, Armstrong D, Baker R, et al. An implementation research agenda. *Implement Sci.* April 7, 2009;4:18.

> *Documents results of an expert panel convened to develop an agenda for research in implementation science in the UK.*

Estabrooks CA, Derksen L, Winther C, et al. The intellectual structure and substance of the knowledge utilization field: a longitudinal author co-citation analysis, 1945 to 2004. *Implement Sci.* November 13, 2008;3:49.

> *Describes the content and evolution of several subfields closely related to, and overlapping with, the field of implementation science. Provides a useful introduction and overview of these fields.*

McKibbon KA, Lokker C, Wilczynski NL, et al. A cross-sectional study of the number and frequency of terms used to refer to knowledge translation in a body of health literature in 2006: a Tower of Babel? *Implement Sci.* February 12, 2010;5:16.

> *Documents the range of labels employed in published articles within the field of implementation research and its related fields and subfields. Together with the Estabrooks et al. article listed above, it provides a valuable roadmap or inventory of labels, fields, and subfields employed by researchers studying implementation phenomena, facilitating other researchers' access to this literature.*

Remme JH, Adam T, Becerra-Posada F, et al. Defining research to improve health systems. *PLoS Med.* November 16, 2010;7(11):e1001000.

> *Offers an overview and description of implementation research and related fields of research intended to improve health systems, health care, and public health from a global perspective.*

SELECTED WEBSITES AND TOOLS

http://ktclearinghouse.ca/
The KT Clearinghouse is a repository of implementation research (or "knowledge translation") resources and tools. Individual components with in the Clearinghouse include a Knowledge Base listing training resources, research frameworks, a glossary and other items, a KT Tools section listing specific tools for locating and using evidence and evidence-based programs, and links to related resources.

http://www.queri.research.va.gov/clearinghouse/
The VA QUERI Implementation Research Resource Clearinghouse is a repository of implementation research frameworks, annotated bibliographies, listings of key stakeholder organizations and programs (funding programs, research centers, advocacy and partner organizations), and listings of key activities and resources (conferences, training programs, journals, seminar series).

http://conferences.thehillgroup.com/obssr/DI2011/index.html
The Annual NIH Conference on the Science of Dissemination and Implementation (2007, 2009, 2010, 2011, and planned for 2012) represents the largest annual gathering of dissemination and implementation researchers and research activity in the United States and internationally. The website for each year's conference offers copies of the agenda, participant list, presentations, and selected session summaries and videos. Links to prior years' materials are contained on the "Resources" page within the 2011 conference website.

http://www.kusp.ualberta.ca/en/KnowledgeUtilizationColloquia.aspx
The Knowledge Utilization Colloquia Archive provides materials from the annual Knowledge Utilization Colloquium (convened annually from 2001 to 2011 with planned continuation) and the occasional Knowledge Translation Forum. The Colloquium is a relatively small but intensive conference encompassing implementation research and practice in the fields of nursing research and broader domains of health and health care.

■ REFERENCES

1. Eisenberg JM. *Doctors' Decisions and the Cost of Medical Care: The Reasons for Doctors' Practice Patterns and Ways to Change Them.* Ann Arbor, MI: Health Administration Press; 1986.

2. Smith WR. Evidence for the effectiveness of techniques to change physician behavior. *Chest.* August 2000;118(2 Suppl):8S–17S.

3. Davis DA, Thomson MA, Oxman AD, Haynes RB. Evidence for the effectiveness of CME. A review of 50 randomized controlled trials. *JAMA.* September 2, 1992;268(9):1111–1117.

4. Davis DA, Thomson MA, Oxman AD, Haynes RB. Changing physician performance. A systematic review of the effect of continuing medical education strategies. *JAMA.* September 6, 1995;274(9):700–705.

5. McDonald CJ, Wilson GA, McCabe GP Jr. Physician response to computer reminders. *JAMA.* October 3, 1980;244(14):1579–1581.

6. Burack RC, Gimotty PA, George J, et al. How reminders given to patients and physicians affected pap smear use in a health maintenance organization: results of a randomized controlled trial. *Cancer.* June 15, 1998;82(12):2391–2400.

7. Greer AL. The state of the art versus the state of the science. The diffusion of new medical technologies into practice. *Int J Technol Assess Health Care.* 1988;4(1):5–26.

8. Kanouse DE, Jacoby I. When does information change practitioners' behavior? *Int J Technol Assess Health Care.* 1988;4(1):27–33.

9. Eddy DM. Variations in physician practice: the role of uncertainty. *Health Aff* 1984 Summer;3(2):74–89.

10. Lomas J, Enkin M, Anderson GM, Hannah WJ, Vayda E, Singer J. Opinion leaders vs audit and feedback to implement practice guidelines. Delivery after previous cesarean section. *JAMA.* May 1, 1991;265(17):2202–2207.

11. Soumerai SB, Avorn J. Principles of educational outreach ("academic detailing") to improve clinical decision making. *JAMA.* January 26, 1990;263(4):549–556.

12. Mittman BS, Tonesk X, Jacobson PD. Implementing clinical practice guidelines: social influence strategies and practitioner behavior change. *QRB Qual Rev Bull.* December 1992;18(12):413–422.

13. McIntosh KA, Maxwell DJ, Pulver LK, et al. A quality improvement initiative to improve adherence to national guidelines for empiric management of community-acquired pneumonia in emergency departments. *Int J Qual Health Care.* 2011;23(2):142–150.

14. Ornstein S, Nemeth LS, Jenkins RG, Nietert PJ. Colorectal cancer screening in primary care: translating research into practice. Med Care. October 2010;48(10):900–906.

15. Wennberg J, Gittelsohn. Small area variations in health care delivery. *Science.* December 14, 1973;182(117):1102–1108.

16. Chassin MR, Kosecoff J, Park RE, et al. Does inappropriate use explain geographic variations in the use of health care services? A study of three procedures. *JAMA.* November 13, 1987;258(18):2533–2537.

17. Donabedian A. Twenty years of research on the quality of medical care: 1964–1984. *Eval Health Prof.* September 1985;8(3):243–265.

18. Donabedian A. The quality of care. How can it be assessed? *JAMA.* September 23–30, 1988;260(12):1743–1748.

19. Dubois RW, Brook RH, Rogers WH. Adjusted hospital death rates: a potential screen for quality of medical care. *Am J Public Health*. September 1987;77(9):1162–1166.
20. Schuster MA, McGlynn EA, Brook RH. How good is the quality of health care in the United States? *Milbank Q*. 1998;76(4):517–563, 509.
21. Institute of Medicine. *Crossing the Quality Chasm: A New Health System for the 21st Century*. Washington DC: National Academy Press; 2001.
22. McGlynn EA, Asch SM, Adams J, et al. The quality of health care delivered to adults in the United States. *N Engl J Med*. June 26, 2003;348(26):2635–2645.
23. Hussey PS, Anderson GF, Osborn R, et al. How does the quality of care compare in five countries? *Health Aff*. May–June 2004;23(3):89–99.
24. Brook RH, Chassin MR, Fink A, Solomon DH, Kosecoff J, Park RE. A method for the detailed assessment of the appropriateness of medical technologies. *Int J Technol Assess Health Care*. 1986;2(1):53–63.
25. Woolf SH. Practice guidelines: a new reality in medicine. I. Recent developments. Arch Intern Med. September 1990;150(9):1811–1818.
26. Field MJ, Lohr KN. *Clinical Practice Guidelines: Directions for a New Program*. Washington DC: National Academies Press, 1990.
27. Kelly JT, Swartwout JE. Development of practice parameters by physician organizations. *QRB Qual Rev Bull*. February 1990;16(2):54–57.
28. Sackett DL, Rosenberg WM, Gray JA, Haynes RB, Richardson WS. Evidence based medicine: what it is and what it isn't. *BMJ*. January 13, 1996;312(7023):71–72.
29. Lomas J. Words without action? The production, dissemination, and impact of consensus recommendations. *Annu Rev Public Health*. 1991;12:41–65.
30. Grimshaw JM, Thomas RE, MacLennan G, et al. Effectiveness and efficiency of guideline dissemination and implementation strategies. *Health Technol Assess*. February 2004;8(6):iii–iv, 1–72.
31. Lineker SC, Husted JA. Educational interventions for implementation of arthritis clinical practice guidelines in primary care: effects on health professional behavior. *J Rheumatol*. August 1, 2010;37(8):1562–1569.
32. Naik AD, Petersen LA. The neglected purpose of comparative-effectiveness research. May 7, 2009;360(19):1929–1931.
33. Bonham AC, Solomon MZ. Moving comparative effectiveness research into practice: implementation science and the role of academic medicine. *Health Aff*. October 2010;29(10):1901–1905.
34. Ratner R, Eden J, Wolman D, Greenfield S, Sox H, eds.; Institute of Medicine. *Initial national priorities for comparative effectiveness research*. Washington, DC: National Academies Press; 2009.
35. Berwick DM. Continuous improvement as an ideal in health care. *N Engl J Med*. January 5, 1989;320(1):53–56.
36. Kritchevsky SB, Simmons BP. Continuous quality improvement. Concepts and applications for physician care. *JAMA*. October 2, 1991;266(13):1817–1823.
37. Ash J. Organizational factors that influence information technology diffusion in academic health sciences centers. *J Am Med Inform Assoc*. March–April 1997;4(2):102–111.
38. Rosenheck R. Stages in the implementation of innovative clinical programs in complex organizations. *J Nerv Ment Dis*. December 2001;189(12):812–821.
39. Sheaff R, Pilgrim D. Can learning organizations survive in the newer NHS? *Implement Sci*. October 30, 2006;1:27.

40. Weiner BJ. A theory of organizational readiness for change. *Implement Sci.* October 19, 2009;4:67.
41. Simpson DD, Flynn PM. Moving innovations into treatment: a stage-based approach to program change. *J Subst Abuse Treat.* September 2007;33(2):111–120.
42. Lukas CV, Holmes SK, Cohen AB, et al. Transformational change in health care systems: an organizational model. *Health Care Manage Rev.* October–December 2007;32(4):309–320.
43. Michie S, Johnston M, Abraham C, Lawton R, Parker D, Walker A; "Psychological Theory" Group. Making psychological theory useful for implementing evidence based practice: a consensus approach. *Qual Saf Health Care.* February 2005;14(1): 26–33.
44. Godin G, Belanger-Gravel A, Eccles M, Grimshaw J. Healthcare professionals' intentions and behaviours: a systematic review of studies based on social cognitive theories. *Implement Sci.* July 16, 2008;3:36.
45. Gardner B, Whittington C, McAteer J, Eccles MP, Michie S. Using theory to synthesise evidence from behaviour change interventions: the example of audit and feedback. *Soc Sci Med.* May 2010;70(10):1618–1625.
46. Rogers EM. *Diffusion of Innovations.* 5th ed. New York: Free Press; 2003.
47. Greenhalgh T, Robert G, Macfarlane F, Bate P, Kyriakidou O. Diffusion of innovations in service organizations: systematic review and recommendations. *Milbank Q.* 2004;82(4):581–629.
48. Rycroft-Malone J, Kitson A, Harvey G, et al. Ingredients for change: revisiting a conceptual framework. *Qual Saf Health Care.* June 2002;11(2):174–180.
49. Green LW, Kreuter MW. Health Program Planning: An Educational and Ecological Approach. 4th ed. NY: McGraw-Hill Higher Education; 2005.
50. Glasgow RE, Vogt TM, Boles SM. Evaluating the public health impact of health promotion interventions: the RE-AIM framework. *Am J Public Health.* September 1999;89(9):1322–1327.
51. Stetler CB. Research utilization: defining the concept. *Image J Nurs Sch.* 1985 Spring;17(2):40–44.
52. Champion VL, Leach A. Variables related to research utilization in nursing: an empirical investigation. *J Adv Nurs.* September 1989;14(9):705–710.
53. Brown BS. Reducing impediments to technology transfer in drug abuse programming. *NIDA Res Monogr.* 1995;155:169–185.
54. Remme JH, Adam T, Becerra-Posada F, et al. Defining research to improve health systems. *PLoS Med.* November 16, 2010;7(11):e1001000.
55. McKibbon KA, Lokker C, Wilczynski NL, et al. A cross-sectional study of the number and frequency of terms used to refer to knowledge translation in a body of health literature in 2006: a Tower of Babel? *Implement Sci.* February 12, 2010;5:16.
56. Sung NS, Crowley WF Jr, Genel M, et al. Central challenges facing the national clinical research enterprise. *JAMA.* March 12, 2003;289(10):1278–1287.
57. Crowley WF Jr, Sherwood L, Salber P, et al. Clinical research in the United States at a crossroads: proposal for a novel public-private partnership to establish a national clinical research enterprise. *JAMA.* March 3, 2004;291(9):1120–1126.
58. Zerhouni E. Medicine. The NIH Roadmap. *Science.* October 3, 2003;302(5642): 63–72.
59. Zerhouni EA. Translational and clinical science—time for a new vision. *N Engl J Med.* October 13, 2005;353(15):1621–1623.

60. Baker R, Camosso-Stefinovic J, Gillies C, et al. Tailored interventions to overcome identified barriers to change: effects on professional practice and health care outcomes. *Cochrane Database Syst Rev.* March 17, 2010;(3):CD005470.
61. Stetler CB, Mittman BS, Francis J. Overview of the VA Quality Enhancement Research Initiative (QUERI) and QUERI theme articles: QUERI Series. *Implement Sci.* February 15, 2008;3:8.
62. Grol R, Wensing M, Eccles M. *Improving Patient Care: The Implementation of Change in Clinical Practice.* Oxford: Elsevier; 2004.
63. Sales A, Smith J, Curran G, Kochevar L. Models, strategies, and tools. Theory in implementing evidence-based findings into health care practice. *J Gen Intern Med.* February 2006;21 (Suppl 2):S43–S49.
64. Grol RP, Bosch MC, Hulscher ME, Eccles MP, Wensing M. Planning and studying improvement in patient care: the use of theoretical perspectives. *Milbank Q.* 2007;85(1):93–138.
65. Improved Clinical Effectiveness through Behavioural Research Group (ICEBeRG). Designing theoretically-informed implementation interventions. *Implement Sci.* February 23, 2006;1:4.
66. Stetler CB, Legro MW, Wallace CM, et al. The role of formative evaluation in implementation research and the QUERI experience. *J Gen Intern Med.* February 2006;21 (Suppl 2):S1–S8.
67. Cochrane Effective Practice and Organisation of Care Group http://epoc.cochrane.org. Accessed December 21, 2010.
68. Evidence-based Practice Centers. Agency for Healthcare Research and Quality. http://www.ahrq.gov/clinic/epc. Accessed October 2010.
69. Data Collection Checklist. Cochrane Effective Organisation of Care Review Group. http://epoc.cochrane.org/sites/epoc.cochrane.org/files/uploads/datacollection checklist.pdf. Accessed December 28, 2010.
70. Stone EG, Morton SC, Hulscher ME, et al. Interventions that increase use of adult immunization and cancer screening services: a meta-analysis. *Ann Intern Med.* May 7, 2002;136(9):641–651.
71. Cabana MD, Rand CS, Powe NR, et al. Why don't physicians follow clinical practice guidelines? A framework for improvement. *JAMA.* October 20, 1999;282(15): 1458–1465.
72. Tunis SR, Hayward RS, Wilson MC, et al. Internists' attitudes about clinical practice guidelines. *Ann Intern Med.* June 1, 1994;120(11):956–963.
73. Hayward RS, Guyatt GH, Moore KA, McKibbon KA, Carter AO. Canadian physicians' attitudes about and preferences regarding clinical practice guidelines. *CMAJ.* June 15, 1997;156(12):1715–1723.
74. Mintzberg H. Organizational design, fashion or fit? *Harv Bus Rev* 1981;59(1): 103–116.
75. Ross L. The intuitive psychologist and his shortcomings: distortions in the attribution process. *Advances in Experimental Social Psychology.* 1977;10:173–220.
76. Phillips LS, Branch WT, Cook CB, et al. Clinical inertia. *Ann Intern Med.* November 6, 2001;135(9):825–834.
77. Altman DG. The scandal of poor medical research. *BMJ.* January 29, 1994;308(6924): 283–284.
78. Ioannidis JP. Why most published research findings are false. *PLoS Med.* August 2005;2(8):e124.

79. Ferlie, EB, Shortell, SM. Improving the quality of health care in the United Kingdom and the United States: a framework for change. *Milbank Q.* 2001; 79(2):281–315.

80. Mechanic D. Improving the quality of health care in the United States of America: the need for a multi-level approach. *J Health Serv Res Policy.* July 2002;7(Suppl 1): S35–S39.

81. Berwick DM. A user's manual for the IOM's "Quality Chasm" report. *Health Aff* May–June 2002;21(3):80–90.

82. Aligning Forces for Quality. Robert Wood Johnson Foundation. www.forces4 quality.org.

83. Grol R, Wensing M, Eccles M. *Improving Patient Care: The Implementation of Change in Clinical Practice.* Edinburgh: Elsevier; 2005.

84. Straus SE, Tetroe J, Graham ID. *Knowledge Translation in Health Care: Moving from Evidence to Practice.* West Sussex: Blackwell; 2009.

85. Young AS, Sullivan G, Burnam MA, Brook RH. Measuring the quality of outpatient treatment for schizophrenia. *Arch Gen Psychiatry.* July 1998;55(7):611–617.

86. Lehman AF. Quality of care in mental health: the case of schizophrenia. *Health Aff.* 1999;18:52–65.

87. Young AS, Sullivan G, Duan N. Patient, provider, and treatment factors associated with poor-quality care for schizophrenia. *Ment Health Serv Res.* December 1999;1(4):201–211.

88. Young AS, Niv N, Cohen AN, Kessler C, McNagny K. The appropriateness of routine medication treatment for schizophrenia. *Schizophr Bull.* July 2010;36(4): 732–739.

89. Rost K, Hsieh YP, Xu S, Menachemi N, Young AS. Potential disparities in the management of schizophrenia in the United States. *Psychiatr Serv.* June 2011;62(6):613–618.

90. Young AS. Evaluating and improving the appropriateness of treatment for schizophrenia. *Harv Rev Psychiatry.* July–August 1999;7(2):114–118.

91. Henderson C, Jackson C, Slade M, Young AS, Strauss JL. How should we implement psychiatric advance directives? Views of consumers, caregivers, mental health providers and researchers. *Adm Policy Ment Health.* November 2010;37(6): 447–458.

92. Young AS, Niv N, Chinman M, et al. Routine outcomes monitoring to support improving care for schizophrenia: report from the VA Mental Health QUERI. *Community Ment Health J.* April 2011;47(2):123–135.

93. Cradock J, Young AS, Sullivan G. The accuracy of medical record documentation in schizophrenia. *J Behav Health Serv Res.* November 2001;28(4):456–465.

94. Chinman M, Young AS, Rowe M, Forquer S, Knight E, Miller A. An instrument to assess competencies of providers treating severe mental illness. *Ment Health Serv Res.* June 2003;5(2):97–108.

95. Chinman M, Hassell J, Magnabosco J, Nowlin-Finch N, Marusak S, Young AS. The feasibility of computerized patient self-assessment at mental health clinics. *Adm Policy Ment Health.* July 2007;34(4):401–409.

96. Young AS, Mintz J, Cohen AN, Chinman MJ. A network-based system to improve care for schizophrenia: the Medical Informatics Network Tool (MINT). *J Am Med Inform Assoc.* September–October 2004;11(5):358–367.

97. Young AS, Chinman M, Forquer SL, et al. Use of a consumer-led intervention to improve provider competencies. *Psychiatr Serv.* August 2005;56(8):967–975.

98. Cohen AN, Glynn SM, Hamilton AB, Young AS. Implementation of a family intervention for individuals with schizophrenia. *J Gen Intern Med.* January 2010;25 (Suppl 1):32–37.

99. Brown AH, Cohen AN, Chinman MJ, Kessler C, Young AS. EQUIP: implementing chronic care principles and applying formative evaluation methods to improve care for schizophrenia: QUERI Series. *Implement Sci.* February 15, 2008;3:9.

100. Hamilton AB, Cohen AN, Young AS. Organizational readiness in specialty mental health care. *J Gen Intern Med.* January 2010;25 (Suppl 1):27–31.

101. Eccles MP, Armstrong D, Baker R, et al. An implementation research agenda. *Implement Sci.* April 7, 2009;4:18.

102. Argote L, Epple D. Learning curves in manufacturing. *Science.* February 23, 1990:247(4945):920–924.

103. Huber G. Organizational learning. *Organization Science.* 1991;2(1):88–115.

104. Campbell NC, Murray E, Darbyshire J, et al. Designing and evaluating complex interventions to improve health care. *BMJ.* March 3, 2007;334(7591):455–459.

105. Eccles M, Grimshaw J, Campbell M, Ramsay C. Research designs for studies evaluating the effectiveness of change and improvement strategies. *Qual Saf Health Care.* February 2003;12(1):47–52.

106. Speroff T, O'Connor GT. Study designs for PDSA quality improvement research. *Qual Manag Health Care.* January–March 2004;13(1):17–32.

107. Ovretveit JC, Shekelle PG, Dy SM, et al. How does context affect interventions to improve patient safety? An assessment of evidence from studies of five patient safety practices and proposals for research. *BMJ Qual Saf.* July 2011;20(7):604–610.

108. Kaplan HC, Brady PW, Dritz MC, et al. The influence of context on quality improvement success in health care: a systematic review of the literature. *Milbank Q.* December 2010;88(4):500–559.

109. Taylor SL, Dy S, Foy R, et al. What context features might be important determinants of the effectiveness of patient safety practice interventions? *BMJ Qual Saf.* July 2011;20(7):611–617.

110. Shekelle PG, Pronovost PJ, Wachter RM, et al. Advancing the science of patient safety. *Ann Intern Med.* May 17, 2011;154(10):693–696.

111. Walshe K, Freeman T. Effectiveness of quality improvement: learning from evaluations. *Qual Saf Health Care.* March 2002;11(1):85–87.

112. Walshe K. Understanding what works—and why—in quality improvement: the need for theory-driven evaluation. *Int J Qual Health Care.* April 2007;19(2):57–59.

113. Berwick DM. The stories beneath. *Med Care.* December 2007;45(12):1123–1125.

20 Health Dissemination and Implementation within Schools

■ REBEKKA LEE AND
STEVEN GORTMAKER

■ INTRODUCTION

Schools hold great promise for the promotion of health. In much of the world, individuals spend the majority of their formative years within school settings. Thus, schools are ideal places to initiate healthy behaviors early on to promote life-long health. A healthy school environment can promote norms about foods and beverages children consume, physical activity participation, and appropriate social behavior. These healthy environments can be created by local school practices or mandated by top-down policies. In addition to providing healthy environmental cues, schools are optimal settings for disseminating health education messages discouraging risk-taking behaviors (e.g., smoking, drinking, drug use, or unprotected sex) and can be an important place for delivering basic preventive services (e.g., vaccines, vision screening, mental health assessments). Elementary, middle, and high schools as well as preschools and afterschool programs are fundamental settings for establishing healthy habits early in life for optimal prevention of childhood health risks as well as chronic disease later in life. With sound implementation, schools have the potential for tremendous reach and impact. That being said, research on public health dissemination and implementation in schools is in an early stage of development.

Careful study is necessary to ensure that the full promise of schools for health promotion is reached, especially considering the important public health objective of narrowing health disparities. Education, in and of itself, has been targeted as a key factor for future health and poverty reduction across the global. In fact, one of the United Nations' eight Millennium Development Goals is to achieve universal primary education by 2015.[1] Moreover, the World Health Organization has identified the school setting as particularly important for promoting intersectoral action to address child and adolescent health.[2] In the United States, education has been considered a public good since it became mandatory at the close of World War I.[3] On the other hand, while deliberate health promotion by the state has been encouraged since the 1800s, countries today vary dramatically in their role as provider of health services and preventive programs to their citizens.[4,5] By weaving health promotion, above and beyond the delivery of health services, into the public school agenda, there is the opportunity to reach the whole population, including underserved groups (e.g., rural, low income, people of color), with health messages and services that other settings may miss. Moreover, the amount of time that children spend in school is incomparable to other settings such as primary care. Consider, for instance, the difference between the 30 minutes a doctor might spend with a child at an annual well visit exam compared with the roughly 75,600 minutes (7 hours/day over 180 days) children spend within school walls each year. Thus, promoting health within schools has the potential to reinforce the messages of health professionals in a sustained manner, changing norms and everyday behaviors with accumulating effects across the early years of life (Table 20–1).

However, there is a flipside to this potential. Roughly half of funding for schools in the United States comes from local sources.[6] This translates into differences in public school resources and quality. Without careful planning and attention to issues of implementation and dissemination, situating health promotion efforts in schools could actually exacerbate health disparities because communities with fewer resources may not be able to afford to implement health interventions. The excitement of translating public health research findings into practice should be balanced by the realities of the educational system and the implementation barriers and facilitators specific to schools. Future school-based dissemination and implementation research cannot overestimate the importance of developing strategies that are compatible with the primary aims of schools: promoting learning through reading, writing, math, and so on. Equally important is considering policy and environmental change strategies at the national, state, and district level to promote health within schools. Policies that make use of existing personnel and infrastructure can

TABLE 20–1. *Typology of Health Intervention Implemented and Disseminated within Schools*

Type	Definition	Examples
Health-promoting policies	Regulations implemented at the national, state, district, or school level intended to promote children's health within schools	• District wellness policies • State law mandating physical activity time • School rule mandating access to potable drinking water via working drinking fountains or water coolers
Environmental change strategies	School practices that are intended to create healthy environments for children	• Healthy options through school food service in vending machines on school grounds • Classroom-based social skills development (e.g., Responsive Classroom)
Health education messages	Health lessons and messages designed to lay the foundation for lifelong health	• Physical education • Sexual health education • Classroom-based nutrition and physical activity curricula (e.g., Planet Health) • Substance use prevention lessons • Healthy messaging directed toward students, staff, and parents on posters, newsletters, etc.
Health programs and services	Delivery of prevention and treatment within the school setting	• School food service • After-school sports • Immunization • Vision, body mass index, and scoliosis screening • Mental health assessment and counseling

be particularly cost-effective.[7] Finally, increased attention should be paid toward selecting low-cost solutions for schools and families that will be most acceptable and feasible for dissemination across schools with varying resources. Although there is still much to be learned about which interventions (e.g., policies, practices, services, and curricula) are best to implement and disseminate within schools, as well as by whom, when, and how; this chapter seeks to review the school-based dissemination and implementation evidence base and discuss the specific challenges that schools face in their quest to promote health.

■ EVIDENCE BASE AND THEORY

Current State of School-Based Dissemination and Implementation

In addition to the World Health Organization's recognition of schools as excellent spaces for promoting health, the Centers for Disease Control and Schools for Health in Europe have specifically endorsed the idea that evidence-based health programming should be disseminated and implemented within schools. These organizations have set forth guidance for how schools can best create healthy school environments and integrate health promotion services, education, and programs for children.

The Centers for Disease Control (CDC) recommends Coordinated School Health Programs as a means for achieving better health for students. Coordinated School Health consists of eight components: health education, physical education, health services, nutrition services, counseling and psychological services, healthy school environment, staff health promotion, and family/community involvement.[8] Major areas of focus include healthy eating, physical activity, tobacco prevention, asthma management, and STI/HIV prevention. The CDC also helps schools implement and disseminate effective, low-cost programming with their school guidance documents for topics such as tobacco and skin cancer prevention, mental health, and healthy eating as well as self-assessments (e.g., School Health Index and Physical Education Curriculum Analysis Tool).[9]

Similar school-based health guidance was introduced in Europe through the European Network of Health Promoting Schools (ENHPS), now under the name of Schools for Health in Europe (SHE) network.[10,11] Projects are designed to move beyond single-issue educational programs, with the aim to achieve healthy lifestyles for school populations through supportive environments. Five categories of intervention were initially proposed to comprise the ENHPS: improvements to schools' physical environments, improvements to programs addressing health-related topics, building democracy in schools (i.e., giving students a voice in school decision making), development of policies and materials for teacher training on healthy education, and teacher skills development such as communication and active teaching.[10] Today, SHE's health-promoting school approach emphasizes the values of educational and health equity, sustainability, inclusion, empowerment, and democracy to encourage school, health, and social services sectors to collaborate toward optimal child health.[11]

Although these guidelines for school-based health promotion have been disseminated broadly, there remains a large gap between the program, policies, curricula, and services that are suggested as best practices and those that are currently being implemented within schools. In 2006, the School Health Programs and Policies Study (SHPPS) estimated the following: only 61% of schools require health education in at least one specific grade; 78% of schools require students to take some physical education, but less than 10% require daily physical education across the school year; 86% of schools have a school nurse, yet only 14% of schools provide immunizations and less than 5% of high schools make condoms available to students.[12-14] There is also evidence that "junk food" is easily available in high school vending machines—50% have chocolate candy and 78% soda or fruit drinks for purchase.[15] There is much research on the efficacy of specific school-based health interventions that has not been replicated or taken to scale. Some evidence exists for health interventions such as programs designed to address mental and emotional health, substance use, healthy eating and nutrition, and sexual health.[16-27] School-based health policies have not been as widely evaluated, but results show that they are likely effective.[28-30] The broad adoption of DARE (Drug Abuse Resistance Education) over more effective interactive prevention programs is an illustration of how the dissemination and implementation gap can work in reverse. Although this program showed little to no efficacy for preventing substance use behavior, it was the only curriculum endorsed in the 1986 Drug-Free Schools and Communities Act and has been disseminated to over half of U.S. school districts, costing at least $1 billion each year.[31,32] While one step toward creating schools that promote health is to continue to build the evidence base for efficacy of new interventions, addressing the dissemination and innovation gap is essential for future public health research.

One excellent place to start bridging this gap includes the replication of cost-effective interventions with diverse populations in a variety of settings. Considering the constant presence of school in children's lives for over 12 years, it is also important to conduct research that promotes programs that can work together across the life course to promote health and how schools can help to link children to services beyond the school walls.[33] Evaluations within schools should also investigate the factors that influence quality of implementation and assess the impact of interventions that have been adapted to local contexts and to accommodate real-world barriers.

Theory Base

With school-based public health implementation and dissemination research still in its development, the majority of literature to date lacks an explicit theoretical framework. That being said, two key frameworks—the RE-AIM framework and diffusion of innovations—have been repeatedly and successfully applied to dissemination and implementation research within schools. Additionally, social-ecological models are useful for thinking through the appropriate level at which to intervene within schools, and considerations for cost should be made as interventions are designed to be feasibly delivered in real-world settings.[34-36]

The RE-AIM framework, developed by Glasgow and colleagues in 1999, has been effectively (if only seldom) used as a guide for evaluating implementation within the school context.[37-39] RE-AIM identifies five elements that are key for measuring the success of interventions in real-world settings—reach, efficacy, adoption, implementation, and maintenance.[37] In the context of school-based health promotion, reach would refer to the number of children who are served water or fruits and vegetables every day in the school cafeteria or how many children participate in physical education class. Efficacy, the standard measure of success in most public health research, refers to changes in children's behavior (beverage or fruit and vegetable consumption or physical activity level) that can be attributable to a given intervention. Adoption would refer to the number of schools that order water coolers to promote water consumption, change their lunch menus, or schedule more hours of physical education. Implementation, although closely linked to adoption, refers specifically to whether planned changes in practice or policy are translated into action: for example, if foods and beverages served match those on menus or if scheduled physical activity blocks run successfully. The final construct, maintenance, refers to the degree to which initiatives like more nutritious offerings at lunch and improved physical education continue over time.[38] While the RE-AIM framework and constructs have been infrequently used in school-based research, they can help to highlight the importance of external validity and identify where implementation and dissemination starts to unravel differentially across school contexts.[39]

Everett Rogers's *Diffusion of Innovations*, first published in 1962, aims to describe how ideas or practices perceived as new (e.g., policies, practices, curricula, or services) are communicated through a variety of channels over time among members of a social system.[40] The framework emphasizes the stages through which innovations are developed and spread over traditional efficacy research that focuses on the end result of behavior change.[40] For example, researchers following diffusion of innovation would measure the initial adoption of a new physical education curricula (e.g., ordering new materials or equipment), the planned effort to introduce the new curricula within a given number of schools, the maintenance of the practices across multiple school years, the sustainability of the curriculum after initial funding is used up, and its institutionalization within all physical education classes in a given school district. While much of its early application stemmed from the fields of rural sociology and anthropology, diffusion of innovations describes the multitude of factors that can influence the likelihood of implementation and dissemination of health interventions within schools as it has been successfully applied within education and health fields for decades.[40] These factors include characteristics of the innovation (e.g., relative advantage over current practice, compatibility with current values, trialability, and observability) and characteristics of the setting (e.g., geography, culture, and politics).[40] Diffusion of innovations also implicitly points to the role of cost in the implementation and dissemination of new interventions. Applying diffusion of innovations to school settings encourages research on the factors that inhibit or facilitate schools to implement and disseminate health-promoting initiatives, an important domain of study for the investigation of health disparities.

Ecological theories of change are unique in their consideration of the many levels of influence on human behavior. They share the common assumption that the best public health solutions include behavior-specific intervention for *both* the individual and the environment.[41] Stokols articulated these concepts in his social-ecological model, which points to interpersonal, intrapersonal, organizational, community, and policy as different levels at which behavior change can occur.[42] This theoretical orientation is important for deciding the appropriate level or levels of intervention for implementation and dissemination research within schools.

■ DISSEMINATION AND IMPLEMENTATION CHALLENGES SPECIFIC TO SCHOOL SETTINGS

Adapting Interventions to Diverse School Settings

As researchers choose their targets for implementation and dissemination research within schools, it is essential that they be designed with enough flexibility that they can adapt to have local relevance and account for the norms and culture within schools. Examples of adaptations to diverse communities would be considering regional differences in the availability of fruits and vegetables, inaccessibility to drinking fountains due to lead piping, or differences in weather and facilities that would impact physical education curricula or policy changes. Interventions that explicitly seek to identify and change local norms about children's food preferences, the safety of drinking water, or the importance of physical activity will also have a greater chance to be implemented and sustained as they will be more relevant to teachers, children, parents and members of the community. While school priorities and cultures will vary across space and time, one key factor to keep in mind as researchers develop school-based interventions is the importance of aligning with the primary mission of learning. Thus, all policies, environmental change strategies, health education, programs, and services should be designed to fit easily into current school practices and, if possible, aim to promote academic as well as health objectives.

Considering Economic Cost and Impacts beyond Health

School-based health promotion research has seldom explicitly applied economic concepts to investigate issues of dissemination and implementation. Cost is a major factor that influences implementation, especially within public schools where budgets are tight and resources have to be allocated carefully. Although Levin started to apply cost-effectiveness within education in the 1970s and 1980s, few studies have applied the strategy to compare the relative costs and effects of interventions in schools.[34,43,44] Within the health field, Weinstein was among the first to develop cost-effectiveness guidelines to inform resource distribution decisions.[45,46] Although only recently applied to health promotion costs within the school setting, Carter and the ACE (Assessing Cost Effectiveness) team developed a cost-effectiveness model for priority setting of health interventions using an economic approach.[36,47] This strategy costs out all resources used in provision and use of an intervention, including personnel (e.g., wages and additional time for teachers, administrators, and volunteers), equipment (e.g., curriculum, water coolers, parent newsletters), and travel. These costs are partitioned out in terms of costs to the health sector, costs to government sectors (in this case, education), and costs incurred by children, families, and staff.[35,48,49] Finding cost-effective strategies is particularly important for making health promotion appealing to education leaders, teachers, policymakers, and tax payers. A recent report designed to direct available resources in Australia ranked 160 health interventions and found that policies that have a broad reach and make use of existing personnel and infrastructure can be particularly cost-effective and may even be cost-saving in the long run.[7]

Providing evidence for cost-effectiveness and benefits beyond health can be important for achieving buy-in and continuing support since academics are the number one priority for schools. Policies and practices that do not require extra staff and limited training and equipment are appealing to administrators as they keep costs down and can be more easily maintained once a research project is complete. Planet Health, for instance, was able to keep costs low by incorporating the curriculum into existing class time, requiring just one book per teacher, and calling for minimal extra materials in lessons (see Planet Health case study for more details).[23] In the realm of school health services, while all interventions may seem beneficial on the surface they could vary greatly in their cost-effectiveness. For example, there is evidence supporting the cost-effectiveness of providing Hepatitis B vaccinations in schools versus through HMOs; however, vision and hearing screenings in schools may be largely duplicate efforts and end up being cost inefficient.[50] A nutrition curriculum that includes grade- and subject-specific academic lessons, a physical activity program that provides 10 minute classroom activity breaks, or a water campaign that combines messages about environmental responsibility are a few examples of innovative approaches that consider the multitude of priorities within the school setting.

Targeting Multiple Levels of Change

Careful consideration of the level of change is also important in the design of interventions that are to be successfully implemented within the school setting.[42] School-based health promotion interventions could be implemented at a national, state, or district policy level; as a change in school practice; or via one-on-one services delivered by teachers, counselors, nurses, and others. Each of these strategies has different implications for the reach, dose, and cost of implementation. For instance, a district wellness policy may be able to be disseminated broadly across a large school system. This change would likely cost very little and reach a large number of children with a small change for each child. School food services changing to provide more fruits and vegetables during lunches across a district would have similar reach with perhaps a higher cost to implement but a larger gain to each individual child. As interventions rely more on teachers and counselors, training and implementation time and costs increase; in this case, reach is likely to decrease but the potential benefit to an individual may be larger. This is all to say that weighing the level of intervention with the costs linked to that strategy is key for designing policies, programs, and curricula that can be easily implemented and disseminated within schools.

Overcoming Challenges: Strategies for Designing School-Based Health Interventions

Developing partnerships with teachers and administrators via community-based participatory research (CBPR) strategies is key for developing initial buy-in for interventions, institutionalizing new school policies, sustaining curricula usage, or maintaining healthy school environments.[51-53] Employing CBPR means including key stakeholders in all stages of the research process—the development of research questions, the choice of intervention strategies and measurement decisions, and the review of findings in a manner that can be useful for future planning and intervention. By engaging classroom teachers, superintendents, physical education teachers, counselors, and school food service personnel, school-based health interventions are likely to be implemented with greater attention to the real-world barriers to change within schools and be better sustained once any formal study of the intervention is complete.

Beyond designing interventions that can be implemented and sustained, researchers should ensure that they can be disseminated with ease once efficacy is established. In the end, what's the good of creating a health-promoting policy, environmental change, curriculum, or service that can never be replicated? Again, formative research with teachers and administrators is key; understanding the ways that education policies are made within a district or teacher's preferred strategies for adopting new curricula can make or break the ultimate success of school-based interventions. Costs also play a major role here, as initial implementation of a service is one way that schools may have a marginal financial impact, but hiring new personnel to carry it out across a city or state could be expensive. Conversely, implementing policies via school board mandates or programs via low-cost training programs will likely bode well for large-scale dissemination. Finally, dissemination cannot be undertaken by a researcher alone. Collaboration with school or health organizations, publishers, and community groups can help to promote successful interventions more broadly.

Choosing the appropriate study design is essential for researchers to conduct sound dissemination and implementation research. As diffusion of innovations and the RE-AIM framework emphasize, it is important to conduct a thorough process evaluation concurrent with a traditional outcome evaluation in order to look beyond what changes can be attributable to the intervention and understand *how* interventions work in real-world settings. While randomized control trials are the most rigorous study designs to investigate the efficacy and effectiveness of interventions within schools, natural and quasi-experimental designs can also produce valuable results.[54]

Care should be taken to develop reliable and valid measures of implementation processes and health outcomes, regardless of study design (see also Chapter 13).[27,54] There are benefits and drawbacks to the variety of measurement strategies that are currently utilized in school-based implementation research. Whenever possible, it is beneficial to collect data on the implementation process prospectively to avoid collecting retrospective data that could be influenced by the experience of the participation in the intervention. Most school implementation studies to date rely on self-reports of implementation barriers and facilitators via questionnaire to determine the factors that influence successful change. These self-reports can provide insight into the perceptions of those who are responsible for implementing the interventions, but could be subject to selection bias. Researchers should consider whom they are collecting reports from when they develop questionnaires to ensure they understand the realities of implementation within the school. For instance, classroom teachers and principals may have differing perspectives of the barriers they face in implementation of a nutrition curriculum—teachers may emphasize resistance from students while administrators focus more on the costs to their budget. Observations and in-depth interviews may lend important information to measurement in implementation for future studies.[55] The stages or levels of implementation are also generally self-reported, although they could also come from more objective sources such as purchasing reports for curricula, attendance at trainings, online reporting systems, or purchases made through school food service. Finally, the measurement of costs has great potential for prioritizing school-based health solutions; however, more research is needed to assess the validity and reliability of these measurement strategies.

■ OVERVIEW AND SUMMARY OF EMPIRICAL DISSEMINATION AND IMPLEMENTATION RESEARCH REGARDING EFFECTIVE D&I STRATEGIES IN SCHOOL SETTINGS

A range of policies, environmental change strategies, curricula, and services within schools have been shown to be effective for creating health change.[16-30] A number of these interventions provide evidence for cost-effectiveness and, as such, are optimal choices for widespread implementation and dissemination.[50,56-58] However, the gap between determining efficacy within the research setting and effectiveness in the real world is substantial, and much research is still needed to investigate how interventions can be effectively implemented and sustained within schools. Here, we turn to the limited research to date on specific factors that influence the success of interventions within school settings.

Provider characteristics such as age, years of experience, education, personality, expectations and attitudes about a given intervention, coping style, self-efficacy, motivation to implement, and leadership experience are common factors hypothesized to influence effective implementation of interventions within schools.[59,60-62] Also linked to the influence of providers is the impact of teacher turnover on implementation success. Interventions at the interpersonal level would be more likely to be influenced by individual differences among teachers or counselors, whereas policy and practices changes would rely more on initial strong leadership and a system for accountability thereafter.

Factors related to the intervention itself have also been investigated as they relate to real-world effectiveness in schools. These attributes include standardization of a particular curriculum or service, the degree of integration within the school day, and the cost and time associated with the intervention.[61] The quality and quantity of training associated with intervention implementation have also been investigated, but little attention has been paid to the time and cost associated with these trainings that may make sustainability over time difficult.[61,62] Using existing staff to deliver school health interventions may be one way to balance these cost and training concerns.

Finally, school climate (e.g., organizational capacity, size, support from principals and superintendents, competing demands), and external community factors (e.g., poverty) have also been studied in their relation to implementation success.[59–61,63] Payne's recent article considered these implementation factors in conjunction with one another, determining that structural influences predict quality implementation over factors related to personnel or school and community climate.[61]

■ RESEARCH GAPS AND DIRECTIONS FOR THE FUTURE

In sum, there is much need for more research in the field of school-based implementation and dissemination. While there is solid evidence for the efficacy of interventions and policies that are designed to promote health in schools, few have been translated from "best practice" to "common practice." Investigating the factors that influence the implementation and dissemination of efficacious interventions into real-world settings should be a top research priority. While a handful of studies have attempted to tease out the different influences of personnel, setting, and intervention features on intervention effectiveness, this research is limited in scope. Similar to the inconsistent measurement of implementation and dissemination processes, these moderating factors that make or break the success of an intervention within schools are infrequently measured.[27] When assessed, they vary considerably in how they are operationalized within studies. One major step toward addressing this research gap is for investigators to broaden the traditional intervention effectiveness study that narrowly focuses on short-term behavioral and attitudinal outcomes to include more rigorous study of the intervention implementation process and the factors that positively and negatively affect uptake at each stage. These studies should be rooted in comprehensive theories, such as Diffusion of Innovations and RE-AIM, and employ strong study designs. Finally, in order to take advantage of the potential schools have as settings for narrowing health disparities, research should focus on developing strong school and community partnerships and emphasize the importance cost-effective strategies for health promotion.

■ PLANET HEALTH CASE STUDY

Background

The prevalence of childhood obesity in the United States has tripled over the past 20 years. Today, 32% of children and adolescents are considered obese or overweight.[64] Moreover, higher rates of obesity occur among of minority and economically disadvantaged youth. Increases in trends between the 1980s and 1990s were particularly large among African-American and Hispanic children.[65] Obesity is associated with significant health problems in early life, including high cholesterol and hypertension, and is a significant risk factor for adult morbidity and mortality.[66]

Context

Interventions designed to increase physical activity and improve nutrition are a promising solution for curbing obesity among children.[22,24] Planet Health, conducted in the mid-1990s, was the first field trial of a middle school–based obesity prevention program.[23] It aimed to move beyond the evidence for efficacy of obesity prevention interventions to show effectiveness within a "real-world" context. Moreover, process evaluations of Planet Health helped to investigate how the program was implemented and disseminated within schools.[53,67]

The intervention had a group-randomized design with 10 middle schools matched on area characteristics (e.g., mean income) and then randomized to receive the intervention. [23] The communities in the sample had a mean income similar to the U.S. average, and the intervention followed boys and girls in grades 6–8 over 2 school years. The primary end point for the intervention was obesity prevalence. Secondary end points included moderate and vigorous physical activity, TV viewing, dietary intake of fat, fruits, and vegetables, and total energy intake. The interdisciplinary curriculum took a population approach to disease prevention and was guided by behavioral choice and social cognitive theories. Intervention components included staff trainings, classroom lesson plans, materials for physical education teachers, staff wellness sessions, and small funds to put toward fitness improvements.

Findings and Lessons Learned

Intervention effectiveness

The 2-year Planet Health intervention was effective across a range of outcomes. It reduced TV watching among boys and girls as well as decreased obesity prevalence, decreased daily calories consumed, and increased fruit and vegetable intake among girls.[23] Girls in the intervention were also less likely to report weight control behavior disorders.[68]

Evidence for Successful Dissemination and Implementation

After the program was shown to be effective, the Boston Public Schools expressed interest in disseminating Planet Health. In a process evaluation of this dissemination effort, teachers delivered the program at intended levels, indicating that Planet Health can be implemented at the intended dose over 3 school years.[53] Despite reported challenges of planning time and conflicts with school meals programs, vending machines, and home environments, over 75% of teachers planned to continue teaching Planet Health the next year and self-reported feasibility and acceptability were high.[53] Collecting theory-based process measures of feasibility, acceptability, and sustainability in the dissemination phase of Planet Health helped to show the promise of how similar interventions can be implemented and sustained within a school system.[53] Following this successful dissemination effort, as of 2010, more than 10,000 copies of Planet Health have been purchased in all 50 states and more than 20 countries. Moreover, the program has been show to be cost-effective for reducing obesity in middle-school age youth and has been recommended by Cancer Control P.L.A.N.E.T. and the Guide to Community Preventive Services as an effective intervention for reducing screen time and improving weight-related outcomes.[58]

Lesson #1: School context is challenging for study design and measurement

The Planet Health intervention faced numerous research challenges due to the unique context of the school setting. First, like many school-based interventions, measurement of health behaviors was limited to self-report.[23] This strategy is often more feasible for a field trial but has limited reliability and validity, especially among children. Evaluation of school-based programs is also complicated due to the difficulty of tracking changes over time. Planet Health investigators were careful to select of a sample of students that would be relatively stable over time and chose implementation measures that would withstand any school or personnel changes over a two-year time period. Although the study did face these design challenges, the benefits of evaluating the intervention for effectiveness in a "real-world" setting outweigh these limitations.

Lesson #2: Benefits of adapting interventions to diverse school settings

Considering the various competing demands within school was important to ensure that the curriculum appealed to teachers and administrators and was implemented as intended. Accordingly, lesson evaluations and focus groups were conducted with teachers during the development of the units.[23] One finding from this formative research was that teachers preferred text books to web-based materials. Producing a curriculum that teachers are likely to perceive as advantageous and easy to utilize may seem like an obvious step; however, most research does not build in time to discover these implementation preferences and could miss similar factors and end up developing a program that would not be readily adopted by schools and teachers.

Researchers also spent years building authentic school and community partnerships that help to explain the effectiveness of the intervention in the middle-school setting and the positive process evaluation finding. The importance of developing partnerships and working within a community-based participatory research framework also stands out as crucial for moving Planet Health beyond a field trial to dissemination throughout the state and across the country.[53]

Lesson #3: Benefits of considering economic cost and impacts beyond health

Researchers took an interdisciplinary approach that incorporates subject and grade-specific learning objectives in the development of Planet Health. The design of the intervention also considered the limited resources available to schools for health promotion. Its low-cost, population approach weaves nutrition and physical activity messaging into math, English, science, and social studies material with existing classroom teachers.[23,67] Each lesson is designed to promote literacy, and the curriculum aligns with the Massachusetts Department of Education Curriculum Frameworks, which is consistent with learning standards in many other states.[69] In addition to the curriculum, the intervention provided small Fitness Funds to purchase items that would help to sustain changes beyond the study period.[23] By designing a curriculum that was inexpensive and supported the school's primary objective, researchers made the curriculum more appealing to teachers and administrators and likely aided initial implementation, maintenance, and dissemination.

■ CONCLUSION

The findings from Planet Health hold several key implications for teachers, policymakers, and researchers. First, the importance of building partnerships with schools cannot be overstated. If researchers want to develop programs that will outlive their evaluation, they must collaborate with the people who will be responsible for delivery down the road from the onset. Specific factors that are likely to carry over to other school-based programs are those that are low cost and easy to integrate into existing classroom practices. These principles have also been adopted in the development of the Harvard Prevention Research Center Food & Fun Afterschool curriculum. Developed in collaboration with the largest provider of afterschool programming, the YMCA of the USA, these free nutrition and physical activity lessons are designed to be easily integrated into a variety of out-of-school time programs.

SUGGESTED READINGS

Estabrooks P, Dzewaltowski DA, Glasgow RE, Klesges LM. Reporting of validity from school health promotion studies published in 12 leading journals, 1996–2000. *J Sch Health.* 2003;73(1):21–28.

The authors of this study used the RE-AIM framework to evaluate school-based studies emphasizing good nutrition, physical activity, and smoking prevention published over a four-year period. The article recommends more frequent reporting of representativeness criteria in order to increase applicability outside of the research setting.

Haby MM, Vos T, Carter R, et al. A new approach to assessing the health benefit from obesity interventions in children and adolescents: the assessing cost-effectiveness in obesity project. *Int J Obes (Lond).* Oct 2006;30(10):1463–1475.

This paper describes the ACE modeling approach used in assessing the cost effectiveness of interventions. Investigators apply these methods to 13 policy or programmatic interventions targeted at preventing childhood obesity to determine their relative health benefits.

Klimes-Dougan B, August GJ, Lee C-YS , et al. Practitioner and site characteristics that relate to fidelity of implementation: the early risers prevention program in a going-to-scale intervention trial. *Prof Psychol Res Pr.* 2009;40(5):467–475.

Authors of this study examine the influence of practitioner characteristics (e.g., experience, personality, beliefs, coping) and perceived school climate/culture on implementation fidelity among 27 elementary schools taking a prevention program to scale. The study demonstrates how researchers can operationalize and systematically investigate the influence of a variety of contextual factors on intervention success in the real world.

Payne AA, Eckert R. The relative importance of provider, program, school, and community predictors of the implementation quality of school-based prevention programs. *Prev Sci.* 2010;11(2):126–141.

This study examines implementation factors such as program structure, school climate, and community structure in school-based prevention programs. Using national data from over 500 schools, the authors concluded that program structure characteristics (e.g., supervision, use of standardized materials, high quality training) had the greatest impact on program quality.

Rabin BA, Glasgow RE, Kerner JF, Klump MP, Brownson RC. Dissemination and implementation research on community-based cancer prevention: a systematic review. *Am J Prev Med.* 2010;38(4):443–456.

A systematic review of recent dissemination and implementation research of evidence-based interventions in smoking, healthy diet, physical activity, and sun protection. This review highlights, among other recommendations, the need for studies that cover a broader range of populations and settings, more consistent terminology use, more practice-based evidence, and measures with higher validity and reliability.

Stokols D. Translating social ecological theory into guidelines for community health promotion. *Am J Health Promot.* Mar–Apr 1996;10(4):282–298.

This article describes how the core principles of social-ecological theory can be translated into practical guidelines for research conducted in real-world settings. The author describes how researchers can intervene within organizations to achieve optimal implementation, emphasizes the importance of creating change at multiple levels of influence, and highlights the need for more assessment of intervention sustainability over time.

SELECTED WEBSITES AND TOOLS

Centers for Disease Control and Prevention Adolescent and School Health http://www.cdc.gov/healthyyouth/
The CDC Adolescent and School Health page provides links to a series of guidelines documents that identify the school health program strategies most likely to be effective in promoting healthy behaviors among young people. Based on extensive reviews of research literature, the guidelines were developed by CDC in collaboration with other federal agencies, state agencies, universities, voluntary organizations, and professional organizations.

Schools for Health in Europe http://www.schoolsforhealth.eu/
Schools for Health in Europe aims to support organizations and professionals to further develop and sustain school health promotion by providing the European platform for school health promotion. The network is coordinated by the Netherlands Institute for Health Promotion, as a WHO Collaborating Centre for School Health Promotion.

Harvard School of Public Health Prevention Research Center http://www.hsph.harvard.edu/research/prc/
The Harvard School of Public Health Prevention Research Center website includes links to sample lessons from Planet Health and Eat Well and Keep Moving (a similar curriculum designed for elementary grades). The HPRC Food and Fun Afterschool materials

also include planning tools designed to improve implementation of nutrition and physical activity changes in resource-tight settings.

REFERENCES

1. United Nations. Millennium Project. http://www.unmillenniumproject.org/. Accessed July 14, 2010.
2. WHO. *European Strategy for Child and Adolescent Health and Development*. Copenhagen: WHO Regional Office for Europe; 2008.
3. National Conference of State Legislatures. Compulsory Education. http://www.ncsl. org/IssuesResearch/Education/CompulsoryEducationOverview/tabid/12943/ Default.aspx. Accessed July 15, 2010.
4. Young I. Health promotion in schools—a historical perspective. *Promot Educ.* 2005;12(3–4):112–117, 184–190, 205–111.
5. Chadwick E. *Report of the Sanitary Conditions of the Labouring Population of Great Britain.* London: Poor Law Commission; 1842.
6. Kenyon DA. *The Property Tax-School Funding Dilemma.* Cambridge, MA: Lincoln Institute of Land Policy; 2007.
7. Vos T, Carter R, Barendregt J, et al. *Assessing Cost-Effectiveness in Prevention (ACE-Prevention): Final Report.* University of Queensland, Brisbane, and Deakin University, Melbourne; 2010.
8. Centers for Disease Control and Prevention. Coordinated School Health Program. September 24, 2008; http://www.cdc.gov/HealthyYouth/CSHP/. Accessed July 14, 2010.
9. Centers for Disease Control and Prevention. Adolescent and School Health. October 21, 2011; http://www.cdc.gov/HealthyYouth/. Accessed November 8, 2011.
10. Burgher MS, Rasmussen VB, Rivett D. *The European Network of Health Promoting Schools: The Alliance of Education and Health.* Copenhagen, Denmark: The European Network of Health Promoting Schools; 1999.
11. Schools for Health in Europe. http://www.schoolsforhealth.eu/. Accessed July 14, 2010.
12. Kann L, TellJohann, Wooley SF. Health education: results from the School Health Policies and Programs Study 2006. *J Sch Health.* 2007;77(8):408–434.
13. Brener ND, Weist M, Adelman H, Taylor L, Vernon-Smiley M. Mental health and social services: results from the School Health Policies and Programs Study 2006. *J Sch Health.* Oct 2007;77(8):486–499.
14. Lee SM, Burgeson CR, Fulton JE, Spain CG. Physical education and physical activity: results from the School Health Policies and Programs Study 2006. *J Sch Health.* Oct 2007;77(8):435–463.
15. O'Toole TP, Anderson S, Miller C, Guthrie J. Nutrition services and foods and beverages available at school: results from the School Health Policies and Programs Study 2006. *J Sch Health.* 2007;77(8):500–521.
16. Wilson SJ, Lipsey MW, Derzon JH. The effects of school-based intervention programs on aggressive behavior: a meta-analysis. *J Consult Clin Psychol.* 2003;71(1): 136–149.
17. Neil AL, Christensen H. Efficacy and effectiveness of school-based prevention and early intervention programs for anxiety. *Clin Psychol Rev.* 2009;29(3):208–215.

18. Botvin GJ, Baker E, Dusenbury L, Botvin EM, Diaz T. Long-term follow-up results of a randomized drug abuse prevention trial in a white middle-class population. *JAMA.* April 12, 1995;273(14):1106–1112.

19. Thomas RE. PR. School-based programmes for preventing smoking (Review). *The Cochrane Library.* 2008(4): 1–185.

20. Faggiano F. Vigna-Taglianti F, Versino E, Zambon A., Borraccino A., Lemma P. School-based prevention for illicit drugs' use (Review). *The Cochrane Library.* 2008(3):1–69.

21. Mytton JA, DiGuiseppi C, Gough D, Taylor RS, Logan S. School-based secondary prevention programmes for preventing violence (Review). *The Cochrane Library.* 2009(4):1–54.

22. Luepker RV, Perry CL, McKinlay SM, et al. Outcomes of a field trial to improve children's dietary patterns and physical activity. The Child and Adolescent Trial for Cardiovascular Health. CATCH collaborative group. *JAMA.* March 13, 1996; 275(10):768–776.

23. Gortmaker SL, Peterson K, Wiecha J, et al. Reducing obesity via a school-based inter-disciplinary intervention among youth: Planet Health. *Arch Pediatr Adolesc Med.* Apr 1999;153(4):409–418.

24. Dobbins M. DeCorby K, Robeson P, Husson H, Tirilis D. School-based physical activity programs for promoting physical activity and fitness in children and adolescents aged 6–18 (Review). *The Cochrane Library.* 2009(3): 1–76.

25. Oringanje C, Meremikwu MM, Eko H, Esu E, Meremikwu A, Ehir iJE. Interventions for preventing unintended pregnancies among adolescents (Review). *The Cochrane Library.* 2010(1): 1–69.

26. Institute of Medicine. *Bridging the Evidence Gap in Obesity Prevention: A Framework to Inform Decision Making.* Washington DC: The National Academies Press; 2010.

27. Rabin BA, Glasgow RE, Kerner JF, Klump MP, Brownson RC. Dissemination and implementation research on community-based cancer prevention: a systematic review. *Am J Prev Med.* 2010;38(4):443–456.

28. Evans-Whipp T, Beyers JM, Lloyd S, et al. A review of school drug policies and their impact on youth substance use. *Health Promot. Int.* June 1, 2004;19(2):227–234.

29. Jaime PC, Lock K. Do school based food and nutrition policies improve diet and reduce obesity? *Prev Med.* 2009;48(1):45–53.

30. Kahn EB, Ramsey LT, Brownson RC, et al. The effectiveness of interventions to increase physical activity: a systematic review. *Am J Prev Med.* 2002; 22(4, Supplement 1): 73–107.

31. Ennett ST, Tobler NS, Ringwalt CL, Flewelling RL. How effective is drug abuse resistance education? A meta-analysis of Project DARE outcome evaluations. *Am J Public Health.* September 1, 1994;84(9):1394–1401.

32. Shepard EM. *The Economic Costs of D.AR.E.* Syracuse, NY: Institute of Industrial Relations; 2001.

33. Greenberg MT. Current and future challenges in school-based prevention: the researcher perspective. *Prev Sci.* Mar 2004;5(1):5–13.

34. Levin HM. Waiting for Godot: cost-effectiveness analysis in education. *New Directions for Evaluation.* 2001;90:55–68.

35. Haby MM, Vos T, Carter R, et al. A new approach to assessing the health benefit from obesity interventions in children and adolescents: the assessing cost-effectiveness in obesity project. *Int J Obes (Lond).* Oct 2006;30(10):1463–1475.

36. Carter R, Moodie M, Markwick A, et al. Assessing Cost-Effectiveness in Obesity (ACE-Obesity): an overview of the ACE approach, economic methods and cost results. *BMC Public Health.* 2009;9(1):419.
37. Glasgow RE, Vogt TM, Boles SM. Evaluating the public health impact of health promotion interventions: the RE-AIM framework. *Am J Public Health.* 1999;89(9): 1322–1327.
38. Dunton GF, Lagloire R, Robertson T. Using the RE-AIM framework to evaluate the statewide dissemination of a school-based physical activity and nutrition curriculum: "Exercise Your Options." *Am J Health Promot.* Mar–Apr 2009;23(4):229–232.
39. Estabrooks P, Dzewaltowski DA, Glasgow RE, Klesges LM. Reporting of validity from school health promotion studies published in 12 leading journals, 1996–2000. *J School Health.* Jan 2003;73(1):21–28.
40. Rogers EM. *Diffusion of Innovations.* 5th ed. New York: Free Press; 2003.
41. Sallis JF, Owen N, Fisher EB. Ecological Models of Health Behavior. In: Glanz K, Rimer BK, Viswanath K, eds. *Health Behavior and Health Education: Theory, Research, and Practice.* 4th ed. San Francisco, CA: Jossey-Bass; 2008:465–482.
42. Stokols D. Translating social ecological theory into guidelines for community health promotion. *Am J Health Promot.* Mar–Apr 1996;10(4):282–298.
43. Levin HM, Glass GV, Meister GR. Cost-effectiveness of computer-assisted instruction. *Eval Rev.* February 1, 1987; 11:50–72.
44. Hummel-Rossi B, Ashdown J. The state of cost-benefit and cost-effectiveness analyses in education. *Rev Educ Res.* 2002;72(1):1–30.
45. Weinstein MC, Siegel JE, Gold MR, Kamlet MS, Russell LB. Recommendations of the Panel on Cost-effectiveness in Health and Medicine. *JAMA.* October 16, 1996;276(15):1253–1258.
46. Mandelblatt JS, Fryback DG, Weinstein MC, Russell LB, Gold MR. Assessing the effectiveness of health interventions for cost-effectiveness analysis. Panel on Cost-Effectiveness in Health and Medicine. *J Gen Intern Med.* Sep 1997;12(9):551–558.
47. Carter RC. A macro approach to economic appraisal in the health sector. *Aust Econ Rev.* 1994;27(2):105–112.
48. Moodie M, Haby M, Galvin L, Swinburn B, Carter R. Cost-effectiveness of active transport for primary school children—Walking School Bus program. *Int J Behav Nutr Phys Act.* 2009;6:63.
49. Moodie ML, Carter RC, Swinburn BA, Haby MM. The cost-effectiveness of Australia's Active After-school Communities Program. *Obesity (Silver Spring).* 2010;18(8):1585–1592.
50. Deuson RR, Hoekstra EJ, Sedjo R, et al. The Denver school-based adolescent hepatitis B vaccination program: a cost analysis with risk simulation. *Am J Public Health.* Nov 1999;89(11):1722–1727.
51. Israel BA, Schulz AJ, Parker EA, Becker AB. Review of community-based research: assessing partnership approaches to improve public health. *Annu Rev Public Health.* 1998;19:173–202.
52. Leung MW, Yen IH, Minkler M. Community based participatory research: a promising approach for increasing epidemiology's relevance in the 21st century. *Int J Epidemiol.* Jun 2004;33(3):499–506.
53. Wiecha JL, El Ayadi AM, Fuemmeler BF, et al. Diffusion of an integrated health education program in an urban school system: planet health. *J Pediatr Psychol.* Sep 2004;29(6):467–474.

54. Shadish WR, Cook TD, Campbell DT. *Experimental and Quasi-Experimental Designs for Generalized Causal Inference*. Boston, MA: Houghton Mifflin Company; 2002.

55. Resnicow K, Davis M, Smith M, et al. How best to measure implementation of school health curricula: a comparison of three measures. *Health Educ Res.* Jun 1998;13(2): 239–250.

56. Wang LY, Crossett LS, Lowry R, Sussman S, Dent CW. Cost-effectiveness of a school-based tobacco-use prevention program. *Arch Pediatr Adolesc Med.* Sep 2001;155(9): 1043–1050.

57. Wang LY, Davis M, Robin L, Collins J, Coyle K, Baumler E. Economic evaluation of Safer Choices: a school-based human immunodeficiency virus, other sexually transmitted diseases, and pregnancy prevention program. *Arch Pediatr Adolesc Med.* Oct 2000;154(10):1017–1024.

58. Wang LY, Yang Q, Lowry R, Wechsler H. Economic analysis of a school-based obesity prevention program. *Obes Res.* 2003;11(11):1313–1324.

59. Klimes-Dougan B, August GJ., Lee C-Y S, et al. Practitioner and site characteristics that relate to fidelity of implementation: the Early Risers Prevention Program in a going-to-scale intervention trial. *Prof Psychol Res Pr.* 2009;40(5):467–475.

60. Ransford C, Greenberg MT, Domitrovich CE, Small M, and Jacobson L. The role of teachers' psychological experiences and perceptions of curriculum supports on the implementation of a social and emotional learning curriculum. *School Psych Rev.* 2009;38(4):510–532.

61. Payne AA, Eckert R. The relative importance of provider, program, school, and community predictors of the implementation quality of school-based prevention programs. *Prev Sci.* Jun 2010;11(2):126–141.

62. Rohrbach LA, D'Onofrio CN, Backer TE, Montgomery SB. Diffusion of school-based substance abuse prevention programs. *Am Behav Sci.* 1996;39:919–934.

63. Hoyle TB, Bartee RT, Allensworth DD. Applying the process of health promotion in schools: a commentary. *J Sch Health.* Apr;80(4):163–166.

64. Ogden CL, Carroll MD, Curtin LR, Lamb MM, Flegal KM. Prevalence of high body mass index in US children and adolescents, 2007–2008. *JAMA.* 2010;303(3): 242–249.

65. Strauss RS, Pollack HA. Epidemic increase in childhood overweight, 1986–1998. *JAMA.* December 12, 2001;286(22):2845–2848.

66. Freedman DS, Dietz WH, Srinivasan SR, Berenson GS. The relation of overweight to cardiovascular risk factors among children and adolescents: the Bogalusa Heart Study. *Pediatrics.* Jun 1999;103(6 Pt 1):1175–1182.

67. Franks A, Kelder SH, Dino GA et al. School-based programs: lessons learned from CATCH, Planet Health, and Not-On-Tobacco. *Prev Chronic Dis.* April 2007; 4(2):A33.

68. Austin SB, Field AE, Wiecha J, Peterson KE, Gortmaker SL. The impact of a school-based obesity prevention trial on disordered weight-control behaviors in early adolescent girls. *Arch Pediatr Adolesc Med.* Mar 2005;159(3):225–230.

69. Carter J, Wiecha JL, Peterson KE, Nobrega S, Gortmaker SL. *Planet Health: An Interdisciplinary Curriculum for Teaching Middle School Nutrition and Physical activity.* 2nd ed. Champaign, IL: Human Kinetics; 2007.

21 Policy Dissemination Research

■ ELIZABETH A. DODSON,
ROSS C. BROWNSON,
AND STEPHEN M. WEISS

■ INTRODUCTION

Public health policy, in the form of laws, regulations, and guidelines, has a profound effect on health status. For example, a review of the 10 great public health achievements of the 20th century[1] shows that each of them was influenced by policy change, such as seat belt laws or regulations governing permissible workplace exposures. Health policies can be broad in scope (e.g., a state clean indoor air law) or may involve smaller-scale organizational practices (e.g., a private worksite ban on smoking). As with any decision-making process in public health practice or health care delivery, formulation of health policies is complex and depends on a variety of scientific, economic, social, and political forces.[2]

A goal for dissemination and implementation (D&I) researchers can be to measure and understand the adoption of evidence-based policy. To improve public health outcomes, evidence-based policy is developed through a continuous process that uses the best available quantitative and qualitative evidence.[3] In defining evidence-based policy, it is important to consider three key domains: the policy process, content, and outcomes. Many factors affect the *policy process*, including successful advocacy and skills in communication. In studying social movements, progress hinges on the standing of those articulating an issue and the presence of a policy "sparkplug."[4,5] *Policy content* focuses on identifying the specific policy elements that are likely to be effective. Both quantitative and qualitative data can be used by policymakers to determine the appropriate policy content. Documenting the effects of implemented policies (*policy outcome*) is equally important in supporting evidence-based policy. Policy evaluations are critical to understanding the impact of policies on community- and individual-level behavior changes. They should include "upstream" (e.g., presence of zoning policies supportive of physical activity), "midstream" (e.g., enrollment in walking clubs), and "downstream" (e.g., rate of physical activity) factors.[6,7]

To conduct policy dissemination research, it is also important to understand the various policy systems and players. Governmental policy systems vary widely in their structure and scope, ranging from totalitarian to democratic governments. In this chapter, the descriptions of evidence-based policy are focused primarily on multicentric (democratic) governments, which are more common in middle- and upper-income countries. Whether at a local, state, or federal level, the purpose of a representative body is to enact rules, laws, or ordinances that are in turn implemented by executive or administrative agents. Although there is overlap, this chapter focuses primarily on "big P" policies (formal laws, rules, regulations enacted by elected officials) as contrasted with "small p" policies (organizational guidelines, internal agency decisions/memoranda, social norms guiding behavior).[8,9] The term "policymaker" in this chapter primarily refers to elected officials (e.g., city council members, state legislators). There is considerable overlap between the roles and impacts of health policymakers and administrators (e.g., program and agency leaders in the executive branch of government). For example, the director of a state health department makes decisions about how resources are allocated and where an agency's emphasis should be placed when carrying out various health policies. Legislative staff members also play key roles in policy development. Differences among various policy-making audiences are myriad. One example is that executive branch officials can spend more time on a fewer number of issues than legislative staff or elected officials.

There are several overarching issues related to how policy dissemination research differs from inquiry on programs or behavioral interventions. In many types of research, the investigator is able to control or manipulate the exposure (the independent variable). This is often difficult in policy research because the policy process can be unpredictable and complex. Therefore, policy evaluations may employ both qualitative and quantitative methodologies and may make use of "natural experiments" surrounding the adoption and implementation of the policy. These evaluations involve naturally occurring circumstances where different populations are exposed or not exposed to a potentially causal factor (e.g., a new policy) such that it resembles a true experiment in which study participants are assigned to exposed and unexposed groups. While many public health practitioners receive training in key content areas (e.g., epidemiology, behavioral science), a major competency that is lacking involves how to effectively communicate and translate research into policy.[10] And finally, researchers, practitioners, and intermediaries who affect the policy process have unclear roles in how to disseminate evidence-based interventions. While all recognize the importance of dissemination, no one group tends to take responsibility for making it happen.[11]

This chapter will outline key issues of evidence-based theories and frameworks for policy dissemination research, discuss policy intervention design, and specify potential challenges that may be faced in policy dissemination research. We provide entry points into a rapidly growing and widely dispersed literature that crosses multiple disciplines, including public health, political science, and economics. Because the field of D&I research is so new, the "implementation" literature on setting-specific evidence-based interventions is sparse; therefore, the remainder of this chapter will focus instead on policy dissemination research.

■ THEORY, EVIDENCE BASE, AND METHODS

Theory Base/Conceptual Framework

Several other chapters in this book have discussed the value and applicability of both the RE-AIM framework and the Diffusion of Innovations theory for D&I research (in particular, Chapters 3 and 16); they are comparably useful for dissemination research in policy settings.[12] However, for policy settings, in particular, well-established theory about dissemination research is still under development. Two models are currently available. One is useful for thinking about the policy process, which can be applied to research about policy change and policy dissemination. This framework comes from the work of Kingdon, who illustrates a model borrowed from political science (Figure 21–1). When populated with public health data, information, and players, this model can serve as a means of understanding how policy change often occurs in the real world.

According to Kingdon's model, the policy itself and the policy process are both important.[13] He argues that policies move forward when elements of three "streams" come together. These streams are very distinct and when coupled together, increase the odds of a policy being adopted. The first of these is the definition of the problem (e.g., a high diabetes rate). The second is the development of potential policies to solve that problem (e.g., identification of policy measures to achieve an effective diabetes prevention strategy). Both of these streams are concerned with agenda setting and how certain problems or conditions come to be regarded as problems worthy of governmental intervention and the alternative policy approaches that may be taken to address those problems. Finally, there is the role of politics and public opinion, factors both inside and outside of government that influence the policy-making process (e.g., interest groups supporting or opposing the policy). Policy change occurs when a "window of opportunity" opens and the three streams push policy change through.[13] Thus, public policies not only need to be "technically sound, but also politically and administratively feasible."[14] The study of these streams and their participants may help researchers understand, communicate, and collaborate with policymakers.

Another framework that may be useful for policy dissemination research is shown in Figure 21–2. Each phase of this framework has specific characteristics that are important for effective dissemination. Carefully assessing the phase of each target population can help target dissemination activities. Further, the components of each phase may inform policy dissemination research questions. The framework starts with the definition of evidence-based policies (EBPs) and then

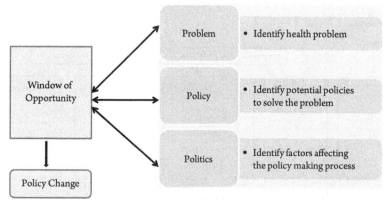

Figure 21–1. Three streams of the policy process. Adapted from Kingdon.[13]

illustrates how both active and passive dissemination may take place. In the innovation development phase, members from the target audience provide critical feedback on policies, and the rationale is built for EBPs. The awareness stage defines the actions taken to make target audiences aware of the innovative policies across sites and settings.[15,16] Adoption can be defined as "a decision to make full use of an innovation as the best course of action available."[17] The adoption phase examines factors that influence the decision to undertake the innovation by an individual or organization.[16] Implementation can be defined as the extent to which an innovation is carried out with completeness and fidelity. This phase involves improving the skills of adopters through training and technical assistance. Maintenance refers to the extent to which an innovation, such as a program, becomes embedded into the normal operation of an organization.[18] This phase also involves ensuring policy enforcement. This framework provides a helpful guide to studying various steps in the policy dissemination research process.

Evidence Base

An evaluation of the existing evidence base for policy dissemination research reveals that while public health policy has vast potential to influence population health, there is limited evidence on how precisely it may do so. In this way, it illustrates the "inverse evidence law," which states that those interventions most likely to influence whole populations (e.g., policy change) are least valued in an evidence matrix emphasizing randomized designs.[19,20] For example, knowledge is growing about the ways policy can be used to facilitate healthy decision making and reduce

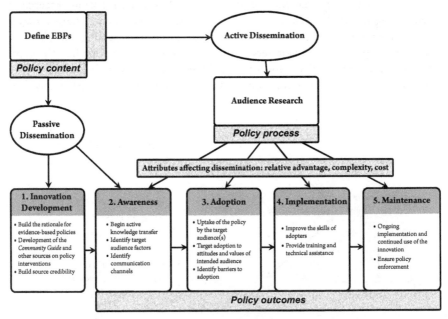

Figure 21–2. A framework for dissemination of evidence-based policies.

risk of obesity.[14,21] There is still much more to learn about which policies work and which do not, how policies should be developed and implemented, and the best ways to combine quantitative and qualitative methods for evaluation of so-called "upstream" risk factors.[6] These methods are unlikely to involve randomized designs but more likely will use quasi-experimental methods.[22] Yet, as this chapter notes, policies have potential for enormous impact.

Nonetheless, there is an array of evidence-based policy interventions currently available, which may be applied in a variety of settings (e.g., schools, worksites, communities) to address a range of topics (e.g., tobacco cessation, increasing physical activity, reducing risk of skin cancer). While these studies may not demonstrate an evidence base according to standards common in randomized, controlled trials, they constitute the best of what is currently available. Because policy interventions often do not lend themselves to the designs and evaluation of other scientific interventions, a more appropriate way of considering the evidence base for policy dissemination interventions is necessary.

To this end, Brennan and colleagues propose a four-level evidence typology that incorporates a range of evidence levels that can include the highest-quality systematic reviews, research and evaluation reports, and new innovations.[23] The first level includes "Tier 1" effective strategies. Leading sources for such information include the Community Guide[24] and the Cochrane Review,[25] which consist of a range of interventions that have been evaluated by systematic review. The second level includes "Tier 2" effective strategies, which include published, peer-reviewed studies indicating considerable health impacts. The third level of evidence includes promising strategies, which may show important, probable health outcomes in published or unpublished studies. The fourth evidence level includes emerging strategies, which come from innovative, untested interventions with some face validity. Applying this typology to existing policy interventions can help dissemination researchers appropriately identify those worthy of further examination.

Policy Dissemination Research Methods

The primary goal of policy dissemination research is to identify the methods that are most effective in promoting the uptake and utilization of evidence-based interventions into community and clinical practice settings. While research is often conducted in an isolated and controlled environment, policy dissemination research typically involves close collaborations with stakeholders, such as decision makers in health departments or legislatures.[26] To distinguish this type of research, it may be helpful to outline some important steps to follow when considering dissemination research ideas. First, to engage in this type of work, one might identify a policy intervention (e.g., local clean indoor air ordinances to reduce exposure to secondhand tobacco smoke). It would then be important to conduct formative research on the policy intervention, and to search and assimilate the literature to find out what works, paying special attention to systematic reviews. This is also an important time to engage local stakeholders.

Next, one would consider various methods of disseminating to policy audiences the idea of clean indoor air ordinances as a means of addressing tobacco (e.g., creating policy briefs, visits with city council members). At this stage one should examine existing research on how best to reach local policymakers, identify trusted spokes-people willing to work on the issue, and search for local data to properly frame the issue for local policy audiences. Finally, one would select the best means of evaluating the effects of these methods on the target audiences (e.g., Did they receive, read, understand, or use the policy briefs?). These methods could include surveying local policymakers about what they found useful in the policy briefs or conducting surveillance of local, clean indoor air laws.

As noted in the chapter introduction, those interested in conducting policy dissemination research face unique challenges uncommon in other types of dissemination research in health. There are emerging methods, however, that can provide valuable insights into the processes of disseminating policy information. Dissemination researchers may participate in each stage of the process described above and ideally would design their research program to include methods of evaluating the dissemination of their study materials and effects.

Alternatively, one may encounter a natural experiment, which facilitates the study of an occurrence in which one group is exposed to a new policy and another, comparable group is not (a comparable group may not always be available). In such instances, the policy research seeks to understand the impact(s) of a particular policy following enactment. In these studies, quasi-experimental designs (e.g., ecologic, before and after, time series study designs) are likely to be more useful than randomized experiments. A key issue in the evaluation of the impacts of policies is whether there is adequate variation in policy exposure among the target population.[27]

Other common methods used in policy dissemination research are designed to study the policy process. Often, case studies can be a powerful tool for doing so, though they are more often used in political science than in public health research. Other means of studying the policy process might involve conducting key informant interviews with policymakers on their use of research evidence in decision making or the primary sources from which they seek information when making decisions. Further, it is often informative to interview decision makers after a public health-related policy has passed in the legislature to learn about the barriers and facilitators affecting the policy-making process.[28] Such qualitative methods may also be combined with more quantitative methods. This can include conducting surveillance of policy introduction and enactment relevant to a specific topic or issue, and can be done at the local, state, or federal level. The range of study types for policy dissemination research shows that multi-method approaches are likely to be the most useful (Table 21–1).

Increasingly, policy surveillance can be carried out through the use of several online resources that are available to the public. Some of the most useful national and international sources include the National Conference of State Legislatures, The Yale Rudd Center for Food Policy and Obesity, Thomas.gov (a site detailing the activities of Congress), the National Cancer Institute's State Cancer Legislative Database, the World Health Organization's Health for All Database, the Canadian Partnership Against Cancer's Cancer View Canada database, and individual state legislative websites.

Finally, it is vital to policy dissemination research that the work be conducted by a team of people representing multiple disciplines and stakeholders.[29] Ideally, such a team would be comprised of policymakers, practitioners, and researchers from

TABLE 21–1. *Types of Studies in Health Policy Research*

Study Type	Purpose	Methods
Policy-making studies	To identify factors influencing the likelihood that health policy will be adopted, the nature of policies adopted, and the process through which they are adopted	Multivariate regression Key informant interviews Content analysis of transcripts, rule-making notices, memos, and other policy materials Surveys of policymakers
Mapping studies	To analyze the state of the law or the legal terrain and the application of policies surrounding a particular health topic	Content analysis of statutes, administrative Regulations, and formal policy statements Key informant interviews Surveys of state and local policymakers
Implementation studies	To examine how and to what extent the "policy on the books" is implemented and enforced	Content analysis of administrative agency Documents, including public communications Key informant interviews Direct observation of enforcement actions Examination of business records of regulated entities Surveys of regulators, regulated entities, and the public
Intervention studies	To assess the effect of a policy intervention on health outcomes or mediating factors that influence health outcomes	Descriptive analysis of outcomes data Multivariate regression Case/control designs Controlled experiments Simulations Surveys of persons targeted by the law
Mechanism studies	To examine the specific mechanisms through which the policy affects environments, behaviors, or health outcomes	Controlled experiments Surveys, focus groups, or interviews of persons targeted by the law

Source: Adapted from Burris et al.[105]

multiple disciplines, who can each work to ensure that the research is relevant to and representative of their sectors. This is rarely done, and investigators often are unsure of how best to create such collaborations.[30] However, an excellent example of such teamwork exists in the creation of CLASPs (Coalitions Linking Action and Science for Prevention) by the Canadian Partnership against Cancer, which is described in Chapter 17 of this book. Other relevant work includes that by Stokols and colleagues, who study the science of team science. This work examines how interdisciplinary teams collaborate and how these collaborations can enhance the translation of research findings into practice and policy settings.[31,32]

■ D&I RESEARCH CHALLENGES IN POLICY SETTINGS

There are substantial challenges in developing, implementing, and evaluating evidence-based policies. Others have written about these in detail.[33–37] In part, these challenges reflect what has been learned from Diffusion Theory (Table 21–2).[17]

TABLE 21-2.   *Policy Attributes that Affect Dissemination*

Characteristic	Description/rationale
Relative advantage	More beneficial than available alternatives
Complexity	The more easily communicated, the better
Comparability	More consistent with the new environment or setting
Flexibility	Policy is robust to modification, or can be subdivided, and still be effective
Reversibility	For a policy that is not working, the old approach can be resumed
Risk	The less the uncertainty about the results of the policy, the better
Cost	Benefits of the policy outweigh the costs

Source: Adapted from King et al.[39]

While these attributes have been applied to multiple disciplines (e.g., agriculture, business)[38] and some public health programs,[39,40] their use in policy settings is limited. Building on these attributes, this section highlights several challenges most relevant for D&I research in policy settings.

Clash of Cultures

Perhaps most importantly, the cultures and decision-making processes for researchers and policymakers are significantly different. Researchers rely on experimental and observational studies to test specific hypotheses in a systematic way. Their influence is based on their specialized knowledge, and their timelines to action are long. On the other hand, policy making is built on a history of related policies and demands from stakeholders.[41] Policymakers have to sell, argue, advocate, and get reelected in light of the available political capital. Decisions are often the result of compromise. Their interests are often shorter term and keyed to an election cycle, leaving little room for interaction with the slower, calculated pace of researchers.

Poor Timing

Scientific studies are not always conducted at the right time to influence policy decisions. Research tends to progress at a deliberate, although not always predictable, pace. Frequently, research projects take 3–6 years to complete, and as many as 8–10 years may pass from the time of the initial hypothesis or research question to publication and dissemination of findings. Contrast this with the policy process, which moves much more quickly, and where public officials are elected every 2–6 years and often are dealing with hundreds of policy issues in a single legislative cycle. By the time that research findings are sufficient to support policy changes, the political and social climates may not be receptive, or the issues/problems may have subsided or disappeared from public concern.

Ambiguous Findings

Policymakers often become frustrated with the ambiguity of findings that researchers present (e.g., "confidence intervals" around their estimates). Policymakers prefer "point estimates" (e.g., a precise estimate) of the effect. For example, while projections of budget numbers for health programs, such as the numbers of persons that will be enrolled in these programs, are uncertain, policymakers often vote on the precise estimate of the number of people affected. The Congressional Budget Office, which is charged by the Congress to project future changes in the budget, has for years documented the difficulty in projecting the future health costs of Medicare and explained that their projections are uncertain. Nevertheless, when Congress passed the Medicare Modernization Act, they passed the policy with one point estimate of the budget costs, not a range of budget estimates.

Balancing Objectivity and Advocacy

There has been considerable dialogue and disagreement among researchers regarding the degree to which scientists should be involved in the policy-making process. Largely, the differences focus on the role of scientists as advocates. Even the definition of advocacy is ambiguous,[42] ranging from raising awareness of an issue, to communicating research results to policymakers, to actively lobbying for a particular policy. Some argue that researchers who take a public stance on a given health policy issue may face real or perceived loss of objectivity that may adversely affect their research.[43] Objectivity implies that a researcher seeks to observe things as they are, without falsifying observations to match some preconceived view. Objectivity may be influenced by the research questions in which a researcher is personally interested.[44] Even if a D&I researcher is not involved in all stages along the advocacy continuum, she/he can still study the policy process and raise awareness of important health policy issues.

Information Overload

Multiple legislative and nonlegislative demands compete for the time of a policymaker, and the number of demands has grown at a steady pace over the years. A fundamental tenet of the communication process is that people are limited in how much information they can process. A policymaker in the United States is typically exposed to hundreds of messages from multiple sources on a daily basis. A study of 292 state policymakers supported the notion that much of the information provided to policymakers is not assimilated. Among surveyed policymakers, 27% read the information they receive in detail, 53% skim the information for general content, and 35% "never get to" material.[45] Some have suggested that many policymakers "read people" not written reports.[46] In addition, scientists may be ill equipped to communicate complex information to policymakers in effective ways.[47]

Lack of Relevant Data

Data can be powerful in shaping policy decisions, yet the type of evidence needed often varies across research and policy audiences.[48,49] Epidemiologic data, whether from etiologic research or from surveillance systems, are often not in the form most useful for policymakers. Many datasets provide disease or risk factor data at the national, state, or county level. Surveillance data are often compiled in reports that can be hundreds of pages in length. In a study of directors of applied research organizations in Canada, 67% of organizations reported targeting policymakers with their research knowledge.[30] Among these groups, only 49% tailored materials to specific policy audiences. Policymakers often look for data that: (1) show public support for a particular issue; (2) demonstrate priority for an issue over many others; (3) show relevance at the local (voting district) level; and (4) personalize an issue by telling a compelling story of how peoples' lives are affected. In a political setting, a good anecdote or intuitive argument may carry more weight than a plethora of statistics or research results. Anecdotes are especially persuasive to the audiences policymakers speak with (their constituents), who often are not sophisticated consumers of statistical evidence.[50]

The Mismatch of Randomized Thinking with Nonrandom Situations

In biomedical research, the most rigorous design for hypothesis testing is the randomized controlled trial;[51] thus, systematic reviews (e.g., Cochrane Review) tend to favor such designs. As such, randomized controlled trials are often more likely to be funded, and their results are more likely to be published. However, well-designed observational studies can also be powerful tools by which to estimate risk and understand disease.[52,53] Further, a randomized design is seldom useful in policy-related dissemination research because the scientist cannot randomly assign exposure (the policy), and problems are often qualitative—thus, alternative research designs are often superior in framing policy-relevant questions.

■ OVERVIEW OF EXISTING POLICY DISSEMINATION RESEARCH

While there is not an extensive collection of existing policy dissemination research to date, some helpful work has been published recently. For example, researchers in Canada have conducted studies comparing the effectiveness of different dissemination or knowledge translation strategies that are used to communicate research findings into public health practice.[54,55] Dobbins and colleagues evaluated the influence of systematic reviews on decision making in public health units. They found that 50% of respondents perceived systematic reviews to be influential in program-planning decisions, but only 16% found them useful in policy development decisions.[56] Another study sought to identify public health decision makers' preferred means of receiving research evidence to inform decisions. This work revealed that respondents value systematic reviews, research summaries, and clear, concise explanations of real-world research implications.[57] Such research helps to build the evidence base for effective policy dissemination strategies.

Another set of studies has examined the relative effectiveness of policy dissemination through various communication methods. Sorian and Baugh reported on a survey of nearly 300 state government policymakers that sought to understand their methods of obtaining information about policy topics. Respondents in this study discussed being overwhelmed with information and therefore never even reading 35% of what they receive.[45] Policymakers also reported finding summaries and brief reports more useful than e-mail lists, conferences, and press releases. State policymakers in this survey were divided regarding preferred information media, with younger (under age 30) respondents reporting much more frequent use of electronic information compared to the hard-copy materials preferred by older officials.[45]

Mitton and colleagues conducted a review of D&I (or knowledge translation and exchange) literature in health policy settings. They reported that only 20% of the studies examined included practical applications of dissemination strategies and that only a fraction of those strategies had been evaluated. The authors argue for primary research to build an evidence base of policy dissemination strategies that have been formally evaluated.[58] Other studies are available that have examined the conceptual foundations for dissemination research specific to certain types of interventions, such as several targeting physical activity, that have been successfully disseminated.[29] This work also examined policies that have potential to enhance D&I.

Finally, Brownson and colleagues explored the factors that influence the likelihood that state-level policymakers would find a policy brief understandable, credible, and useful, by comparing narrative-based policy briefs to those containing primarily statistical information. Their findings suggested that the likelihood of using these briefs was generally greater among women, those who identify themselves as socially liberal, respondents over age 52, and those without graduate education. They concluded that a "one-size-fits-all" approach to communicating with policymakers is less effective than one that considers the differences in communication preferences of legislators, staff, and executive branch administrative decision makers.[59] These studies represent the small but growing empirical literature on policy D&I research.

■ CASE STUDY: TRANSLATING SCIENCE INTO PUBLIC HEALTH STRATEGY: MALE CIRCUMCISION IN ZAMBIA

Background

Ample scientific evidence indicates that male circumcision (MC) reduces the risk of acquiring HIV through heterosexual intercourse in males in sub-Saharan Africa by approximately 51 to 60%,[60-65] providing "unequivocal evidence that circumcision plays a causal role in reducing the risk of HIV infection among men."[66] This evidence was so compelling that three randomized, controlled, clinical trials were halted early due to positive preliminary results.[61-63] In March 2007, the WHO and the Joint United Nations Programme on HIV/AIDS held a technical consultation on MC and concluded that MC should be recognized as an effective intervention for the prevention of heterosexually acquired HIV infection in men.[67,68]

Context

With a population of nearly 12 million, Zambia has high HIV/AIDS prevalence (19.7% urban) and incidence (4% urban) and a low rate (12%) of MC.[69,70] The public health recommendations of the Joint Programme on HIV/AIDS for scaling up national circumcision programs have been embraced by the Zambian Ministry of Health and codified into a 10-year plan, the National Male Circumcision Strategy and Implementation Plan 2010–2020, with the goal of performing 2.5 million circumcisions by 2020, or 250,000 circumcisions per year. To reach this goal, the National Plan proposes to train and certify up to 1,500 additional health care providers to perform circumcisions. Although 400 health care providers have been trained thus far, only 40,000 circumcisions have been performed during the first program year, reaching only 16% of the goal of the National Plan.

Attaining this goal clearly will require increasing the availability (*supply*) of circumcision services through training additional health care personnel. However, the Plan assumes there will be an appropriate reservoir of men willing to undergo the procedure (*demand*). The initial enthusiasm for MC stimulated long waiting lines of prospective patients at hospitals and community health centers. The recent Zambia Sexual Behaviour Survey (2010) paints a less optimistic portrait of MC acceptability. Although studies conducted in several sub-Saharan African countries have found at least 50% of the men expressing willingness to be circumcised,[71] the population-based Zambian survey indicated that over 80% of uncircumcised men questioned had *no* interest in considering MC as an HIV prevention option. In fact, circumcision rates have *decreased* over the past 5 years in Zambia, from 15% in 2005 to 12% of the present survey respondents. Their concerns about endorsing MC to reduce HIV risk included fear of pain, cost, concerns about postsurgical sexual performance and satisfaction, cultural values, and partner preferences.

It is instructive to note that these perceived barriers are not supported by the empirical data on MC, when performed by trained health care providers. Penile sensitivity,[72,73] sexual function,[72,74–76] sexual satisfaction,[74] ejaculatory latency,[77] erectile function,[78] and partner satisfaction[79–82] have typically improved following MC. The disconnect between these findings and the perceptions of uncircumcised Zambians suggests the need for a more comprehensive public health approach to achieving **acceptability** as well as **availability** of circumcision in Zambia.

To achieve the National Circumcision Plan goals, it has become obvious that "scaling up" the training of health care providers is essential, but not sufficient. Equally important is the development and implementation of an evidence-based strategy to dispel the myths associated with MC as part of a comprehensive sexual risk reduction/circumcision promotion program. Gruskin noted that the positive outcomes of circumcision were significantly enhanced by the availability and intensity of sexual risk reduction counseling, referring to counseling as "an absolutely vital component of any male circumcision service package."[83]

It has become clear that to increase the availability of MC services (*supply*) without addressing the issue of acceptability (*demand*) would waste scarce time and financial and human resources. Conversely, to increase demand through effective circumcision promotion strategies without an adequate supply of trained medical service providers would be equally unfortunate and could lay the groundwork for abuses by unqualified "practitioners."[84-86] Policymakers need to be made aware that both components must be melded into a "biobehavioral" partnership combining evidence-based biomedical and behavioral interventions to simultaneously expand both supply and demand to meet the goals of the National Plan.

Policy implementation also must be coupled with a resource plan: Who is going to pay for it? A critical part of this plan should include cost-effectiveness analyses to address how this program compares with other national health care priorities. Such analyses are also essential in seeking support from donor countries.

In Zambia, the U.S. Agency for International Development conducted a cost-effectiveness analysis on male circumcision,[87] including projections of how the scaling up of male circumcision would affect the national epidemic over the next 12 years (2008–2020). The unit cost of a comprehensive package of MC services was estimated at U.S. $46.82. Based on the cost analysis, the epidemiological impact and cost effectiveness of scaling up MC among males (ages 15–49) to 58.5% coverage (i.e., to reduce the number of uncircumcised men by half) between 2008 and 2020 were projected for Zambia. It was estimated that one HIV infection will be averted for every eight circumcisions performed and that the cost per infection averted will be U.S. $313.

How sensitive are the cost-effectiveness results to assumptions about behavioral responses to MC? For example, the impact of male circumcision would be smaller than shown here if those who are circumcised adopt riskier behaviors because they think they are fully protected by the circumcision. A 25% reduction in condom use among those who are circumcised would reduce the impact by about 20%. These results underscore the critical importance of locating the surgical provision of MC within a broader set of effective prevention interventions.

Lessons Learned

As a work in progress, this case study illustrates that the "translation" pathway bringing important scientific findings into the real world (population level) must ultimately align with policy and resources in addition to the personal, social, and cultural values of the target population to take full advantage of scientific discovery.

What constitutes sufficient evidence generates much debate. For example, in the case of circumcision being considered an effective HIV prevention strategy, several cross-sectional and retrospective studies in the late 1990s had identified a consistent inverse relationship between HIV infection and circumcision prevalence (**efficacy**),[64,88,89] but the level of evidence necessary to support policy action was not attained until the results of three prospective randomized, controlled, clinical trials were published in 2005–2007 (**effectiveness**).[61-63] Following these reports, the WHO and policymakers in high–HIV incidence countries promulgated national policies encouraging large-scale circumcision programs (**dissemination and implementation**).

Such policy support is unquestionably necessary, but is it sufficient? It must be remembered that circumcision is only 50–60% protective: it is not a "permanent condom." In the case of Zambia and the "rollout" of circumcision on a national scale, MC must be promoted as part of a comprehensive sexual risk reduction program to gain the support and participation of the target population and to achieve the ultimate goal of containing the spread of HIV (**impact**).[90,91]

Finally, one must also address the issue of external validity whereby generalizations from one series of studies must be cautiously considered when applying the findings to other populations (Chapter 15). For example, disease prevalence and incidence in the study populations may limit the salience of such findings when applying the intervention to other prospective recipient populations (e.g., Green et al.).[92] The risk of HIV infection varies even within Africa (e.g., in Western and Northern Africa, HIV prevalence and incidence are much lower than Eastern and Southern Africa).[93] Therefore, as encouraging as the findings from the three major randomized trials regarding the protective effect of MC may be, the similarity (or differences) between the study populations and potential recipient populations must be analyzed carefully by policymakers in other countries to determine whether MC is likely to achieve similar findings in their at-risk populations.

■ DIRECTIONS FOR FUTURE RESEARCH

Because policy dissemination research is a new and emerging field, many research gaps exist, creating ample opportunities for future studies. Several of the most important areas are summarized below.

Developing the Appropriate Measures

High-quality measures are essential for all types of health research.[94] In policy research, metrics for describing the process and outcomes of laws, rules, and regulations are largely missing.[7] Much of the effect of public health policy on health behaviors and outcomes occurs locally, and in most jurisdictions high-quality data are lacking at the city, county, and metropolitan levels. Certain topics (e.g., cardiovascular disease,[95] obesity prevention,[96] asthma[97]) are making progress in identifying and tracking local indicators, but a set of reliable and valid policy metrics needs to be developed (Chapter 13). Such metrics might include those proposed for implementation research,[98] some of which are used in this chapter's case study (e.g., acceptability). Finally, policy metric frameworks need to track both intended and unintended consequences (e.g., criminal laws aimed at controlling illicit drug use may increase the risk of users acquiring HIV[99]).

Developing New Methods for Policy Dissemination and Implementation Research

New and enhanced methods for policy dissemination research would be a valuable contribution to the field. Policy dissemination researchers would benefit from the development of a taxonomy of dissemination outcomes. An excellent example of such a taxonomy exists for implementation research and includes such items as level of analysis, theoretical basis, and applicable forms of measurement for implementation outcomes.[98] Additionally, as noted in this chapter, the field of policy implementation research is young. Future research should build upon and expand existing evidence-based policy implementation research.

Finding New and Better Ways of Communication

The process of policy development and adoption should be further studied to enhance understanding of how policies are created.[100] Also, as researchers better comprehend the process of policy development, they should examine the best ways to enhance their communication with policymakers (e.g., Which methods and modes of communication are most effective?). This work will be especially enhanced by diverse teams of researchers, policymakers, practitioners, and advocates.

Building the Evidence on the External Validity of Policy

Similar to the needs for stronger evidence on external validity across a variety of health issues, as outlined in Chapter 15, policymakers often need to know how a policy intervention will work in a particular setting.[101] Jilcott and colleagues have shown that frameworks such as RE-AIM can be applied to policy research.[12] Use of frameworks such as RE-AIM should improve researchers' understanding of the external validity of policy.

Conducting "Rapid-Response" Research

There is need for the development and testing of rapid methods for studying policy dissemination, which may be more applicable to real-world settings and facilitate the effective use of natural experiments when policy change occurs. Some funders, such as the Robert Wood Johnson programs in Healthy Eating Research and Active Living Research and the Canadian Institute for Health Research have developed rapid-response initiatives that provide support for time-sensitive, natural experiments on environmental and policy change.

Applying Methods from Outside the Health Arena

For progress on D&I research in health policy, methods and frameworks from other disciplines and sectors show promise. This chapter has already shown how the Kingdon model can be applied to policy dissemination research (Figure 21–1). As another example, institutional theory has been used mainly in business, economics, and political science.[102-104] It can help inform a conceptual framework, the dissemination process, and the bidirectionality of institutional change (i.e., organizations influence policies and the reverse).

■ CONCLUSION

Among the settings for D&I covered in this book, research on policy dissemination is perhaps the least developed. To improve these programs and to further evidence-based policy, researchers need to use the best available evidence and expand the role of researchers and practitioners to communicate evidence packaged appropriately for various policy audiences; to understand and engage all three streams[13] (problem, policy, politics) to implement an evidence-based policy process; to develop content based on specific policy elements that are most likely to be effective; and to document outcomes to improve, expand, or terminate policy.

SUGGESTED READINGS

Brownson RC, Royer C, Ewing R, McBride TD. Researchers and policymakers: travelers in parallel universes. *Am J Prev Med.* Feb 2006;30(2):164–172.

Examines reasons why public health research may not be effectively translated into policy. Compares and contrasts the complex worlds of research and policy making.

Glasgow RE, Emmons KM. How can we increase translation of research into practice? Types of evidence needed. *Ann Rev Public Health* 2007;28:413–433.

Summary and review of what is needed to facilitate more and faster uptake of research. Uses the RE-AIM model and community partnership perspectives to discuss current status and future needs.

Kerner J, Rimer B, Emmons K. Introduction to the special section on dissemination: dissemination research and research dissemination: how can we close the gap? *Health Psychol.* Sep 2005;24(5):443–446.

Highlights the vital importance of disseminating evidence-based interventions into public health practice. Makes a case for enhanced dissemination research efforts.

Kingdon JW. *Agendas, Alternatives, and Public Policies.* New York: Addison-Wesley Educational Publishers, Inc.; 2003.

Kingdon's seminal work on agenda setting and policy formation is informed by interviews with individuals working in and around the U.S. government.

Zaza S, Briss PA, Harris KW, eds. *The Guide to Community Preventive Services: What Works to Promote Health?* New York: Oxford University Press; 2005.

Summary and evaluation of vast evidence on a variety of health topics (e.g., risk factors: tobacco, physical activity; diseases: diabetes, cancer). Recommendations provided where evidence is sufficient.

SELECTED WEBSITES AND TOOLS

Cancer Control P.L.A.N.E.T. <http://cancercontrolplanet.cancer.gov>. Cancer Control P.L.A.N.E.T. acts as a portal to provide access to data and resources for designing, implementing, and evaluating evidence-based cancer control programs. The site provides five steps (with links) for developing a comprehensive cancer control plan or program.

National Conference of State Legislatures <http://ncsl.org>. The NCSL is a bipartisan organization providing resources, technical assistance, and other services to the legislators and staffs of all 50 state governments. Their website offers extensive resources, such as information on myriad topics, webinars, networks, and access to policy specialists.

THOMAS <http://thomas.gov>. A site detailing the daily activities of the United States Congress. THOMAS was launched under the leadership of the 104th Congress, when it instructed the Library of Congress to make federal legislative information publicly available. THOMAS now includes information about bills and resolutions, Congressional activity, committees, schedules, and so on.

World Health Organization's European Health for All Database <http://www.euro.who. int/en/what-we-do>. This database includes core health statistics covering demographics, disease determinants, and health care utilization and expenditures for the 53 member states. Data are updated twice annually.

The Canadian Partnership Against Cancer's Cancer View Canada Prevention Policies Directory <www.cancerview.ca/preventionpolicies>. This searchable catalogue includes Canadian policies and legislation regarding primary modifiable risk factors for cancer and relevant chronic diseases. The database is based on environmental scans tracking policies and legislation from 1997 to the present.

■ REFERENCES

1. Centers for Disease Control and Prevention. Ten great public health achievements—United States, 1900–1999. *MMWR Morb Mortal Wkly Rep.* April 2, 1999;48(12):241–243.
2. Spasoff RA. *Epidemiologic Methods for Health Policy.* New York: Oxford University Press; 1999.
3. Brownson RC, Chriqui JF, Stamatakis KA. Understanding evidence-based public health policy. *Am J Public Health.* Sep 2009;99(9):1576–1583.
4. Benford RD, Snow DA. Framing processes and social movements: An overview and assessment. *Annu Rev Sociol.* 2000;26:611–639.
5. Economos CD, Brownson RC, DeAngelis MA, et al. What lessons have been learned from other attempts to guide social change? *Nutr Rev.* Mar 2001;59(3 Pt 2):S40–S56; discussion S57–S65.
6. McKinlay JB. Paradigmatic obstacles to improving the health of populations—implications for health policy. *Salud Publica Mex.* Jul–Aug 1998;40(4):369–379.
7. Brownson RC, Seiler R, Eyler AA. Measuring the impact of public health policy. *Prev Chronic Dis.* Jul 2010;7(4):A77.
8. Milio N. Glossary: healthy public policy. *J Epidemiol Community Health.* Sep 2001; 55(9):622–623.
9. Schmid TL, Pratt M, Howze E. Policy as intervention: environmental and policy approaches to the prevention of cardiovascular disease. *Am J Public Health.* 1995;85(9):1207–1211.
10. Dodson EA, Baker EA, Brownson RC. Personal and Organizational Barriers to Evidence-based Decision Making among U.S. Chronic Disease Practitioners. Presented at Cultivating Healthy Communities: 20th National Conference on Chronic Disease Prevention and Control, Washington, DC. February, 2009.
11. Kerner J, Rimer B, Emmons K. Introduction to the special section on dissemination: dissemination research and research dissemination: how can we close the gap? *Health Psychol.* Sep 2005;24(5):443–446.

12. Jilcott S, Ammerman A, Sommers J, Glasgow RE. Applying the RE-AIM framework to assess the public health impact of policy change. *Ann Behav Med.* Sep–Oct 2007;34(2):105–114.
13. Kingdon JW. *Agendas, Alternatives, and Public Policies.* New York: Addison-Wesley Educational Publishers, Inc.; 2003.
14. Sallis JF, Cervero RB, Ascher W, Henderson KA, Kraft MK, Kerr J. An ecological approach to creating active living communities. *Annu Rev Public Health.* 2006;27:297–322.
15. Kar SB. Implications of diffusion research for planned change. *Int J Health Educ.* 1976;17:192–220.
16. McCormick LK, Steckler AB, McLeroy KR. Diffusion of innovations in schools: a study of adoption and implementation of school-based tobacco prevention curricula. *Am J Health Promot.* Jan–Feb 1995;9(3):210–219.
17. Rogers EM. *Diffusion of Innovations.* 5th ed. New York: Free Press; 2003.
18. Goodman RM, Tenney M, Smith DW, Steckler A. The adoption process for health curriculum innovations in schools: a case study. *J Health Educ.* 1992;23:215–220.
19. Nutbeam D. How does evidence influence public health policy? Tackling health inequalities in England. *Health Promot J Aust.* 2003;14:154–158.
20. Ogilvie D, Egan M, Hamilton V, Petticrew M. Systematic reviews of health effects of social interventions: 2. Best available evidence: how low should you go? *J Epidemiol Community Health.* Oct 2005;59(10):886–892.
21. Story M, Kaphingst KM, Robinson-O'Brien R, Glanz K. Creating healthy food and eating environments: policy and environmental approaches. *Annu Rev Public Health.* 2008;29:253–272.
22. Wholey J, Hatry H, Newcomer K, eds. *Handbook of Practical Program Evaluation.* 2nd ed. San Francisco: Jossey-Bass; 2004.
23. Brennan L, Castro S, Brownson RC, Claus J, Orleans CT. Accelerating evidence reviews and broadening evidence standards to identify effective, promising, and emerging policy and environmental strategies for childhood obesity prevention. *Annu Rev Public Health.* 2011;32:199–223.
24. Zaza S, Briss PA, Harris KW, eds. *The Guide to Community Preventive Services: What Works to Promote Health?* New York: Oxford University Press; 2005.
25. The Cochrane Collaboration. http://www.cochrane.org/. Accessed August 28, 2010.
26. Remington PL, Moberg DP, Booske BC, Ceraso M, Friedsam D, Kindig DA. Dissemination research: the University of Wisconsin Population Health Institute. *WMJ.* Aug 2009;108(5):236–239, 255.
27. Koepsell TD, Weiss NS. *Epidemiologic Methods. Studying the Occurrence of Illness.* New York: Oxford University Press; 2003.
28. Dodson EA, Fleming C, Boehmer TK, Haire-Joshu D, Luke DA, Brownson RC. Preventing childhood obesity through state policy: qualitative assessment of enablers and barriers. *J Public Health Policy.* 2009;30(Suppl 1):S161–S176.
29. Owen N, Glanz K, Sallis JF, Kelder SH. Evidence-based approaches to dissemination and diffusion of physical activity interventions. *Am J Prev Med.* Oct 2006; 31(4 Suppl):S35–S44.
30. Lavis JN, Robertson D, Woodside JM, McLeod CB, Abelson J. How can research organizations more effectively transfer research knowledge to decision makers? *Milbank Q.* 2003;81(2):221–248, 171–222.
31. Stokols D. Toward a science of transdisciplinary action research. *Am J Community Psychol.* Sep 2006;38(1–2):63–77.

32. Stokols D, Hall KL, Taylor BK, Moser RP. The science of team science: overview of the field and introduction to the supplement. *Am J Prev Med.* Aug 2008; 35(2 Suppl):S77–S89.

33. Brownson RC, Royer C, Ewing R, McBride TD. Researchers and policymakers: travelers in parallel universes. *Am J Prev Med.* Feb 2006;30(2):164–172.

34. Feldman PH, Nadash P, Gursen M. Improving communication between researchers and policy makers in long-term care: or, researchers are from Mars; policy makers are from Venus. *Gerontologist.* Jun 2001;41(3):312–321.

35. Lavis JN, Posada FB, Haines A, Osei E. Use of research to inform public policymaking. *Lancet.* October 3–November 5, 2004;364(9445):1615–1621.

36. Hennink M, Stephenson R. Using research to inform health policy: barriers and strategies in developing countries. *J Health Commun.* Mar 2005;10(2):163–180.

37. Jewell CJ, Bero LA. "Developing good taste in evidence": facilitators of and hindrances to evidence-informed health policymaking in state government. *Milbank Q.* Jun 2008;86(2):177–208.

38. Dearing J. Evolution of diffusion and dissemination theory. *J Public Health Manag Pract.* 2008;14(2):99–108.

39. King L, Hawe P, Wise M. Making dissemination a two-way process. *Health Promot Int.* 1998;13(3):237–244.

40. Dearing JW. Improving the state of health programming by using diffusion theory. *J Health Commun.* 2004;9(Suppl 1):21–36.

41. Choi BC, Pang T, Lin V, et al. Can scientists and policy makers work together? *J Epidemiol Community Health.* Aug 2005;59(8):632–637.

42. Stoto MA, Hermalin AI, Li R, Martin L, Wallace RB, Weed DL. Advocacy in epidemiology and demography. *Ann N Y Acad Sci.* Dec 2001;954:76–87.

43. Poole C, Rothman KJ. Epidemiologic science and public health policy. *J Clin Epidemiol.* 1990;43(11):1270–1271.

44. Zalta E. *Stanford Encyclopedia of Philosophy.* Palo Alto, CA: Stanford University; 2005.

45. Sorian R, Baugh T. Power of information: closing the gap between research and policy. When it comes to conveying complex information to busy policy-makers, a picture is truly worth a thousand words. *Health Aff (Millwood).* Mar–Apr 2002;21(2):264–273.

46. Weiss C. Congressional committees as users of analysis. *J Policy Anal Manage.* 1989;8:411–431.

47. Matanoski GM, Boice JD, Jr., Brown SL, Gilbert ES, Puskin JS, O'Toole T. Radiation exposure and cancer: case study. *Am J Epidemiol.* December 15, 2001;154(12 Suppl): S91–S98.

48. Green LW, Ottoson JM, Garcia C, Hiatt RA. Diffusion theory, and knowledge dissemination, utilization, and integration in public health. *Annu Rev Public Health.* 2009;30:151–174.

49. Kerner JF. Integrating research, practice, and policy: what we see depends on where we stand. *J Public Health Manag Pract.* Mar–Apr 2008;14(2):193–198.

50. Peterson M. How health policy information is used in Congress. In: Mann T, Ornstein N, eds. *Intensive Care.* Washington, DC: Brookings Institution; 1995.

51. Porta M, ed. *A Dictionary of Epidemiology.* 5th ed. New York: Oxford University Press; 2008.

52. Concato J, Shah N, Horwitz RI. Randomized, controlled trials, observational studies, and the hierarchy of research designs. *N Engl J Med.* 2000;342:1887–1892.

53. Colditz GA, Taylor PR. Prevention trials: their place in how we understand the value of prevention strategies. *Annu Rev Public Health*. Apr 21;31:105–120.

54. Dobbins M, Hanna SE, Ciliska D, et al. A randomized controlled trial evaluating the impact of knowledge translation and exchange strategies. *Implement Sci*. 2009;4:61.

55. Dobbins M, Robeson P, Ciliska D, et al. A description of a knowledge broker role implemented as part of a randomized controlled trial evaluating three knowledge translation strategies. *Implement Sci*. 2009;4:23.

56. Dobbins M, Cockerill R, Barnsley J, Ciliska D. Factors of the innovation, organization, environment, and individual that predict the influence five systematic reviews had on public health decisions. *Int J Technol Assess Health Care*. Fall 2001;17(4):467–478.

57. Dobbins M, Jack S, Thomas H, Kothari A. Public health decision-makers' informational needs and preferences for receiving research evidence. *Worldviews Evid Based Nurs*. 2007;4(3):156–163.

58. Mitton C, Adair CE, McKenzie E, Patten SB, Waye Perry B. Knowledge transfer and exchange: review and synthesis of the literature. *Milbank Q*. Dec 2007;85(4): 729–768.

59. Brownson R, Dodson E, Stamatakis K, et al. Communicating evidence-based information on cancer prevention to state-level policy makers. *JNCI*. 2011;103:1–11.

60. Warner L, Ghanem KG, Newman DR, Macaluso M, Sullivan PS, Erbelding EJ. Male circumcision and risk of HIV infection among heterosexual African American men attending Baltimore sexually transmitted disease clinics. *J Infect Dis*. January 1, 2009;199(1):59–65.

61. Auvert B, Taljaard D, Lagarde E, Sobngwi-Tambekou J, Sitta R, Puren A. Randomized, controlled intervention trial of male circumcision for reduction of HIV infection risk: the ANRS 1265 Trial. *PLoS Med*. Nov 2005;2(11):e298.

62. Bailey RC, Moses S, Parker CB, et al. Male circumcision for HIV prevention in young men in Kisumu, Kenya: a randomised controlled trial. *Lancet*. February 24, 2007;369(9562):643–656.

63. Gray RH, Kigozi G, Serwadda D, et al. Male circumcision for HIV prevention in men in Rakai, Uganda: a randomised trial. *Lancet*. February 24, 2007;369(9562):657–666.

64. Lavreys L, Rakwar JP, Thompson ML, et al. Effect of circumcision on incidence of human immunodeficiency virus type 1 and other sexually transmitted diseases: a prospective cohort study of trucking company employees in Kenya. *J Infect Dis*. Aug 1999;180(2):330–336.

65. Reynolds SJ, Shepherd ME, Risbud AR, et al. Male circumcision and risk of HIV-1 and other sexually transmitted infections in India. *Lancet*. March 27, 2004;363(9414):1039–1040.

66. Byakika-Tusiime J. Circumcision and HIV infection: assessment of causality. *AIDS Behav*. Nov 2008;12(6):835–841.

67. Weiss HA, Halperin D, Bailey RC, Hayes RJ, Schmid G, Hankins CA. Male circumcision for HIV prevention: from evidence to action? *AIDS*. March 12, 2008;22(5):567–574.

68. World Health Organization. *WHO and UNAIDS announce recommendations from expert consultation on male circumcision for HIV prevention*. Available at: http://www.who.int/hiv/mediacentre/news68/en/index.html; 2007.

69. Ministry of Health. *Zambia Demographic and Health Survey*. Lusaka, Zambia: Central Statistics Office; 2009.

70. Ministry of Health. *Zambia Sexual Behavior Survey, 2009*. Lusaka, Zambia: Central Statistics Office, University of Zambia. 2010.

71. Westercamp N, Bailey RC. Acceptability of male circumcision for prevention of HIV/AIDS in sub-Saharan Africa: a review. *AIDS Behav*. May 2007;11(3):341–355.

72. Krieger JN, Mehta SD, Bailey RC, et al. Adult male circumcision: effects on sexual function and sexual satisfaction in Kisumu, Kenya. *J Sex Med*. Nov 2008;5(11): 2610–2622.

73. Payne K, Thaler L, Kukkonen T, Carrier S, Binik Y. Sensation and sexual arousal in circumcised and uncircumcised men. *J Sex Med*. May 2007;4(3):667–674.

74. Kigozi G, Watya S, Polis CB, et al. The effect of male circumcision on sexual satisfaction and function, results from a randomized trial of male circumcision for human immunodeficiency virus prevention, Rakai, Uganda. *BJU Int*. Jan 2008;101(1): 65–70.

75. Collins S, Upshaw J, Rutchik S, Ohannessian C, Ortenberg J, Albertsen P. Effects of circumcision on male sexual function: debunking a myth? *J Urol*. May 2002;167(5): 2111–2112.

76. Fink KS, Carson CC, DeVellis RF. Adult circumcision outcomes study: effect on erectile function, penile sensitivity, sexual activity and satisfaction. *J Urol*. May 2002;167(5):2113–2116.

77. Senkul T, Iser IC, sen B, Karademlr K, Saracoglu F, Erden D. Circumcision in adults: effect on sexual function. *Urology*. Jan 2004;63(1):155–158.

78. Shen Z, Chen S, Zhu C, Wan Q, Chen Z. [Erectile function evaluation after adult circumcision]. *Zhonghua Nan Ke Xue*. Jan 2004;10(1):18–19.

79. O'Hara K, O'Hara J. The effect of male circumcision on the sexual enjoyment of the female partner. *BJU Int*. Jan 1999;83(Suppl 1):79–84.

80. Bailey RC, Muga R, Poulussen R, Abicht H. The acceptability of male circumcision to reduce HIV infections in Nyanza Province, Kenya. *AIDS Care*. Feb 2002;14(1):27–40.

81. Kebaabetswe P, Lockman S, Mogwe S, et al. Male circumcision: an acceptable strategy for HIV prevention in Botswana. *Sex Transm Infect*. Jun 2003;79(3):214–219.

82. Kigozi G, Lukabwe I, Kagaayi J, et al. Sexual satisfaction of women partners of circumcised men in a randomized trial of male circumcision in Rakai, Uganda. *BJU Int*. Dec 2009;104(11):1698–1701.

83. Gruskin S. Male circumcision, in so many words. *Reprod Health Matters*. May 2007;15(29):49–52.

84. Peltzer K, Nqeketo A, Petros G, Kanta X. Evaluation of a safer male circumcision training programme for traditional surgeons and nurses in the Eastern Cape, South Africa. *Afr J Tradit Complement Altern Med*. 2008;5(4):346–354.

85. Crabb C. Male circumcision to prevent heterosexual HIV transmission gets (another) green light, but traditional circumcision in Africa has "shocking" number of complications. *AIDS*. January 2, 2010;24(1):N1–N2.

86. de Bruyn G, Martinson NA, Gray GE. Male circumcision for HIV prevention: developments from sub-Saharan Africa. *Expert Rev Anti Infect Ther*. 2010;8(1):23–31.

87. USAID. Costing male circumcision in Zambia and implications for the cost effectiveness of circumcision as an HIV intervention. *USAID Health Policy Initiative Task Order 1*. 2007:1–39.

88. Bongaarts J, Reining P, Way P, Conant F. The relationship between male circumcision and HIV infection in African populations. *AIDS*. Jun 1989;3(6):373–377.

89. Jessamine PG, Plummer FA, Ndinya Achola JO, et al. Human immunodeficiency virus, genital ulcers and the male foreskin: synergism in HIV-1 transmission. *Scand J Infect Dis Suppl.* 1990;69:181–186.

90. Karim QA. Prevention of HIV by Male Circumcision. *BMJ.* 2007;335:4–5.

91. Vermund SH, Allen KL, Karim QA. HIV-prevention science at a crossroads: advances in reducing sexual risk. *Curr Opin HIV AIDS.* Jul 2009;4(4):266–273.

92. Green LW, Travis JW, McAllister RG, Peterson KW, Vardanyan AN, Craig A. Male circumcision and HIV prevention: insufficient evidence and neglected external validity. *Am J Prev Med.* Nov;39(5):479–482.

93. UN Joint Programme on HIV/AIDS, *Global Report: UNAIDS Report on the Global AIDS Epidemic: 2010,* December 2010, ISBN 978–92-9173–871-7, available at: http://www.unhcr.org/refworld/docid/4cfca9c62.html.

94. Sallis JF, Owen N, Fotheringham MJ. Behavioral epidemiology: a systematic framework to classify phases of research on health promotion and disease prevention. *Ann Behav Med.* 2000;22(4):294–298.

95. Cheadle A, Sterling TD, Schmid TL, Fawcett SB. Promising community-level indicators for evaluating cardiovascular health-promotion programs. *Health Educ Res.* 2000;15(1):109–116.

96. Haire-Joshu D, Elliott M, Schermbeck R, Taricone E, Green S, Brownson RC. Surveillance of obesity-related policies in multiple environments: the Missouri Obesity, Nutrition, and Activity Policy Database, 2007–2009. *Prev Chronic Dis.* Jul;7(4):A80.

97. Lyon-Callo SK, Boss LP, Lara M. A review of potential state and local policies to reduce asthma disparities. *Chest.* Nov 2007;132(5 Suppl):840S–852S.

98. Proctor E, Silmere H, Raghavan R, et al. Outcomes for implementation research: conceptual distinctions, measurement challenges, and research agenda. *Adm Policy Ment Health.* 2011;38(2):65–76.

99. Friedman SR, Cooper HL, Tempalski B, et al. Relationships of deterrence and law enforcement to drug-related harms among drug injectors in US metropolitan areas. *AIDS.* January 2, 2006;20(1):93–99.

100. Schmid T, Pratt M, Witmer L. A framework for physical activity policy research. *Phys Act Health.* 2006;3(Suppl 1):S20–S29.

101. Atkins D, Siegel J, Slutsky J. Making policy when the evidence is in dispute. *Health Aff (Millwood).* Jan–Feb 2005;24(1):102–113.

102. Hall P, Taylor R. Political science and the three new institutionalisms. *Polit Stud.* 1996;44:936–958.

103. March J, Olsen J. The new institutionalism: organizational factors in political life. *Am Polit Sci Rev.* 1984;78:734–749.

104. North D. *Institutions, Institutional Change and Economic Performance.* Cambridge, UK: Cambridge University Press; 1990.

105. Burris S, Wagenaar AC, Swanson J, Ibrahim JK, Wood J, Mello MM. Making the case for laws that improve health: a framework for public health law research. *Milbank Q.* Jun;88(2):169–210.

22 Dissemination and Implementation Research in Populations with Health Disparities

■ ANTRONETTE (TONI) YANCEY,
BETH A. GLENN,
LASHAWNTA BELL-LEWIS,
AND CHANDRA L. FORD

■ INTRODUCTION

Over the past 100 years, the health of the U.S. population has improved substantially as evidenced by a 30-year increase in average life expectancy.[1] Despite these gains, ethnic minorities lag behind the general population on many health metrics including incidence and mortality rates for chronic diseases, life expectancy, and disease risk and quality-of-life indicators.[2] As explained by the WHO's Commission on Social Determinants of Health, avoidable, societal inequities constitute the root causes of persistent health disparities among vulnerable populations.[3] In the United States, race and ethnicity are key axes along which societal inequities occur; thus, racial/ethnic minorities experience disproportionately high rates of morbidity and mortality.[4] Health inequities predicated upon slavery and subsequent Jim Crow laws, which restricted African Americans' access to basic goods and services such as medical care, property ownership, voting rights, fair trials, and quality education, continue to impose a burden on the health of this population.[5] American Indian populations subjected to extreme isolation and exploitation have lagged behind on multiple health indices, and disparities are growing.[6] Immigration trends over the past century have also played a role in the population's health.[7] Although in the past, "selective migration" has prevailed (i.e., immigrants to the United States were healthier than their host country counterparts), more recent immigrants may not have such health advantages. Immigrants are substantially less likely to have access to medical care in the United States, particularly preventive services, and may reside in health-compromising environments.[8,9] Furthermore, a growing body of evidence demonstrates that risk for common diseases increases over time, paralleling adoption of unhealthy American lifestyle behaviors and exposure to negative aspects of the social environment (e.g., racial discrimination).[10-12]

Public health efforts aimed at preventing chronic disease have been insufficient for the population as a whole and have infrequently targeted ethnic minority groups. Utilization of randomized designs with strict protocols and narrow eligibility criteria has yielded results that have limited applicability to ethnic minorities or to the population as a whole.[13] Relatively little is known about how best to culturally adapt existing interventions to new settings, outside of language translation. Issues related to cultural adaptation are discussed in more detail in Chapters 14 and 23. In general, however, the dissemination of interventions developed in nonmainstream cultures is rarely systematically evaluated and disseminated.[14]

This chapter is a focused narrative review that describes dissemination and implementation (D&I) efforts among vulnerable populations in key areas of prevention and proposes future directions for moving the field forward. The chapter begins with a discussion of models that can be used to conceptualize and guide the process of D&I efforts in racially/ethnically diverse contexts such as the United States, goes on to discuss challenges specific to D&I in underserved groups, summarizes the literature in six prevention areas (physical activity/obesity, nutrition, tobacco, cancer screening, HIV/STIs, immunizations), and presents a successful case study of D&I in ethnic minority and underserved populations.

■ MODELS FOR CONCEPTUALIZING D&I IN DISADVANTAGED GROUPS

There are few existing models that specifically aim to explain the process of D&I within diverse and vulnerable populations. Existing and emerging models that can be used to conceptualize the process of D&I in disadvantaged groups are described below. In general, these models are heuristics to assist in understanding how the dissemination process may occur and provide points of entry for interventions to improve these efforts. These models are often broad and, by nature, not designed to be tested within any particular study. Therefore, the summaries below illustrate how these models may apply to D&I research in special populations; they do not evaluate the models based on empirical evidence. Although the lack of disparities-specific D&I models may be considered a limitation by some, it may be equally valuable to consider how broad D&I models that are widely used can be modified to guide D&I work with diverse and vulnerable populations.

Established Models

Socioecologic frameworks, Community-Based Participatory Research (CBPR), and culturally targeted approaches derived from Social Cognitive Theory (SCT) or social marketing campaigns have been used to guide intervention research in disease prevention in vulnerable populations and will continue to be valuable in conceptualizing the process of D&I in these groups. Socioecologic frameworks emphasize the synergy between environmental-level change and individual-level change; therefore, they are preferred over individual-level models that typically do not acknowledge the powerful influence of the environment (i.e., policy, social, built, political) on health.[15-18] Environmental influences may play an even more important role in D&I research than in traditional efficacy and effectiveness studies. For example, building trust within a community in order to carry out a particular study can be difficult but does not compare to the challenge of attempting to implement effective prevention strategies across the entire population.

The CBPR paradigm recalls the historical roots of public health, where problems were identified and addressed through collaboration with the "public" or community for the common good[19] (covered in more detail in Chapter 17). Group members play an integral role in shaping the research process, the content of interventions, the scope of evaluation, and the dissemination of findings. Because it emerges from the affected community as much as from the academic research team, CBPR research is culturally appropriate for and congruent with the needs and values of the community.

By developing strong, respectful partnerships with communities, researchers can foster the trust and mutual respect necessary for true participation in the development and evaluation of interventions (Figure 22–1).[20] A true partnership—shared decision making, resources and recognition or "credit" with "cultural insider" key informants, marketing messengers, and investigators or research team members—creates a foundation for institutionalizing the organizational support necessary for intervention sustainability.[21] CBPR partnerships also cultivate leadership by training group members in research skills and assisting them in developing collaborations that reach beyond the initial research goals. A key component of CBPR is direct intervention or the incorporation of research findings into community change efforts.[19] CBPR has been integral in guiding health disparities research across a variety of contexts and continues to be highly relevant for D&I research efforts.

Social marketing or client-centered approaches derived from commercial marketing are consistent with CBPR approaches.[22] They take into account individual and organizational considerations. For example, participating in physical activity may be framed as fun, nonstrenuous, and enjoyable versus demanding and high-exertion; promotional materials targeting employers may focus on improved productivity, enhanced morale (averting attrition costs such as training of new employees),

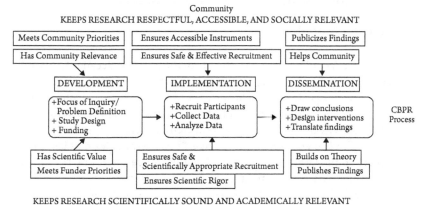

Figure 22–1. The community-based participatory research process.
Source: 2010 Academic Autistic Spectrum Partnership in Research and Education. www.aaspire.org/about/cbpr.html.

or lowered rates of injury and illness (decreasing costs of absenteeism, disability) versus "common good" messages more salient to the public health community.

SCT posits, among other assertions, that learning occurs through observation and imitation of role models, individuals perceived as worthy of emulation.[23] A key premise of the theory is that certain sociodemographic similarities exist between individuals and their role model choices; for example, they may share ethnic, socio-economic status (SES), and/or gender backgrounds. Another central construct is self-efficacy, which refers to one's self-confidence about being able to perform specific behaviors. Observing others with similar sociodemographic characteristics carrying out a desired behavior has been shown to increase one's own self-efficacy regarding similar behaviors. Experiential learning ("enactive mastery") such as recognizing and tasting healthier foods at a church picnic, sampling short bouts of moderate intensity aerobic dance in a classroom, or participating in a walking meeting with coworkers, as well as sociocultural norm change via leadership and role modeling ("vicarious experience") by high-status individuals within the hierarchy, are also critical elements of effective intervention supported by SCT. These approaches are designed to take into account the specific characteristics of the community targeted and thus can be easily applied to work with diverse and vulnerable populations.

Emerging Models

Inclusiveness, cultural appropriateness, equity, and diversity are common themes in emerging models of population-level prevention, though each model's focus is slightly different. The Meta-Volition Model (MVM) illuminates the processes by which innovations may be taken to scale; the Health Impact Pyramid specifies a hierarchy in which interventions influencing socioeconomic determinants of health are most sustainable and scalable. The Public Health Critical Race praxis explores how society's racial inequities contribute to health disparities.

Meta-Volition Model

The MVM dissects public health movements of the past few decades to discern the critical elements and sequencing of efforts driving their success. In these recent public health successes—for example, tobacco control, reducing alcohol consumption and driving, instituting seat restraints while driving, and promoting breast-feeding--social environmental change as reflected in social norm change preceded and catalyzed physical environmental change. "Push" strategies that identified the behavioral economic levers and made the healthy choice easier and the unhealthy choice more difficult were prominent features.[24] Organizational settings permit a ready means of delivering targeted messages and a "microenvironment" or community, both physically and socioculturally, that may be malleable by one or a few leaders and permit more rapid change than does the broader societal milieu.

The model also recognizes the weaknesses and gaps in these movements, for example, the persistent smoking prevalence disparities in low-income and immigrant populations. MVM embeds an intrinsic cultural proficiency in aligning public health aims with those of a diversity of organizations, necessitating building interdisciplinary and intersectoral understanding of and ongoing attention to and working through differing motivators, barriers and facilitators. The model recognizes that cultural contexts and values are critical to success in driving change, from the outset of movement building. This shifts the frame from problems and deficits seen through the research lens, while capturing and explaining the impetus to seek out, identify and introduce cultural assets–based intervention approaches "bubbling up" from diverse communities and settings, rather than attempting to impose or adapt those developed for affluent mainstream audiences. For example, in physical activity promotion, the content area for which the model is most fully developed, structured group activity breaks are advanced because they resonate culturally for the sedentary majority, for example, women, less affluent people, ethnic minority groups,[25] the less fit and agile, and overweight or obese individuals.

Meta-volition refers to leaders' and decision makers' motivation to innovate in driving behavior change as a way of protecting or enhancing the interests of their own organizations. The MVM posits that population-wide behavior change will occur only by shifting the primary driver of change from individual motivation and self-efficacy (the focus of most health promotion models) to a collective and overarching volition (meta-volition) and efficacy.

The MVM is dynamic rather than static, integrating biological influences with psychological factors, and sociocultural influences with organizational and larger societal processes. The model specifies a sequence of six levels or orders of dissemination: initiating (leader–leader), catalyzing (organization–individual), viral marketing (individual–organization), accelerating (organization–organization), anchoring (organization–community), and institutionalizing (community–individual). These levels can be used as points of entry for efforts to facilitate dissemination of interventions across a variety of health content areas. The model has been most completely explicated for physical activity, in proposing brief bouts of activity incorporated into organizational routine as the equivalent of smoking bans in spurring tobacco control.

Health Impact Pyramid

The Health Impact Pyramid is a five-tiered hierarchical schematic capturing the impact of different types of public health interventions.[26] Given the importance of social determinants of health in causing health disparities, interventions aimed at influencing socioeconomic factors appear at the base of the pyramid, reflecting the promise of these strategies to promote health equity. In ascending order, reflecting decreasing impact, are interventions that change the context to make individuals' default decisions healthy, clinical interventions that require limited contact but confer long-term protection, ongoing direct clinical care, and health education and counseling. Approaches concentrated at the lower levels of the pyramid tend to be more sustainable and have a greater impact because they reach broader segments of society, require less individual effort, and may be more likely to reduce health disparities.

Critical Race Theory

The Public Health Critical Race praxis (PHCR) emphasizes the need to understand and address specific ways that racism and racial inequities contribute to health disparities. [27] Grounded in Critical Race Theory, it employs social justice and racial equity orientations in targeting racial inequities.[28]

PHCR encourages the use of race consciousness in studying racial inequities in health. Race consciousness means to understand and acknowledge the workings of racial dynamics both in one's personal life and in the social environment. PHCR considers the perspectives of marginalized communities more central than those of the mainstream for understanding and, most importantly, addressing the fundamental causes of health disparities.

PHCR is praxis (i.e., an iterative methodology) that combines theory, experiential knowledge, science, and action to actively counter inequities. It may be used as a standalone framework guiding research or combined with other theories or methods. Community members play an important role in developing and implementing interventions that address the root causes of identified disparities. These interventions may aim to change community factors or challenge disciplinary conventions typically used to study the problem (e.g., the tendency to view minority populations from a deficits perspective).

As the evidence base for D&I research in marginalized communities expands, additional models will emerge and existing models will continue to be refined. Researchers should draw on these models and seek to expand use of existing models not specifically developed to address disparities.

■ DISSEMINATION AND IMPLEMENTATION CHALLENGES IN WORKING IN ETHNIC MINORITY COMMUNITIES

Ethnic minority, lower-income, rural, aged, and other socioeconomically marginalized populations groups have generally been considered "hard to reach" by public health researchers because of their nonresponsiveness to audiovisual and print health promotion materials and messages targeting "general" (i.e., younger, white, urban, affluent audiences).[13,29] Reasons underlying poor representation of ethnic minority populations in D&I research studies fall into several general categories:

- Conscious nonparticipation by group members. Disinterest in or suspicion about participating in research among people in underserved groups may arise from mistrust engendered by past exploitation.[30,31] These attitudes are common even when the incidents engendering mistrust occurred in the distant past. A contemporary example is the disproportionately low uptake of influenza vaccine in black communities in which health departments do not adequately allay concerns rooted in knowledge of the Tuskegee Study and similarly egregious instances of exploitation. Poor framing of disease prevention efforts may contribute to perceptions of disproportionately high costs incurred compared with benefits received or perceived irrelevance to a particular population. Messages insufficiently targeted to the values and contexts of the lives of their intended audiences compete with pervasive and well-designed commercial communications.[32] Pressing priorities of meeting daily survival needs and obligations may overshadow future-oriented concerns. In addition, incentives may be inadequate to offset the difficulties of participating in research when, for example, transportation is unreliable or time away from work is uncompensated.

- Lack of capacity or infrastructure to absorb opportunity or transactional costs among organizations that serve disadvantaged populations. An unsuitably trained workforce, inadequate space and staffing for the workload, unstable financing, outdated information technology, no resources for staff wellness promotion or professional development, and a poorly maintained surrounding built-environment are all examples of challenges faced by organizations in low-resource communities.

- Investigators' failure to engage these populations. Research and management hierarchies that do not reflect the cultural diversity of targeted population may create perceptions of—or actual lack of—relevance and inclusiveness. Recruitment, implementation, and evaluation success requires long-term relationship-building activities, and these investments of time and energy are poorly rewarded by the academy.[13,33-36]

- Use of research methods that are not culturally appropriate. Modification of research methods may be necessary to engage disadvantaged and ethnic minority communities. This may include altering the process of administering surveys (e.g., interviewer administered vs. self-administered for low-literacy populations), oversampling subgroups of interest, and modifying existing data collection instruments, beyond simple translation, to be more appropriate for special populations. Failure to consider the specific needs of the population of interest may lead to low-quality data or alienation of the community under study.

■ THE IMPORTANCE OF TRUST AND COMMUNITY PARTNERSHIPS FOR DISSEMINATION AND IMPLEMENTATION EFFORTS IN ETHNIC MINORITY POPULATIONS

Although it is important to establish trust when working with any community, it is particularly important to do so when working with underserved, racial/ethnic minority communities. Both the message and the messenger are important when reaching out to underserved communities, which, though frequently targeted for research, may receive few lasting benefits of participation. Levels of distrust of the government, of providers, and of the biomedical sector can be high in these communities.[37,38] How long it takes to establish trust varies from project to project. In general, however, the greater the potential for an intervention to stigmatize communities (e.g., because they involve stigmatized diseases such as HIV/AIDS or populations such as sex workers) or the more invasive the approach, the more resistance can be expected. Ford et al.[39] reported spending more than a year building rapport with the community for an HIV/STD prevention project, and this duration of time was similar to that reported by other HIV prevention researchers.[39] Matching outreach workers by race or ethnicity can boost community members' levels of trust, but researchers will still have to address any intraracial power dynamics (e.g., due to SES differences) that remain. Further, even ethnically matched investigators may require training to ensure their work is culturally relevant and responsive.

Partnering with communities in their ongoing efforts may enhance trust and reach. Innovative settings for health promotion (e.g., churches; Ys; Women, Infants and Children [WIC] clinics; barbers and beauty shops) broaden reach by connecting people where they are, including those with higher levels of need who may be less likely to seek out services. Ethnic minority media, including newspapers, television, magazines and newsletters, radio, websites and LISTSERVs are established institutions with credibility among priority populations.

■ OVERVIEW AND SYNTHESIS OF EMPIRICAL DISSEMINATION AND IMPLEMENTATION RESEARCH

As noted in a number of reviews, relatively little D&I research has been conducted in settings with large proportions of ethnic minority and other underserved populations.[13,14,22,40-44] In this section, community-based D&I efforts are summarized in six prevention areas (physical activity/obesity, nutrition, tobacco, cancer screening, HIV/STIs, immunizations) with a specific focus on describing work within ethnic minority and marginalized communities. Given the sparseness of the literature, the goal was mainly to provide a snapshot of the efforts in these areas to date rather than to provide a critique of individual studies.

Physical Activity and Obesity

Few studies have documented the dissemination of evidence-based physical activity interventions in the population at large,[45-50] much less in underserved communities.[14] The Child and Adolescent Trial for Cardiovascular Health (CATCH) is a comprehensive school-based intervention that focuses on decreasing sodium and fat intake, and increasing moderate-to-vigorous activity during and outside of school hours.[51-54] CATCH was pilot tested and then implemented in 96 schools in four ethnically diverse states.[51,52] Low-income schools were included in the sample; however, there were not a substantial number of African Americans.[51,52] Implementation of CATCH increased minutes of moderate-to-vigorous physical activity[52] and curtailed the rate of increase in overweight among Latino children grades 3 to 5.[55]

Integrating 10-minute physical activity bouts into school routine is an evidence-based policy enjoying increasingly widespread adoption.[56] Several studies have assessed the effectiveness of this intervention in ethnic minority students— Instant Recess®, Take 10! and Energizers.[57-60] For example, Tsai and colleagues[57] implemented Take 10! in a Chicago public urban elementary school with 92% low-income, Hispanic children, increasing students' physical activity knowledge and concentration on coursework. The positive intervention outcomes subsequently resulted in supplementary in-class physical activities such as yoga breaks.[56]

VERB, a nationwide social marketing campaign, disseminated recommendations for physical activity to youth using culturally targeted messages and events showcasing culturally relevant images, fashions, and music.[61] VERB increased physical activity awareness and participation across groups, but its effect first emerged in African-American girls.[61]

Other studies have primarily employed "evidence-informed" or "practice-based" interventions versus evidence-based interventions reflecting scientific consensus because of: (1) stakeholders' limited access to credible sources of scientific evidence,[49,62] (2) the lack of interventions reporting outcomes that have been adapted for practical use in multiethnic populations,[14,63] and (3) the dearth of research studies (e.g., efficacy trials) that include a representative sample of individuals from disadvantaged groups (i.e., low external validity).[13,35,36]

Nutrition

Among the few studies of the dissemination of community-based nutrition interventions in underserved populations, most applied in community settings were school-based initiatives. Examples include comprehensive whole-school interventions such as CATCH,[51-54] which reduced the fat content of school lunches and dietary fat intake in children,[52] and Action Schools! BC, which increased healthy eating activities and practices in the classroom.[64,65] Assessments have been conducted examining the effectiveness of large-scale initiatives, such as 5 A Day For Better Health, in underserved and low-socioeconomic communities.[66] Churches have been utilized in targeting adults and families, for example, Body and Soul, which increased fruit and vegetable consumption among African Americans by 1.4 servings per day.[67]

Community-based nutrition efforts have been designed not only to influence individuals' behaviors, but also to modify the surrounding food environment. Environmental-level changes have included: (1) eliminating advertisements for unhealthy foods and beverages,[68-70] (2) creating community gardens, (3) increasing farmers' markets events, (4) increasing the availability of fresh fruits and vegetables in grocery stores,[70,71] (5) building supermarkets and organic and whole food stores,[71-73] and (6) reducing the cost of healthy food items.

Tobacco Control

A fair amount of D&I research has been conducted in the area of tobacco cessation relative to other disease prevention areas, though many have been descriptive in nature, and conducted in clinical settings. One of the most promising dissemination strategies outside of clinical settings is the promotion of tobacco cessation quitlines or telephone hotlines. A number of dissemination studies aimed at referring study participants to quitlines specifically focused on ethnic minorities. Boyd and colleagues[74] evaluated the use of television and radio commercials as well as direct community outreach to increase the number of callers to the Cancer Information Service (CIS) in African-American communities. Marin and colleagues evaluated the effect of media strategies to increase awareness and use of smoking cessation services among Latinos in San Francisco.[75–77] Although these studies provide important information to inform future dissemination activities, many did not yield data about quit rates among the population of users of these services or were unable to compare quit rates among users and nonusers.

For youth-focused prevention, recent systematic reviews have found sufficient evidence to support the effectiveness of school-based programs in preventing tobacco use among youth in the short term[78]; however, many questions remain about their long-term effectiveness.[79] Although most of these studies were not specifically focused on the underserved, school-based interventions may be more inclusive of low-income and ethnic minorities than studies conducted within clinical settings. These studies have compared the effects of different methods of training teachers and others involved in delivering the interventions and have examined factors related to program compliance, level of adoption, and changes in knowledge and attitudes.[80–84]

Another effective tobacco control strategy has been the passage of clean–indoor air laws.[85] This type of policy-level intervention holds the promise of reducing health disparities given its intention to provide benefit to the greater population and make the unhealthy choice (i.e., smoking) more difficult. However, there is evidence to suggest that disadvantaged communities may have weaker or less restrictive ordinances,[86] which is likely to reduce the benefit for these groups. Future research is needed to assess enforcement of clean air policies, which is likely not uniform across communities.

Cancer Screening

Interest in dissemination, implementation, and translational research in cancer screening promotion has grown dramatically over the past 10 years.[87,88] The evidence base from efficacy studies for the promotion of breast and cervical cancer screening, conducted in both clinical and community settings, is quite robust, based on a relatively large number of randomized trials conducted over several decades.[89,90] Data regarding the most effective methods of promoting colorectal cancer screening and informed decision making regarding prostate cancer screening is expanding, although more limited at this time. Representation of ethnic minorities in efficacy studies has varied by group, with increasing inclusion of African Americans and Latinos over time, but fewer studies in Native Americans or Asian populations.

The CDC-funded *National Breast and Cervical Cancer Early Detection Program* is one of the few federal dissemination initiatives to provide low-income, uninsured, and underserved women access to low-cost or free breast and cervical cancer screening.[91] The program has placed increasing emphasis on evaluating the best strategies to increase both effectiveness and reach of the program. The CDC recently expanded this initiative to include access to colorectal cancer screening in the 22 states and four tribal territories. To date, however, relatively few of the interventions have been evaluated.

There are also a growing number of D&I research projects conducted at the state and local level. Several recent studies were conducted in community settings focused on vulnerable populations. Slater and colleagues[92] described the process by which an effective multicomponent intervention, developed through an NCI-funded trial, was adapted by the American Cancer Society (ACS) to increase mammography use among women living throughout the state of Minnesota. Bencivenga and colleagues[93] found that disseminating an evidence-based intervention through collaborations with food pantries and other community-based organizations in rural Appalachia was effective in increasing mammography rates. Kreuter and colleagues[94] tracked patterns of use and characteristics of users of computer kiosks, located in 40 different St. Louis community sites, generating individually tailored breast health education. This method had been shown in prior studies to be effective in increasing mammography rates. Although the study was not designed to evaluate the effect of kiosk use, results suggest that laundromats may be a promising location for cancer screening promotion activities for urban, African-American women.

HIV/STIs

The CDC's Diffusion of Effective Behavioral Interventions (DEBI) initiative packages and distributes theory-based HIV interventions proven effective through randomized efficacy trials.[95] The packages are intended to be implemented with few or no changes, which ensures that implementation occurs with fidelity to the proven models. Sometimes adaptations are necessary to improve the fit for specific communities. If intervention results are unexpected, however, it can be difficult to determine whether this reflects lack of fidelity to the proven intervention, poor fit to the new population or context, or failure of an appropriate and correctly implemented intervention to have an impact.[95,96] The CDC's Replicating Effective Programs (REP) framework helps to address these challenges by guiding the process by which researchers decide whether to keep an intervention exactly as designed or adapt it per local needs.[97]

HIV/STI interventions occur in three main types of settings. Street outreach is used to contact "hidden" populations (e.g., homeless persons, injection drug users).[39] Clinical settings (e.g., STI clinics, needle exchange sites, and emergency departments) are used to efficiently access both high-HIV/STI prevalence groups and some lower-risk ones. Organizational settings (e.g., community centers, churches) extend prevention efforts to lower-risk subpopulations.[98] Community-wide implementation and dissemination can bolster intervention effectiveness and sustainability. It builds community capacity to provide HIV/STI services, increases awareness of disparities, may improve rates of screening, and may reduce HIV/STI stigma. For example, the National Black HIV Testing Day promotes HIV testing without regard to actual or perceived risk and helps reduce HIV stigma. Whether community-wide implementation and dissemination affect condom use, incident infections, and numbers of sexual partners remains unclear.

Many interventions targeting racial/ethnic minorities are gender specific. Those developed for women have been demonstrated to improve HIV knowledge, self-efficacy, and risk reduction behaviors (e.g., condom use) in sexual partnerships. Many efforts among men target those who self-identify as heterosexual but engage in sexual risk behaviors with other men.[99,100] The greatest challenge to HIV/STI prevention in this population is that it remains hidden and stigmatized. Strategies for reaching these men include intercepting them online (e.g., in chat rooms where men go to meet other men for sex), using respondent-driven sampling to reach members of a social network, and targeting places (e.g., parties) where they gather. Given the limited extent of intervention implementation and dissemination research in this population, the impact on preventive outcomes is still unclear; nevertheless, studies have established that interventions and prevention messages developed for or disseminated via the white gay community are ineffectual for minority men.[101]

HIV prevention interventions rely on a wide range of psychosocial and behavioral theories. Most interventions aim to change individual-level psychosocial factors (e.g., HIV knowledge) or behaviors (e.g., unprotected sex). Others aim to diffuse effects through social/sexual networks or communities. These approaches draw on the resources within and characteristics of networks or communities, and the capacity of peers (e.g., lay health workers) or leaders (e.g., ministers), to influence members of their networks. Few interventions target structural inequities and the social determinants of health. SISTA, which was developed for use among African-American and, more recently, Latina women, acknowledges social determinants of health but focuses on individual-level behavior change. By addressing how race and gender oppression influence women's lives, SISTA aims to empower women to make decisions and take actions that reduce their risk of HIV transmission.[102]

Immunization/Vaccination

Universal coverage programs for childhood vaccinations have been in place since the 1940s in the United States.[103] Coverage rates have increased over time and remain quite high (>90%) across most childhood vaccines with the exception of the flu vaccine.[104,105] The high level of vaccine coverage was achieved through a combination of activities, primarily at the policy level, including coordinated efforts at the federal, state, and local level to promote vaccination, state-based immunization registries, recommendations from professional organizations regarding the importance of vaccination, systematic collection of data to measure coverage, and prioritization of immunizations by governmental and professional bodies.[103,106,107] However, gaps in immunization rates between white and ethnic minority children were first identified in the 1970s and continue to persist today.[104–107] Policy-level efforts specifically aimed at improving vaccination rates in underserved populations have included federal funding for low-cost or free vaccine through the Vaccines for Children Program, linkages between WIC and immunization activities, enhancement of payment for immunization services for children covered by Medicaid, and partnerships with minority health organizations.[107]

However, relatively few studies have rigorously evaluated vaccine promotion efforts targeting ethnic minority communities, within the larger context of vaccine promotion activities at the local, state, and national level; thus, the evidence base is somewhat limited, which may serve as a barrier to D&I research. Examples of interventions aimed at increasing vaccination coverage within underserved populations within nonclinical settings have included several randomized trials among families enrolled in WIC programs, which found that both linking food vouchers to immunization and escorting a child to a local vaccination clinic led to significant increases in vaccination coverage.[108,109] The New York State Department of Health found that their efforts to partner with community-based organizations to outreach to underimmunized children were successful in increasing vaccination in New York City.[110] Although promising, relatively few intervention efforts have been "taken to scale" or disseminated to the broader population. A recent review by Galea and colleagues[107] noted that without moving beyond trials to implementation and dissemination studies, sustainable increases in vaccination rates among underserved and ethnic minority populations will not occur.

Although the majority of vaccine promotion efforts have focused on childhood vaccination, increasing emphasis has been placed on vaccines targeted to the adolescent with recent additions of the HPV, tetanus/diphtheria/pertussis (Tdap), and the meningococcal vaccines as well as catch-up vaccinations for hepatitis B.[111,112] Efforts have also intensified to increase uptake of the seasonal flu vaccine among adults, particularly the elderly, although most interventions to date have been conducted within clinical settings.[113] Evidence suggests that ethnic and socioeconomic disparities are likely more pronounced in vaccine coverage among adolescents and adults than in children.[112,114]

■ SUMMARY

The evidence base on D&I of interventions for racial/ethnic minority communities is expanding rapidly. While the nature of the evidence varies depending upon the health outcome, some general trends are apparent. Key lessons include that cultural appropriateness enhances community "buy-in" of interventions. Increasingly, interventions are expected to be culturally appropriate. This requires that both the message and the messenger are well suited for the community. Targeting captive audiences, which reduces the cost to the individual of participating, and utilizing culturally valued and ubiquitous settings are also associated with success. CBPR approaches that share power and decision making are also gaining in prominence. They suggest that intervention sustainability is enhanced when community members are actively involved in all phases of research, implementation, and dissemination. Efforts that account for place characteristics (e.g., neighborhood geography, intervention setting) can also improve the uptake of interventions. In contrast to the individually focused models of early prevention efforts, emerging approaches target social networks or whole communities and attempt to address macro-level factors that may influence multiple health outcomes. For example, despite impressive advances in dissemination of effective HIV prevention interventions, disparities persist. One reason may be that interventions primarily target proximal factors (e.g., condom use). As concluded by the WHO Commission on the Social Determinants of Health, the eradication of health disparities is possible; however, it requires that the effects of structural influences (e.g., policies) on societal inequities be addressed. These factors fundamentally shape all individual-level risk factors.[115]

■ DIRECTIONS FOR FUTURE RESEARCH

Clearly much remains to be studied in order to advance health equity at a population level. Future research should explore how to adapt effective interventions to improve the fit for communities without losing fidelity to the elements or kernels of the original model producing its effects, and seek to better identify and evaluate promising practice-based interventions emerging from communities experiencing disparities. Future research should also clarify the strategies to use for intervention sequencing and prioritization. For example, demand generation should generally precede supply creation.

Many of these issues are reflected in a comparison of the levels of mammography screening achieved across ethnic groups, as the following case study illustrates.

■ CASE STUDY

Background

Breast cancer is the most common cause of cancer among women in the United States. Incidence rates of breast cancer are highest among non-Latino white women.[116] Although they are less likely to get the disease than non-Latino white women, African-American women are more likely to die of the disease than any other ethnic group. Furthermore, evidence is accumulating that risk for breast cancer may increase with acculturation to a U.S. lifestyle among immigrants to this country.[117,118] Mammography has been considered an important tool in reducing the burden of breast cancer, and differential uptake of mammography screening has been identified as a major contributor to ethnic disparities in breast cancer mortality.[119,120] As a result, promoting uptake among all women has been a central goal of cancer prevention and control efforts in the United States over the past several decades.

Recent data collected through the Behavioral Risk Factor Surveillance Survey show that rates of having had a mammography within the past 2 years among women between the ages of 50 and 74 are nearly equal for white, African-American, Asian-Pacific Islander, and Latina women, hovering around 80% for each group.[116] Rates among Alaskan Native/American Indian women continue to lag behind, with only around 70% of Native women having had a mammogram within the same time frame. Despite this notable exception, the narrowing of the gap in mammography use between ethnic minority and white women represents a success story in the diffusion of effective prevention strategies among ethnic minorities in the United States. A number of factors have likely contributed to this success, including national policy-level initiatives, advocacy efforts at the national, state, and local level, and active and passive diffusion of effective strategies to promote mammography that have emerged from randomized trials.

Context

Efforts to promote mammography were initiated in the early 1990s after data first suggested that mammography was an effective strategy in lowering mortality from breast cancer. The National Breast and Cervical Cancer Early Detection Program (NBCCEDP) was created in 1990, by the Centers for Disease Control, following the passage of the Breast and Cervical Cancer Mortality Prevention Act, to provide funding for low-income, uninsured women to receive breast and cervical cancer screening for free or at a low cost. In 2000, the passage of the Breast and Cervical Cancer Prevention and Treatment Act allowed funds to be made available to help these same women access needed follow-up and treatment resources following screening. Although likely an important contributor to reducing ethnic disparities in mammography use, evidence to support the unique contribution of this program in eliminating disparities is not available. Dovetailing with the mission of the NBCCEDP, increasing mammography rates has long been a central goal of the Healthy People initiative, increasing awareness of the importance of mammography and providing guidance to local and state efforts. Many states have supplemented national funds received through the NBCCEDP to increase the number of women served and to implement outreach efforts to reach priority populations within their state. Increasing use of mammography is also a central goal of most, if not all, states' comprehensive cancer control plans.

As described earlier in this chapter, a large number of randomized trials have evaluated strategies to increase use of mammography starting in the late 1980s and continuing today. A number of effective strategies have emerged from these trials, including strategies primarily implemented in clinical settings (reminder strategies) as well as a number of strategies that have been implemented in community settings (small media, U.S. Preventive Services Task Force). Relatively few randomized trials have evaluated the best ways of disseminating effective strategies that emerged from efficacy trials. However, it is likely that passive diffusion has led to uptake of successful strategies over time. This is particularly the case in clinical settings where reminder systems have been increasingly implemented to enhance delivery of a number of services, including mammography.

Numerous community-based initiatives at the national (ACS "Tell a Friend"), state, and local level have attempted to use messaging and social networks to promote use of mammography among underserved and ethnic minority women. Efforts have included outreach at community venues such as churches, beauty salons, community-based organizations, and health fairs, often linking women reached through community venues to existing low-cost or free mammography services or bringing mammograms to the community through use of mobile mammography vans. All of these efforts have taken place against the backdrop of aggressive advocacy aimed at reducing deaths from breast cancer that has taken place at the national, state, and local levels over the past several decades. These efforts have been led by large nonprofit organizations such as the American Cancer Society, the Susan G. Komen Foundation, Avon Foundation, and countless smaller nonprofit foundations, and have been pioneered by an engaged, enthusiastic, and growing population of breast cancer survivors.

Findings and Lessons Learned

The case of diffusion of mammography use in underserved and ethnic minority women is somewhat unique and thus poses challenges when trying to apply "lessons learned" to other priority health areas. It is unlikely that a conscious decision can be made to use advocacy to precipitate similar successes for other preventive health strategies given the culmination forces that led to the breast cancer advocacy movement. However, as has been previously documented, widespread policy-level efforts to increase access and reduce barriers to receiving mammograms has been an integral part of reducing disparities in mammography use and suggest directions for increasing use of other preventive health services. Opportunism in involving leaders personally affected by a disease or condition is certainly a common springboard for broad-based action. Furthermore, the success of community-based efforts to promote mammography, a service that can only be accessed by interfacing with a clinical setting and through use of specialized equipment, speaks to the potential impact of preventive health strategies that can be delivered in less restrictive settings such as immunizations, chronic disease screenings (glucose, blood pressure, cholesterol), and the promotion of lifestyle behaviors (physical activity and nutrition).

Recent data suggest that mammography rates may have plateaued and begun to decline in recent years.[121] This trend may have been amplified, especially among underserved and ethnic minority women, by the recent economic downturn. Given these observations, it will be particularly important to continue to expand efforts to disseminate effective strategies to increase use of mammography, particularly in community settings where the most vulnerable and needy women can be reached.

Implications

The importance of inclusivity and equity in public health efforts to prevent and control disease is paramount. The participation of ethnic minority and other underserved populations in leadership and as targets of such research and service efforts must be central, rather than marginal, weak, and fragmented. The provisions of the health care reform legislation present a rare opportunity for a substantial infusion of resources into prevention. The best way to achieve social justice *and* improve the health of the entire population is to ensure that the strategies most effective in preventing disease are disseminated within the populations at greatest risk. Maximizing external validity is critical to the goals of disseminating evidence-based protocols to broader audiences and understanding public health impacts in terms of population reach as well as representativeness.[122]

SUGGESTED READINGS

Israel BA, Schulz AJ, Parker EA, Becker AB. Review of community-based research: assessing partnership approaches to improve public health. *Annu Rev Public Health.* 1998;19:173–202.

The single most cited paper on Community-Based Participatory Research (CBPR) in the health field. This paper introduces CBPR, its core principles, as well as some of the challenges entailed in their implementation. In addition to providing a review of the literature, this work uses early lessons of the Detroit Community-Academic Research Center to explicate CBPR principles and their implementation.

Kreuter M, Black W, Friend L, et al. Use of computer kiosks for breast cancer education in five community settings. *Health Educ Behav.* 2006 Oct;33(5):625–642.

This paper describes the results of a study that tracked patterns of use and characteristics of users of computer kiosks placed in community settings in St. Louis, Missouri, to provide breast cancer education. Significant differences were found in rates and patterns of kiosk use and user characteristics when comparing across community settings, including beauty salons, churches, health centers, laundromats, and social service agencies. Findings can inform dissemination efforts in underserved community settings.

Ford CL, Airhihenbuwa CO. The public health critical race methodology: praxis for anti-racism research. *Soc Sci Med.* 2010;71(8):1390–1398.

Introduces the Public Health Critical Race praxis (PHCR), developed by the authors as an aid for studying modern-day racial concerns. This model provides potential tools for finding and eradicating race-based health disparities.

Frieden T. A framework for public health action: the health impact pyramid. *Am J Public Health.* 2010 Apr;100(4):590–595.

Describes a framework that uses a five-tier pyramid to prioritize public health interventions with regard to their potential impact on population health and health disparities. Authors suggest that interventions at each level are needed to maximize sustainable population health benefits.

Welch V, Tugwell P, Petticrew M, et al. How effects on health equity are assessed in systematic reviews of interventions. Cochrane Database Syst Rev. 2010;Issue 12: Art No. MR000028. DOI: 10.1002/14651858.MR000028.pub2.

A systematic review of methods to assess effects of health equity within systematic reviews of effectiveness of health care interventions. The authors propose clarifying the definition of health equity in order to accurately report health equity effects in systematic reviews.

Yancey A. The meta-volition model: organizational leadership is the key ingredient in getting society moving, literally! *Prev Med.* 2009 Oct;49(4):342–351.

Introduces a dynamic population health behavior change conceptual model (MVM) derived from key drivers of successful social movements. The model specifies a cascade of changes from initiation to institutionalization that must be sparked by "healthy by default" organizational practices and policies such as smoking bans, inpatient postnatal breastfeeding support and elimination of formula distribution, and structural integration of brief physical activity bouts.

SELECTED WEBSITES AND TOOLS

Cancer Control—Plan, Link, Act, Network with Evidence-based Tools (P.L.A.N.E.T.). http://cancercontrolplanet.cancer.gov/

World Health Organization Commission on the Social Determinants of Health. http://whqlibdoc.who.int/publications/2008/9789241563703_eng.pdf

National Breast and Cervical Cancer Early Detection Program (NBCCEDP). http://www.cdc.gov/cancer/nbccedp/

DEBI: Diffusion of Effective Behavioral Interventions. http://effectiveinterventions.org/en/home.aspx

Guide to Community Preventive Services. http://www.thecommunityguide.org/index.html

REFERENCES

1. National Center for Health Statistics (U.S.). *Health, United States, 2004.* Atlanta: Centers for Disease Control and Prevention; 2004.

2. Harper S, Lynch J, Burris S, Davey Smith G. Trends in the black-white life expectancy gap in the United States, 1983–2003. *JAMA*. Mar 2007;297(11):1224–1232.

3. Commission on Social Determinants of Health. *Achieving Health Equity: From Root Causes to Fair Outcomes*. Geneva, Switzerland: World Health Organization; 2007.

4. Ford CL, Harawa NT. A new conceptualization of ethnicity for social epidemiologic and health equity research. *Soc Sci Med*. Jul 2010;71(2):251–258.

5. Byrd W, Clayton L. *An American Health Dilemma: Race, Medicine, and Health Care in the United States*. New York: Routledge; 2002.

6. Jones D. The persistence of American Indian health disparities. *Am J Public Health*. Dec 2006;96(12):2122–2134.

7. Gee G, Ford C. Structural racism and health inequities: old issues, new directions. *Du Bois Rev*. 2011;8(1):115–132.

8. Derose K, Escarce J, Lurie N. Immigrants and health care: sources of vulnerability. *Health Aff (Millwood)*. 2007 Sep–Oct 2007;26(5):1258–1268.

9. Osypuk T, Roux A, Hadley C, Kandula N. Are immigrant enclaves healthy places to live? The Multi-ethnic Study of Atherosclerosis. *Soc Sci Med*. Jul 2009;69(1):110–120.

10. Koya D, Egede L. Association between length of residence and cardiovascular disease risk factors among an ethnically diverse group of United States immigrants. *J Gen Intern Med*. Jun 2007;22(6):841–846.

11. Williams DR. The health of U.S. racial and ethnic populations. *J Gerontol B Psychol Sci Soc Sci*. Oct 2005;60 Spec No 2:53–62.

12. Viruell-Fuentes EA. Beyond acculturation: immigration, discrimination, and health research among Mexicans in the United States. *Soc Sci Med*. Oct 2007;65(7): 1524–1535.

13. Yancey A, Ortega A, Kumanyika S. Effective recruitment and retention of minority research participants. *Annu Rev Public Health*. 2006;27:1–28.

14. Yancey A, Ory M, Davis S. Dissemination of physical activity promotion interventions in underserved populations. *Am J Prev Med*. Oct 2006;31(4 Suppl):S82–S91.

15. Matson-Koffman DM, Brownstein JN, Neiner JA, Greaney ML. A site-specific literature review of policy and environmental interventions that promote physical activity and nutrition for cardiovascular health: what works? *Am J Health Promot*. Jan–Feb 2005;19(3):167–193.

16. Lobstein T, Baur L, Uauy R. Obesity in children and young people: a crisis in public health. *Obes Rev*. May 2004;5(Suppl 1):4–104.

17. Kersh R, Morone J. The politics of obesity: seven steps to government action. *Health Aff (Millwood)*. Nov–Dec 2002;21(6):142–153.

18. Stokols D, Grzywacz J, McMahan S, Phillips K. Increasing the health promotive capacity of human environments. *Am J Health Promot*. Sep–Oct 2003;18(1):4–13.

19. Israel BA, Schulz AJ, Parker EA, Becker AB. Review of community-based research: assessing partnership approaches to improve public health. *Annu Rev Public Health*. 1998;19:173–202.

20. Green L, Daniel M, Novick L. Partnerships and coalitions for community-based research. *Public Health Rep*. 2001;116(Suppl 1):20–31.

21. Yancey A, Miles O, Jordan A. Organizational characteristics facilitating initiation and institutionalization of physical activity programs in a multi-ethnic, urban community. *J Health Educ*. March/April 1999;30(2):S44–S51.

22. Grier S, Bryant CA. Social marketing in public health. *Annu Rev Public Health*. 2005;26:319–339.

23. Bandura A. *Social Foundations of Thought and Action: A Social Cognitive Theory.* Englewood Cliffs, NJ: Prentice-Hall; 1986.
24. Yancey A. The meta-volition model: organizational leadership is the key ingredient in getting society moving, literally! *Prev Med.* Oct 2009;49(4):342–351.
25. Yancey T. *Instant Recess: Building a Fit Nation 10 Minutes at a Time.* Berkeley, CA: University of California press, 2010.
26. Frieden T. A framework for public health action: the health impact pyramid. *Am J Public Health.* Apr 2010;100(4):590–595.
27. Ford C, Airhihenbuwa C. The public health critical race methodology: praxis for antiracism research. *Soc Sci Med.* 2010;71(8):1390–1398.
28. Ford CL, Airhihenbuwa CO. Critical Race Theory, race equity, and public health: toward antiracism praxis. *Am J Public Health.* Apr 2010;100(Suppl 1):S30–S35.
29. Freimuth VS, Mettger W. Is there a hard-to-reach audience? *Public Health Rep.* May–Jun 1990;105(3):232–238.
30. Bell L, Butler T, Herring R, Yancey A, Fraser G. Recruiting blacks to the Adventist health study: Do follow-up phone calls increase response rates? *Ann Epidemiol.* Oct 2005;15(9):667–672.
31. Thomas S, Curran J. Tuskegee: from science to conspiracy to metaphor. *American Journal of Medical Sciences.* 1999;317(1):1–4.
32. Yancey A, Cole B, Brown R, et al. A cross-sectional prevalence study of ethnically targeted and general audience outdoor obesity-related advertising. *Milbank Q.* Mar 2009;87(1):155–184.
33. Ory M, Kinney Hoffman M, Hawkins M, Sanner B, Mockenhaupt R. Challenging aging stereotypes: strategies for creating a more active society. *Am J Prev Med.* Oct 2003;25(3Suppl 2):164–171.
34. Yancey AK. Building capacity to prevent and control chronic disease in underserved communities: expanding the wisdom of WISEWOMAN in intervening at the environmental level. *J Womens Health (Larchmt).* Jun 2004;13(5):644–649.
35. Yancey A, Kumanyika S, Ponce N, et al. Population-based interventions engaging communities of color in healthy eating and active living: a review. *Prev Chronic Dis.* Jan 2004;1(1):A09.
36. Herring P, Montgomery S, Yancey AK, Williams D, Fraser G. Understanding the challenges in recruiting blacks to a longitudinal cohort study: the Adventist health study. *Ethn Dis.* Summer 2004;14(3):423–430.
37. Herek GM, Capitanio JP. Conspiracies, contagion, and compassion: trust and public reactions to AIDS. *AIDS Educ Prev.* 1994;6(4):365–375.
38. Corbie-Smith G, Ford CL. Distrust and poor self-reported health. Canaries in the coal mine? *J Gen Intern Med.* Apr 2006;21(4):395–397.
39. Ford CL, Miller WC, Smurzynski M, Leone PA. Key components of a theory-guided HIV prevention outreach model: pre-outreach preparation, community assessment, and a network of key informants. *AIDS Educ Prev.* Apr 2007;19(2):173–186.
40. Rabin B, Glasgow R, Kerner J, Klump M, Brownson R. Dissemination and implementation research on community-based cancer prevention: a systematic review. *Am J Prev Med.* Apr 2010;38(4):443–456.
41. Aisenberg E. Evidence-based practice in mental health care to ethnic minority communities: has its practice fallen short of its evidence? *Soc Work.* Oct 2008;53(4):297–306.

42. Whitt-Glover M, Kumanyika S. Systematic review of interventions to increase physical activity and physical fitness in African-Americans. *Am J Health Promot.* 2009 Jul–Aug 2009;23(6):S33–S56.

43. Yancey A, Tomiyama A. Physical activity as primary prevention to address cancer disparities. *Semin Oncol Nurs.* Nov 2007;23(4):253–263.

44. Agency for Healthcare Research and Quality. *Diffusion and Dissemination of Evidence-based Cancer Control Interventions.* 2003. Summary, Evidence Report/Technology Assessment: Number 79. Available at: http://www.ahrq.gov/clinic/epcsums/canconsum.pdf. Accessed on November 8, 2011.

45. Oldenburg B, Sallis J, Ffrench M, Owen N. Health promotion research and the diffusion and institutionalization of interventions. *Health Educ Res.* Feb 1999;14(1):121–130.

46. Orleans C, Gruman J, Ulmer C, Emont S, Hollendonner J. Rating our progress in population health promotion: report card on six behaviors. *Am J Health Promot.* Nov–Dec 1999;14(2):75–82.

47. Bauman A, Sallis J, Dzewaltowski D, Owen N. Toward a better understanding of the influences on physical activity: the role of determinants, correlates, causal variables, mediators, moderators, and confounders. *Am J Prev Med.* Aug 2002; 23(2 Suppl):5–14.

48. Dzewaltowski D, Estabrooks P, Klesges L, Bull S, Glasgow R. Behavior change intervention research in community settings: how generalizable are the results? *Health Promot Int.* Jun 2004;19(2):235–245.

49. Owen N, Glanz K, Sallis J, Kelder S. Evidence-based approaches to dissemination and diffusion of physical activity interventions. *Am J Prev Med.* Oct 2006; 31(4 Suppl):S35–S44.

50. Rabin B, Brownson R, Kerner J, Glasgow R. Methodologic challenges in disseminating evidence-based interventions to promote physical activity. *Am J Prev Med.* Oct 2006;31(4 Suppl):S24–S34.

51. Perry C, Stone E, Parcel G, et al. School-based cardiovascular health promotion: the child and adolescent trial for cardiovascular health (CATCH). *J Sch Health.* Oct 1990;60(8):406–413.

52. Luepker R, Perry C, McKinlay S, et al. Outcomes of a field trial to improve children's dietary patterns and physical activity. The child and adolescent trial for cardiovascular health (CATCH). *JAMA.* 1996;275(10):768–776.

53. McKenzie T, Nader P, Strikmiller P, et al. School physical education: effect of the child and adolescent trial for cardiovascular health. *Prev Med.* 1996;25(4): 423–431.

54. Perry C, Sellers D, Johnson C, et al. The child and adolescent trial for cardiovascular health (CATCH): intervention, implementation, and feasibility for elementary schools in the United States. *Health Educ Behav.* 1997;24(6):716–735.

55. Coleman K, Tiller C, Sanchez J, et al. Prevention of the epidemic increase in child risk of overweight in low-income schools: the El Paso coordinated approach to child health. *Arch Pediatr Adolesc Med.* Mar 2005;159(3):217–224.

56. Whitt-Glover M, Alexander R, Creecy J, Tate A, Yancey A. *Do Physical Activity Breaks in Classrooms Work? Active Living Research Policy Brief.* Princeton, NJ: RWJF. 2012.

57. Tsai P, Boonpleng W, McElmurry B, Park C, McCreary L. Lessons learned in using TAKE 10! with Hispanic children. *J Sch Nurs.* 2009;25(2):163–172.

58. Kibbe DL, Hackett J, Hurley M, McFarland A, Schubert KG, Schultz A, Harris S. Ten Years of TAKE 10!(*): Integrating physical activity with academic concepts in elementary school classrooms. *Prev Med.* 2011;52(Suppl 1):S43–50.

59. Mahar M. Impact of short bouts of physical activity on attention-to-task in elementary school children. *Prev Med.* 2011;52:S60–64.

60. Whitt-Glover M, Ham SA, Yancey A. Instant Recess®: A practical tool for increasing physical activity during the school day. *Prog Comm Health Partn.* In press, 2011.

61. Huhman M, Berkowitz J, Wong F, et al. The VERB campaign's strategy for reaching African-American, Hispanic, Asian, and American Indian children and parents. *Am J Prev Med.* Jun 2008;34(6 Suppl):S194–S209.

62. Hazel K, Onaga E. Experimental social innovation and dissemination: the promise and its delivery. *Am J Community Psychol.* Dec 2003;32(3–4):285–294.

63. Mummery W, Schofield G, Hinchliffe A, Joyner K, Brown W. Dissemination of a community-based physical activity project: the case of 10,000 steps. *J Sci Med Sport.* Oct 2006;9(5):424–430.

64. Naylor P, Macdonald H, Reed K, McKay H. Action Schools! BC: a socioecological approach to modifying chronic disease risk factors in elementary school children. *Prev Chronic Dis.* Apr 2006;3(2):A60.

65. Naylor P, Scott J, Drummond J, Bridgewater L, McKay H, Panagiotopoulos C. Implementing a whole school physical activity and healthy eating model in rural and remote first nations schools: a process evaluation of action schools! BC. *Rural Remote Health.* 2010 Apr–Jun 2010;10(2):1296.

66. Stables G, Young E, Howerton M, et al. Small school-based effectiveness trials increase vegetable and fruit consumption among youth. *J Am Diet Assoc.* Feb 2005;105(2): 252–256.

67. Resnicow K, Campbell M, Carr C, et al. Body and soul. A dietary intervention conducted through African-American churches. *Am J Prev Med.* Aug 2004;27(2):97–105.

68. Grier S, Mensinger J, Huang S, Kumanyika S, Stettler N. Fast-food marketing and children's fast-food consumption: exploring parents' influences in an ethnically diverse sample. 2007;26(2):221–235.

69. Grier S, Kumanyika S. The context for choice: health implications of targeted food and beverage marketing to African Americans. *Am J Public Health.* Sep 2008;98(9): 1616–1629.

70. Grier S, Kumanyika S. Targeted marketing and public health. *Annu Rev Public Health.* Apr 2010;31:349–369.

71. Galvez M, Morland K, Raines C, et al. Race and food store availability in an inner-city neighbourhood. *Public Health Nutr.* Jun 2008;11(6):624–631.

72. Powell L, Slater S, Mirtcheva D, Bao Y, Chaloupka F. Food store availability and neighborhood characteristics in the United States. *Prev Med.* Mar 2007;44(3):189–195.

73. Ford P, Dzewaltowski D. Disparities in obesity prevalence due to variation in the retail food environment: three testable hypotheses. *Nutr Rev.* Apr 2008;66(4):216–228.

74. Boyd N, Sutton C, Orleans C, et al. Quit Today! A targeted communications campaign to increase use of the cancer information service by African American smokers. *Prev Med.* Sep–Oct 1998;27(5 Pt 2):S50–S60.

75. Marín G, Marín B, Pérez-Stable E, Sabogal F, Otero-Sabogal R. Changes in information as a function of a culturally appropriate smoking cessation community intervention for Hispanics. *Am J Community Psychol.* Dec 1990;18(6):847–864.

76. Marín G, Pérez-Stable E. Effectiveness of disseminating culturally appropriate smoking-cessation information: Programa Latino Para Dejar de Fumar. *J Natl Cancer Inst Monogr.* 1995(18):155–163.

77. Pérez-Stable E, Marín B, Marín G. A comprehensive smoking cessation program for the San Francisco Bay Area Latino community: Programa Latino Para Dejar de Fumar. *Am J Health Promot.* Jul–Aug 1993;7(6):430–442, 475.

78. Dobbins M, DeCorby K, Manske S, Goldblatt E. Effective practices for school-based tobacco use prevention. *Prev Med.* Apr 2008;46(4):289–297.

79. Wiehe S, Garrison M, Christakis D, Ebel B, Rivara F. A systematic review of school-based smoking prevention trials with long-term follow-up. *J Adolesc Health.* Mar 2005;36(3):162–169.

80. Basen-Engquist K, O'Hara-Tompkins N, Lovato C, Lewis M, Parcel G, Gingiss P. The effect of two types of teacher training on implementation of Smart Choices: a tobacco prevention curriculum. *J Sch Health.* Oct 1994;64(8):334–339.

81. Perry C, Murray D, Griffin G. Evaluating the statewide dissemination of smoking prevention curricula: factors in teacher compliance. *J Sch Health.* Dec 1990;60(10):501–504.

82. Parcel G, Eriksen M, Lovato C, Gottlieb N, Brink S, Green L. The diffusion of school-based tobacco-use prevention programs: project description and baseline data. *Health Educ Res.* 1989;4:111–124.

83. Parcel G, O'Hara-Tompkins N, Harrist R, et al. Diffusion of an effective tobacco prevention program. Part II: Evaluation of the adoption phase. *Health Educ Res.* Sep 1995;10(3):297–307.

84. Brink S, Basen-Engquist K, O'Hara-Tompkins N, Parcel G, Gottlieb N, Lovato C. Diffusion of an effective tobacco prevention program. Part I: Evaluation of the dissemination phase. *Health Educ Res.* Sep 1995;10(3):283–295.

85. Levy D, Chaloupka F, Gitchell J. The effects of tobacco control policies on smoking rates: a tobacco control scorecard. *J Public Health Manag Pract.* 2004;10(4):338–353.

86. Ferketich A, Liber A, Pennell M, Nealy D, Hammer J, Berman M. Clean indoor air ordinance coverage in the Appalachian region of the United States. *Am J Public Health.* Jul 2010;100(7):1313–1318.

87. Glasgow R, Marcus A, Bull S, Wilson K. Disseminating effective cancer screening interventions. *Cancer.* Sep 2004;101(5 Suppl):1239–1250.

88. Bowen D, Sorensen G, Weiner B, Campbell M, Emmons K, Melvin C. Dissemination research in cancer control: where are we and where should we go? *Cancer Causes Control.* May 2009;20(4):473–485.

89. Baron R, Rimer B, Coates R, et al. Client-directed interventions to increase community access to breast, cervical, and colorectal cancer screening: a systematic review. *Am J Prev Med.* Jul 2008;35(1 Suppl):S56–S66.

90. Centers for Disease Control and Prevention. Guide to community preventive services. Cancer prevention and control: client-oriented screening interventions. Available at: www.thecommunityguide.org/cancer/screening/client-oriented/index.html. Last updated: June 27, 2011. Accessed on November 8, 2011.

91. Centers for Disease Control and Prevention. National Breast and Cervical Cancer Early Detection Program (NBCCEDP). Available at: http://www.cdc.gov/cancer/nbccedp/. Last updated: July 25, 2011. Accessed on November 8, 2011.

92. Slater J, Finnegan JJ, Madigan S. Incorporation of a successful community-based mammography intervention: dissemination beyond a community trial. *Health Psychol.* Sep 2005;24(5):463–469.

93. Bencivenga M, DeRubis S, Leach P, Lotito L, Shoemaker C, Lengerich E. Community partnerships, food pantries, and an evidence-based intervention to increase mammography among rural women. *J Rural Health.* 2008;24(1):91–95.

94. Kreuter M, Black W, Friend L, et al. Use of computer kiosks for breast cancer education in five community settings. *Health Educ Behav.* Oct 2006;33(5):625–642.

95. Dworkin S, Pinto R, Hunter J, Rapkin B, Remien R. Keeping the spirit of community partnerships alive in the scale up of HIV/AIDS prevention: critical reflections on the roll out of DEBI (Diffusion of Effective Behavioral Interventions). *Am J Community Psychol.* Sep 2008;42(1–2):51–59.

96. Norton W, Amico K, Cornman D, Fisher W, Fisher J. An agenda for advancing the science of implementation of evidence-based HIV prevention interventions. *AIDS Behav.* Jun 2009;13(3):424–429.

97. Kilbourne A, Neumann M, Pincus H, Bauer M, Stall R. Implementing evidence-based interventions in health care: application of the replicating effective programs framework. *Implement Sci.* 2007;2:42.

98. Stallworth J, Andía J, Burgess R, Alvarez M, Collins C. Diffusion of effective behavioral interventions and Hispanic/Latino populations. *AIDS Educ Prev.* Oct 2009;21(5 Suppl):152–163.

99. Mays V, Cochran S, Zamudio A. HIV prevention research: are we meeting the needs of African American men who have sex with men? *J Black Psychol.* 2004;30(1):78–105.

100. Ford C, Whetten K, Hall S, Kaufman J, Thrasher A. Black sexuality, social construction, and research targeting "The Down Low" ("The DL"). *Ann Epidemiol.* Mar 2007;17(3):209–216.

101. Goldbaum G, Perdue T, Wolitski R, et al. Differences in risk behavior and sources of AIDS information among gay, bisexual, and straight-identified men who have sex with men. *AIDS Behav.* 1998;2(1):13–21.

102. Prather C, Fuller T, King W, et al. Diffusing an HIV prevention intervention for African American Women: integrating afrocentric components into the SISTA Diffusion Strategy. *AIDS Educ Prev.* Aug 2006;18(4 Suppl A):149–160.

103. Freed G, Bordley W, DeFriese G. Childhood immunization programs: an analysis of policy issues. *Milbank Q.* 1993;71(1):65–96.

104. Centers for Disease Control and Prevention. Influenza vaccination coverage among children and adults—United States, 2008–09 influenza season. *MMWR Morb Mortal Wkly Rep.* Oct 2009;58(39):1091–1095.

105. Centers for Disease Control and Prevention. National, state and local are vaccination coverage among children aged 19–35 months-United States, 2008. *Morb Mortal Wkly Rep.* 2009;58(33):921–926.

106. Hutchins S, Jiles R, Bernier R. Elimination of measles and of disparities in measles childhood vaccine coverage among racial and ethnic minority populations in the United States. *J Infect Dis.* May 2004;189(Suppl 1):S146–S152.

107. Galea S, Sisco S, Vlahov D. Reducing disparities in vaccination rates between different racial/ethnic and socioeconomic groups: the potential of community-based multilevel interventions. *J Ambul Care Manage.* 2005 Jan–Mar 2005;28(1):49–59.

108. Hoekstra E, LeBaron C, Megaloeconomou Y, et al. Impact of a large-scale immunization initiative in the Special Supplemental Nutrition Program for Women, Infants, and Children (WIC). *JAMA.* Oct 1998;280(13):1143–1147.

109. Birkhead G, LeBaron C, Parsons P, et al. The immunization of children enrolled in the Special Supplemental Food Program for Women, Infants, and Children (WIC). The impact of different strategies. *JAMA.* Jul 1995;274(4):312–316.

110. Rosenberg Z, Findley S, McPhillips S, Penachio M, Silver P. Community-based strategies for immunizing the "hard-to-reach" child: the New York State immunization and primary health care initiative. *Am J Prev Med.* May–Jun 1995; 11(3 Suppl):14–20.

111. Brabin L, Greenberg D, Hessel L, Hyer R, Ivanoff B, Van Damme P. Current issues in adolescent immunization. *Vaccine.* Aug 2008;26(33):4120–4134.

112. Centers for Disease Control and Prevention. Vaccination coverage among adolescents aged 13–17 years—United States, 2008. *Morbid Mortal Wkly Rep.* 2009;38(36):997–1001.

113. Ompad D, Galea S, Vlahov D. Distribution of influenza vaccine to high-risk groups. *Epidemiol Rev.* 2006;28:54–70.

114. Lu P, Bridges C, Euler G, Singleton J. Influenza vaccination of recommended adult populations, U.S., 1989–2005. *Vaccine.* Mar 2008;26(14):1786–1793.

115. Friedman SR, Cooper HL, Osborne AH. Structural and social contexts of HIV risk Among African Americans. *Am J Public Health.* Jun 2009;99(6):1002–1008.

116. Centers for Disease Control and Prevention. Vital signs: breast cancer screening among women aged 50–74 years—United States, 2008. *Morb Mortal Wkly Rep.* 2010;59(26):813–818.

117. Gomez S, Quach T, Horn-Ross P, et al. Hidden breast cancer disparities in Asian women: disaggregating incidence rates by ethnicity and migrant status. *Am J Public Health.* Apr 2010;100(Suppl 1):S125–S131.

118. Krieger N, Chen J, Waterman P, Rehkopf D, Yin R, Coull B. Race/ethnicity and changing US socioeconomic gradients in breast cancer incidence: California and Massachusetts, 1978–2002 (United States). *Cancer Causes Control.* Mar 2006;17(2): 217–226.

119. Sassi F, Luft H, Guadagnoli E. Reducing racial/ethnic disparities in female breast cancer: screening rates and stage at diagnosis. *Am J Public Health.* Dec 2006;96(12): 2165–2172.

120. Blackman D, Masi C. Racial and ethnic disparities in breast cancer mortality: are we doing enough to address the root causes? *J Clin Oncol.* May 2006;24(14): 2170–2178.

121. Breen N, A Cronin K, Meissner H, et al. Reported drop in mammography: is this cause for concern? *Cancer.* Jun 2007;109(12):2405–2409.

122. Dzewaltowski D, Estabrooks P, Glasgow R. The future of physical activity behavior change research: what is needed to improve translation of research into health promotion practice? *Exerc Sport Sci Rev.* Apr 2004;32(2):57–63.

23 Considering the Multiple Service Contexts in Cultural Adaptations of Evidence-Based Practice

■ LUIS H. ZAYAS,
JENNIFER L. BELLAMY,
AND ENOLA K. PROCTOR

■ INTRODUCTION

During the past decade and a half, increasing attention has been given to adapting empirically supported interventions for use with ethnic, cultural, and racial minority groups who were not part of the original intervention development process. The work of adapting has been intended to make interventions responsive and resonant to underrepresented groups, reflecting their cultural norms, values, beliefs, and parent practices (see Chapter 22). Among adaptation specialists, it has become axiomatic that the more attention given to the cultural adaptation of extant and new empirically supported treatments (ESTs), the closer interventions will approximate the characteristics of clients to be served.[1,2] Cultural adaptations of evidence-based interventions must be included as part of the dissemination and implementation process. The National Institutes of Health's Program Announcement on Dissemination and Implementation Research in Health (PAR-10–038) calls for research on adapting existing practices to optimize their benefits.

■ EVIDENCE BASE AND THEORY

This chapter argues that one of the shortcomings in the cultural adaptation literature is the inattention to the multiple service contexts that influence the implementation of interventions, and the critical features that enhance the uptake of interventions and services: availability, accessibility, accommodation, affordability, and acceptability.[3] The mismatch between interventions and the realities of service contexts is an oft-cited reason for the limited use of ESTs in practice. The literature on cultural adaptation indicates that shaping interventions to the needs of cultural groups increases their impact. This chapter addresses this issue, using parenting intervention with Hispanic families as a case in point.

We argue that contextual and cultural adaptations cannot be considered in isolation. As the implementation of ESTs move out of the controlled environment of clinical trials and are applied in multiple service contexts, the features of service settings must also be addressed (NIH PA 10–038). An integrated approach, which includes the careful consideration of both the service context as well as the cultural diversity represented among families and children, is essential to success-ful intervention adaptation. The multiple contexts that must be considered include the service sectors that segregate social problems and needs into categories (e.g., child welfare, education, juvenile justice, medical), the regional and geographic contexts (e.g., urban, rural, remote/isolated), and the organizations and institutions that deliver the services (e.g., agencies, hospital, clinics, health centers).

Although efficacious parenting interventions continue to be developed and rigorously tested, adding to the supply of ESTs,[4,5] the failure to implement those evidence-based interventions remains a widely recognized problem.[6,7] Much of the literature on cultural adaptation organizes its arguments around the acknowledg-ment and integration of the values, beliefs, norms, and associated behavioral prac-tices of specific ethnic, racial, and cultural groups. The implicit assumption is that culturally adapting the intervention or service completes the process. However, there are larger contextual factors, in addition to sociocultural factors, that must be considered in the adaptation process such as the different service contexts in which interventions are implemented and the multiple types of modifications required at different levels of the service delivery and implementation chain. In each con-text, cultural adaptations must be differently conceptualized and operationalized. Indeed, adaptation is required across service contexts that serve culturally similar clients. ESTs are commonly developed with a target population in mind, and just as often within a particular, and usually narrowly defined, service context. Moving interventions to other populations and settings will often require alterations. For example, Parent–Child Interaction Therapy (PCIT) was developed to treat "dis-ruptive behaviors of Caucasian preschoolers"[8(p.199)] and needs to be adapted for use with different populations.

An EST,s efficacy comes from its design for and use with a specific population (e.g., age or ethnocultural group) and a specific problem (e.g., disruptive pre-schoolers; older children with conduct disorders).[9] When ESTs are adapted to the characteristics and needs of diverse sociocultural groups, they often retain their effectiveness.[10] Although empirical studies directly testing adapted ESTs against standard ESTs are limited in number, adapted ESTs may be more effective with particular sociocultural groups than nonadapted treatments would be. For exam-ple, one study of a cultural adaptation to Cognitive Behavioral Therapy (CBT) found that adapting CBT to include case management services and culturally tailored services for Spanish-speaking patients (including bilingual/bicultural providers, materials in Spanish, and allowing warmer and more personalized interactions) resulted in better functioning for Latino patients than CBT alone.[11] There is also agreement among intervention developers and adaptation special-ists that any implementation must keep intact the core or active ingredients, that is, those aspects of the EST that constitute the mechanisms by which the intervention effects change in people.[8,12,13]

However, it is not enough to assume that an EST that is relevant to diverse populations and communities can be implemented equally well across service set-tings. There are many considerations to be made: we must deal with organizational and client cultures, the capacity of communities and organizations to adapt and implement ESTs, and the policy environment. The potency of the service setting's effects on client participation, whether the service is willingly sought by clients or mandated on them by a court or other external authority, cannot be overlooked. Therefore, it is important to distinguish between the *culture of the client* (i.e., the social norms, beliefs, and values that guide the client's worldview and lifeways) and the *culture of the agency* (i.e., the orientation that the organization operates in when it comes to selecting, delivering, and evaluating the effectiveness of its services).[14] Both types of culture must be considered in adapting treatments in order to increase the success of their implementation. Three algorithms are possible: (1) to adapt for reasons associated with the clients' culture or cultures, (2) to adapt the intervention according to the different service settings, or (3) to adapt interventions when both conditions of client culture and organizational culture and structure call for it. These hypothetical considerations can be empirically tested through research.

Efforts to implement adapted treatments must also consider the capacity needed to select and deliver ESTs and other evidence-based services.[14,15] Capacity refers to those factors that increase implementation success and is comprised of three levels. First, a community's capacity to deliver ESTs is related to the community's awareness of the problem, how it defines the problem, its readiness to address problems, and the resources, social capital, and community leadership that the community can mobilize for service implementation. Second, capacity at the organizational level speaks to an agency's leadership, vision, commitment, size, and structure. No amount of community capacity and readiness can be easily harnessed without the presence, will, and expertise of service organizations in its midst. Third, individual-level capacity refers to the attitudes of the providers (and the agency hierarchy), their skills and knowledge of the selected ESTs, and their motivation to adapt and implement them. It is often the case that organizations hire well-trained staff, but they may lack capacities to serve specific client populations. This is often the case in long-standing agencies whose client communities change over time, with new emerging populations bringing unique consideration and needs. Each of these capacity levels affects the adaptation and implementation process.

Another contextual perspective on implementation is the "policy ecology," that is, the importance of taking into account the effects of policy action across the many contexts and levels in which interventions and services are delivered so as to achieve widespread and sustained uptake of evidence-based systems.[16] There is the policy ecology of the organization rendering the service, the policy ecology at the payer and regulatory level, and the policy ecology at the political level. The influences of these policy ecologies can range from dramatic (e.g., sudden funding and legal changes, organizational redirection) to gradually and nearly imperceptible (e.g., erosion of funding opportunities or support and confidence of funders and regulators).

Failure to address the capacity and contextual issues in service delivery systems may undermine—or invalidate—the effectiveness of ESTs, even when they have been thoughtfully and appropriately culturally adapted for particular client groups. Without adequate attention to the contextual levels of real-world service delivery systems, the result may be an unwitting undermining of what researchers and providers are trying to achieve through adaptation, possibly invalidating the interventions. Dissemination and implementation will be enhanced by a more systematic and contextually inclusive view of adaptation, just as consideration of client cultural factors in treatment will benefit from a broader consideration of dissemination and implementation. The field needs more, not less, guidance about how to implement culturally adapted interventions into the multifaceted ecological contexts of community practice.[17,18] In the case study that follows, the many contextual levels for adaptation using parenting and family interventions and their adaptation for Hispanic families are illustrated.

■ CASE STUDY: ETHNIC AND CULTURAL ADAPTATION IN PARENTING INTERVENTIONS

Background

Cultural and ethnic minority psychology has the distinction of being arguably the field in which conceptualizations and model building for adapting interventions originated and have continued to the present. Early on, arguments were made that traditional treatments could be made accessible to Hispanic groups by modifying these treatments through the identification, extraction, and integration of cultural features from the target culture.[19] Available therapies and services could also be selected for use according to their proximity to the culture of the ethnocultural minority group. These two approaches are still the most viable approaches to implementing ESTs for Hispanic and other cultural and ethnic minority families. Alternatively, treatments could also be created based on the culture of the group, an approach that reflected an expensive, labor-intensive approach with limited generalizability, although possibly very successful.[20] (There are also recent developments in "community-derived evidence," often programs develop indigenously by practitioners and community groups.) Since those seminal works, the adaptation literature on Hispanic groups has focused on cultural features for recommending adaptations.[21] The field still needs to develop models and methods to empirically isolate a client group's cultural features before adapting interventions.

Context

Within the parent and family intervention field, there is some research that shows that more specificity in terms of the impact of particular cultural features on the intervention process is required. For example, a review of 21 parenting interventions for Hispanic families shows that most studies identified one or more pan-Hispanic values but offered no citations or other information "to substantiate the validity of these values."[22(p.215)] Similarly, others have generated lists of potential modifications to a parenting intervention for Mexican parents without extending it to a methodological approach.[23] There is no "gold standard," empirically tested, methodological model to guide cultural adaptation. Moreover, the modifications range from rather modest ones (e.g., increasing the number of fathers recruited by using testimonials from fathers who participated in the training) to bolder ones (e.g., reframing parenting behaviors). It seems likely that a variety of methods are needed in order to address the varied extent and nature of adaptations—to move them from drawing on impressionistic data to empirically derived results.[2,13,24]

Targeting and tailoring parenting and family interventions to Hispanic clients' unique cultural features and circumstances will certainly enhance the appeal, accessibility, and acceptability of interventions while leaving intact the core elements (active ingredients) of the interventions. However, when adaptation occurs there is an inherent tension that emerges between fidelity to the intervention and the fit to the cultural group, a dynamic tension that must be balanced.[25] Multiple stakeholders have an interest in adaptation research and practice. From the individual client who is seeking services that fit with personal needs, preferences, and circumstances to the policymakers who seek to fund, mandate, and monitor the use of cost-effective treatments, stakeholders are found at every contextual level: clients, providers, agencies, treatment developers, policymakers, and funders. A parent management intervention can be adapted, for instance, by keeping many of the core elements of the treatment while tailoring and creating some components to reflect the culturally and community-relevant experiences of the target families.[26,27,28]

However, some writers question whether a community-specific adaptation erodes the effectiveness of the intervention.[29] One answer to this critique is that deriving scientific evidence about the adaptation helps in *selectively* identifying the specific problems of given communities that should drive the cultural adaptation of the treatment.[30] The selection argument urges that the cultural adaptations of interventions should not be decided or based on surface characteristics such as ethnicity (i.e., making one cultural adaptation for all Hispanic subgroups), but rather on contextually driven data (e.g., populations and communities with identifiable problems where an intervention has not been favorable). It is not enough to attend to culture and community alone in the intervention adaptation and implementation process. In addition, the specific organizational or service setting must also be considered. This perspective then changes the question of, "Does the intervention work in the real world?"[31] to "How does the intervention work in the real world of different cultural contexts and diverse service settings?"

A balance between community needs and scientific integrity can be achieved through the participation of three key stakeholders: researchers, community opinion leaders, and members of the target community. Each stakeholder represents a particular perspective that permits achieving a common understanding about the community's needs and what it can reasonably accept and integrate, allowing the intervention to be taken to scale and tested in other contexts. Thus, adaptation, targeting, and tailoring are informed by the input of multiple stakeholders. This technology transfer to agencies and providers serving ethnic minorities incorporates the service context in which ESTs will be implemented, and also encompasses provider characteristics and organizational structures that impede or facilitate the adoption of the interventions.[32]

■ DESIGNING FOR IMPLEMENTATION: A MODEL FOR CULTURAL ADAPTATION

Cultural adaptations are necessary, but they are not sufficient for reducing the social and health disparities that are mostly visited on disadvantaged ethnic and cultural minorities. Adaptation must occur within the many contextual levels that influence the ultimate delivery of the service to the client. Figure 23–1 depicts the levels of service delivery contexts and includes the issues of policy ecology, levels of capacity, and organizational and client cultures. The flow from left to right in the figure represents the directionality of influences. (Feedback in the figure would move from right to left, that is, from clients to providers and programs; from providers and programs to organizations; and organizations to sectors of service; and so on. To avoid visual clutter in the model, feedback arrows are omitted, but they should be assumed to be operating.)

It is helpful to define how the terms *adaptation, targeting,* and *tailoring* are used in this chapter to organize the discussion and map onto the conceptual framework. *Adaptation* represents the broadest term used to describe adjustments and modifications made to interventions. Adaptation occurs naturally as interventions are adopted and implemented into real-world contexts without necessarily changing the intervention's internal logic or *core elements*.[33,34,35] At one level of adaptation, the adjustments that are made to ESTs are called *targeting.* Here changes are made to interventions and services at the group- or population- rather than individual level. Targeting involves the adaptation of an intervention or service for a defined subpopulation subgroup that takes into account characteristics shared by the subgroup's members,[36] for example, adapting parenting interventions for Mexican parents or adapting substance abuse programs for women. These adapted interventions could presumably be subsequently targeted to other communities and subpopulations (e.g., incarcerated youth with substance abuse disorders, adolescent mothers in a maltreatment prevention program). Adaptation and targeting may also be conceptualized at the organizational level as adaptations conducted to meet the specific needs and conditions of a given setting of care.[35] For example, when an organization adopts an intervention developed in another setting, adaptations are generally necessary so that the intervention can be implemented to the peculiarities of a specific service organization. These peculiarities might include billing procedures, staffing, or other organizational characteristics that, as a whole, impact the procedures related to the EST.

Tailoring, by contrast, refers to adaptation that is intended to address variation at an individual level. It is defined as changes in the focus or style of delivery of an established treatment that is based on adjustments made to interventions to reflect the unique features of individual cases, where cases can be an individual, family, or small group.[8,23] Tailoring for individuals is distinct from targeting in that adaptations of this nature are not meant to adapt interventions for a subgroup identified by common characteristics but are, rather, responsive to the unique constellation of needs of that individual, in effect "personalizing" their care. This view of tailoring is defined as "any combination of information or change strategies intended to reach one specific person, based on characteristics that are unique

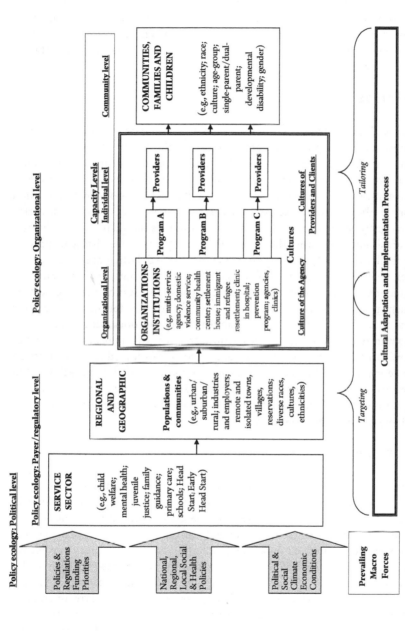

Figure 23–1. Conceptual pathways to implementation and sources of influence: cultural adaptation, targeting and tailoring from sector of care to provider and recipients of care.

to that person, related to the outcome of interest, and have been derived from an individual assessment."[36(p.1)] It is at this level that clinical judgment is most evident in the delivery of the intervention. Clinicians regularly engage in tailoring where clinical judgment, experience, and knowledge join to make adjustments to treatments based on individual characteristics, which can be referred to as *clinical tailoring*. These conceptual distinctions provide a lens for viewing the adaptation process across multiple service contexts.

Macro Forces

The broadest, least controllable level of influence on contexts and the implementation process are broad, prevailing, political, economic, social, and historic macro forces that are typically beyond any institution's or groups of institutions' abilities to control or influence. Thus, for example, an economic recession that affects governmental revenues and corporate profits will affect decisions by funding and regulatory bodies. Other cataclysmic natural disasters (e.g., hurricanes, earthquakes, oil spills) spur major changes in, say, how homes should be built or disaster services are aligned. But from these natural events, families are displaced, parents severely challenged, and parenting quality compromised. Different service sectors must then meet the needs of these families, such as in schools, mental health and family guidance services, and child welfare. An austere fiscal climate dictated by government policies and economic conditions affect deeply, for instance, funding levels that dictate how much adaptation can realistically be done with available staff resources and training, or whether residential treatment (versus day programs or outpatient care) can continue to be an option for localities. In short, adaptation is not done merely along cultural lines, without contextualizing the real world in which services or interventions will be applied. These shifting influences necessitate adaptations that are often as difficult to foresee as they are to control; therefore, their influence must be acknowledged.

Sectors of Care

At the overarching level of service system context stands the *service sector* in which interventions are delivered for specific groups of people with social problems or needs (e.g., child welfare, primary care, juvenile justice, preventive services, community mental health, drug rehabilitation, education). These sectors of care represent "industries" dedicated to combating specific human social and health problems. A sector's mandate is based on the social problem it is dedicated to, such as, for example, child welfare, which encompasses many different aspects from protective and preventive services to foster and adoptive care, residential treatment, and others. Notable, too, is that sectors can overlap, say, in circumstances in which child welfare may provide residential care that is intended for youth with severe mental illness. Sectors of care are typically represented by many organizations, regional and local, with a variety of funders and regulators. The unique collection of regulators and payers influence services, type of providers delivering services, and other important elements of interventions that may or may not impact the treatment effectiveness.[6,16] Each sector then considers adaptations of ESTs to match its social mission and service array, often in response to legislative, economic, and regulatory policy mandates.

Regional and Geographic Contexts: Population and Communities

At the next level of contextualization are *regional* or *geographic* variations, such as demographic and population groups, local policies, regulatory jurisdictions, and local and regional funding sources. Communities and their populations tend to determine what is needed. Therefore, rural communities will have distinct needs from those that are urban; Appalachian families will need a different set of services, or at least different service delivery modes than, say, an isolated and remote American Indian community. Adaptation efforts at this level *target* subgroups identified by the intersection of racial or ethnic group membership and urbanicity. Alternatively, in a single community, it may be necessary to adjust existing youth programs that reduce their risk for criminality and drug use through introduction of vocational skills development adapted to the peculiar landscape of community employment opportunities.

Geographic dispersal results in specific service contexts, organizations, and institutions that can range from chronic or long-term institutionalization, to short-term residential care, to day programs, to outpatient programs and home-based services. Interventions may likewise be targeted to each of these service contexts, or tailored to meet the needs of a single entity. For example, an intervention developed for use in primary care may be adapted for use in a nonspecialty service setting, such as a youth development agency. Note that targeting is used as the adaptation at this level of service context.

Service Organizations and Institutions

Service organizations and institutions are typically locally or regionally licensed institutions within one or more care sectors that deliver interventions and services to regional and demographic communities. These institutions often have multiple sites in the geographic area to which clients come (e.g., community health center, after-school drop-in center) or from which they are served (e.g., visiting nurse services, in-home prevention programs), or both. One agency providing services to different communities in rural, urban, and suburban areas requires that it marshal the selection of services and interventions—and the targeting of interventions—in order to reflect each community's needs.

Programs and Providers: "Where the Rubber Meets the Road"

Within agencies and clinics are *programs* that deliver the interventions and services and are staffed by *providers*. At this level, tailoring is possible since program and clinicians are often more intimately acquainted with the clientele, local community, referring sources, and service networks than other levels of the organization or regulators. Often within service settings, multiple programs operate under one agency umbrella, sometimes within the same building and sometimes across sites. Such programs may target different subpopulations of their communities. Thus, for example, a multiservice agency may have a prevention program for children and parents, one for adolescent parenting, a mental health clinic, and after-school program. Each of these programs may need to conduct the same or similar interventions, requiring tailoring to its specific population and program objectives. The implementation process at this level also includes the consideration of what was done to make the climate or culture of the program or organization ready and receptive to use of the EST.[17,37] Indeed, this issue spans the levels of organization and programs.

Often omitted in the calculus for culturally adapting and implementing the intervention is such essential information as the type of agency and organization sponsoring the adaptation, the programs in which the culturally adapted intervention is lodged, and the programs and providers who ultimately apply evidence-based practices to their clients. At this point program administrators and clinical staff have to give balanced attention to the service context that includes, as examples, the makeup of the client population, local geography and neighborhood, and the agency's capacity to deliver evidence-based service.[32] In addition, there are considerations of providers' characteristics and their collective knowledge of the service populations. Take, for example, an urban free clinic (primary care) staffed by volunteer physicians, dentists, mental health professionals, and some paid paraprofessionals that is adapting evidence-based trauma services for undocumented Latin American immigrants. The free clinic must consider budget constraints, service limitations, and episodic help seeking by its clients in targeting and tailoring the intervention. Adaptation and implementation processes in this context contrast vastly from a large, well-funded preventive service agency (e.g., child welfare) with a cadre of veteran service professionals adapting the same evidence-based trauma service to abused children in foster care.

Each of the levels just outlined incorporates three critical elements: structural elements (e.g., sectors of care need sufficient number of institutions to address major social problems in their regions; agencies determine the number of trained clinicians), procedural elements (e.g., agencies and their programs seek to improve clinicians' practice), and outcomes (e.g., client engagement, retention, and improvements; efficient, cost-effective agency and provider activities).[16]

■ RESEARCH GAPS AND FUTURE DIRECTIONS

The growth in the field of cultural adaptation has proceeded despite a lingering question as to whether interventions can be sufficiently effective without adaptation for cultural groups. There is evidence to suggest that cultural adaptation has a beneficial impact ranging from moderate to strong effects.[10] Interventions delivered in the clients' native language can be more effective than those in the nonnative language, and interventions targeted at a specific cultural group can show higher effectiveness than when delivered to a group made up of varied cultural backgrounds. Scientific exploration and experimentation must proceed in order to advance the state of intervention science and reduce the disparities in care that have been widely documented. Adapting and testing ESTs in both traditional and nontraditional delivery settings can enhance their accessibility and uptake in communities with underserved special populations while maintaining the critical ingredients of care.[12]

This chapter has argued that adapting and publishing results, without regard to the sector of care, service delivery institutions, its programs, and providers falls short in guiding clinicians and researchers. One recommendation for reporting on adaptations of ESTs in professional journals is to identify and describe the service context, thereby giving readers a more nuanced contextual understanding of the process of adaptation. As pointed out in this chapter, knowing the sector of care, the nature of the institution in which the effectiveness of the adaptation was tested, the nature of the adaptation level (e.g., targeting and tailoring), and the characteristics of programs and providers makes clear something about the generalizability of the adaptation and its utility to others in similar or dissimilar situations. At each level—sector, community, institution, program, and provider—adapting interventions and services makes them more accessible, acceptable, responsive, and available to stakeholders.

The added benefit of considering and reporting each level of the implementation context is that, with more experience in adapting and testing of interventions across different groups and settings, it will become increasingly possible to generate conceptual and methodological approaches for adaptation to guide the field. Thus, effective interventions can be made increasingly available across these very same contexts and groups of service recipients. The argument is, in short, that when considering adaptations and targeting or tailoring of interventions and services for multiethnic client populations, much more than cultural factors has to be considered. While culture undoubtedly guides the adaptation, other contexts dictate in many ways how adaptations occur. The perspective taken in this chapter requires that providers be aware of prevailing macro, service sector, regional, and organizational trends, resources, and constraints and become proficient in adapting interventions accordingly in their clinical work with clients.

SUGGESTED READINGS

Bernal G, Bonilla J, Bellido C. Ecological validity and cultural sensitivity for outcome research: Issues for the cultural adaptation and development of psychosocial treatments with Hispanics. *J Abnorm Child Psychol*.1995;23(1):67–82.

The authors present a culturally sensitive perspective so as to enhance the ecological validity of treatment research. After reviewing the relationships among external validity, ecological validity, and culturally sensitive research, the authors present a framework that consists of eight dimensions of treatment interventions (language, persons, metaphors, content, concepts, goals, methods, and context). Following these dimensions can guide the adaptation and development of culturally sensitive treatments for specific ethnic minority groups.

Mendel P, Meredith L, Schoenbaum M, Sherbourne C, Wells, K. Interventions in organizational and community context: A framework for building evidence on dissemination and implementation in health services research. *Adm Policy Ment Health*. 2008;35:21–37.

This paper presents a framework developed by the UCLA/RAND NIMH Center to (1) provide a theoretically grounded understanding of the multilayered nature of community and health care contexts and the mechanisms by which new practices and programs diffuse within these settings; (2) distinguish among key components of the diffusion process— including contextual factors, adoption, implementation, and sustainment of interventions; (3) facilitate the identification of new strategies for adapting, disseminating, and implementing relatively complex, evidence-based health care and improvement interventions; and (4) enhance the ability to meaningfully generalize findings across varied interventions and settings to build an evidence base on successful dissemination and implementation strategies.

Guerra N, Knox L. How culture impacts the dissemination and implementation of innovation: A case study of the Families and Schools Together Program (FAST). *Amer J Community Psychol.* 2008;41(3–4):304–313.

> *This paper focuses on the culture of the client and the culture of the agency implementing selected programs in communities with ethnic and cultural minority groups. The authors look at the impact of cultural characteristics on the translation into practice at the community level, relying on an interactive systems framework.*

Lau A. Making the case for selective and directed cultural adaptations of evidence-based treatments: Examples from parent training. *Clin Psychol Sci Pr.* 2006;13(4):295–310.

> *Our concern with the generalizability of evidence-based treatments (EBTs) in real-world practice settings has also increased our attention to cultural adaptations of treatments to ensure fit. But most EBTs have not been disseminated or evaluated with minority populations. Lau discusses a framework (a) for identifying instances where cultural adaptation of EBTs may be most indicated, and (b) for using research to direct the development of treatment adaptations to ensure community engagement and the contextual relevance of treatment content.*

Harshbarger, C., Simmons, G., Coelho, H., Sloop, K., Collins, C. An empirical assessment of implementation, adaptation, and tailoring: the evaluations of the CDC's national diffusion of VOICES/VOCES. *AIDS Educ Prev.* 2006;18(Suppl A):184–197.

> *Based on the Centers for Disease Control and Prevention's Diffusion of Effective Behavioral Interventions (DEBI) program, 260 agencies were trained on VOICES/VOCES. In this report, the authors discuss diffusion, adoption, adaptation, and implementation, and needs for ongoing proactive technical assistance. While most agencies implemented VOICES/ VOCES with fidelity to the core elements and some agencies successfully adapted the intervention to make it more appealing to target populations, TA was needed for interventions to be successfully adapted and implemented with fidelity to the core elements, and to ensure program sustainability.*

Kreuter M, Skinner C. Tailoring, what's in a name? *Health Educ Res.* 2000;15:1–4.

> *Based on work with Hispanic women in San Francisco to raise the level of breast and cervical cancer screening, the authors carefully delineate the distinctions among adapting, tailoring, and targeting.*

SELECTED WEBSITES AND TOOLS

Parent–Child Interaction Therapy. http://pcit.phhp.ufl.edu/ provides information on PCIT.

Parent management training. http://www.oslc.org/projects/projects.html. *The Oregon Social Learning Center has numerous projects testing the effectiveness of parent management training. One example is The Kids in Transition to School—Early Childhood Special Education Program is a randomized efficacy trial of a preventive intervention to enhance psychosocial and academic school readiness in children with developmental disabilities and behavior or social difficulties who are entering kindergarten. Others include older and younger populations and ethnic and racial minority families.*

The Incredible Years curriculum. http://www.incredibleyears.com/About/about.asp. *This website is dedicated to the Incredible Years curriculum that includes training programs, intervention manuals, and instructional DVDs for use by trained therapists, teachers, and group leaders. The program promotes children's social competence, emotional regulation, and problem solving skills and reduces their behavior problems by focusing on helping parents and teachers provide young children (0–12 years) with a strong emotional, social, and academic foundation. The program is intended to reduce development of depression, school dropout, violence, drug abuse, and delinquency in later years.*

■ REFERENCES

1. Bernal G, Bonilla J, Bellido C. Ecological validity and cultural sensitivity for outcome research: Issues for the cultural adaptation and development of psychosocial treatments with Hispanics. *J Abnorm Child Psychol.*1995;23(1):67–82.
2. Borrego J. Introduction to special series: Culturally responsive cognitive and behavioral practice with Latino families. *Cogn Behav Pract.* 2010;17:154–156.
3. Penchansky R, Thomas J. The concept of access: Definition and relationship to consumer satisfaction. *Med Care.* 1981;19:127–140.
4. McCue Horwitz S, Chamberlain P, Landsverk J, Mullican C. Improving the mental health of children in child welfare through the implementation of evidence-based parenting interventions. *Adm Policy Ment Health.* 2010;37:27–39.
5. Wyatt G, Kaminski J, Valle L, Filene J, Boyle C. A meta-analytic review of components associated with parent training program effectiveness. *J Abnorm Child Psychol.* 2008;35:567–589.
6. Mendel P, Meredith L, Schoenbaum M, Sherbourne C, Wells, K. Interventions in organizational and community context: A framework for building evidence on dissemination and implementation in health services research. *Adm Policy Ment Health.* 2008;35:21–37.
7. Proctor E, Landsverk J, Aarons G, Chambers D, Glisson C, Mittman B. Implementation research in mental health services: An emerging science with conceptual, methodological, and training challenges. *Adm Policy Ment Health.* 2009;36:24–34.
8. Eyberg S. Tailoring and adapting Parent-Child Interaction Therapy to new populations. *Education Treatment of Children.* 2005;28(2):197–201.
9. Chambless D, Hollon S. Defining empirically supported therapies. *J Consult Clin Psychol.*1998;66(1):7–18.
10. Griner D, Smith T. Culturally adapted mental health interventions: A meta-analytic review. *Psychother Theor Res.* 2006;43(4):531–548.
11. Miranda J, Azocar F, Organista K, Dwyer E, Arean P. Treatment of depression among impoverished primary care patients from ethnic minority groups. *Psychiatr Serv.* 2003;54(2):219–225.
12. Miranda J, Bernal G, Lau A, Kohn L, Hwang W, La Fromboise T. State of the science on psychosocial interventions for ethnic minorities. *Annu Rev Clin Psychol.* 2005;1(1):113–142.
13. Zayas LH. Seeking models and methods for cultural adaptation of interventions: Commentary on the special section. *Cogn Behav Pract.* 2010;17:198–202.
14. Guerra N, Knox L. How culture impacts the dissemination and implementation of innovation: A case study of the Families and Schools Together Program (FAST). *Amer J Community Psychol.* 2008;41(3–4):304–313.

15. Wandersman A, Duffy J, Flaspohler P, et al. Bridging the gap between prevention science and practice: The interactive systems framework for dissemination and implementation. *Amer J Community Psychol.* June 2008;41(3–4):171–181.

16. Raghavan R, Bright C, Shadoin A. Toward a policy ecology of implementation of evidence-based practices in public mental health settings. *Implement Sci.* 2008 May 16;3:26.

17. Glisson C, Schoenwald S. The ARC organizational and community intervention strategy for implementing evidence-based children's mental health treatments. *Ment Health Serv Res.* 2005;7(4):243–259.

18. Rabin B, Brownson R, Haire-Joshu D, Kreuter M, Weaver N. A glossary for dissemination and implementation research in health. *J Public Health Manag Pract.* 2008;14: 117–123.

19. Rogler L, Malgady R, Constantino G, Blumenthal R. What do culturally sensitive mental health services mean? The case of Hispanics. *Am Psychol.* 1987;42(6):565–570.

20. Costantino G, Malgady R. Culturally sensitive treatment: Cuento and hero/heroine modeling therapies for Hispanic children and adolescents. *Psychosocial Treatments for Children and Adolescent Disorders: Empirically Based Strategies for Clinical Practice.* Washington, DC: American Psychological Association; 1996:639–669.

21. Barker C, Cook K, Borrego J. Addressing cultural variables in parent training programs with Latino families. *Cogn Behav Pract.* 2010;17:157–166.

22. Dumka L, Lopez V, Carter S. Parenting interventions adapted for Hispanic families: Progress and prospects. *Latino Children and Families in the United States: Current Research and Future Directions.* Westport, CT: Praeger Publishers/Greenwood Publishing Group; 2002:203–231.

23. McCabe K, Yeh M, Garland A, Lau A, Chavez G. The GANA program: A tailoring approach to adapting parent child interaction therapy for Mexican Americans. *Education Treatment of Children.* 2005;28(2):111–129.

24. Calzada EJ. Bringing culture into parent training with Latinos. *Cogn Behav Pract.* 2010;17:167–175.

25. Castro F, Barrera M, Martinez C. The cultural adaptation of prevention interventions: Resolving tensions between fidelity and fit. *Prev Sci.* 2004;5(1):41–45.

26. Martinez C, Eddy M. Effects of culturally adapted parent management training on Hispanic youth behavioral health outcomes. *J Consult Clin Psychol.* 2005;73(5): 841–851.

27. Harachi TW, Catalano RF, Hawkins JD. Effective recruitment for parenting programs within ethnic minority communities. *Child Adolesc Soc Work J.* 1997;14(1):23–39.

28. Kumpfer K, Alvarado R, Smith P, Bellamy N. Cultural sensitivity and adaptation in family-based prevention interventions. *Prev Sci.* 2002;3(3):241–246.

29. Elliott D, Mihalic S. Issues in disseminating and replicating effective prevention programs. *Prev Sci.* 2004;5(1):47–52.

30. Lau A. Making the case for selective and directed cultural adaptations of evidence-based treatments: Examples from parent training. *Clin Psychol Sci Pr.* 2006;13(4):295–310.

31. Domenech-Rodriguez M, Wieling E. Developing culturally appropriate, evidence-based treatments for interventions with ethnic minority populations. *Voices of Color: First-Person Accounts of Ethnic Minority Therapists.* Thousand Oaks, CA: Sage; 2004:313–33.

32. Santisteban D, Vega R., Suarez-Morales L. Utilizing dissemination findings to help understand and bridge the research and practice gap in the treatment of substance abuse disorders in Hispanic populations. *Drug Alcohol Depend.* 2006;84(Suppl 1): S94–S101.

33. Rogers EM. (1995). *Diffusion of Innovations.* (4th ed.). New York: The Free Press; 1995.

34. Eyberg S, Graham-Pole J. Mindfulness and behavioral parent training: Commentary. *J Clin Child Adol Psychol.* 2005;34(4):792–794.

35. Harshbarger C, Simmons G, Coelho H, Sloop K, Collins C. An empirical assessment of implementation, adaptation, and tailoring: the evaluations of the CDC's national diffusion of VOICES/VOCES. *AIDS Educ Prev.* 2006;18(Suppl A):184–197.

36. Kreuter M, Skinner C. Tailoring, what's in a name? *Health Educ Res.* 2000;15:1–4.

37. Zayas LH, Borrego J, Domenech Rodríguez M. (2009). Parenting interventions for Latino families and children. *Handbook of Latino Psychology: Developmental and Community Based Perspectives.* Los Angeles: Sage; 2009:291–307

24 The Path Forward in Dissemination and Implementation Research

■ ROSS C. BROWNSON,
MARIAH DREISINGER,
GRAHAM A. COLDITZ,
AND ENOLA K. PROCTOR

■ INTRODUCTION

Two converging bodies of knowledge hold promise for bridging the gap between discovery of new research findings and application in public health and health care settings. First, the concept of evidence-based practice (in medicine, public health, and other related disciplines) is growing in prominence due in part to a larger body of intervention research on what works to improve patient care or population health (e.g., the Clinical Guide[1] or Community Guide[2] recommendations on effective interventions).[3,4] Second, effective methods of dissemination and implementation (D&I) are needed to put evidence to work in "real-world" settings.

Particularly related to this second point, this book provides a foundation in and strives to catalyze further knowledge development in the nascent science of D&I research. While we continue to accumulate an evidence base on how to improve population health and patient care, knowledge about how to apply and evaluate the evidence is lacking for many settings and populations. This large gap can be filled by a growing investment in and lessons learned from D&I research, which elucidates the processes and factors that lead to widespread use of an evidence-based intervention by a particular population (e.g., youth, ethnic minorities) or within a certain setting (e.g., worksite, school).[5] This research has begun to identify a number of important factors that enhance the uptake of evidence-based interventions in both practice (e.g., a primary care clinic) and policy (e.g., a state legislature) settings.

In this chapter, we highlight several research topics that we believe are the most pressing areas for future inquiry. In large part, our list was developed from the recommendations contained within the previous 23 chapters. The issues covered are not meant to be exhaustive; rather, we seek to identify the most promising areas that will move D&I science forward most quickly given the current state of the research and funding opportunities.

■ TERMINOLOGY AND THEORY

Developing the Terminology

For any field of scientific inquiry to thrive, consistent terminology is needed. Because D&I research in the health field has emerged from research traditions in diverse disciplines ranging from agriculture to education, there are numerous inconsistencies in the use and meaning of terms and main concepts.[5] While Chapter 2 presents what we believe is a reasonable current snapshot of terminology for D&I research, further work is needed to standardize the terminology and to include more concepts from outside of health (e.g., D&I terms from business or organizational psychology). A particular concern is that the term "translation" is now being used for everything from cellular and molecular research to global health.[6]

Making Use of Theory and Frameworks

Theories and models explain behavior and suggest ways to achieve behavior change. A theory is a set of interrelated concepts that present a systematic view of events by specifying relations among variables in order to explain and predict events.[7] As illustrated in this book, D&I research can be enhanced by the use of theory, systematic-planning frameworks, and logic models. The most common theories in D&I research are Diffusion of Innovations, persuasive communication, and social marketing.[8] Future research is needed to better understand which theories are best suited for various settings (schools, worksites, communities) and levels (policy, organizational change) and how theories might need to be adapted for D&I research on health disparities.

The most common frameworks for D&I planning and evaluation have been PRECEDE-PROCEED (an acronym for: Predisposing, Reinforcing, and Enabling Constructs in Educational/environmental Diagnosis and Evaluation, with its implementation phase: Policy, Regulatory and Organizational Constructs in Educational and Environmental Development)[9] and RE-AIM (an acronym for: Reach, Effectiveness, Adoption, Implementation, and Maintenance).[10] But several new models and attempts at integrating different models are receiving increased attention.[11,12] Described in detail in Chapter 16, the earliest uses of RE-AIM focused on individualized behavioral interventions (e.g., a primary care intervention to improve diabetes management). An area deserving more research involves recent attempts to apply frameworks like RE-AIM to population-level interventions such as policy dissemination and environmental change research.[13] Individual chapters should spark the development and testing of further frameworks and models, as needed, to lay out the complex array of factors required for successful dissemination of information and implementation of evidence-based programs in specific health care and public health settings.

■ METHODS AND MEASUREMENT

Developing New and Improved Measures

A public health and quality improvement adage is "what gets measured, gets done."[14] Successful progress of D&I science will require the development of practical measures of outcomes that are both reliable and valid. These enable empirical testing of the success of D&I efforts. While we have built many excellent surveillance systems for measuring long-term change (e.g., behavioral risk factors, mortality, cancer incidence), most of these are only partially helpful for D&I research, where a greater focus is needed on "midstream" and "upstream" factors.[15,16] Currently, there are very few measures designed to focus on D&I research at the population level; most are relevant for interventions addressing acute patient care. Moreover, most existing measures focus on ultimate outcomes, such as change in health status. Proximal measures of dissemination and implementation processes and outcomes are sorely needed. As new measures are developed (or existing metrics adapted), some key considerations include: which outcomes should be tracked and how long it will take to show progress; how implementation fidelity and adaptation can best be measured across a broad range of D&I studies; how to best determine criterion validity (how a measure compares with some "gold standard"); how to best measure moderating factors across a range of settings (e.g., schools, worksites); and how common, practical measures can be developed and shared so researchers are not constantly reinventing measures.

Understanding How to Benefit from Comparative Effectiveness Research

As described in Chapter 4, D&I research can be improved by drawing on new techniques and findings from comparative effectiveness research (CER), defined as "the conduct and synthesis of research comparing the benefits and harms of different interventions and strategies to prevent, diagnose, treat and monitor health conditions in "real-world" settings."[17] The growth of CER with a translational focus (so-called CER-T) provides new research opportunities, as outlined by Glasgow and Steiner in Chapter 4. Among the areas needing inquiry are: (1) understanding whether studies that are efficacious in research studies will translate to specific groups (e.g., low income, minority, economically disadvantaged), (2) applying CER-T methods to emerging issues such as public health genomics and policy dissemination, (3) finding better ways to conduct CER-T studies with new innovations such as electronic medical records or rapid learning research networks, and (4) finding ways to better integrate primary care and public health. The benefits of CER require that D&I researchers develop effective methods of disseminating and implementing the interventions that emerge from CER as "best."

Moving from Theory to Evidence-Based D&I Strategies

Our knowledge base about *how to* disseminate or *how to* implement lags far behind our knowledge base of *what to* disseminate or *what to* implement. That is, we have a growing repertoire of evidence-based interventions, programs, and policies, but few dissemination or implementation strategies that have been tested and shown to be effective. Therefore, as noted in numerous chapters, we need well-designed studies to develop and test D&I strategies.

Understanding Fidelity and Its Connection to D&I Research

Fidelity, defined in Chapter 14 as the "extent to which the intervention was delivered as planned,"[18] is currently not well understood within the realm of D&I research. Key to the concept of fidelity is also the concept of adaptability, or the ability of the target audience to adapt the intervention to its own population. Striking a balance between adaptability and fidelity is challenging, but there are several models currently in place that have been able to strike this balance. The challenge in the future is to develop a means of evaluating these models in a way that helps determine their utility across myriad settings, populations, and health outcomes. Another key need is for more transparent reporting of program implementation and consistency of implementation across settings, staff, target groups, and time.

Several important topics can help inform our knowledge on fidelity and D&I research. Researchers should collaborate to design interventions and develop measures that assess and maximize the fidelity of the intervention. Practitioners should identify the evidence-based interventions that would be best suited for their populations and settings and assess how successfully the interventions are delivered. By doing this, practice-based evidence can be developed. Policymakers should be involved in the creation of the infrastructure needed to open up the lines of communication between researchers, practitioners, and intervention developers. Finally, the reviewers and editors of professional journals should make a greater effort to increase (and not punish) transparent reporting of issues around program implementation and adaptation.

Building the Evidence on External Validity

As described in this book, there are numerous forms of evidence. Some types of evidence inform our knowledge about the etiology of disease.[4] Other evidence demonstrates the relative effectiveness of specific interventions to address a particular health condition. However, what is fundamental to D&I research and is often missing is a body of evidence that can help to determine the generalizability of an intervention from one population and/or setting to another, that is, the core concepts of external validity (described in Chapter 15).[19] There are many remaining research questions related to external validity, for example: Which factors need to be taken into account when an internally valid program or policy is implemented in a different setting or with a different population subgroup? How does one balance the concepts of fidelity and adaptation (reinvention)? If the adaptation process changes the original intervention to such an extent that the original efficacy data may no longer apply, then the program may be viewed as a new intervention under very different contextual conditions. How might we efficiently and effectively measure external validity across a wide range of intervention studies? How can systematic reviews more fully incorporate concepts of external validity? Green has recommended that the implementation of evidence-based approaches requires careful consideration of the "best processes" needed when generalizing research to alternate populations, places, and times.[20] This greater attention to external validity has many benefits, including greater relevance and enhanced credibility of findings from D&I research for practitioners and policymakers and a better understanding of what constitutes an "effective" intervention (i.e., based solely on whether it worked in a narrowly defined population or a broader understanding of the key factors needed for replication or "scaling up"[21]). At the earliest stages, D&I research could benefit from more consistent application of what is being called "exploratory evaluation" or "evaluability assessment." (i.e., a preevaluation activity designed to maximize the chances that any subsequent evaluation will result in useful information).[22]

Understanding the Contributions of Economic Evaluation

As noted in Chapter 5, economic evaluation is an important tool for D&I research. It can provide information to help assess the relative value of alternative expenditures on health services and public health programs. For example, cost-effectiveness analysis (CEA) can suggest the relative value of alternative interventions (i.e., health return on dollars invested), and can play key roles in a whole range of D&I studies. While CEA has been increasingly applied to medical and public health interventions, it is seldom used in a systematic manner for D&I research.

Improving the Knowledge Base on Sustainability

Sustainability describes the extent to which an evidence-based intervention can deliver its intended benefits over an extended period of time after external support from the donor agency is terminated.[23] Rarely do studies assess long-term sustainability of practice changes, even when implementation of effective practices is successful. This is a priority area for research, as the inability to overcome barriers to sustainability and scalability prevents population-wide benefits of new health care and public health discoveries. Most implementation practice and research focuses on initial uptake, by early adopters, of one health intervention at a time. It is important that D&I research begin to tackle later-stage challenges of scaling up and sustaining evidence-supported interventions in complex community settings that serve vulnerable populations.

Documenting the Public Health Impact of D&I Research

It is critical that D&I researchers document the incremental advances in improved health care that result from dissemination and implementation. In many studies, the success of the implementation is assumed and evaluated from data on clinical outcomes alone. This may obscure D&I's unique value added to the quality of health care and public health. Woolf asserts that later-stage translation research can do more to decrease morbidity and mortality than a new imaging device or class of drugs.[24] Indeed, some studies show that health care can be improved as much as 68% through educational outreach and social marketing and by 250% through clinician performance feedback.[25–27] Dissemination and implementation researchers should find the confidence to propose and strive toward these kinds of measurable impacts. We need methods and data to demonstrate the potential of D&I research to ultimately reduce the burden of disease and improve the quality of lives.

■ STRATEGIES AND POPULATIONS

Conducting Research in High-Risk Populations and Low-Resource Health Systems

As noted in Chapter 22, despite enormous gains in health over the past century, several populations lag behind in realizing these gains in life years and quality of life (ethnic minorities, low-income and low-literacy populations). Moreover, under-resourced settings lag behind in the capacity to implement and sustain good care. This leads to a great urgency for D&I approaches among high-risk populations and low-resource systems where health disparities exist. There are several priorities for research. Perhaps most fundamental, we need to better understand how evidence-based interventions can be adapted and replicated successfully in low-income, minority, low–health literacy, and disadvantaged groups. Second, more inquiry is needed to understand how to maintain cultural appropriateness as a means of increasing "buy-in" from the target population. As was discussed in Chapter 23, there are several key strategies for improving the cultural adaptation of interventions, including tailoring the intervention to the target audience. This emphasizes a need for delivery of interventions in the native language of the population and targeting specific cultural groups rather than trying to implement an intervention across several cultural backgrounds. Third, following on the principles of participatory research,[28] we need to balance "top-down" (researcher-driven) approaches with "bottom-up" approaches that closely involve the populations suffering from health disparities in the research process. Finally, we need cost-efficient methods to disseminate, train, implement, and monitor quality in underresourced health settings.

Understanding How to Design for Dissemination

As described in Chapter 6, effective dissemination and implementation of evidence-based interventions is a formidable challenge. In part, this is due to differing priorities. For researchers, the priority is often on discovery (not application) of new knowledge, whereas for practitioners and policymakers, the priority is often on practical ways for applying these discoveries for their setting. Research on how to disseminate evidence-based interventions has now taught us several important lessons: (1) dissemination generally does not occur spontaneously, (2) passive approaches to dissemination are largely ineffective, and (3) single-source prevention messages are generally less effective than comprehensive approaches. Similarly, we have learned several important lessons on how to implement evidence-based interventions: (1) multicomponent, active strategies need to target several "layers" or levels of health systems; (2) leadership matters but is not sufficient; (3) provider behavior is hard to change, and changed health care is even harder to sustain; and (4) systems are complex and change is recursive. Yet most of these lessons have been learned from studies with early adopters in high-resource settings. We have yet to learn the lessons of how to change health care in more challenging settings.

We have also learned that researchers should identify dissemination and implementation partners prior to conducting discovery research, so that those who might adopt the discoveries will see results in a collaborative manner. This suggests several areas where additional research is warranted: how to place a greater emphasis on building strategic partnerships early in the D&I process; new and more rapid methods for determining when a new program or policy is ready for adoption in a nonresearch setting (e.g., exploratory evaluation[22]); and ways of ensuring that the intervention is developed in ways that match well with adopters' needs, assets, and time frame. Many of these challenges need particular attention in settings with high health disparities, where the system constraints may be the greatest and the delivery systems are underdeveloped. Ultimately, we need to better understand how to design interventions with the elements most critical for external validity in mind, addressing these issues during early developmental phases, not near the end of a project.

■ PARTNERSHIPS

Applying Transdisciplinary Approaches

Transdisciplinary research provides valuable opportunities to collaborate on interventions to improve the health and well-being of both individuals and communities.[29-31] For example, tobacco research and control efforts and more recently, physical activity projects, have been successful in facilitating cooperation among disciplines such as advertising, policy, business, economics, medical science, and behavioral science. Research activities within multidisciplinary tobacco networks try to fill the gaps between scientific discovery and research translation by engaging a wide range of stakeholders.[32-34] Progress in D&I research will depend not only on fields like medicine or public health, but importantly on other disciplines such as law, business, economics, agriculture, marketing, transportation, urban planning, and education. Moreover, unlike tobacco control, disseminating and implementing interventions to address other public health problems (e.g., obesity) will necessarily involve partnerships among government, nongovernmental organizations, and academic and private sectors. We have begun to identify factors that facilitate transdisciplinary research in basic sciences, etiologic research, and intervention trials, including the breadths of disciplines involved, prior work together among researchers, spatial proximity of researchers, face-to-face interaction, and support from leadership.[35,36] There is sparse understanding of how best to facilitate transdisciplinary D&I research as "best practice," making this a research priority.

Building Knowledge on Participatory Approaches

As noted in Chapter 10, participatory research methods have the potential to improve D&I research by involving community members and stakeholders in the decision-making processes, thus enhancing the relevance and overall quality of research. Within community and public health settings, participatory research builds trust, respect, capacity, empowerment, accountability, and sustainability,[28,37,38] all of which are critical to enhancing the success of D&I efforts down the road. This has tremendous potential for the successful dissemination of research findings and also for conducting D&I research. Community engagement and participation can play roles in D&I research across a wide spectrum, ranging from engaging consumers, patients, or practitioners as advisors, to hiring research staff from communities being targeted, to full participation from community members in all research activities. An important future D&I research area is to understand how to best link the needs of community members' or practitioners' participation with the objectives of researchers.

■ TRAINING AND SUPPORT

Developing Training Programs

As the field of D&I research advances, increasing opportunities for training becomes essential to meeting the full potential of the discipline to improve population health in an efficient and timely manner. While in the United States the National Institute of Mental Health has funded the Implementation Research Institute (IRI) to support training among researchers across the United States,[39] there are few other opportunities to engage scholars in mentored training. The IRI focuses on mental health services, and goals include training the next generation of D&I scholars and the development and dissemination of a D&I research course module for use by other mental health research training programs. Clearly the module may serve as a starting point for application in other clinical and public health areas. More broadly the structure of this training institute may serve as a model and catalyst for other NIH and CDC areas of focus to initiate parallel training programs. For example, the NIH Training Institute for Dissemination and Implementation Research in Health was launched in August 2011. In Canada, initiatives include the Knowledge Translation training workshops and a Canadian Institutes of Health Research Strategic Training Initiative in Health Research, which funds a knowledge utilization studies program at the University of Alberta. This new training program aims to provide advanced training in the science of knowledge translation research, link trainees and mentors, and partner with national and international research groups to promote knowledge translation training and research. From funded initiatives such as these, we hope to see new, shared curriculum developed. The scope of material offered in these chapters should advance methods for design, improve standards for reporting, and provide examples of applications of D&I research methods.

Developing Resources and Academic Incentives

To further advance the field, the growing emphasis on funding D&I research must withstand competitive pressures for funding resources within numerous federal agencies (e.g., NIH, CDC, AHRQ, VA), and at the same time we need foundations and other funding agencies to embrace the principles of D&I research to make this area a top priority. Given the lean budget years ahead, creative approaches to funding are needed, including cofunding between federal agencies and foundations. Importantly as we move along the discovery to application pipeline, there is a need to include an emphasis on many issues covered in these chapters (e.g., funding to better understand the role of fidelity, support for more research on organizational factors). More generally, additional funding resources for methods research that can grow out of the applications of D&I research projects will broaden the science base on which we build a sustainable field of scientific research. Increasing emphasis is needed on how to develop resources and sustain implementation after the research funding has ended. This can be particularly challenging in settings with limited resources.

As noted in Chapter 1, in parallel with funding for research studies, our institutions must develop career paths for promotion and tenure of faculty who engage in D&I research. Simply put, systems changes are needed in our academic institutions so that D&I research and the time commitments needed to build relationships and knowledge users are recognized and more highly valued and rewarded. As we look forward to the future of D&I research, each health sector and government research and practice funding agency will need to evaluate priorities and determine its interest in funding collaborative initiatives. Since the field of D&I research often involves projects with long time horizons and numerous disciplines, junior investigators will need to be afforded adequate support and time to show progress and ways to provide credit and incentives within the many disciplinary "silos."

■ CONCLUSION

There is enormous potential to advance the health of patients and the community through greater focus on implementing what we already know, and through greater application of the methods outlined in this book—D&I research. More simply put, taking what we know about improving health and putting it into practice must be our highest priority.[31]

This chapter has highlighted just a sample of the many rich areas for D&I research that will assist us in shortening the gap between discovery and practice, thus beginning to realize the benefits of research for patients, families, and communities. Greater emphasis on implementation in challenging settings, including lower- and middle-income countries and underresourced urban and rural settings in higher-income countries will add to the lessons we must learn to fully reap the benefit of our advances in D&I research methods. Moreover, collaboration and multidisciplinary approaches to D&I research will help to make efforts more consistent and more effective moving forward. Thus, we will be better able to identify knowledge gaps that need to be addressed in future D&I research, ultimately informing the practice and policies of clinical care and public health services.

■ ACKNOWLEDGMENTS

The authors are grateful for helpful input on this chapter from Drs. David Chambers, Russ Glasgow, and Jon Kerner.

■ REFERENCES

1. US Preventive Services Task Force. Guide to Clinical Preventive Services. 3rd ed. http://www.uspreventiveservicestaskforce.org/recommendations.htm. Accessed July 30, 2011, 2011.
2. Zaza S, Briss PA, Harris KW, eds. *The Guide to Community Preventive Services: What Works to Promote Health?* New York: Oxford University Press; 2005.
3. Satterfield JM, Spring B, Brownson RC, et al. Toward a transdisciplinary model of evidence-based practice. *Milbank Q.* Jun 2009;87(2):368–390.
4. Brownson RC, Baker EA, Leet TL, Gillespie KN, True WR. *Evidence-Based Public Health.* 2nd ed. New York: Oxford University Press; 2011.

5. Rabin BA, Brownson RC, Haire-Joshu D, Kreuter MW, Weaver NL. A glossary for dissemination and implementation research in health. *J Public Health Manag Pract.* Mar–Apr 2008;14(2):117–123.

6. Kerner JF. Integrating research, practice, and policy: what we see depends on where we stand. *J Public Health Manag Pract.* Mar–Apr 2008;14(2):193–198.

7. Glanz K, Bishop DB. The role of behavioral science theory in development and implementation of public health interventions. *Annu Rev Public Health.* April 21, 2010;31:399–418.

8. Wilson PM, Petticrew M, Calnan MW, Nazareth I. Disseminating research findings: what should researchers do? A systematic scoping review of conceptual frameworks. *Implement Sci.* 2010;5:91.

9. Green LW, Kreuter MW. *Health Promotion Planning: An Educational and Ecological Approach.* 4th ed. New York: McGraw Hill; 2005.

10. Glasgow RE, Vogt TM, Boles SM. Evaluating the public health impact of health promotion interventions: the RE-AIM framework. *Am J Public Health.* Sep 1999;89(9): 1322–1327.

11. Greenhalgh T, Robert G, Macfarlane F, Bate P, Kyriakidou O. Diffusion of innovations in service organizations: systematic review and recommendations. *Milbank Q.* 2004;82(4):581–629.

12. Wandersman A, Duffy J, Flaspohler P, et al. Bridging the gap between prevention research and practice: the interactive systems framework for dissemination and implementation. *Am J Community Psychol.* Jun 2008;41(3–4):171–181.

13. Jilcott S, Ammerman A, Sommers J, Glasgow RE. Applying the RE-AIM framework to assess the public health impact of policy change. *Ann Behav Med.* Sep–Oct 2007;34(2):105–114.

14. Thacker SB. Public health surveillance and the prevention of injuries in sports: what gets measured gets done. *J Athl Train.* Apr–Jun 2007;42(2):171–172.

15. Brownson RC, Jones E. Bridging the gap: translating research into policy and practice. *Prev Med.* Oct 2009;49(4):313–315.

16. McKinlay JB. Paradigmatic obstacles to improving the health of populations—implications for health policy. *Salud Publica Mex.* Jul–Aug 1998;40(4):369–379.

17. Institute of Medicine. *Initial National Priorities for Comparative Effectiveness Research.* Washington DC: Institute of Medicine of The National Academies; 2009.

18. Linnan L, Steckler A. Process evaluation and public health interventions: an overview. In: Steckler A, Linnan L, eds. *Process Evaluation in Public Health Interventions and Research.* San Francisco: Jossey-Bass; 2002:1–24.

19. Green LW, Glasgow RE. Evaluating the relevance, generalization, and applicability of research: issues in external validation and translation methodology. *Eval Health Prof.* Mar 2006;29(1):126–153.

20. Green LW. From research to "best practices" in other settings and populations. *Am J Health Behav.* May–Jun 2001;25(3):165–178.

21. Norton W, Mittman B. *Scaling up Health Promotion/Disease Prevention Programs in Community Settings: Barriers, Facilitators, and Initial Recommendations.* Hartford, CT: Patrick and Catherine Weldon Donaghue Medical Research Foundation; 2010.

22. Leviton LC, Khan LK, Rog D, Dawkins N, Cotton D. Evaluability assessment to improve public health policies, programs, and practices. *Annu Rev Public Health.* April 21, 2010;31:213–233.

23. Shediac-Rizkallah MC, Bone LR. Planning for the sustainability of community-based health programs: conceptual frameworks and future directions for research, practice and policy. *Health Educ Res*. Mar 1998;13(1):87–108.

24. Woolf SH. The meaning of translational research and why it matters. *JAMA*. January 9, 2008;299(2):211–213.

25. Bennett JW, Glasziou PP. Computerised reminders and feedback in medication management: a systematic review of randomised controlled trials. *Med J Aust*. March 3, 2003;178(5):217–222.

26. Thomson O'Brien MA, Oxman AD, Davis DA, Haynes RB, Freemantle N, Harvey EL. Educational outreach visits: effects on professional practice and health care outcomes. *Cochrane Database Syst Rev*. 2000(2):CD000409.

27. Woolf SH, Johnson RE. The break-even point: when medical advances are less important than improving the fidelity with which they are delivered. *Ann Fam Med*. Nov–Dec 2005;3(6):545–552.

28. Minkler M, Wallerstein N. *Community-Based Participatory Research for Health: From Process to Outcomes*. 2nd ed. San Francisco: Jossey-Bass; 2008.

29. Harper GW, Neubauer LC, Bangi AK, Francisco VT. Transdisciplinary research and evaluation for community health initiatives. *Health Promot Pract*. Oct 2008;9(4): 328–337.

30. Stokols D. Toward a science of transdisciplinary action research. *Am J Community Psychol*. Sep 2006;38(1–2):63–77.

31. Colditz GA, Emmons KM, Vishwanath K, Kerner JF. Translating science to practice: community and academic perspectives. *J Public Health Manag Pract*. Mar–Apr 2008;14(2):144–149.

32. Kobus K, Mermelstein R. Bridging basic and clinical science with policy studies: the Partners with Transdisciplinary Tobacco Use Research Centers experience. *Nicotine Tob Res*. May 2009;11(5):467–474.

33. Kobus K, Mermelstein R, Ponkshe P. Communications strategies to broaden the reach of tobacco use research: examples from the Transdisciplinary Tobacco Use Research Centers. *Nicotine Tob Res*. Nov 2007;9 (Suppl 4):S571–S582.

34. Morgan GD, Kobus K, Gerlach KK, et al. Facilitating transdisciplinary research: the experience of the transdisciplinary tobacco use research centers. *Nicotine Tob Res*. Dec 2003;5 (Suppl 1):S11–S19.

35. Stokols D, Harvey R, Gress J, Fuqua J, Phillips K. In vivo studies of transdisciplinary scientific collaboration: lessons learned and implications for active living research. *Am J Prev Med*. Feb 2005;28(2 Suppl 2):202–213.

36. Emmons KM, Viswanath K, Colditz GA. The role of transdisciplinary collaboration in translating and disseminating health research: lessons learned and exemplars of success. *Am J Prev Med*. Aug 2008;35(2 Suppl):S204–S210.

37. Cargo M, Mercer SL. The value and challenges of participatory research: strengthening its practice. *Annu Rev Public Health*. April 21, 2008;29:325–350.

38. Israel BA, Schulz AJ, Parker EA, Becker AB. Review of community-based research: assessing partnership approaches to improve public health. *Annu Rev Public Health*. 1998;19:173–202.

39. Center for Mental Health Services Research. Implementation Research Institute (IRI). http://cmhsr.wustl.edu/Training/IRI/Pages/ImplementationResearchTraining.aspx. Accessed July 24, 2011.

■ INDEX